MATERNITY
NURSING
TODAY

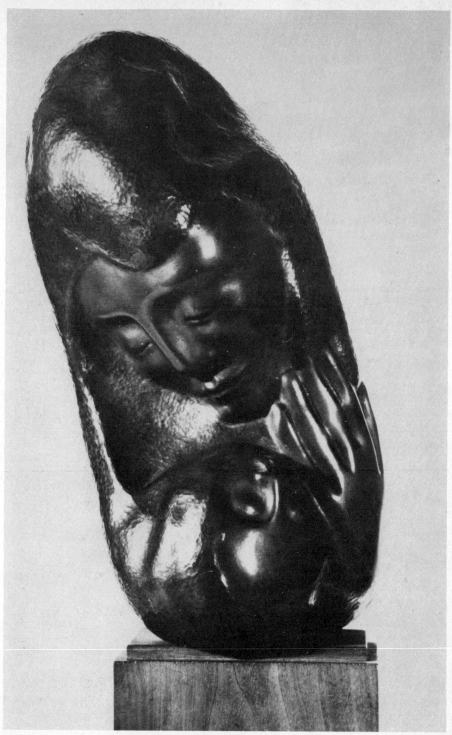

Not Yet. A twentieth century American sculpture by John Flannagan (1895-1942).
Reproduced with the permission of the Minneapolis Institute of Arts and the Francesca Winston Fund.

MATERNITY NURSING TODAY

JOY PRINCETON CLAUSEN, B.S., M.S.
Assistant Professor
Continuing Education Services
University of Colorado School of Nursing

MARGARET HEMP FLOOK, B.S., M.S.
Assistant Professor
Continuing Education Services
University of Colorado School of Nursing

BOONIE FORD, B.A., B.S., M.A.
Associate Professor, Acting Chairman
Maternal Child Nursing
University of Colorado School of Nursing

MARILYN M. GREEN, B.S., M.S.
Doctoral Student, Nursing of Children
University of Pittsburgh

ELDA S. POPIEL, B.S., M.S.
Professor, Assistant Dean
Continuing Education Services
University of Colorado School of Nursing

McGRAW-HILL BOOK COMPANY
A Blakiston Publication

New York   St. Louis   San Francisco   Düsseldorf
Johannesburg   Kuala Lumpur   London   Mexico
Montreal   New Delhi   Panama
Rio de Janeiro   Singapore   Sydney   Toronto

Library of Congress Cataloging in Publication Data
Main entry under title:

Maternity nursing today.

   "A Blakiston publication."
   Includes bibliographies.
   1. Obstetrical nursing. I. Clausen, Joy Princeton,
1935–   ed. [DNLM: 1. Obstetrical nursing.
2. Pediatric nursing. WY 157 M425 1973]
RG951.M33   610.73'678   72-11786
ISBN 0-07-011283-5

MATERNITY NURSING TODAY

4 5 6 7 8 9 – M A M B – 7 6 5 4

This book was set in Palatino by Monotype Composition Company, Inc.
The editors were Cathy Dilworth and Sally Mobley;
the designer was Nicholas Krenitsky;
and the production supervisor was Sally Ellyson.
The drawings were done by Vantage Art, Inc.
The printer was Halliday Lithograph Corporation;
the binder, The Maple Press Company.

CONTENTS

LIST OF
CONTRIBUTORS

ROSIE L. ACTON, R.N., B.S.N., M.S.
Nursing Audit Consultant
University of Minnesota Hospitals and
    Northlands Regional Medical Program
Minneapolis, Minnesota

PATRICIA A. BANASIAK,
    R.N., B.S., M.S., C.A.G.S.
Associate Professor
Boston University School of Nursing
Boston, Massachusetts

SANDRA L. BERRY,
    R.N., B.S., M.S.N., M.S.P.H
Assistant Professor
University of North Carolina School of
    Nursing
Chapel Hill, North Carolina

JANE M. BRIGHTMAN, R.N., B.S., M.S.
Master Nurse Clinician, Maternal Infant
    Care
St. Luke's Hospital
New Bedford, Massachusetts

SYLVIA J. BRUCE, R.N., S.B., M.S.,
    C.A.G.S., Ed.D.
Assistant Dean, Faculty and Academic
    Affairs
Boston University School of Nursing
Boston, Massachusetts

BARBARA CABELA, R.N., B.S., M.S.
Nursing Consultant
Colorado Department of Health
Denver, Colorado

JOAN E. CARTER, B.S., M.P.H.
Regional Nutrition Consultant
Health Service and Mental Health
    Administration
Department of Health, Education and
    Welfare
Denver, Colorado

FRED CARVELL, B.A., M.A.
Vice-President
Tadlock Associates, Inc.
Los Altos, California

JOAN CARVELL, B.A.
Research Associate
Tadlock Associates, Inc.
Los Altos, California

MARILYN A. CHARD, R.N., B.S.,
  Ed.M., M.S.
Associate Professor
Boston University School of Nursing
Boston, Massachusetts

STEPHANIE CLATWORTHY,
  R.N., B.S., M.S.
Instructor
Boston University School of Nursing
Boston, Massachusetts

MARYA M. CORCORAN, R.N., B.S., M.S.
Professor of Nursing
Boston University School of Nursing
Boston, Massachusetts

MILDRED A. DISBROW, R.N., C.N.M.,
  B.S., M. Litt., Ph.D.
Professor of Maternal and Child Nursing
University of Washington School of
  Nursing
Seattle, Washington

ELIZABETH M. EDMANDS,
  R.N., B.S., M.A.
Associate Professor
Maternal and Child Health and Public
  Health Nursing
University of North Carolina School of
Public Health
Chapel Hill, North Carolina

DAVID M. FULCOMER, B.A., M.A., Ph.D.
Director
Family Studies Center
Temple Buell College
Denver, Colorado

BEVERLY M. HORN, R.N., B.S.N., M.N.
Predoctoral Intermediate Student
Individual Ph.D. Program in Nursing,
  Anthropology, and Sociology
University of Washington
Seattle, Washington

MARY B. JOHNSON, R.N., B.S.N.
Formerly Head Nurse Obstetrics and
  Gynecology Outpatient Department
University of Minnesota Hospitals
Minneapolis, Minnesota

SHARON SERENA JOSEPH, R.N.,
  B.S., M.S.
Clinical Nurse Specialist
Denver Women's Clinic
Denver, Colorado

JOANNE M. JUHASZ, R.N., B.S., M.S.N.,
  C.N.M.
Clinical Nursing Specialist,
  Maternal-Infant Health
Good Samaritan Hospital
Phoenix, Arizona

KARYN SMITH KAUFMAN, R.N., B.S.N.,
  M.S., C.N.M.
Instructor
University of Toronto School of Nursing
Toronto, Ontario
Canada

ROSEMARY CANNON KILKER, R.N.,
  B.S., M.S.
Assistant Professor
Department of Nursing Education
University of Kansas Medical Center
Kansas City, Kansas

VIRGINIA GRAMZOW KINNICK,
  B.S.N., M.S.N., C.N.M.
Inservice Coordinator, Maternity and
  Pediatric Nursing
Weld County General Hospital
Greeley, Colorado

RUTH ANN LAMBERT, R.N., B.S., M.S.
Assistant Professor
Boston University School of Nursing
Boston, Massachusetts

ROSE S. LeROUX, R.N., B.S., M.S.
Doctoral Candidate
University of Denver
Denver, Colorado

VIVIAN LITTLEFIELD, R.N., B.S., M.S.
Chairman Level I and Assistant Professor
University of Colorado School of Nursing
Denver, Colorado

MIRIAM T. MANISOFF, R.N., B.A., M.A.
Director, Professional Educational
Planned Parenthood–World Population
New York, New York

KATHARINE A. McCARTY, R.N., B.S.,
  M.S., C.A.G.S.
Associate Professor, Maternal and Child
  Health Nursing
Boston University School of Nursing
Boston, Massachusetts

ELLEN J. MEVIS, B.A.
Newborn Service, Division of Perinatal
  Medicine
Department of Medical Social Service
University of Colorado Medical Center
Denver, Colorado

RANA LIMBO PECK, R.N., B.S.N., M.S.
Clinical Instructor and Permanent Team
  Leader
University of Colorado Medical Center
Denver, Colorado

GLADYS M. SCIPIEN, R.N., B.S., M.S.
Assistant Professor
Boston University School of Nursing
Boston, Massachusetts

ANN NOORDENBOS SMITH, R.N., B.S.,
  M.S.
Graduate Student, Department of Sociology
University of Colorado
Boulder, Colorado

MARNA STEINBRONER, B.R.E., R.N.,
  B.S., M.S.
Instructor
Boston University School of Nursing
Boston, Massachusetts

JANET M. STEWART, M.D.
Assistant Professor, Department of
  Pediatrics
University of Colorado Medical Center
Denver, Colorado

ELIZABETH W. STURROCK, R.N., B.S.,
  M.S., C.N.M.
Nurse-Midwife Clinical Specialist III
Henry Grady Memorial Hospital
Atlanta, Georgia

DAVID S. TORBETT, Ph.D.
Assistant Professor of Sociology and
  Family Studies
Temple Buell College
Denver, Colorado

ERNESTINE WIEDENBACH, R.N., B.A.,
  M.A., C.N.M.
Associate Professor Emeritus of Maternal
  and Newborn Health Nursing
Yale University
New Haven, Connecticut

BETTY L. WILKERSON, R.N., B.S., M.A.
Assistant Professor, Nursing Education
University of Kansas Medical Center
Kansas City, Kansas

ELIZABETH J. WORTHY, R.N.,
  B.S., M.N.
Assistant Professor
University of Washington School of
  Nursing
Seattle, Washington

SHIRLEY STRATTON YEE,
  R.N., B.S., M.S.
Assistant Professor
University of Colorado Medical Center
Denver, Colorado

SALLY ANN YEOMANS, R.N., B.A.,
  M.S.N., C.N.M.
Instructor
University of Utah College of Nursing
Salt Lake City, Utah

PREFACE

As concepts of the family and family roles have changed in recent years, so too have the concept and practice of maternity nursing. Family patterns such as single parenthood and communal living and social issues such as abortion and family planning have challenged the traditionally narrow focus of maternity nursing and made most of the existing textbooks obsolete. In this book the authors identify and deal with these recent changes and the concomitant changes in nursing practice. In viewing the maternity patient and everyone involved with her and her child as important individuals worthy of intelligent, high-level concern, the authors hope to suggest the new satisfaction and purpose awaiting nurses today who are making family-centered maternity care a reality.

Nurses whose specialty is maternal and child health, sociologists, ecologists, a social worker, a nutritionist, and a geneticist have all combined their knowledge and expertise in writing this book, discussing the pertinent issues related to and inherent in the interdisciplinary care of families. These authors emphasize the person in the nurse and the person in the patient and other family members. They stress the use of self by the nurse in giving effective care. Nursing today, more than ever before, is a profession for both men and women. Therefore, we believe that the word *nurse* should not carry the feminine gender exclusively. In this book we have attempted to avoid naming gender in reference to the nurse. There are instances, however, in which the feminine gender has been used, such as in Chapter 3, because the author intends to individualize concepts about *a* nurse rather than nurses in general.

The book is organized into five parts. The first, Perspectives in Maternity Nursing, examines current definitions of "family," changing roles of individuals within various types of families, and the relation of these differences to the nursing process and to the nurse's role as a teacher and counselor. Part II, Planning the Family: Childbearing and Childrearing, provides the nurse with the background necessary for effective counseling in family planning. Such factors as family income, size, and spacing, as well as problems of infertility, are discussed. Part III, Childbearing and the Nursing Process, applies the preceding two parts to normal pregnancy, labor, and delivery. Meeting the biological, psychosocial, and cultural needs of the total family is stressed. Part IV, Childrearing and the Nursing Process, applies the contents of Parts I and II in describing the impact on the family of the presence of a new member. Characteristics, appraisal, and needs of the newborn are covered here. Finally, Part V, Complications of Childbearing and Childrearing, explores the effects of physiological and psychological complications on the fetus, mother, and family and on the role of the nurse.

Pertinent information from the social sciences is included throughout the book, particularly as it relates to the childbearing and childrearing periods in the life of the family from preconception through the first six weeks postpartum. The nursing process is a central theme of the book. It is related to maternity care by the various authors either in discussing the steps of identification, ministration, validation, and coordination or those of assessment, development of a plan of action, implementation, and evaluation. Although an understanding of basic anatomy and physiology is prerequisite, the specific principles of physiology necessary for the practice of maternity care are explained.

This book is designed as a textbook for students in diploma, baccalaureate, and associate-degree programs in nursing and for practicing nurses who wish to keep abreast of current knowledge and practice and to improve their care of maternity patients and their families. Inactive nurses seeking information about new developments and current practice will find the book useful as well.

The editors wish to acknowledge with gratitude and appreciation the secretarial assistance of Mrs. Janet Genow, whose efficiency and patience with our directions, changes, and rewriting made our job easier and the book a reality.

Joy Princeton Clausen, Margaret Hemp Flook,
Boonie Ford, Marilyn M. Green, Elda S. Popiel

PART I

PERSPECTIVES IN MATERNITY NURSING

For many years maternity care has been described and carried out in various ways because the specific emphasis in the definition or the type of service performed in maternity care depended upon the person, group, or health discipline speaking or acting. Some believe that the major objective of maternity care should be to ensure that every expectant mother maintains good health, has a normal delivery, bears healthy children, and learns skillful child care. To others, maternity care should consist of the appropriate care of the pregnant woman, the safe delivery of her child, her postpartum examination, and the care of her newly born infant. Still others believe that maternity care should begin much earlier and be aimed at promoting the health and well-being of young people who are potential parents. The focus of this philosophy is on helping them develop healthy approaches to family life and recognize the importance of being active, contributing citizens in the community. Parent and expectant parent education and family planning, including limiting the size of the family and treating certain problems associated with infertility, have gradually evolved as significant components of maternity care.

Recently, maternity care has been defined as services provided by people for families. This definition places the focus of the plan of care on the needs of the family. For too long the health professionals identified, planned, and offered the health care in behalf of the pregnant woman, but they did not necessarily involve her or her husband or other family members in the deliberations, decisions, and plans. Health workers are recognizing that providing services is a two-way street; sometimes they may know what is best for families, and sometimes family members know best. In addition to involving families in the plan of care, emphasis is placed on the personal attributes of the health practitioners providing the services as well as the quality of their relationship with the families whom they serve. The educational preparation of health personnel is not questioned by families. Most families are not aware of the increase in the number of new health workers in the health care system. Their concern is for health workers to translate their professional knowledge into services perceived by families as being personal, meaningful, and, therefore, satisfying.

Part I contains a comprehensive discussion of the changing roles and self-concepts of people and, more specifically, the changing roles of the maternity nurse. The need for the nurse to be confident and competent in performing these roles is of the utmost importance. The maternity nurse of today is expected to be many things—knowledgeable, kind, understanding, and compassionate—and, with commitment, to be able to express these qualities skillfully and effectively. The nursing process, which includes the steps of perceiving, assessing, planning, implementing, and evaluating, is explained as it relates to maternity nursing and to the physical and emotional relationship of the nurse with the expectant woman and her family.

The specific family constellations discussed in Part I are the single-parent family, the commune, the extended family, and the nuclear family. The need for the nurse to understand and, therefore, to consider the cultural, religious, ethnic, educational, economic, and social background of each family structure in all nursing interactions is also emphasized. No two families are alike. The way individual families identify their unique roles and responsibilities influences their approach to and expectations of health services. Knowledge of current concepts of individuals and families is essential to the practice of maternity nursing today. These concepts are related to the nursing process and to the goals and standards of maternity care.

Maternity nursing today is exciting and challenging because of the dynamic roles and individual opportunities the nurse has to utilize her professional and personal qualities. There is an important place in health care for the nurse who wishes to accept the responsibilities that contribute to the development of healthy, happy parents and families of today and tomorrow.

UNIT A
MATERNITY NURSING CARE

1 | CHANGING ROLES AND SELF-CONCEPTS OF PEOPLE

Mildred A. Disbrow

At first consideration the concept *role* might appear to be a clear-cut, unambiguous term which refers to what a person does in a given situation or position. Further consideration, however, begins to raise questions which cast doubt on the clarity of the term. Is role what a person actually does or what he should do? Are these two behaviors necessarily different? Who decides what one should do? Do all persons who occupy the same position behave in the same way? Is there consensus even on a particular behavior when it is observed by several persons present at the same time? We might cite as an example an actor's role for a particular part in a play. What he *should* do was first written by the author, then interpreted by the actor and director, and perhaps reinterpreted by both. What he *does* do may be influenced by how he views himself, his past experiences with similar roles in life or in the theater, and what he perceives as cues from his coactors, the director, and the audience. The audience's and critics' *perceptions* of his behavior depend on their own personal experiences, their familiarity with the author's work, and their expectations of the play. If we multiply this one example by all the different actors, directors, critics, and audiences who have been or will be involved with any one play, we can see that the actor's role for this part is not clear and unambiguous. There are many interpretations of the role of the actor cited here, and we would expect even more equivocation about the roles of persons in less structured positions or situations.

Role, then, is behavior. The term role may refer to the behavior which the person himself and/or others expect or believe to be appropriate or ideal —the *prescribed role*; it may refer to the behavior actually being emitted— the *enacted role*; or it may refer to how the person thinks he behaved or how others view his behavior—the *perceived role*. How one actually does behave, how he and others perceive the behavior, and what is deemed appropriate all depend on the *self-concept* of actor and of the others with whom he interacts.

The self-concept is developed through interaction with others, a special kind of interaction called *role taking*. To take the role of another is to put oneself in the place of the other person and, using his cues, to look at oneself as the other person would do so. Those others whose roles a person would want to assume in order to evaluate his own behavior are significant others, or *reference persons*. When the three categories of behavior—the ideal, the actual, and the perceived—are the same, there should be little or no difficulty.

If, however, there is deviance in any one of these categories, *role conflict* will result. Role conflict may also be experienced when one's different reference persons are not in agreement on the prescribed role. Since each person may occupy many positions concurrently, such as wife, mother, daughter, student, and editor of the school paper, then role conflict may also be experienced when incongruent sets of behavior are required of one person for the different positions he occupies. In the process of resolving role conflict, behaviors are altered and roles change. This chapter will be concerned with the interrelationships of self-concept, reference persons, and role conflict as they pertain to role acquisition and role change.

THE SELF-CONCEPT

The *self*, that conception one has of himself, is very important. It has been called the self-image, the self-concept, the body image, self-esteem, identity, character, and the "real" person. How one's image of oneself is thought to influence his behavior can be seen in examples such as the saleswoman who tells the customer, "Now that's really you," in an attempt to sell her a dress; the student refusing to take on the chairmanship of a committee who says, "I could never do that"; or the new mother who tells the nurse, "I can't believe that I'm really a mother." What the saleswoman wants the customer to believe is that wearing that particular dress will influence how she acts, and it may do just that. The student refusing to chair a committee may feel that the qualities of a committee chairman are different from those which he possesses; therefore, what the chairman would have to do cannot be part of his repertoire of behavior. The new mother may be thinking that since she does not yet see herself as a mother, she may not be able to behave like one.

Contributions to the literature on self span more than three quarters of a century, starting with the writings of William James in 1892 and continuing to the present. A brief look at some of these contributions might help to clarify just what the self is, how it develops, and how it affects the person's role.

William James dichotomized the self into the "self as known" and the "self as knower."[1] He divided the known or empirical self into the *material self*, the *social self*, and the *spiritual self*. Each of these was viewed in terms of either *self-seeking* or *self-estimating*. Self-seeking had a goal of preservation, and self-esteem was based on a ratio of success to pretentions. For example, manifestations of self-seeking with respect to the social self could include a desire to please, to be noticed, or to be admired, as in the case of the new father who uses cigars as a means of eliciting the attention and congratulations of others. Self-estimation for the material self could be reflected through personal vanity, pride of wealth, or fear of poverty. Both the hoarder and the conspicuous consumer fit this pattern.

Baldwin emphasized the influence of social interaction on the development of the self-concept.[2] He called the "give and take" between a person and his associates the "dialectic of personal growth." There were three stages to this: the first, or projective, stage was the one in which the infant adapted to individual variations of others; in the second, or subjective, stage he became aware of himself, not adapting to others but assimilating them into himself as part of him; and the third, or ejective, stage was one in which he saw himself in relation to others who assimilated themselves to him. This third stage was the beginning of the social self.

Some of James' formulation was carried further by Cooley who introduced the "looking glass self" through which he emphasized the importance of the person's interpretations of others' judgments of him in the development of his self-conception.[3] This was James' "self as known." The three elements of Cooley's construct of self were one's imagination of his appearance to others, one's imagination of others' judgment of that appearance, and some sort of self-feeling such as pride or mortification. It was the imputed sentiment of the other, that which the person imagined the other thought, that caused the pride or mortification. One might, however, experience both types of feeling with respect to the same act. For example, a youth might brag about his sexual prowess to a friend but be ashamed of it in terms of what his mother might think. Cooley pointed out also the relationship between love and self. One takes on values, attitudes, and attributes of persons whom he loves, and these become part of the self. Thus, love can be seen as necessary for a healthy self. Conversely, since it was felt that one's behavior is consistent with his self, a substantial self would be necessary if a person were to be capable of loving another person and maintaining the relationship over time. Just as Cooley felt that love was necessary for a healthy self-concept, Coopersmith found that acceptance (a part of loving) was one of the conditions necessary for the development of the "self-esteem" dimension of the self in adolescents. [4]

Mead also followed James' model of dichotomizing the self. [5] Mead's "I" was the portion of the self which reacted to his "me," or reflected portion. The me was reflected in that it came into being through the person's *taking the role of the other* and thus defining the situation as the other would define it. In doing this, the person could look at himself as an object just as the other person looked at him. *Role taking*, as Mead used it, was evaluating one's own behavior by looking at it through the eyes of another person. This same process was used as part of Rubin's "taking *in* of the maternal role." [6] In Rubin's introjection-projection-rejection operation the mothers tried out bits of the maternal role and used role taking to determine whether or not these bits of behavior "fit" them as reflected in the words and gestures of others.

Mead's main contribution was the introduction of the *generalized other*. The generalized other can be the perceived reactions of many others at one time or in one situation, or it can be the perceived reactions of multitudes of others with whom the person has interacted over time. The latter and more global type of generalized other has been the more acceptable of the two. For example, Brim's "me" in his "I-me" type of relationship is analogous to the generalized other generated from interaction with many others over time. [7]

Schilder extended the body image beyond the body itself to include clothes, the voice, and bodily secretions and excretions. [8] It is this part of Schilder's conceptual framework which could be used as a rationale for today's advertising copy for cosmetics and hygiene products. Schilder suggested that while a change in body image may follow a change in bodily appearance, it was not necessarily a lasting change unless it was congruent with the "psychic attitude" of the person. One's psychic attitude is influenced by the attitudes of others and by the person's projected mirror image. Thus, a physical impairment may change the body image negatively, but it can be rebuilt again. In the same way, a person with a negative body image may have cosmetic surgery to alter a disliked physical appearance, but unless the surgery is accompanied by a positive projected mirror image and by changed attitudes of others, the resulting body image may not be an improved one.

Schilder's work is pertinent when thinking of the alterations of bodily contour which accompany pregnancy. For some women this is a traumatic part of pregnancy, for others it is passively accepted; and for some it becomes a badge to wear with pride. How each person reacts is largely influenced by previous experience and by the attitudes of peers, parents, and husbands. Treat found that women whom she interviewed in the sixth month of pregnancy were passively accepting of most of the changes accompanying pregnancy but, when given an opportunity to discuss them, concentrated mainly on physical changes, altered body images, and feelings about themselves as feminine.[9] Since most of the body changes due to pregnancy do not persist beyond the puerperium, one would expect any body change to be reversible.

The development of moral judgments about the self was suggested by Cooley and explored further by Sullivan.[10] Sullivan categorized person-other interactions into three types: those which resulted in rewards; those which produced anxiety; and those which inflicted severe anxiety. A different self-concept emerged as a consequence of each type of interaction. The *good-me*, or positive conception, developed out of rewards, such as when a mother rewarded a child for behavior that pleased her. A person would be good-me when he does things which he perceives would please the rewarder. A *bad-me*, or negative self-concept, is a result of anxiety induced when disapproval of one's actions is manifested or when certain behavior is forbidden. The woman who has been socialized to believe that there is something shameful about the sexual organs and that "nice" women do not enjoy coital relations could see herself as a bad-me when sexually aroused. She therefore tries to avoid stimuli which could produce that feeling or, once aroused, could become frigid. The "too tired" wife or the wife who manages to find emergency ironing to do at bedtime could be protecting herself against the bad-me. The *non-me* does things of which the "me" could have no knowledge. It may be dream behavior, or it may be behavior regarded as dreadful enough to be loathed. The non-me results from experiences which induce anxiety so intense as to obliterate the conscious emitting of such behavior. Examples of the non-me behavior could be the frigidity mentioned above, amnesic behavior when something intolerable is repressed, or the behavior seen in some types of psychoses.

Allport's self was an all-encompassing construct which he called a *proprium*, that which is central to our sense of existence.[11] At first Allport dichotomized the self as James did into the known self and the knowing self. Later he discarded the subjective portion, the knower, which he said he had then consigned to philosophy.[12] Allport's known self, was a material self with seven dimensions and functions. These included the bodily self described by Schilder, but without the bodily extensions, and the self-seeking and self-esteem dimensions of James' self. To these Allport added *ego extension* (composed of people, pets, things, ideas, and beliefs which a person could consider his own), a rational facet for problem solving, and a dimension which included one's evaluation of his abilities today versus what he wanted to become. He also added something which he called *propriate striving* in which the person resisted equilibrium and maintained the tension necessary for accomplishing things. This last dimension was seen as similar to Maslow's "self actualizing people."[13] Allport offered more cues for detecting manifestations of the self empirically than did others before him.

Turner differentiated between self-images and the self-concept.[14] He viewed the self-image as the picture of oneself that one sees at any given time. It may be one shifting image which is easily changed, or there may be many self-images presenting themselves concurrently. The self-concept, on the other hand, is more stable and emerges from interaction between the person's goals and values and his many self-images. The self-concept is influenced more by what the person would like to be or is trying to be than by self-images. Images may be communicated directly or may be inferred from how one thinks he would appear to someone else. For example, one self-image of a new mother bathing her baby could be inferred from how she thinks she would appear to her absent mother were she present and watching the performance. Other images could be obtained through direct communication with her husband, with a nurse, or with a neighbor, all actually present. These four possible self-images might all be present at the same time and might or might not be congruent. Whether any of these self-images would be a threat to the mother's self-concept would depend on her values, goals, previous experience, and how highly she valued the opinions of these four persons. If she placed a high value on her ability to develop skill in the procedures necessary for caring for her baby, a self-image of herself as inept might be a real threat.

In a study in Los Angeles, breast-feeding primiparas apparently committed themselves to breast-feeding by putting motherhood up as a side bet.[15] This conception of commitment, putting up as a side bet something one does not dare lose, has been suggested by Becker.[16] What this means is that by aligning success in breast-feeding with success in mothering, the woman who failed in the feeding situation would also then have failed in mothering. This kind of failure was intolerable and inadmissible. The mother's image of herself as a failure in this instance would be a threat to her self-concept. A negative self-image may be more of a threat to the self-concept if the person from whose cues the mother detects her self-image is one with whom she will need to continue interaction, such as her husband. This is one of the reasons why the husband's support is so important for the new mother.

In spite of the fact that most of the authors cited so far have pointed out that the social self is both developed and altered through social interaction, there is a tendency to consider the self as an entity or thing. Gordon has reemphasized the point that the self is a process, not a thing.[17] He suggested that each person has a structure of multiple selves of temporal nature: the selves of the past, the selves of the present, and the potential or prospective selves of the future. The comprehensive self must include both social identity and personal attributes. Identity is composed of certain social types, described by nouns. The social types—mother, daughter, wife, church member, and lawyer—may comprise one woman's identity. Her personal attributes, manifested as adjectives, could be pretty, creative, gregarious, and sensitive.

Most of the authors whose contributions have been discussed have at least recognized a dichotomized self, one part knower and one part as known.

However, more emphasis in recent years has been on the known or reflected self. Much of the criticism about the James and Mead approaches to self has been aimed at the difficulty or impossibility of testing or measuring something as subjective as the knowing self. There is consensus that the self is primarily social and arises from social interaction. This is of prime importance when working with socially deprived persons, or with social isolates who never learned to take the role of the other. These people are not accustomed to anticipating feedback from others or considering the effect of their behavior on others. If one accepts empathy as a synonym of role taking (and the author does), then one would expect that social isolates would be lacking in empathic capacity.

Empathic persons grow up in an atmosphere of acceptance, one which promotes trust and confidence. Most of the action in their lives has been interaction. This has been true at home, in school, and with peers at play. It has been proposed that primary group interaction with peers during the crucial period from the age of five to the early teens is necessary if the individual is to learn to make accurate interpretations of the meanings of the reactions of others.[18] This is because children are frank with one another and criticize freely without worrying about hurting one another or being hurt in the process. Children learn this also at home, but in the home the freedom to reciprocate may be hampered by inequities in power distribution. Adults seldom have opportunity for that easy give-and-take which was part of childhood. With adults, criticism is likely to be offered to other adults not so much with intent to help the other person, but more to let him know that he is interfering with another's goals.

Use of this type of communication, voiced criticism of another's behavior, was found in problem-solving groups only when one member of the group was holding up the group's progress.[19] This can be empirically documented in various daily life situations. Examples of this can be seen when a driver ties up traffic at an intersection, when someone in a supermarket brings his entire weekly grocery order to be checked out between five and six in the evening when commuters are stopping off for one or two items on the way home, or when a patient takes "more than his share" of the nurse's or physician's time. Unless other adults are infringing upon one's rights, it is customary to avoid those whose behavior is not acceptable. Thus, the person who has not learned to correctly interpret others' reactions by the time he becomes an adult will most likely continue to have difficulty in interaction with others throughout his life.

The tragedy of a lack of empathic capacity in social isolates is not restricted to how it affects their lives. When these people become parents, the child's life also is affected. Parents who abuse or batter their children have been found to be lacking in empathic capacity.[20, 21] (Morris and Gould deny that this is lack of role-taking ability, but unrealistic expectations of children cannot be divorced from a role-taking ability which provides cues for expectations.) Abusive parents are usually socially isolated persons who have themselves been abused and/or reared in a manner to preclude their developing role-taking ability. It follows, then, that the abused children will probably rear their own children as they were reared themselves unless provided with some alternatives to broaden their perspectives.

In maternity nursing, we have an opportunity to work with new parents of all kinds before they have established their own patterns of childrearing through actual practice. How much can be done at this time to promote empathy in a person who has reached adulthood without developing such capacity is questionable, but screening for potential problems and seeking resources for them should be part of the nursing role. Nursing as a profession is not without members who are low in empathic behavior. Ware and Chelgren illustrated this with an incident about nurses who attempted to remove a patient's hands from the bedside rails and in so doing frightened the patient even more.[22] The patient was disoriented and afraid and felt that she was being sent down a slide into a sardine can. One nurse, not knowing of the delusion but recognizing the fear, suggested that the patient hold on to her and assured the patient that she would not let anything hurt her. Similar examples certainly could be drawn from labor and delivery situations.

Since the reactions of other people, obtained either through role taking or through direct communication, are so influential in the development and altering of the self-concept, and since those others whose reactions can have influence are *significant others*, it might be advisable to consider these significant others, or reference persons, in more detail.

REFERENCE PERSONS

Reference persons are significant others—individuals or groups—whose attitudes, values, and opinions have enough salience to influence another person's behavior. Just as one's conception of self develops and changes according to feedback, or perceived feedback, from important others, so also does one's conception of the behavior appropriate for him at any given time develop and change as he makes use of reference persons.

The term reference group was invented by Hyman in 1942 when, in studying socioeconomic status, he found that he could not accurately predict a person's status without taking into consideration the social groups the person used as comparisons for self-appraisal.[23] Prior to that time both Cooley and Mead introduced the idea of referents. Cooley's suggestion that a person takes pride or feels mortification based on how he thinks he appears to others[24] and Mead's "generalized other" or "me" which acts as a conscience to the "I" or acting self[25] imply that such feedback is utilized as a frame of reference.

Many psychologists and sociologists have contributed to reference group literature. Kelly distinguished between two kinds of functions for reference groups: (1) providing values which the person assimilates and (2) serving as a standard of comparison for self-evaluation.[26] Merton and Kitt introduced the concept of "relative deprivation," in which a person evaluates his own condition against that of a reference group which he uses as a standard.[27] Shibutani's definition of a reference group was one whose outlook was used by the actor for a frame of reference for organizing his own perceptual field. He also introduced the imaginary reference group as might be used by the artist who was "born ahead of his time."[28] Turner reorganized some of these ideas and renamed the groups as an identification group, which was a source of values; a valuation group, whose influence depended upon the valuation which his basic orientations allowed him to place on the group; and an audience group, which observed and evaluated his performance.[29] Eisenstadt made a contribution that was somewhat different from the rest in that he saw the norm itself as the frame of reference to which one oriented himself and that it was only in specific situations that the norm would be tied to a specific group.[30]

Kemper alone attempted to present this material in the form of a limited theory with reference groups as social mechanisms by which individual achievement was effected.[31] Kemper categorized reference groups into *normative, comparative,* and *audience* groups. Normative referents are persons or groups who establish norms and state values congruent with those norms. These are the individuals or groups to whom one looks to learn what behavior is appropriate for his given position and situation.

If one perceives the referent individuals or groups as positive referents, he will comply with their norms and internalize their values. However, normative referents may not always be positive. *Negative reference groups*, a term introduced by Newcomb,[32] are individuals or groups whose norms are not only unacceptable to one but which precipitate his setting up counter norms.

Comparative referents offer a frame of reference by which one can compare himself with others. The most common of the comparative referents are role models through which one learns how to enact his role. Comparative referents can also be used to determine the equity of one's fate. When a person perceives his fate as unfair in relation to his particular reference groups at a particular time and place, such unfairness is called relative deprivation.[33] Homans referred to this same phenomenon as status incongruence.[34]

Another comparative referent group is composed of persons that give legitimacy to one's attitude or behavior. The ubiquitous "they" and "everyone" fit into this category which one uses to give face validity to what he wants to do.[35]

Audience reference groups vary somewhat from the other two types in that they are composed of individuals or groups to whom one has attributed values and norms which he then uses to guide his behavior. These referents may have espoused the values he attributes to them and may have made them known in some way. They could be persons with whom he has interacted, public figures in the news, or authors whose publications he has read. On the other hand, they may be persons whose values are not known but only imputed to them by the one who utilizes them as referents. Conformity to the imputed values and norms may in itself be rewarding.

Audience referents may be living persons, heroes from the past, or imaginary characters. This last classification might be illustrated in a study of parents who abused their children.[36] The abusers were social isolates who did not make use of the reference persons normally used by others for help in childrearing such as parents, spouses, neighbors, friends, teachers, or church members. Rather, they imputed to an unknown collectivity of living people their own behavior as the norm. That is, they felt that there were living persons like themselves who, if faced with what the abusers had been faced, would think it appropriate to do what they had done. When questioned about this, they said that they were glad that there were others like themselves. This could be interpreted as support.

Normative reference groups usually make their prescriptions known and impose punishment if there is not compliance. An example of this would be the increasing number of long-haired naturalists, earth people, or hippies—there seems to be no agreement on names, only rejection of type casting by the persons so typed—who want to deliver their babies at home against the advice of some nurses and physicians. When things go wrong, lacerations for example, these persons have hesitated to go to the hospital for assistance because they say they are lectured about the impropriety of their behavior. One couple told of the husband calling the hospital to report that he was bringing his wife in for repair of a perineal laceration. When they arrived at the hospital, they said they were met with statements like, "Oh, you're the one who wanted to have a home delivery." The couple changed their story to one of having planned to come to the hospital but not getting there in time. The attitudes of the hospital personnel changed immediately from punitive to sympathetic.[37] It is often difficult to refrain from making statements like, "I was afraid this would happen" or "I told you so" when the consequences of a person's behavior are serious enough to provoke worry. The deviants themselves may be role models for others. Normative referents seldom reward for compliance except with negative reinforcement, the avoidance of punishing behavior. Rewards come from audience referents.

Physicians have usually been audience referents for their maternity patients as have the women's own mothers, friends, and other women whom they have met in the physician's office or clinic.[38] Nurses are more often seen as normative or comparative referents than audience referents. In a study on breast-feeding, women were asked what their physicians felt about their choice of breast-feeding. Many responded, "He approves," or "He said 'good.'"[39] It turned out that none of the physicians involved were trying to influence the patients with respect to type of feeding. Usually they were telling them that they were glad they had made a decision regardless of which decision. The patients, however, chose to accept their physicians as audience referents. When these same women were asked what the nurses felt about their choice of feeding their infants, most replied that they did not know or that it did not matter to the nurse. They were not putting the nurses in the role of audience referents.

This does not mean that nurses cannot be audience reference persons. This type of referent depends largely upon image. The image of the physician as one who knows what is best for his patients has a long tradition. Even today with criticism of methods of delivery of health services, little criticism is being leveled at the knowledge or capability of the physician per se. Nursing's image in society has not been the same. The image of the nurse has been one of giving comfort, providing emotional support, and following the physician's orders. An example of this can be found in Dalen's study comparing newly delivered maternity patients' and nurses' role expectations for maternity nurses.[40] This image is changing, but to establish the kind of rapport necessary to perceive the nurse as an audience referent takes time. Public health nurses who carry case loads over time, clinic nurses who see the same patients on a regular basis, nurse-midwives who carry their own case loads of pregnant women, students who follow a pregnant woman and her family throughout pregnancy, labor and delivery, and into the puerperium and at home, and some office nurses have achieved this kind of rapport and respect.[41, 42]

When the maternity patient has a different nurse on each clinic visit, several different nurses during labor and delivery, and different nurses during her two or three postpartum days in the hospital, this kind of rapport does not develop. Usually nurses are seen as normative reference persons who tell patients what they should do and sometimes as comparative referents who show by example how to do something.

The comparative referent, or role model, has an essential quality. He or she "possesses skills and displays techniques which the actor lacks (or thinks he lacks) and from whom, by observation and comparison with his own performance, the actor can learn."[43] Rubin found that maternal grandmothers were not utilized by new mothers as role models. Peers were models. The patients' mothers "seemed too competent, too masochistic, too knowledgeable and too overwhelming to be comfortable models for sustained periods."[44] It would seem unlikely that the new mother would consider the nurse as a role model for the same reasons she rejects her own mother as one. It is familiar to hear the new mother tell the nurse, "You do that so well. I could never handle the baby the way you do."

We might think that exceptions to the rejection of the nurse as a role model would be the nurse who helps the mother manually express milk from her breast after feeding her infant, who demonstrates breathing techniques in a prenatal class or while the patient is in labor, or the nurse who demonstrates how to bathe the baby. These, however, are not role model behaviors;

rather, they are what would be expected of a normative referent, one who tells the patient what he or she should do. When the patient asks the nurse if she has children, how she handles certain problems with her own children, or what she, the nurse, had as an anesthetic, then the patient is attempting to use the nurse as a role model.

Kemper has proposed that in order to achieve, in this case role enactment, one needs all three types of referents—normative, comparative, and audience. He further suggests what might happen if one or more of the types of referents were missing.[45] When there are both normative and comparative reference persons but no audience groups, there is no inducement to achieve. Many women who plan for psychoprophylactic childbirth find they are unable to carry it through if there is no one present to give support and reward them when they attempt to follow what they have been taught. Obese persons of either sex are more successful in weight loss when there is an appreciative audience to notice the results and commend them. Infants themselves have been used as audience referents through emphasis on infant satisfaction with positioning, type of feeding, or type of holding.

When normative and audience referents are present but comparative types are missing, the person may know *what* to do and may be *motivated* but may not know *how* to do what is appropriate. This is one of the difficulties with the very young mother who does not have peers who are currently involved in behavior like her own. Most aspects of human behavior, unlike that of lower animals, are not guided by instinct.

Whether or not the absence of normative reference persons is serious when both comparative and audience referents are available depends upon the type of behavior involved. Infants face this kind of situation when they first learn imitation for which they are rewarded. However, until norms are set and the infant is mature enough to learn and internalize them, he cannot think for himself, use logic, or make decisions about solving complicated problems. Ethical problems concerning some types of behavior control such as brainwashing fall into this category.

We have seen how one's concept of self influences his perception of his role, how he actually performs, and how he perceives himself performing. We have also considered how the presence or absence of significant others influences both the self-concept and one's ability to recognize his role and to enact it. Now let us consider what happens when various significant others are in disagreement or when one person's many roles are not congruent. These are the two main forms of role conflict.

ROLE CONFLICT

Two other concepts must be included before beginning the discussion of role conflict. One is *role set* and the other is *reference set*. Role set, introduced by Merton, refers to that "complement of role relationships which a person has by virtue of occupying a particular social status."[46] A role set is composed of the *behavioral relationships* of the persons (not the persons themselves) with whom one comes in contact. This is an important point, since a raised eyebrow, an unanswered question, or a hurried response from an otherwise warm and supporting person might change a person's self-image and, in turn, his behavior or his future reflections on this time of his life.

For example, a few years ago the author was present when a woman returned to her room from the delivery room of a large metropolitan hospital. The husband had been with his wife when she delivered even though she had been heavily anesthetized and was not able to consciously share the birth experience with him. His first words to her were, "You were a perfect lady at all times." I thought this a rather peculiar opening comment, but apparently one of the real worries she had voiced had been whether or not she would lose self-control. Her self-image through his eyes was very important to her and may have influenced whether or not she would have wanted another pregnancy, would have returned to the same hospital, or would have permitted her husband to be present again.

The concept of reference set was coined by Kemper from Merton's role set and the previously mentioned concept, reference group.[47] This set is composed of persons or groups to whom one refers his behavior for his particular role or for his role at some particular time. Again, using the labor and delivery situation, part of the woman's role as a natural mother (as contrasted with an adopting mother) is her behavior during the labor and delivery process. Her role set in this situation may be the role relationships with physicians, nurses, anesthesiologists, the father of the baby, other relatives, and student nurses. These named persons with whom she interacts are not necessarily her reference set for her behavior in labor and delivery. Her reference set may be composed of her own mother (present or absent), a member of her club or church group who at some time described in detail her own experiences, a public health nurse or instructor in a parents' class who tried to prepare her for what to expect and do, her husband, someone she overheard on a bus who sounded convincing, or perhaps someone on television or the movies who was depicted as having a baby or who discussed it on one of the late evening "talk" shows. Intraset conflict in either set—reference or role—could cause ambiguity, frustration, indecision, and trauma for the laboring woman.

Another type of role conflict is that experienced by the person when one or more of the many roles expected of him have prescriptions which are not consistent with the others. When one or other of these kinds of role conflict occurs, the person involved can use bargaining or balancing measures. This may involve (1) ranking the referents according to power, legitimacy, sanctioning ability, or intensity of involvement with the individual referents; (2) engaging the referents themselves in bargaining procedures through which they settle their difficulties or at least make them less visible to the person being influenced by them; or (3) insulating the person himself from stress or strain by physical withdrawal.

The first of the conflict-reducing mechanisms mentioned above, *ranking referents* to determine which to use for a given situation, might use for criteria Merton's suggestion of considering the intensity of the involvement with the referent.[48] Intensity of involvement may be qualitative or quantitative. A graphic description overheard on a bus may have an influence of more intensity than the advice given by the teacher at a parents' class unless the teacher had allowed for discussion of just such encounters.

Gross and associates utilized criteria of the type of a person's orientation—moral, expedient, or moral expediency.[49] The person with a *moral orientation* would give most weight to the referent whom he feels has the most legitimate claim to his opinion. In the case of the laboring woman, she might give more weight to what has been told her by a peer who just had a baby than to what either her male physician or unmarried nurse told her. The person with an *expediency orientation* would place more emphasis on sanctions that could be imposed. If she felt she might be neglected by the nurse or physician by not following their suggestions, she might place high priority on this. There are, of course, positive sanctions also; the desire to have an alert baby rather than one affected by the medication given the mother might be viewed in the category of positive sanction which might influence the laboring woman to insist upon little or no analgesia or anesthesia. The person with a *moral expediency orientation* would weigh the possibility of both positive and negative sanctions and choose the behavior which would show the most profit for her. Since sanctioning in most cases is based on perception which is not necessarily reality, the use of either the expediency or moral expediency orientation is somewhat hard to predict.

The second type of conflict-reducing mechanism, *engaging the referents themselves in settling the difficulties*, has been suggested by Merton.[50] At best, this is a difficult type of solution to use. It is the basis for negotiations when opposing factions strike in the working or business world, and it can be used in patient conferences when the members of the health team get together to discuss and plan care for the patient. For the new mother, however, it is not so easy to get the maternal and paternal grandparents, the nurse, the physician, the neighbors, friends, and newspaper columnists to sit down together and work out the differences of opinion. When the polemics are restricted to conflicting advice given by the physician and nurse, it is simpler to work out, and patients should be instructed to make such differences of opinion known to those involved.

The third type of mechanism used to cope with role conflict, *insulation of the person experiencing the conflict*, is appropriate for use with either intraset conflict in reference or role sets or with intraperson conflict when one's roles require conflicting behavior. Most of these mechanisms have been suggested by Goode,[51] but some of them overlap with suggestions of other people. Unless otherwise stated, the six major coping mechanisms discussed will be Goode's suggestions. He called these mechanisms role bargains which are used as a process of selection among alternate behaviors. *Compartmentalism* occurs when one can separate the behavior expected in different roles according to time or situation. For example, a Catholic mother who wants to be a role model for her daughter with respect to the church's teaching about birth control may find this behavior in conflict with her role as a marital partner who is in agreement with her husband that they want no more children. One mother resolved this conflict by keeping her birth control pills at the neighbors, thus compartmentalizing the two roles.[52] This type of solution is similar to Merton's mechanism of insulating role activities from observation by members of the role set.[53] Goode also suggested *delegation* in which obligation for the conflicting role expectation is transferred to someone else. Nurses frequently suggest that a new mother get someone to help her with her housework but keep the care of the baby for herself. If this is a mother who is quite uncomfortable with helpless infants but enjoys caring for older children, she may decide to resolve the conflict between housework and baby care by delegating the baby care to another and doing her own housework. The conflict between the mother's getting enough sleep and also fulfilling her role of providing nourishment for her baby may be settled by bottle-feeding with the father lending a hand, unless of course the mother's most salient referent is one who encourages breast-feeding.

Setting up obstacles against meeting role requirements is another of the insulating coping mechanisms. Pleading the need for additional income might provide a solution for the woman who really doesn't like housework or child care. She can't be expected to do all of this if she is working. Commitment to a profession into which was invested much money and time and through which one feels an obligation to make far-reaching contributions to a large population might also be given priority over other role requirements, whether they be childrearing, jury duty, participation in political groups, or working on charity drives. *Setting up barriers* to isolate themselves from others is a frequent method of reducing role strain. Breast-feeding mothers who feel they should give their undivided attention to the young infant in the early weeks of breast-feeding often take their telephones off the hook so others cannot reach them at that time. Goode's last two mechanisms, *eliminating role relationships* and *expanding role relationships*, are self-explanatory. Many a rift between young parents and their in-laws results in elimination, and parents of handicapped children who band together for support and increased involvement reflect the expansion.

Regardless of the type of role conflict experienced, some alteration in role usually occurs as a result of the conflict resolution. A method utilized to resolve role conflict or strain in one type of situation at one time may not be the method of choice in the same type of situation at another time. One's role sets and reference sets change over time, and persons who are referents or whose behavior is involved in the role sets are also subject to change within themselves. Social climate is a factor to be considered throughout. Just as the new mother five decades ago would never have considered telling her physician how or where to conduct her delivery, the pregnant woman of today usually feels that it is quite appropriate to make her wishes known and expects to have them considered and, if at all possible, granted. The increasing number of couples wishing to, and succeeding in, delivering their babies at home against the advice of the majority of physicians is a clear example of the changing social climate and its influence on role enactment.

SUMMARY

It has been the intent of this chapter to show that role is the behavior of a person in a particular position, whether that position is an institutionalized one, requiring patterned behavior, or an informal one as a member of a dyad or larger group. Behavior may be what is expected of a person; it may be the behavior actually emitted, or it may be the behavior as it is perceived by the actor or others.

One's conception of himself influences his expectations of how he should behave, how he does behave, and how he thinks he has behaved. The person's self-concept is a social process guided by his perception of what he thinks others think of him and how they perceive him from time to time. A person's self-concept has two main dimensions, the subjective one of himself as a knower and the reflected one as the known. Subdivisions of these dimensions may be physical, social, emotional, and temporal. One's self-concept may be stable for periods, such as the self of yesterday, the self of today, or the projected self of tomorrow, or it may be manifested in fleeting images which may or may not have lasting effect on a more permanent self-concept.

The self-concept is influenced by the person's perceptions of how he appears to others, very important others, sometimes called significant others or reference persons or groups. Reference persons may be living people with whom one interacts, persons once living but now deceased, or they may be imaginary. One's attachment to reference persons may be positive or negative which determines whether there will be compliance with the expectations of the referents or whether there will be overt attempts to be deviant. Reference persons may be utilized as normative referents, role models, or as audiences whose approval one seeks.

Different reference persons may be utilized for different roles or for one role at different times. The collectivity of persons utilized for any given role or role segment is known as a reference set and is to be distinguished from role set, which is made up of relationships, not persons. When there is lack of agreement between persons or behaviors making up a set, role conflict may occur. There may also be role conflict when one person's many different positions place upon him conflicting role expectations. Role conflict, whether intraset or intraperson, may be resolved through bargaining mechanisms which may rank the referents, eliminate deviant referents, engage conflicting referents in bargaining activities themselves, or provide insulation for the person experiencing the conflict. Interacting with or influencing the choice of conflict-reducing mechanisms is the social climate within which the conflict occurs. Role learning, role enactment, and role change are all social processes. Resolution of role conflict is one of the social processes which frequently is successful in effecting role change.

REFERENCES

1 James, William: *Psychology: The Briefer Course*, Henry Holt and Co., New York, 1892.
2 Baldwin, James Mark: *Social and Ethical Interpretations in Mental Development*, Macmillan, New York, 1897.
3 Cooley, Charles Horton: *Human Nature and the Social Order*, Scribner, New York, 1902, p. 184.
4 Coopersmith, Stanley: *The Antecedents of Self Esteem*, Freeman, San Francisco, 1967.
5 Mead, George Herbert: *Mind, Self and Society*, University of Chicago Press, Chicago, 1934, pp. 155–156, 173–178, 254–256, and 360–376.
6 Rubin, Reva: "Attainment of the Maternal Role: Part I, Processes," *Nursing Research*, 16:237–245, 1967.
7 Brim, Orville G., Jr., and Stanton Wheeler: *Socialization after Childhood: Two Essays*, Wiley, New York, 1966, pp. 12–15.
8 Schilder, Paul: *The Image and Appearance of the Human Body*, Kegan Paul, Trench, Trubner and Co., London, 1935, pp. 11–16, 188–194, 201–206, 273–282.
9 Treat, Janet Nell: "A Study of the Feminine Gender Identity Crisis of Pregnancy," unpublished master's thesis, University of Washington, Seattle, 1969.
10 Sullivan, Harry Stack: *The Interpersonal Theory of Psychiatry*, Norton, New York, 1953, pp. 158–171.
11 Allport, Gordon W.: *Becoming*, Yale University Press, New Haven, Conn., 1955, pp. 36–56.
12 Allport, Gordon W.: *Pattern and Growth in Personality*, Holt, New York, 1961.
13 Maslow, A. H.: "Self-actualizing People: A Study of Psychological Health," in W. Wolff (ed.): *Personality Symposium No. 1*, Grune & Stratton, New York, 1950, pp. 11–34.
14 Turner, Ralph H.: "The Self-conception in Social Interaction," in Chad Gordon and Kenneth J. Gergen (eds.): *The Self in Social Interaction*, Wiley, New York, 1968, pp. 93–106.

15 Disbrow, Mildred A.: "Any Woman Who Really Wants to Nurse Her Baby Can Do So???" *Nursing Forum*, 2:39–48, 1963.

16 Becker, Howard S.: "Notes on the Concept of Commitment," *American Journal of Sociology*, 66:32–40, 1960.

17 Gordon, Chad: "Self-conceptions: Configurations of Content," in Chad Gordon and Kenneth J. Gergen (eds.): *The Self in Social Interaction*, Wiley, New York, 1968, pp. 115–136.

18 Faris, Robert E. L.: *Social Psychology*, Ronald, New York, 1952, pp. 161–170.

19 Emerson, Richard M.: "A Theory of Communication in Group Problem Solving," paper presented at the American Sociological Association Meetings, Miami, Florida, 1966.

20 Steele, Brandt F.: "Parental Abuse of Infants and Small Children," in E. James Anthony and Therese Benedek (eds.): *Parenthood*, Little, Brown, Boston, 1970, pp. 449–477.

21 Morris, M. G., and R. W. Gould: "Role Reversal: A Concept in Dealing with the Neglected/Battered Child Syndrome," in *Neglected/Battered Child Syndrome*, Child Welfare League of America, New York, 1963, pp. 29–49.

22 Ware, Alma Miller, and Mary Nofziger Chelgren: "When 'Holding On' Brought Change," *Nursing Clinics of North America*, 6:125–134, March 1971.

23 Hyman, Herbert H.: "The Psychology of Status," *Archives of Psychology*, 269:93, 1942.

24 Cooley: op. cit., p. 104.

25 Mead: op. cit., p. 256.

26 Kelly, Harold H.: "The Two Functions of Reference Groups," in G. E. Swanson, T. M. Newcomb, and Eugene L. Hartley (eds.): *Readings in Social Psychology*, Holt, New York, 1952, pp. 410–414.

27 Merton, Robert K.: "Contributions to the Theory of Reference Group Behavior," in R. K. Merton (ed.): *Social Theory and Social Structure*, Free Press of Glencoe, Glencoe, Ill., 1966, chap. VIII, pp. 225–280.

28 Shibutani, Tamotsu: "Reference Groups as Perspectives," *American Journal of Sociology*, 60:562–569, 1955.

29 Turner, Ralph H.: "Role-taking, Role Standpoint, and Reference-group Behavior," *American Journal of Sociology*, 61:316–328, 1956.

30 Eisenstadt, S. N.: "Studies in Reference Group Behavior," *Human Relations*, 7:191–216, 1954.

31 Kemper, Theodore D.: "Reference Groups, Socialization and Achievement," *American Sociological Review*, 33:31–45, 1968.

32 Newcomb, Theodore M.: *Social Psychology*, Dryden Press, New York, 1950, pp. 139–155.

33 Kemper: op. cit., p. 33.

34 Homans, George Casper: *Social Behavior: Its Elementary Forms*, Harcourt, Brace & World, New York, 1961, p. 248.

35 Kemper: op. cit., p. 33.

36 Disbrow, Mildred A.: "Deviant Behavior and Putative Reference Persons, in *Fifth Nursing Research Conference Reports*, American Nurses' Association, 1969, pp. 322–346.

37 Healy, Ingrid: "A Descriptive Study of the Social Climate Surrounding Home Deliveries from the Viewpoint of Public Health Nurses and Hippie Type Women," unpublished master's thesis, University of Washington, Seattle, 1972.

38 Rubin, Reva: "Attainment of the Maternal Role: Part II, Models and Referents," *Nursing Research*, 16:342–346, 1967.

39 Disbrow: "Any Woman Who Really Wants to Nurse Her Baby Can Do So???"

40 Dalen, Audrey: "A Study of the Relationship of Role Conflict to Effective Communication in a Maternity Care Setting," unpublished master's thesis, University of Washington, Seattle, 1970.

41 Lang, Dorothea M.: "Providing Maternity Care through a Nurse Midwifery Service Program," *Nursing Clinics of North America*, 4:509–520, 1969.

42 Runnerstrom, Lillian: "The Effectiveness of Nurse-Midwifery in a Supervised Hospital Environment," *Bulletin of the American College of Nurse Midwives*, 14:40–52, 1969.

43 Kemper: op. cit., p. 33.

44 Rubin: op. cit., p. 343.

45 Kemper: op. cit., pp. 39–40.

46 Merton, Robert K.: "Instability and Articulation in the Role Set," in Bruce J. Biddle and Edwin J. Thomas (eds.): *Role Theory: Concepts and Research*, Wiley, New York, 1966, pp. 282–287.

47 Kemper, Theodore D.: "The Relationship between Self-concept and the Characteristics and Expectations of Significant Others," unpublished Ph.D. dissertation, New York University, New York, 1963.

48 Merton: "Instability and Articulation in the Role Set," p. 283.

49 Gross, Neal, W. S. Mason, and A. W. McEachern: *Explorations in Role Analysis*, Wiley, New York, 1957.

50 Merton: "Instability and Articulation in the Role Set," p. 285.

51 Goode, William J.: "A Theory of Role Strain," *American Sociological Review*, 25:483–496, 1960.

52 Connell, Elizabeth B.: "What Emotional Problems in Family Planning Do You Encounter?" *Medical Aspects of Human Sexuality*, September 1968, pp. 14–15.

53 Merton: "Instability and Articulation in the Role Set," p. 284.

2 | CHANGING ROLES OF THE MATERNITY NURSE

Sylvia J. Bruce and Marilyn A. Chard

TRENDS AND DIRECTIONS IN PRACTICE

The future of nursing must be determined by nurses. A frightening thought? Indeed it is. There has been a scarcity of outstanding leaders in nursing since the early 1900s, and even today such leaders are rare. Certainly nursing roles are changing, but time and circumstance have done that—*not* nurses. At best, we are keeping up. But with what? Social trends? Institutional demands? Needs of other professions? Patient care?

Nursing has become too isolated. Our behavior is predictable and dependent. As a group we are not risk-takers, nor are we socially perceptive. We need nursing leaders who will demand freedom and accept the responsibilities it entails. There is no future in a closed system. And present-day systems of nursing education and nursing practice are indeed closed, female-based institutions. Virginia Cleland recently stated, "My fear is that a desire for protection will win over a bolder plan involving more calculated risks."[1] Female Uncle Toms have charted the direction of nursing all too long. Without boldness, nursing will continue to be consumed by more aggressive groups.

And who are these aggressive groups? At a recent convention of the American Medical Association a resolution was passed to take whatever action is necessary "to assure preservation of the physician's authority to use and direct allied health personnel." In a growing number of instances professional nursing has been referred to as one of the allied health groups. During this same convention the chairman of the board of trustees called for programs to expand the role of the nurse in the delivery of basic medical care. "But the American Medical Association wants a moratorium on any licensure laws that would give R.N.'s or P.A.'s (physicians' associates) more specific authority than they now have."[2] The American Nurses' Association supports this moratorium.

Patients are also becoming an aggressive group. The public is no longer willing to accept haphazard care. Yet, the public has not sufficiently defined the multitude of roles assigned to the numerous types, varieties, and levels of workers providing services. A person will go wherever the service, not necessarily the care, can be found according to his medical needs and wants. In all too many instances it is the nonprofessional worker who is there to care. Nursing as an organized group is not visible at block meetings, community service center discussions, social action sessions, legislative hearings, housing authority meetings, school committee sessions, or town meetings. Organized nursing does not initiate or lead causes. Parents and lay groups do. So long as we practice isolationism, there will always be groups who can and will determine the future roles of nursing.

Why have neither nursing as an organized unit nor its leaders been able or even willing to determine and maintain their own direction? There is no valid logic or rationale in discussing trends and directions in maternity nursing roles unless there is first an examination of the larger group—professional nursing practitioners—of which maternity nurses are only one small part. A delineation of the basic issues must be established and discussed before predictions of role potential can be offered.

ACCOUNTABILITY AND INDEPENDENCE

Nurses today are struggling with disjuncture—disjuncture derived from a juxtaposition of vastly different and extremely incongruent beliefs, ideas, and practices. Partial definitions, inefficient proposed models of change, insignificant or unreceptive targets, ineffective attempts at solutions, and inappropriate proposed alternatives all point to the same conclusion. Have we become too preoccupied with the idea of change to examine what to change? If we have, our vision of the future will not halt the diverse, incongruent, and conglomerate programs and systems of care and practice called nursing.

Planned change is grounded in clusters of value commitments. But do we know ours? The crucial question that must be raised and faced squarely at this time by the entire nursing profession is: Do we want to change? Appearances would indicate that we do not. We are at a point where decisions must be made and a direction must be taken. The true test of beliefs is in their implementation. Either we believe in what we say—that change is needed and that change must come now—and act, or we must face the reality that we do not want to change.[3, 4]

Model Construction

Role definition and model construction are present-day professional preoccupations. Assuredly, the role of the clinical nursing specialist is not a new one. Discussions about the need for nurses who are prepared clinicians and the potential contribution these specialists could make toward the improvement of nursing practice can be documented in the professional literature as early as 1944.[5] Over a quarter of a century later the role and its potential are still being discussed, not in terms of reporting the results of scientifically controlled research investigations supporting the identified functions of the specialist and not in terms of rigorously formulated control experiments to measure clinician effectiveness in patient or client care management, but still only in terms of potential model formation and speculative conceptions of effectiveness in practice.

There are a number of reasons why progress in the role development of the clinical specialist has been so slow and confined to such a limited sphere of influence in actual practice. Prevailing inappropriate expectations of nursing roles, underutilization of existing qualified practitioners, lack of physician acceptance in the validity of graduate education for professional nurses, administrative misuse of nursing personnel, rigid systems of organizational structure, and traditional forms of bureaucratic management have all made significant contributions toward stifling the progress of research into the development and testing of models of specialist roles in nursing. Certainly, not the least of these obstacles is the resistance of nurses themselves. No one attributable cause can, or should, be isolated to explain the present dilemma confronting today's activists and innovators in nursing education and practice. However, it would be a propitious move on the part of professional nursing to seriously examine the historical basis of this incongruity of stated role potential that is never transformed into service delivered.

Independent Practice

Although the ANA was founded 75 years ago, entrepreneurs are still significantly lacking among the national leaders in nursing. It is conceivable that the national organizations will not be providing the kind of risk-taking leadership that will be needed to plan for the profound changes that are mandatory for the next quarter century of nursing. If significant methodological changes are to occur in systems of health care delivery, nursing can no longer exist as a dependent, for-hire, quasi profession. A new philosophy of professional nursing practice must be developed—a philosophy of accountable, self-governing independence.

Historical Foundations

It is important to examine the evolution of nursing in its close relation to out-group social movements and emancipationist efforts. The ANA can trace its historical development back to an ardent feminist, Lavinia Dock, who developed the bylaws for nursing alumnae groups and later founded the Nurses' Associated Alumnae of the United States and Canada, renamed the American Nurses' Association in 1911.[6] Nursing associations were the "first professional groups to be organized and controlled by women in the United States."[7] The history of nursing has been marked by many firsts, yet the profession seems to benefit least by its own advances. There have been moments of color and humor; yet these events are frequently unknown, misunderstood, or unappreciated by many.

As a dedicated feminist, socialist, and pacifist, Lavinia Dock went to jail three times in her career as part of her campaign to secure women's right to vote.[8] She, perhaps more than any other nursing leader, demonstrated how closely the development of modern nursing was tied to the movements to secure the emancipation of women. She once appeared at a nursing convention with a sign on her chest urging, "vote for women" and, ignoring the topic assigned to her, proceeded to make a "fiery suffrage speech to a somewhat disinterested audience."[9] One of Miss Dock's most bitter disappointments came when the ANA voted to *oppose* the equal rights amendment to the Constitution—the amendment that gives women equality with men under the law.

Many felt that the failure of organized nursing to support the passage of the equal rights amendment was a great mistake. The year 1913 also marked another historical defeat. During the first 25 years of existence the ANA was never able to establish minimum standards of hours and pay for graduate nurses. In California in 1913 the legislature enacted a law to regulate the hours of work for women. At a mass meeting in San Francisco, before the law was passed, large groups of nurses met and reluctantly agreed to the inclusion of student nurses in the provisions of the act but would not agree to the inclusion of any mention of the graduate nurse.[10] Their stand was supported by nursing groups across the country, and as a consequence, graduate nurses were not included in most of the state laws that regulated working hours for women and children.

Over 50 years later the California Nurses Association and the ANA initiated the present wave of today's dissenting nurses. State nurses' associations all over the country followed California's lead in demanding equal employment opportunities and the right to collective bargaining; the ANA was named as the official bargaining agent to begin again the struggle of fair pay and decent working hours. There is no justifiable reason for a profession of over 100 years' standing to have the issue of wages and hours assume any greater importance than it has for any other professional group.

Feminist movements in this country have provided the impetus needed for nursing development, and the present-day women's liberation front is once again opening the doors for nursing. Whether we go through the door or not is a question only history will record; however, the time is ripe, the clinical practitioner's role is established, the need is great, and the technology for change is available.

Decision and Direction

The idea of self-governance will not be easily implemented for at least two reasons. *First*, the tradition of medical and hospital administrative influences on decision making in professional matters is deeply ingrained. It will require patience, persistence, and understanding to convince physicians and administrators of the need for a shift from their authority to complete independence in matters of professional nursing practice. *Second*, self-governance will require a redivision of authority within the profession itself. For example, consider the area of licensure. Licensure only indicates the meeting of minimum standards of preparation and knowledge, and it is not in itself sufficient to predict competence levels required for independent practice—the role demanded of the professional practitioner of nursing. It will be necessary to evaluate current licensure requirements and the focus of State Board Examinations to assess more realistically competence for independent *nursing* practice.

There is one further issue to consider in the area of professional self-governance. Nurses are reluctant to make peer judgments in the public interest. With operative self-governance this would be a mandatory responsibility. It will be necessary to develop a sophisticated understanding of competence, ethics, due process, and public welfare. To assume that nurses today are primarily responsible for the quality of nursing care provided is absurdly naïve. But nurses should and must be held professionally accountable. It will be incumbent upon the ANA to establish standards for practice, systems of governance and accountability for implementation of practice, and procedures of due process and redress for failure to uphold professional standards of practice.

Although the ANA has had its periods of failure, it has also had brief periods of brilliance. One such period was 1965. The now famous position paper essentially supported two types of nursing preparation: the baccalaureate level of preparation for professional nurses, and the associate degree attainment for technical nurses. Unfortunately, this position has not been well received by the majority of current practicing nurses. Since the ANA is more advisory than regulatory in nature, nursing groups have not felt any real pressure to respond actively in setting realistic and urgent targets for implementation. The most serious threat to the viability of nursing as a profession, however, comes from within. Nursing must make of itself, and of its role in the emerging patterns of health services, something much more vital, substantial, and distinctive than it has up to now. Should it neglect this challenge, it may pass quietly from the scene, "a victim of that bad joke of history which, when salvation seems nearest at hand, shuns those who have prayed most fervently and waited most patiently for it, only to bestow the fruits of its promise on them that cared not."[11]

Emerging Roles

Who will be tomorrow's independent practitioners of nursing? We are rapidly and confusingly developing a myriad of roles, programs, and practices which have achieved little but which have drained off a frightening number of nurses from the mainstream of available manpower for providing health services. It is inconceivable that such a hodgepodge of programs for specific role practice have actually made a significant impact upon the improvement of current systems of organizing and delivering services to people. Presently we have clinical nursing specialists, often with ill-defined roles; physicians' assistants, with vague programs for role preparation; master clinicians, with rigid and often unscientific curricula underpinning a weak role performance; and a host of other groups, providing fragmented services to families.

Possibly the most tragic circumstance of all is the unnecessary competition between current programs to prepare small groups of nurses for unrealistic or outdated professional practices. Controversy can be a positive and driving force in the creation of improved services only if differences of opinion, preparation, and practice are rigorously evaluated. Controversy for its own sake, however, is a profession's greatest tragedy. Within present educational systems of role preparation philosophical differences of content emphasis and scope of practice delineations exist not only to the detriment of providing significant numbers of qualified practitioners but, more seriously, to the detriment of the welfare of the very fabric of today's family health.

The present-day maternity nursing role both as it is taught and as it is practiced is definitely obsolete and often ineffective. A maternity nurse whose training, education, and commitment has been confined to the pregnancy cycle alone, minimizing the family's many related needs, cannot be considered within the dimensions of independent nursing practice. All nurses who provide services to families must have both the theory base and the practice experiences encompassing a philosophy of maternal and child health care. A maternity nurse who is not knowledgeable or comfortable in dealing with issues of child development, family life education, and parent development will provide a professionally deficient service. It is no longer feasible to continue to support programs that cannot provide these experiences.

It would seem logical, therefore, to proceed as rapidly as possible to phase out all specialty preparation programs that are so limited in scope as to develop nurses who cannot provide the care and service that parents need to ensure opportunities for understanding the demands of pregnancy, parenthood, and family development. The place of independent schools of midwifery in such a design is highly questionable. Without a base of maternal–child health knowledge and experience they are mere schools of techniques and procedures of medical practice. With a firm base in maternal–child health theory and practice is there a need to maintain separate schools of midwifery or should they be incorporated into existing programs of maternal–child health nursing? Not only must the profession define the parameters of nursing practice, but it must also come to grips with the scope of specialty services and education.

CONFRONTING ISSUES

The trend for health care today is to provide primary care within the community and episodic and exotic care within the hospital setting. With the change in the direction of health care, there is a concomitant change in the direction of nursing. This seems an ideal time to implement the concept of the independent practitioner in maternity nursing. Before the concept of the independent practitioner in maternity nursing can become a reality, the following issues must be explored by the profession as a whole:

1 Professional concepts for practice
2 Changing parameters in practice
3 Institution roles
4 Sociological confrontations

Professional Concepts for Practice

Two sets of concepts need to be examined when contemplating the efficacy of the independent practitioner in nursing. The first set is accountability and self-governance. The second is freedom and authority. Through the utilization of these concepts, the profession of nursing can develop its image.

ACCOUNTABILITY AND SELF-GOVERNANCE

The issue of accountability means that professional nurses are prepared to answer themselves, their colleagues, and their clients in relation to any nursing actions which are based on a *nursing* diagnosis. It presupposes that the nurse can assess *nursing* needs in a given situation, devise and execute a plan of care based on these needs, and evaluate the effectiveness of nursing actions. No longer would the nurse be under the aegis of the physician or the employing institution. Successes and mistakes become the nurse's own. Because the nurse would be liable for actions based on *nursing* assessments, malpractice insurance becomes a practical investment.

If professional nurses are to be accountable for their own actions, then it follows that nursing as a profession must be self-governing. Standards of practice concomitant with independent practice must be established. New legislation must be enacted relative to the Nursing Practice Act. Decisions regarding pay scales, area of practice, and retirement plans would become the responsibility of nursing. Yet, before professional nurses can know those actions for which they are accountable, they must enhance and validate their application of the basic sciences utilized in nursing. In this way nurses can define the parameters of nursing practice. Once this is accomplished, nurses can determine the degree to which they possess the freedom and authority to be self-governing.

FREEDOM AND AUTHORITY

Freedom without authority is anarchy. Authority without freedom is tyranny. The professional nurse has authority because of the knowledge of and the ability to apply the basic sciences in the field of nursing. Nurses possess freedom because they can choose a nursing action from several possible plans based on their authority. The degree of authority and freedom they possess depends upon the degree to which they make themselves available to others and the degree to which they allow others to make themselves useful to nurses. In this way trust is built between the nurse and the patients and their families, the nurse and colleagues within nursing and related fields, and the nurse and the community.

If nurses utilize their knowledge and ability to apply the basic sciences as *expert* authority, they may blind themselves to available resources in other people. This presenting image may depict one who is always willing to give information but never to receive, one who is unable to realize that others with whom one is working are also authorities. Thus, nurses decrease their own and others' freedom to choose appropriate action because of lack of information.

In order to become independent practitioners, professional nurses must communicate their authority and freedom to all with whom they are concerned. This has been accomplished to some degree on an individual basis, but it must be done for nursing as a profession. Nurses must document, evaluate, and communicate what they do. Otherwise, they will never be free to determine their roles. The professional nurse may disappear.

IMAGE DEVELOPMENT

Regardless of role preparation and setting, professional nurses can communicate their authority and freedom through their actions, both verbally and nonverbally. Once they demonstrate their knowledge and ability to provide meaningful health services, they must document and evaluate their actions. This should then be communicated through publication, not only in nursing journals but also in the mass media. As consumers of health care become aware of the nursing services available to them, they will seek these services more freely. As trust is built between client and nurse, the client can provide the nurse with additional evaluation of nursing actions.

Through documentation and evaluation, the existing body of nursing knowledge will be enhanced and validated. Thus, the basis for defining the parameters of nursing practice is established. Once these parameters are defined, professional nurses can determine those actions for which they are accountable, become self-governing, and establish standards concomitant with independent practice.

RESISTANCE

Resistance to independent practice will come from the profession. Change is threatening. It involves a break with tradition. Documentation and evaluation take time and thought. Some duties traditionally performed by nurses will be taken away, and new ones will be added. In order to prepare nurses for independent practice, the profession must provide continuing inservice education.

Those who would utilize the services of the independent practitioner (physicians, employing institutions, health care consumers) may also resist this change. Traditionally, the physician and the institution have had authority. The nurse has carried out the physician's orders and abided by institution policy.

NURSING SPECIALISTS IN PRACTICE

Imagine that Ida Pendent, a clinical specialist in maternal–child health nursing, is working as an independent practitioner with a group of obstetricians. Her parameters of practice include teaching, counseling, history-taking, physical assessment, and recording of findings. Her caseload consists of women who have uncomplicated pregnancies.

Mary Para, according to Miss Pendent's calculations, is in her twenty-second week of pregnancy. Mrs. Para has one child, Tip, who is eighteen months of age and mentally retarded. During an office visit, Mrs. Para had complained about the difficulty she was having in toilet training Tip. Miss Pendent had tried, during two office visits and one home visit, to help Mrs. Para view Tip according to his developmental age. These attempts appeared unsuccessful, and Miss Pendent felt frustrated.

Lucy Freedman is a clinical specialist in maternal–child health nursing working as an independent practitioner with a group of pediatricians. Miss

Pendent, realizing that she was in need of nursing consultation, made an appointment with Miss Freedman. The Para family is known by Miss Freedman, who has been involved with Tip and his family since he was three months old. One month ago, Mrs. Para announced to Miss Freedman that she no longer wished her to provide health care for Tip. Miss Freedman has been unsuccessful in her attempts to discover the reason for this.

During the consultation visit, Miss Freedman explained to Miss Pendent that she thought Mrs. Para had been realistic about Tip's potential until 2 months ago. She had not known of Mrs. Para's pregnancy until the meeting with Miss Pendent. As each clinical specialist shared information regarding the Para family, they identified what they thought was the major problem— Mrs. Para's fear of producing another defective child. She was in the dilemma of not having accepted fully the reality of one defective child and being afraid of producing a second defective child. The clinical specialists felt that she was so afraid of the possibility of a second defective child that she was trying to make the first normal. She had refused help from Miss Freedman in regard to Tip. Now, she was also refusing help from Miss Pendent in regard to her pregnancy consultation. The clinical specialists decided that Miss Pendent would continue to work with Mrs. Para around her fears during pregnancy. She would also consult with Miss Freedman periodically in relation to realistic expectations for Tip and try to help Mrs. Para resolve this problem.

Both Miss Pendent and Miss Freedman demonstrated their authority through their application of the basic sciences to their nursing intervention with the Para family—for instance, anatomy, physiology, psychology. They utilized their freedom to consult with one another and to devise a plan of nursing care from several possible alternatives. They displayed their accountability for their own actions through the consultative process and their decision making. By defining their parameters of practice in working with the Para family, they exhibited their ability to be self-governing.

The authors adjure the readers to attempt to answer these questions. Is this example of independent nursing practice consistent with nurse practice standards? Are there legal implications? Who will stand behind the nurse who sees her commitment to independent practice as a professional right? The ANA? The universities? The public?

Changing Parameters of Practice

MODEL OBSOLESCENCE

Revitalized systems of role-model preparation are mandatory if health services are to be energized and appropriate target programs are to be developed. Tomorrow's independent practitioners of nursing cannot be produced by today's schools of nursing. The 1965 position paper of the ANA was less than a modest beginning. Substantial—but purposeful—change must occur now in the philosophy and value orientation of the faculties of present schools of nursing. Current curricula in nursing education are essentially obsolete and ineffective. Dependent role-model teachers do not produce independent practitioner graduates. Curricula of acquiescence will not develop practitioners of accountability. Teaching medical practices will not produce nursing practitioners.

It is not at all difficult to understand why a profession of 100 years' standing is still attempting to define the art and science of its being. Nursing and nursing care have never really been the central occupation of nursing. Filling vacuums and coordinating a series of independent or isolated services have been nursing's major preoccupation for over a century—and much of that either could or should have been the work of others. It is little wonder that the goals, philosophy, and curricula of nursing are so varied in expectation and production. Designing programs around the unwanted tasks and unmet needs of others does not validate a profession. If nursing is an independent profession, then it should produce persons who can practice the arts of the profession independently. The nurse's service should not be governed, guided, or ordered by another profession; it should be requested or sought just as it is with any other profession.

There seems to be no scientific evidence in the literature to validate continuing the assumption that a doctor and a nurse constitute the core of a health team. Therefore, there is no justifiable reason to assume that the curricula of nursing education or the practices of nursing service should continue to be fashioned after medical models of education and practice. Essentially, medical practice and the preparation of practitioners of medicine focus on illness concepts. On the other hand, the art and science of nursing are viewed by many as being broader and more comprehensive but also more general in intent. Consequently, medical models have been inappropriate images and ineffective vehicles to achieve the objectives of nursing practices. Professional nursing should be concerned primarily with wellness and *then* with services for restoration to wellness levels. It is inconceivable that wellness philosophies and wellness models can come from illness constructs and theories.

Not only are the models of medical education inappropriate for nursing preparation, but so are the models of clinical division. Maternity nurses should not consider themselves competent professional practitioners if their preparation has been only in hospital-based obstetrics. Obstetric and gynecologic services are undoubtedly appropriate clinical units to prepare a medical specialist for practice in these areas, but these services do not prepare a nurse for maternity nursing practice. Although model components certainly can vary, any model that is developed to prepare a maternity nursing specialist for the kinds of health care services and practices that will be demanded in the future must concern itself with theories and experiences related to the care of parents and their children.

Maternity nursing will soon become one of the artifacts of American history unless both the role and the preparation to carry out the role are drastically expanded. Maternity nursing has too long confined itself to the physical care of a physiologic condition. Some academic attention has been given to the forces and dynamics of parenthood which dramatically and significantly affect the pregnancy state. However, little or no attention has been given in most academic programs to experiences involving the care of children or the education of developing parents. Health needs and social concerns now and in the immediate future demand professional groups who are competent as well as responsive. Programs preparing maternity nurses will need to be well grounded in the liberal arts and in the basic sciences before any attention can be given to the specific knowledges required for independent maternity nursing practice.

MODEL PREPARATION

Programs preparing professional nursing practitioners must be housed in university settings, but these programs—as they now exist—will not be adequate for the kind of educational experiences needed for independent practice. Baccalaureate programs should prepare family health nursing practitioners. The philosophical basis will need to change, as will the teaching methodologies required to implement these programs. Integrated content will not ensure integrated thinking processes. Approaches to learning will require a socioanthropological focus with more attention given to such areas as problem-solving methods, directed and independent study, skill development in the analysis of process and content records of interaction activities, and short-term interventive confrontations. Such skills as the assessment procedures for newborn physical examinations, child development and growth scales, and the physiological progress of pregnancy should be taken out of intermediate or stop-gap programs, such as the current maternity and pediatric practitioner or physician's assistant and associate training experiences, and placed where they are more appropriate and effective—in the first-level professional degree program.

Graduate programs at the master's level would prepare beginning clinical nursing specialists in family health practice. The clinical specialist preparation in maternal–child health care would focus on developing first-level practitioners in both maternity and pediatric nursing; however, future programs in specialty areas will need to consider a philosophical reorganization of the preparation needed and the length of time required to produce the independent professional clinician. There are no valid reasons for lengthening the preparation period for first-level specialty practice. Generally, programs are lengthened not because of knowledge explosions but more likely because of faculty ineffectiveness in developing more advanced teaching methodologies. Problems of faculty development should be faced squarely and handled as such, and not at the expense of students. First-level specialty preparation in maternal–child health nursing can be achieved within the limits of a calendar year and yet include a base of midwifery skills, child development, and family life experiences for both maternity and pediatric nurses.

Second-level specialization will come from independent nursing practitioners prepared at the doctoral level in nursing science, the basic disciplines, or the functional processes of teaching and administration. Regardless of the focus of preparation, all programs at the doctoral level should have a balanced distribution of nursing and discipline or cognate-based course work. Doctoral education should not continue to foster a spiraling narrowness— frequently referred to as depth. A specialist should be able to develop depth in nursing practice through breadth in educational preparation. Doctoral programs would serve to produce nursing consultants, researchers, scientists, and process implementers. The senseless argument of which degree is best for nurses should cease. The profession needs entrepreneurs of practice, research, and process; routes should be accessible to all approaches.

MODEL IMPLEMENTATION

Frequent references have been made to a concept of independent practice and the independent practitioner. A review of the literature does not clarify just what might be considered independent activity in nursing. It would seem, however, that the fullest meaning of the term must be considered, not only in its vernacular intent but also in its professional implementation. It is well past the time for nursing to assume the same independence that is expected of and afforded to all other professional practitioners. In this respect, then, the idea of nurses having hospital appointments, office hours, and group practices should not be unbelievable. Maternity nurses in the future will function within just this sort of framework. There is no reason why maternity and pediatric nurses could not open offices for group practice in which the focus of care is on wellness preservation and wellness restoration. Since pregnancy is a wellness concept, it is conceivable that the maternity nurse would make a physical assessment and have a laboratory perform the usual tests to determine the existence of a pregnancy before referring the client to an obstetrician.

During the general course of nursing practice, the maternity nurse might deal with a mother who has a child who is failing to thrive. After consultation with the pediatric family practitioner in group practice, the pediatric nurse might wish to examine the child and possibly admit him to the hospital to rule out any physical causes of his condition. A resident physician on the staff of the hospital would assume responsibility for this diagnostic admission, but the pediatric nurse practitioner would assume the responsibility for the diagnosis and orders during the period of hospitalization. The maternity family practitioner would continue to see the child's mother, who is pregnant and in need of supportive services as well as pregnancy supervision. For the period of hospitalization of the child the pediatric nurse would work directly with the mother or might serve as a consultant to the maternity nurse.

The idea of hospital appointments is not new for many professional groups, but it certainly is for nursing. No legitimate reason exists to preclude this possibility—the obsequious nature of hospital nursing would need to change dramatically, however. Appointments to staff positions in hospital settings would in no way limit or hinder those specialist family health practitioners who will wish the security of working for organizations or institutions. The manner in which they work for the institution would, however, need to be reexamined and reestablished. Any number of possibilities exist for the future independent family health practitioner. The limits will be the visionary limits of nursing.

Institution Roles

With the advent of neighborhood and community health clinics in urban areas, the role of institutions is beginning to change. In the past, hospitals have been primary health care centers. Many planned visits to hospital clinics were never realized. The hospital was quite a distance from the neighborhood. Too much time was spent in traveling to and from the hospital and in waiting to be seen in the clinic. Parents could not be certain that they would be home when their children returned from school. If they had children younger than school age and could not obtain baby-sitters, they would have to bring these children with them to the hospital. This proved to be an exhausting day for both parents and children. For these reasons many parents failed to come to hospital clinics on the appointed day.

EPISODIC, EXOTIC, AND PRIMARY HEALTH CARE

Today neighborhood and community health clinics are centers for primary health care while hospitals provide episodic and exotic care. Thus, the pregnant woman receives prenatal care in a community setting unless complications develop. With complications, such as toxemia of pregnancy, she would be followed in a hospital-based clinic which is designed to meet her needs. Admission to the hospital would be based on unusual diagnoses, experimental care, and the need for intensive care. The pregnant woman might be hospitalized because of the threat of a spontaneous miscarriage or abortion, preeclampsia or eclampsia, or a multiple pregnancy. She would also be hospitalized for the actual delivery of her baby. Postpartum care begins in the hospital and continues in the community setting unless complications are present. If the postpartum course is abnormal, care would be provided in the hospital setting. The type of hospital setting, either inpatient or ambulatory services, would be dependent upon the nature of the postpartum course.

Americans from all strata of society are making known their belief that good health care is a fundamental right of citizenship. Legislators are responding with various national health insurance plans. Prepaid plans would be underwritten federally and/or privately. Federal monies would come from tax revenues. Private monies would be supplied by payroll levies and by private health insurance plans. One danger of national health insurance is the possible decrease of freedom and authority for the health professions due to federal, industrial, and insurance control. Members of all health professions (medicine, nursing, social work, psychology) must work diligently with legislators and industrial and insurance representatives in order to ensure their rights to freedom and authority and to accountability and self-governance.

One way to accomplish this would be to provide for several private community health centers throughout each state, as formulated by Louis P. Bertonazzi, Massachusetts House of Representatives. These clinics would be designed by members of the health professions. The members of each professional group would collaborate with each other and with community representatives in preparing centers which would meet the health care needs of each individual community. Each center would contract with area hospitals to provide episodic and exotic care. Prepaid insurance plans would furnish the financial needs of the centers and the hospitals. The health centers would be primary care centers for people from all strata of society. This would not preclude private practice for members of the health professions. The members of each health profession would enjoy the right to independent practice, but they would be interdependent in their provision of health care to the community. In order to estimate the efficacy of the community clinics as primary health care centers, periodic evaluation by health professionals and consumers would be necessary. The results of such evaluations would be the basis upon which changes would or would not be made.

THE PROFESSIONAL NURSE

Different levels of professional nurses will be needed in private community health centers. There will be a need for family practitioners and clinical specialists. The type of clinical specialists found in the centers will be dependent upon community health needs. The family practitioner will perform health assessments on all family members. As the need arises, appropriate referral will be made to a clinical specialist in maternal–child health nursing, medical-surgical nursing, adult psychiatric nursing, child psychiatric nursing, rehabilitation nursing, or community health nursing. If family problems are not in the realm of nursing, the family practitioner will make the referral to the appropriate health professional.

In the area of maternity nursing, when a family practitioner discovers that a family member is pregnant, a health assessment is first made. Then a clinical specialist in maternal-child nursing is consulted. Together, they can design a plan of care and decide who will implement the care. The pregnant woman may have many questions relative to her pregnancy which have physiological and psychological implications. If she has other children at home, she may want help in preparing them for the advent of a new family member. She may have questions relative to toilet training her two-year-old or methods of preventing her four-year-old's masturbation. The father of the expected infant may have questions in regard to the pregnant woman's mood swings, sexual intercourse during pregnancy, and the growth of the fetus. These are areas in which the clinical specialist can provide teaching and counseling, both on a one-to-one basis and in groups. If parent instruction groups are being led, the parents can be invited to join. The parent groups would be a supplement to individual counseling.

As the clinical specialist in maternal–child health nursing works with the pregnant woman and her family, nursing problems may be discovered with which the nurse is unable to deal. The nurse can then consult with a clinical specialist in the appropriate field, and together they can decide who should work with the family regarding new nursing problems.

The clinical specialist in maternal–child health nursing can also be a liaison between the health center and the hospital. Continuity of care can be ensured by passing the necessary information to hospital personnel when the pregnant woman must utilize their services and by receiving information from hospital personnel when the patient returns to the community. In the community setting, the nurse can provide information to the pediatric personnel who will be furnishing health care to the newborn infant.

Different levels of nursing will also be needed within the hospital. Health consumers will utilize hospital clinic and inpatient services for the purposes of establishing unusual diagnoses, follow-up in specialty clinics, and intensive care. Medical technology will be a very important part of health care in hospitals. Thus, the bulk of nursing care will be technical. The family nurse practitioner would supervise technical nurses in the various hospital settings. The clinical specialist would be available for consultation relating to nursing practice and staff problems.

In maternity nursing there would be family nurse practitioners in all patient care areas—specialty clinics, labor and delivery suites, postpartum and rooming-in units, and high-risk and newborn nurseries—who would supervise technical nurses and coordinate patient care. The clinical specialist would be called if any nursing problems arose which could not be handled by the staff. Inservice education would be provided for coaching laboring parents-to-be, care of high-risk infants, methods of establishing beginning parent-child relationships, and the like. The nurse could also be a liaison between the hospital and the community health centers.

With the advent of medical technology, there is a very grave danger. Those providing health care can become enamored of machines and their intricate workings. A patient's physiology may assume prime importance. Her feelings and her need to know what is happening to and within her may not be recognized or may be ignored. Hopefully, nurses will remember the person and utilize the machines as extensions of themselves.

Sociological Confrontations

THE COUNTER CULTURE

Along with the explosion of knowledge in this century came great technical advances. Because of these advances, technical experts appeared. Many became more interested in things rather than people and seemed to perceive man as an intellectual being whose psychic component was nonexistent. The technocracy had arrived. Roszak defines the technocracy as "that society in which those who govern justify themselves by appeal to technical experts who, in turn, justify themselves by appeal to scientific forms of knowledge. And beyond the authority of science there is no appeal."[12] Among a minority of middle-class youths, a counter culture is evolving. It is "a culture so radically disaffiliated from the mainstream assumptions of our society that it scarcely looks to many as a culture at all, but takes on the alarming appearance of a barbaric intrusion."[13] Its members have sought ways to go "beyond the authority of science." Some have chosen communal patterns of family life; some have evolved their own sexual code; and some have turned to psychedelic experiences through drugs, poetry, music, or bastardized versions of Zen. Many alienated youths utilize sensitivity groups as a means of finding themselves. While the technocracy concentrates on the development of the intellective aspects of the personality, the counter culture seeks to develop the psychic aspects of the personality. These groups possess their own authority and freedom, but they do not seem able to exchange this authority and freedom with one another. While they work at cross-purposes, society as a whole must cope with sociological problems, such as alienation, venereal disease, and drug dependence and addiction.

"Hot lines" in many communities are providing counsel for these problems. Help is also available in venereal disease clinics, drug clinics, hospital-based drug units, and mobile health units. Nurses can be found working in the venereal disease and drug clinics, on the drug units, and with mobile health units. A nurse, as a private citizen, may volunteer time to the hot line. Nursing must accept the fact that alienation, changing sexual codes, and drug dependence and addiction are nursing issues. As independent practitioners, professional nurses will be involved in providing nursing intervention in problems which have arisen as a result of the dichotomy between the technocracy and the counter culture. They *must* be concerned with the broader issues of society in order to define parameters of practice—a practice which will have a more relevant impact on wellness.

SELF-CONCEPT AND THE MATERNITY NURSE

The maternity nurse has the ideal opportunity to begin to equip future generations with the strength to cast aside and conquer alienation. This can be done by fostering parent-child relationships. During the prenatal period, the maternity nurse can encourage parents to discuss their thoughts, feelings, questions, and fantasies regarding their unborn child, their relationship to this future person, sibling relationships, and their own relationships. The nurse can help them to begin to accept the reality of their newborn infant in the delivery room by allowing them to see, touch, hold, and examine the baby. On the postpartum unit, parents can be encouraged to discuss their thoughts, feelings, questions, and fantasies.

An ideal time to observe mother-child relationships is during feeding. How comfortable is the mother? How comfortable is the baby? How does the mother hold her infant, touch him, look at him? What is her facial expression? The answers to these questions give the nurse the necessary data to begin the assessment of mother-child relationships and to provide nursing intervention.

Although the maternity nurse may have provided parents with excellent information which would aid them in preparing their children for the advent of a new family member, this help should be continued on the postpartum unit. One way to do this would be to provide the opportunity for the siblings to come to the hospital. Seeing their mother and the newborn might dispel many of their own fears and fantasies. Many of their questions could be answered during daily visits to the postpartum unit in the hospital.

Traditionally, the maternity nurse's last contact with the parents would be the 6-week postpartum visit. Continuance of the fostering of parent-child relationships can be ensured by providing pertinent information to the pediatric personnel who will be providing health supervision for the infant. Yet, if the maternity nurse is to be concerned with the broader issues of society, the fostering of parent-child relationships encompasses more than the span of time covered in the prenatal through the postpartum periods. The nurse can become involved with parent groups, church groups, community groups, and teachers who are developing education programs in human sexuality (also known as sex education and family-life education). This education begins in the prenatal period and ends with death. It enhances the self-image in relation to oneself and others, as male and female. It teaches self-respect and respect for others. Thus, a person learns to give as well as receive. He becomes capable of experiencing a loving relationship in all human situations. He learns that he possesses not just intellect but a psyche—that feeling, mystical, mind-expanding part of himself which is unmeasurable yet so meaningful to his personality development and status as an individual.

REFERENCES

1 Cleland, Virginia: "Sex Discrimination: Nursing's Most Pervasive Problem," *American Journal of Nursing*, 71:1547, August 1971.
2 Isler, C., S. Rockwell, and B. Shaw: "A Doctor's View of the Nurse: Still a Handmaiden, but . . .," *R.N.*, 34:58, August 1971.
3 Boucher, Rita J.: "Similarities and Differences in Perceptions of the Role of the Clinical Nursing Specialist," vol. I, unpublished doctoral dissertation, Boston University, 1970.
4 Bruce, Sylvia J.: "Valuation of Functions of the Role of the Clinical Nursing Specialist," vol. II, unpublished doctoral dissertation, Boston University, 1970. Materials related to role development and professional independence were drawn from volumes I and II, chapters 1 and 2.
5 Reiter, Frances: "Nurse-Clinician," *American Journal of Nursing*, 66:225, February 1966.
6 Bullough, Vern, and Bonnie Bullough: *The Emergence of Modern Nursing*, Macmillan, New York, 1969, p. 152.
7 Ibid., p. 149.
8 Ibid., p. 154.
9 Ibid., p. 155.
10 Ibid., p. 167.
11 Davis, Fred (ed.): *The Nursing Profession: Five Sociological Essays*, Wiley, New York, 1966, p. 175.
12 Roszak, Theodore: *The Making of a Counter Culture*, Doubleday, Garden City, N.Y., 1969, p. 8.
13 Ibid., p. 42.

3 | THE NURSING PROCESS IN MATERNITY NURSING

Ernestine Wiedenbach

Nursing has always been regarded as a helping service, to be rendered with compassion, skill, and understanding to those in need of care, counsel, and confidence in the area of health.* Its practice comprises a wide variety of services, each directed toward the attainment of one of its three components: (1) identification of the patient's need for help, (2) ministration of help needed, and (3) validation that the help provided was indeed helpful to the patient.

Over the years, however, the outward character of nursing has changed. The setting in which the nurse functions is different today. In times gone by, patients were cared for in large open wards, and the nurse's "station" was a table or desk in the center of the ward or at its end. A patient need never feel alone. He could readily see the nurse and call for help if necessary, and the nurse could as easily see and call to him. Today, on the other hand, in many hospitals, patients are cared for in single, two-, or four-bed units, with the nursing station centrally located in the corridor outside. Contact between nurse and patient may be established via an intercommunication system (in-

---

* Health is defined by the World Health Organization as a state of complete physical, mental, and social well-being and not merely the absence of disease and infirmity.

tercom) by pushing a button in the box on the wall. In former days, too, the nurse cared for all of the patient's needs, assisted the doctor with dressings and treatments, and managed the ward. Today the nurse is apt to delegate direct care of patients to other personnel, such as licensed practical nurses and nursing aides, may make rounds with the doctor, and cooperates with unit managers in administrative duties.

Changes comparable to those in hospitals have taken place in the field of public health nursing, too. In earlier days nurses went afield to knock on doors to find and help those in need or to invite them to well-baby clinics or to classes for mothers. Today a patient is more apt to be referred to a nursing agency by a community doctor, hospital, or other agency and then may be visited by the nurse to assess his needs and arrange for follow-up care. Not too often does the public health nurse provide bedside nursing care for patients in their homes. Rather, members of the family are instructed and encouraged to give it, or such care may be delegated to a nonprofessional member of the staff. The nurse is then free to concentrate on measures for disease prevention, to teach classes for expectant parents, and to cooperate with community agencies in developing health and welfare programs. Thus, opportunities for fostering warm, close relationships between nurse and patient are less common today, whether in the hospital or in the field of public health; yet, the patients' need for care, counsel, and confidence has remained unchanged or, if anything, has increased.

This trend toward impersonalization of nursing care presents problems. Many patients are unhappy about it and frustrated by it. Their experience with nurses—or lack of it—is not in accord with their preconceived image of the nurse as a helping person. Many nurses, too, are dissatisfied and frustrated by this impersonalization. Their desire to give direct care to patients and to meet their needs is as keen as it was when they, as students, entered the nursing world. Pressures, however, due to understaffing, rising patient census, electronics, research, and sophistication of modern hospital management and medical care make it almost impossible for the nurse to develop a close relationship with the patient and derive the satisfactions that result from concerned patient care.

Frustrations exist in the area of maternity nursing, too, particularly in hospitals where most pregnant women are urged to go for care. Except in relatively rare situations in which nursing students have been assigned expectant mothers to follow through their childbearing courses or in which nurse-midwifery programs have been instituted, nurses are unable to give individual mothers the amount of time and attention they know the mothers need. In antepartum and postpartum clinics, on labor and delivery services, and on postpartum units the ratio between number of nurses and number of patients is usually in serious disproportion—especially during the evening and night hours. The lone nurse then is often so overwhelmed by demands made by doctors, telephone calls, students doing research, families of patients, and patient admissions as well as by administrative responsibilities, including tasks such as charting, that it is almost impossible to give uninterrupted attention to mothers who are in need of service.

Yet, in maternity nursing, a close and warm relationship between nurse and patient is of special importance. The childbearing process imposes on the woman physical alterations, often accompanied by discomforts and fears, to a greater degree than do other physiological phenomena. Changes, sometimes disfiguring, and frequently not completely understood by the woman, occur in her body; the certainty of labor is anticipated with varying degrees of apprehension. A new life which she must nurture is growing either within her or in the crib beside her, and marital relationships and responsibilities can induce strains that are hard to deal with, especially if unaccompanied by love and understanding. Many nurses, in their preparation in both basic and graduate schools of nursing, have become poignantly aware of patients' potential problems and have developed the resources—knowledge, judgment, procedural and interaction skills—so essential to resolve them. But how, amidst the realities of today, does the nurse appropriately apply them? How does the nurse bridge the gap between the desire to meet the needs of patients and the availability to effectively meet them?

Two courses of action are suggested for consideration:

1 Develop understanding of the process that determines nursing actions.
2 Incorporate in practice measures that will enhance the effective functioning of the nursing process.

CONCEPTUALIZATION OF THE NURSING PROCESS

To develop understanding of the process that determines one's nursing actions is a self-searching and self-revealing undertaking. Difficult though this may be, it is worth doing. The quality of nursing service is measured by the effectiveness of the nurse's individual actions, that is, by the degree to which the nurse succeeds in eliciting from the patient, behavioral and physiological responses that are in accordance with the physician's plan of treatment and with the nurse's purpose in nursing. Nursing actions, thus, are significant; they contribute to the patient's ability to realize his hopes and his needs for health.

Nursing action may be envisaged as an energized phenomenon that occurs within the realities of the existing situation and is carried on with, or in behalf of, an individual involved with restoration or insurance of his health. It is the visible portion of nursing practice in which the nurse interacts by word, look, manner, or deed with another person—the patient, another member of the staff, or a member of the patient's family—to bring about results that are desired. Nursing actions, however, do not just happen.

There is a series of operations underlying and powering each one that gives import and direction to each nursing act. This series of operations is regarded as the nursing process, and it is an influencing factor in whatever the nurse may do. It may be activated in many different ways—by bright sunrays striking a sleeping baby's face, an expression of fear in a woman's eyes, or a request for medication to help her go to sleep. Such activating situations are interpreted and made more meaningful to nurses by their personal thoughts and feelings which intensify their awareness of them and give them meaning according to the nurses' knowledge, values, and the realities that obtain.

The meaning the nurse attaches to such awareness, however, represents an interpretation that is based solely upon a subjective view of the situation. Three kinds of subjective interpretations may occur in quick succession within the nurse's mind upon contact with an activating situation: sensation or experienced sensory impressions; perception, or interpretation of a sensory impression; and assumption, or the meaning one attaches to one's perception of a situation. These three interpretations represent levels of awareness that are attained through concentration of attention upon the activating situation.

For example, when the nurse, Miss Black, entered the four-bed maternity unit, she experienced a tightening sensation within her as she sensed that something was wrong. Looking about, she perceived a mother lying on her side with her face buried in her pillow and shoulders heaving; her muffled sobs were faintly audible. In a flash, Miss Black recalled that the mother's baby had a congenital deformity, and she assumed that she was crying because of that distressing fact.

These three levels of awareness—sensation, perception, and assumption—are attained without great mental effort and may be said to represent the involuntary phase of the nursing process. In addition, each could also serve as a staging area for action:

When Miss Black sensed that something was wrong, she might have stopped and spontaneously exclaimed, "Hey, what's going on?"

When she perceived that the mother was crying, she could automatically have gone to her bedside and pulled the curtain around her.

And when she assumed that the reason the mother was crying was because her baby was congenitally deformed, her feelings might have prompted her to whisper, "Oh, don't cry! Your baby will be all right!"

Such acts are spontaneous, automatic, or impulsive in character. They occur on the spur of the moment and are precipitated by unchecked, rampant thoughts and feelings. Occasionally, especially in time of emergency, such spontaneous acts may have useful outcomes. For instance, spontaneous actions have been known to be lifesaving; automatic acts sometimes contribute to preventing the spread of disease; and an impulsive act, indicative of love and understanding, might enable a patient to release pent-up feelings and indulge in a good cry. However, the results of such behavior, as a rule, are

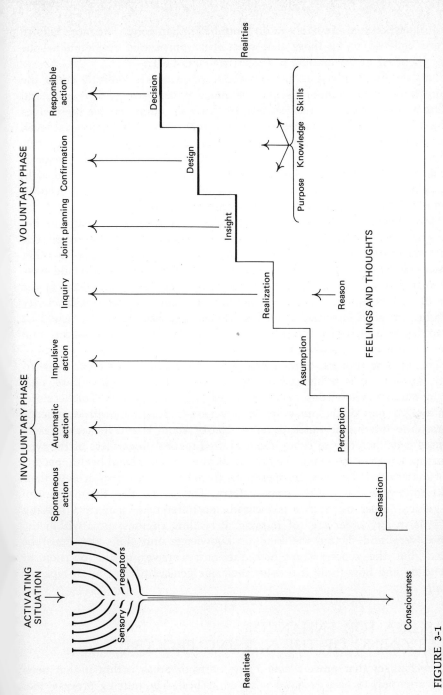

FIGURE 3-1

Conceptualization of the nursing process. Diagrammatic presentation of the influences and forces that raise the consciousness of a situation to higher levels of awareness from each of which a definitive kind of action could result.

open to question and are likely to do more harm than good. The more helpful acts are believed to be those that stem from purposeful deliberation—the voluntary phase of the nursing process. (See Figure 3-1.)

This voluntary phase is brought about when nurses willfully check the random flow of their thoughts and feelings, temper them with reason, and with its aid, bring them under control. In this way, nurses enable themselves to attain a fourth level of awareness, that of realization. It is the crucial level, for it alerts them to the subjective nature of their assumption and to their need to find out from the patient if their interpretation of his behavior is correct. Such validation or clarification then leads successively to the fifth, sixth, and seventh levels of awareness—namely, insight, design, and decision —from which responsible nursing action then can result.

Had Miss Black, for instance, recognized the subjective nature of her assumption that the mother was crying because her baby was deformed, she might well have realized that the mother's crying could be due to other causes. Then, rather than express an unfounded prediction, she would have tried to find out from the mother the reason for her tears. Knowledge of the cause of distress provides insight into her problem, and then, with clarity about her purpose in nursing, her knowledge, and her skills, she would be able to design a plan of responsible action with the patient, if necessary, and make the decision to act upon it.

The nursing process, thus, is essentially an internal, personalized mechanism. As such, it is influenced by the nurse's culture and subculture, purpose in nursing, knowledge, wisdom, sensitivity, and concern. Furthermore, as an integral part of the nurse, its effectiveness increases as, with experience and resolute intent, the nurse develops clarity about it and its many facets and uses it deliberately to bring about desired results. Regardless of the type of nursing engaged in—public health, medical-surgical, mental health, pediatric, or maternity—the series of operations through which nurses achieve their results follows essentially the same pattern. This means that the mechanism that guides nurses in practice is basically no different in maternity nursing than it is in any other area of nursing. Prevailing circumstances within the realities vary and dictate the kind of knowledge and skills that must be applied, but the process by which the nurse arrives at the decision of what to do and how to do it follows the same general pattern in all types of nursing.

MEASURES FOR ENHANCING FUNCTIONING OF THE NURSING PROCESS

Any mechanism that powers action has parts or areas within it that need special attention to keep it functioning at its best. The nursing process, too, has focal points which, if neglected or ignored, will defeat the effectiveness of the nurse's act. They are identified specifically as:

1 The nurse's beliefs and values
2 The nurse's purpose in nursing
3 The nurse's sensitivity to inconsistencies in the immediate reality situation
4 The nurse's access to reason
5 The nurse's application of knowledge and beliefs

These five points may be recognized as personal assets that tend to lie latent in the nurse until they are consciously developed and enhanced. This entails special effort, for first, clarity about them and their significance to practice must be gained. Second, the way in which they may serve best in practice must be ascertained; and third, determination to incorporate them in practice must be sustained.

Beliefs and Values

Beliefs and values supply the energy that motivates the nurse to act, and they determine the attitude displayed in what is done. For example, if the nurse believes the patient has a need, she will try to meet it; and if the nurse regards him as a worthwhile human being, she will treat him with respect and consideration. Together they constitute her value system which is an integral part of the nurse. They develop inconspicuously and may remain unidentified and nebulous unless the nurse takes time to sort them out and make them explicit. Of special importance to her practice are the beliefs she holds about the significance of life; about the worth, individuality, and aspirations of each human being; and about her own responsibilities to both the patient and to herself. By putting these beliefs and values into words, nurses are able to examine them, check their validity, and alter or refine them as their understanding of life, humanity, and themselves is deepened and enlarged. And when the nurse has given expression to them, they enlarge the dimension of her nursing process and become a vital part of it.

The Nurse's Purpose

The nurse's purpose in nursing represents a professional commitment. Although the nurse may have been told by others what it is, it will become a useful part of the nursing process only when the nurse has thought it through introspectively and has formulated a personal understanding. Specifically, the purpose in nursing sets forth (1) the qualities that the nurse will strive consistently to sustain, foster, or bring about in the patient with respect to his condition, attitude, or situation and (2) the special responsibilities that the nurse recognizes as belonging to her in caring for him. The nurse's purpose stems from her beliefs and values and comes into focus when she clarifies them for herself. As with them, the nurse's purpose in nursing will remain vague and ill-defined unless expressed in a clearly set forth statement. Although the nurse will want to reexamine the statement from time to time and possibly refine it as her scope of nursing broadens with experience, the need to have her purpose in nursing readily available in explicit terms becomes ever more apparent. It is the guiding force that sets the direction for the voluntary phase of her nursing process and gives stability to the deliberative thinking that it entails. Thus, when the nurse makes it a conscious part of the nursing process, not only will it set the course for her nursing action, but it will also enable the nurse to determine whether the results which she obtained are desired. Such understanding by the nurse is the basis not only for responsible action, but also for improvement of the quality of nursing care.

Sensitivity

Sensitivity is an attribute which essentially is part of every individual. It is closely associated with the sensory receptors that are located within the eyes, ears, nose, tongue, and somatic sensory areas and may be considered the principal trigger for setting in motion the operations of the nursing process. Sensitivity alerts the nurse to awareness of inconsistencies in the situation that might signify the presence of a problem or need. Since identification of a patient's need for help is one of the objectives of nursing practice, sensitivity is a key factor in contributing to achievement of this goal. The nurse has responsibility to do all that is possible to enhance personal sensitivity and keep it finely tuned. This is of special importance today when the multiplicity of devices that are laborsaving and efficient militate against the heightening of sensitivity.

For example, a monitoring device had been installed in the labor and delivery suite of a large city hospital, enabling the medical and nursing staffs to keep track not only of the baby's condition during the mother's course of labor but also of the frequency and character of the mother's contractions. The viewing box of the monitoring device was located in the nurse's station, thus allowing the staff, particularly the nurse, to engage in other activities while "keeping an eye" on the mother's progress. Mrs. Thompson, who had been admitted to the unit earlier in the day, was feeling increasingly apprehensive and uncomfortable as, with wires attached to her abdomen, she labored alone in her room. She wished the nurse would come and talk to her, rub her back, or listen to the baby's heart as the nurse did when she was in the hospital to have her first baby 2 years ago. But she thought the nurse was probably too busy and was reluctant to call for fear of being considered a nuisance or a weakling. After a while, though, her discomfort overcame her hesitancy, and she mustered enough courage to press the intercom button. A voice from a box on the wall responded, "Yes, Mrs. Thompson, what can I do for you?" The sound of that metallic voice, detached from a visible human being, filled Mrs. Thompson with sudden panic. All she could force herself to say was a whispered, "Could you tell me what time it is, please?"

The voice from the box answered, "Surely. Two o'clock." And that was that.

A nurse who is sensitive and clear about the purpose in nursing might have recognized the shade of anxiety in Mrs. Thompson's whispered question and responded to it rather than directly to the expressed request. The nurse also might have felt a slight surprise at the question itself and geared a response to the discrepancy sensed, especially if a glance at the monitoring device showed that Mrs. Thompson was having strong contractions with only brief intervals between them.

The finer shades of a person's behavior—the brightness of his eye, posture, gestures, mannerisms, or tone of voice—all tend to reflect the thoughts and feelings that are going on inside him, and it is to them that sensitivity needs to be directed. Likewise, sensitivity to discrepancies between behavior a patient may present and that which might be expected can alert the nurse to inner conflict or distress.

Susceptibility to such nuances of behavior is increased when they are allowed to reach the nurse's consciousness via several sensory receptors rather than just one. Had the nurse, for instance, actually been in Mrs. Thompson's presence, her facial expression, the sound and rate of her breathing, and possibly the feel of dampness of her forehead or the firmness of her grip would all have been noted. Such behavioral manifestations are telling indicators of a patient's feelings and condition but may go unnoticed by the nurse who relies primarily upon some electronic or other device to reveal a patient's need.

Effort is required to enhance one's sensitivity. It will not happen of its own accord. Not only does it require determined exposure to a multiplicity of sensory stimuli from the patient whenever possible, but it also necessitates continuous search for discrepancies between the patient's behavior and one's expectation of it. Sensitivity that is keen will impel the nurse to higher levels of awareness of the patient and will contribute to establishment of an empathic relationship from which responsible nursing action can then result.

Reason

Reason is a tempering agent as well as a stimulator of deliberative thought. It enables one to recognize the blinding quality of his feelings and helps him to assuage their intensity so that he can view the situation with greater clarity. At the same time, it enables him to realize the one-sided nature of his assumptions and encourages him to seek their validation. Just as sensitivity alerts awareness to behavioral manifestations in another, so may reason alert the nurse to awareness of inner feelings and assumptions that could cause impulsive actions.

Assumptions are the final level of awareness in the involuntary phase of the nursing process. They result from one's perception of a situation based on his idea of what it means, and they have potential for evoking strong feelings of anger, joy, or distress that may be totally unjustified by fact. They have an insidious quality, too, for their presence all too often is unrecognized, yet they are responsible for the action that is taken. The nurse, for instance, who responded to Mrs. Thompson by giving her the time of day as she requested, acted on the insidious assumption that time of day was what Mrs. Thompson really wanted to know. Had the nurse, however, resorted to reason and allowed it to bring the assumption into proper focus, its one-sidedness might have been recognized, and the response might have been very different.

The insidious quality of assumptions is also apparent in the following incident. A nurse saw a pregnant woman slowly enter the antepartum clinic area at closing time, just as the doctor was about to leave. The nurse recognized the woman as a registered patient and suddenly felt a gush of anger at her late arrival. Consequently the nurse rushed toward her and with a sharp, annoying voice exclaimed, "You know better than to get here at this late hour!" The woman, taken aback, opened her mouth as if to reply, then quickly closed it and dropped despondently onto the clinic bench, tears welling in her eyes.

That nurse let neither sensitivity nor reason preclude the action that brought frustration and unhappiness to a patient—a result the nurse surely would not have wanted to bring about. Instead, a full rein was given to the assumption that the woman had intentionally come late to clinic, and the nurse impulsively chided her for doing so.

Like sensitivity, reason is an attribute with which everyone is to some extent endowed. Furthermore, it complements the awareness to which sensitivity gives rise. Had the nurse in the example noted the nuances in the woman's appearance, manner, or gait, the woman might have been viewed in a clearer light, and reason would probably have helped the nurse realize that the woman was in some sort of distress.

Reason, defined as the ability to think, is a key property of the nursing process. Its introduction elevates awareness to the level of realization which serves as a foundation of deliberative thought. The fact that the nurse has access to reason, however, does not necessarily mean that reason will be utilized. Neither nurse in the two previous examples did. Before effective use can be made of it, the nurse needs to realize the fact that every behavioral manifestation has two aspects: the nurse's view and the view of the other person involved in the situation. When this fact is firmly entrenched in the nurse's mind, then reason can serve as a reminder that assumptions represent a unilateral view of the situation and that to take responsible nursing action the nurse must ascertain the other's view of it. This, too, requires effort to bring about.

Application of a Nurse's Knowledge and Skills

Application of a nurse's knowledge and skills is the substance of the nursing process. The aim of its operations is to enable the nurse to gear nursing action to meet the patient's need. In the field of maternity nursing, most nurses today have acquired the essential knowledge and skills in basic and graduate courses in programs of nursing education. They possess not only theoretic and factual knowledge about parents, their fears and attitudes, and about the childbearing course, but also measures that will contribute to the mother's competence and comfort, promote her health and that of her baby, and safeguard both against illness and distress. Such knowledge and skills represent a tremendous stock of resources for effective functioning, but to have them benefit the patients, nurses must first realize the extent of their knowledge and abilities and then must deliberately apply such skills in their practice.

Timeliness, receptivity, effect, and accountability are four important considerations in the application of a nurse's knowledge and skills.

TIMELINESS

The childbearing course follows an orderly sequence. The first trimester follows conception; the second trimester follows the first; the third follows the second and culminates in delivery, which brings about the baby's birth. Then, postpartum restoration occurs accompanied by lactation and the newborn's growth and development. Each of these periods is characterized by special happenings, hazards, and responsibilities that give rise to needs of which the nurse is well aware and about which parents also may want to know.

Thus, during the first trimester, when realization of pregnancy first comes with hopes, fears, and apprehensions and the developing baby imposes strains on the mother's entire system, parents may want to know when and how to obtain maternity care for the mother, what to do to keep well, and how to deal with curious feelings and symptoms of which the mother may be aware. They also may welcome information about how the baby grows and the demands it may make of her system as well as suggestions regarding adjustments to make in their daily pattern of living.

During the second trimester, when the mother is apt to feel well and buoyant, parents may want to know when classes in preparation for childbearing are held and how to register for them. The mother may appreciate information about the baby's layette as well as suggestions about eating, bathing, exercising, and just keeping well.

During the third trimester, when weight gain often is a problem for the mother, when her tissues are stretched, her muscles strained and she feels pressure everywhere, and when the day for the baby's birth looms closer, information parents may want includes ways for the mother to maintain her appearance and to be more comfortable, foods to eat and to avoid, and preparations she might make for lactation. They also are usually interested in knowing how to recognize the onset of labor, whom to notify when it has begun, when to go to the hospital, and what to expect there.

During labor, when contractions become progressively stronger, comfort measures and reassurance are what parents usually want.

And during the postpartum period, when the mother has many concerns about herself, her baby, and her family, she usually will appreciate a listening ear and answers to questions she may or may not ask. This is true not only while she is in the hospital but also after she is back at home. In addition, she may also welcome guidance and suggestions for doing exercises that will help her to regain her figure, support for her efforts to nurse her baby (especially if she wants to breast-feed), and counsel for giving him the care he actually needs.

Voluntarily offering information and suggestions that are relevant to whichever stage the mother is experiencing in her childbearing course is appropriate nursing action, and nurses would do well to incorporate it deliberately in their practice when giving maternity nursing care. Not only may a mother want and need such information and suggestions, but in offering them and, if wanted, giving them, nurses add to their stature as helping persons. This is especially true in antepartum clinics where the nurse, perhaps because of pressures, is often tempted to abrogate nursing responsibility by referring the patient to another worker without first determining her need. Not infrequently, for instance, when the doctor prescribes a low-calorie, salt-free diet for a pregnant woman, the nurse will immediately refer her to the nutritionist in the clinic for information and suggestions. Yet the nurse probably spent hours during student days calculating low-calorie diets and learning about foods that are low in salt! Likewise, when a young high school girl, pregnant and unmarried, registers with the antepartum clinic, the nurse may refer her to the social worker as soon as the doctor has completed his examination of her. These are unfortunate nursing practices, for by passing on to others the responsibilities that are within the province of nursing and that nurses have been prepared to handle, not only do they render useless much knowledge and skill acquired, but they deny their own ability to help.

RECEPTIVITY

Receptivity, being ready and willing to accept and make the best use of what is offered or is about to be done, is a state of mind to identify or foster in a patient before initiating definitive nursing action. A patient may indicate receptivity in overt form such as a smiling "Yes," an eager reaching out, or a vigorous drawing away that leaves no doubt in the nurse's mind about the acceptability of what is being offered or is about to be done. Many times, however, the patient does not so obviously reveal her acceptance or rejection. At such times, sensitivity to nuances in patient behavior may give the nurse necessary clues which can be explored verbally to discover if the interpretation is in accord with the meaning to the patient. At still other times, the nurse may have to ask the patient how she feels about intended nursing action and pursue the exploration until a credible response is obtained. When it indicates acceptance, the nurse may feel secure in initiating action. When it indicates rejection, however, the nurse must try to establish the reason for the rejection before initiating definitive action. It may be because the patient has no need, or perhaps she does not fully understand or could not easily tolerate the nurse's method of offering aid.

For example, in the antepartum clinic, the nurse discovered that Mrs. Brodish, pregnant for the first time, knew practically nothing about the growth and development of the fetus or the mechanisms of labor. The nurse had a *Birth Atlas* in the office and offered to show it. Mrs. Brodish, however, acted reluctant to accept the offer. However, this rejection was unconvincing to the nurse, who also sensed in Mrs. Brodish a curiosity to see the pictures. When the nurse expressed this quandary about Mrs. Brodish's behavior and asked for help in understanding it Mrs. Brodish then said she would like to see the pictures but not in the nurse's office because she might lose her turn in seeing the doctor. This was an easy adjustment for the nurse to make. The *Atlas* was brought to the clinic area where Mrs. Brodish could give her undivided attention to the pictures and the nurse's explanation of them. Had the nurse not tried to ensure Mrs. Brodish's receptivity but had shown the pictures to her in the office, they would have had little meaning for Mrs. Brodish. Her mind would have been too full of anxiety to be able to comprehend the pictures or the nurse's explanation of them.

EFFECT

The effect of measures initiated either to identify or meet a patient's need for help is also important to ascertain. The nurse's application of nursing knowledge and skills has no particular value unless it produces desired results. Sometimes the effect of nursing action may be immediately discerned, as in the mother who falls asleep shortly after she has been helped to assume the postpartum relaxation position or in the rapt attention Mrs. Brodish manifested when she was shown the *Birth Atlas* pictures. At other times, the effect may not be known until much later. This is true of dietary information an expectant mother may be given. Its effect may not be known until her next clinic visit when she steps upon the scale or when her blood pressure is taken and her extremities are examined for edema. When results are satisfactory, it is a cause for gratification and for rejoicing with the patient; when unsatisfactory, the cause for failure needs to be sought. Rarely does a patient who has placed herself under medical or nursing supervision purposefully disregard suggestions, recommendations, or advice. She usually has a reason for her negative response, such as a lack of understanding, lack of sufficient energy, a serious social problem, or inadequate cooking facilities at home. To scold a patient, as doctors—and nurses, too—have been known to do, serves no useful purpose. It merely alienates the patient. Meaningful application of a nurse's knowledge and skills requires that the cause of unsatisfactory results be sought until uncovered, and then the patient is helped to overcome it. Like Mrs. Brodish, who could not benefit from the *Birth Atlas* pictures until her mind was free of anxiety, so may a patient need help in overcoming whatever may interfere with her ability to respond capably to measures instituted or recommended for her well-being. Therein lies the importance of ascertaining the effect of measures instituted to meet a patient's need for help.

ACCOUNTABILITY

Accountability means to accept responsibility not only for the action that one initiates but also for the results. This presents no problem for the nurse when results are satisfactory. In fact, it is a cause for inner gratification when measures are instituted which provide the beneficial effects that are desired; the nurse is then quite willing to accept responsibility for the consequences of the act. However, when results are disappointing, the nurse may be tempted to blame others or circumstances and thus deny any accountability for what was done. At such times it must be remembered that the action taken represented the nurse's best judgment at the moment; therefore, rather than blame others, the nurse should try to discover how such results were obtained. This can be done by examining the nursing process to determine the level of awareness that was the basis for such judgment. Most likely the nurse will find that it was based on an unvalidated assumption, a level from which effective action seldom results. Such insight is useful. Not only may it suggest what the nurse can do to alter the unsatisfactory results, but it will enable more effective functioning in the future.

SUMMARY

Maternity nursing is a serious and creative as well as a demanding type of service that all too often is not clearly understood. So much has been said in recent years about the normal physiological aspects of the childbearing process that the fears and apprehensions that parents experience are minimized or overlooked. It is true that most pregnant and postpartum women as well as those who are in labor are essentially well individuals with none of the distressing and debilitating conditions that many patients who are sick in hospitals must endure. However, their needs, though different, are as acute and are apt to be more far-reaching, for they often extend well beyond the period defined by their condition, as in the case of illness. They have implications for the development of the family, the basic structure of our society, which today more than ever needs help to be kept intact. Within the professional nurse are the knowledge and the skills with which to provide that help. The nurse has the ability to enable expectant mothers and fathers to increase their competence in assuming their responsibilities; the nurse can help them have a satisfactory childbearing experience and knows how to support them in their efforts to cope with problems that arise along the way.

When the nurse applies nursing knowledge and skills for the benefit of expectant parents whenever opportunity presents, the nurse contributes to the bond of love between parents and between parents and their children and thus adds strength to the family structure. Maternity nursing care is a vital, significant service which must be appreciated by the nurse who, in turn, should help others to appreciate it as well. To realize full professional potential, nurses must respect their knowledge and abilities, offer them voluntarily (not just in response to the doctor's order or to a patient's specific request), and accept responsibility for their acts. Clarity about the nursing process as the implementing power for nursing practice will enable them to do this. And when this is fully realized and the nurse freely gives of nursing knowledge and skills, when appropriate, not only will these services be in demand, but administrative support will be strong for the kind of nursing the nurse both wants and is ready to give. The nurse who is competent and helpful to the patient is a precious asset to any service concerned with patient care.

BIBLIOGRAPHY

Dickoff, James, Patricia James, and Ernestine Wiedenbach: "Theory in a Practice Discipline: Part I. Practice Oriented Theory," *Nursing Research*, 17(5):415, September–October 1968.

——— and ———: "Beliefs and Values: Bases for Curriculum Design," *Nursing Research*, 19(5):415, September–October 1970.

Orlando, Ida J.: *The Dynamic Nurse-Patient Relationship*, Putnam, New York, 1961.

Wiedenbach, Ernestine: *Family-centered Maternity Nursing*, 2d ed., Putnam, New York, 1967.

———: *Clinical Nursing, A Helping Art*, Springer, New York, 1964.

———: *Meeting the Realities in Clinical Teaching*, Springer, New York, 1969.

———: "Nurses' Wisdom in Nursing Theory," *American Journal of Nursing*, 70(5):1057, May 1970.

UNIT B

THE FAMILY
OF TODAY

4 | THE SINGLE-PARENT
FAMILY

David S. Torbett

The family, sociologically speaking, is a group of two or more persons who are united by blood, marriage, or adoption, residing in a common household, wherein they create and maintain a common culture and interact with each other by way of familial roles. The major functions of the family have been and continue to be the production of offspring and the socialization of same. The impact of family life on the individual, group, and society has been well established. We have our most intense life experiences (birth, death, and marriage) within some kind of family system and spend the majority of our early formative years with parents and siblings. Many authors suggest a direct correlation between the rise and fall of civilizations and the stability of the family. Others relegate the family to a rather minor position within the scheme of things and stress the greater importance of political power and economic fluctuations.

However the family is viewed, it has appeared in many forms, ranging from the predominantly patriarchal system with evident power held by males, through matriarchies found in early American Iroquois tribes and black families, to the equalitarian and single-parent families of today. Whatever its form or definition, the family has played and will continue to play an important part in the development of individual identity and group and societal functioning.

THE AMERICAN SCENE

The family of today in the United States is basically a nuclear unit made up of husband, wife, and immediate offspring. The old extended family unit, important during the rural phase of our development when children were economic assets rather than liabilities and survival depended upon cooperation rather than specialization, has given way to a mobile, metropolitanized, and mechanistic unit geared to individualized, industrialized, and immediate gratification. The emergence of a mass-production–oriented society has brought us to a standard of living second to none, while at the same time decreasing the necessity for family interdependence. Today a few persons are able to produce the food and fiber necessary for our continued survival. No longer is marriage in fact necessary as a means to survival. Men and women may, in exchange for money, have their needs met by specialized individuals and groups capable of providing all the necessities of life. Since World War II the movement from the home into industrial positions has increased rapidly, providing the opportunity for women to be self-reliant. In 1970 there were 31,560,000 women, or 43.4 percent of the female population of the United States, holding full-time jobs outside the home, as opposed to 12,845,000 women, or 25.4 percent of the female population in 1940.[1] This economic self-reliance has made it possible for women to take over the financial responsibility for having and rearing their own children outside the usual context of marriage.

THE SOCIALIZATION PROCESS

In order to operate effectively as group members, we must become aware of what is expected of us. The rules of the social game wherein we operate from day to day, often referred to as social norms, are a set of expectations established by others that are then transmitted from parent to child, in turn resulting in a network of established and supported ways of relating. One of our basic social distinctions important to continued family operation is masculinity and femininity. While most of us are born with clear-cut male or female components, the way in which we view our maleness or femaleness to a large extent depends upon the social contexts within which we are reared. The major roles assigned to women have been and continue to be those of seduction, production, and childrearing, while men, simply by way of their biological sex, have been assigned to the power positions within society. Woman is considered to be the helpmate of man, but in our kind of changing society this has really resulted in their being cheated.

The nursing profession itself is an excellent example of how the nurturant role, supported within the American family in the past and at present, is continued outside the home in the clinic, hospital, and health center. The care of children, a most desirable function, prepares some people in our society to care for others outside the home. Present-day nurses, while still rewarded in general for their nuturant care of others, have found themselves on the horns of a dilemma because of the contradictory expectations held for them within the profession. The person oriented toward becoming a nurse finds that the highly specialized, mechanized, and depersonalized hospital or clinic expects an efficient, professional, and highly skilled technician rather than a nurturing, supportive, and humanistically oriented person. For the nurse the result of being expected to do contradictory kinds of things within the profession is feelings of confusion about self, the profession, and those the nurse works with.

Obstetric nurses and those dealing with maternity and child care are further confused by the concerns shared with them by pregnant and delivered women. Within the United States pregnancy and childbirth themselves are experiences entered into by women who are often confused by contradictory messages. On the one hand they are doing their thing in respect to their reproductive role because, for the most part, women are made to feel less adequate if they are not capable of conception and birth. On the other hand they are made to feel that in some way they are paying for Eve's sins in the Garden of Eden. They are caught up in the one-upmanship played by pregnant women to attain status by way of the excruciating experience. Men are prone to talk about their sexual exploits in order to attain a status position with their peers, while women are prone to discuss their birth experiences in much the same way.

Thus we find nurses, themselves the products of contradictory socialization, attempting to deal professionally with a pregnant, birth-oriented woman, who herself is struggling with similar contradictions. The result is often chaos rather than effective professional nurse-patient interrelating. It has been well established that desire of child is of utmost importance in respect to the impact of birth on the delivering mother, the newborn offspring, and the family context within which the mother and child will be involved.

THE CHANGING SCENE

Today we are in a state of transition where rapid change is taking place, especially in respect to family forms. While premarital pregnancies have been around as long as man has existed, the number of premarital pregnancies that are taking place is increasing and also the number of women who are keeping their children and rearing them as a single parent rather than giving them up for adoption or entering into marriage.

MOTIVATIONS AND THE SINGLE-PARENT FAMILY

While the emphasis of this chapter will be on the single-parent family consisting of an unmarried mother and offspring, there are other single-parent families of this type which result from divorce, separation, and death. In this country about 10 million children under the age of eighteen live in one-parent homes, and one of every ten families has a female head, reflecting divorce, separation, or widowhood. It is estimated that there are approximately 1,700,000 females who are legally separated from their husbands in this country. Between a fourth and a third of all marriages in the United States end in divorce, resulting in about 2,100,000 divorced females at the present time. There are approximately 9 million widows, with an annual increase of about 100,000.[2]

The ability to produce a child and rear that child outside marriage reflects the change in attitude held by society. In the past the stigma of being a parent outside marriage would have been so great that the social pressures would have made it nearly impossible for this to take place in any kind of fashion that would be construed by society as acceptable. However, today, while the stigma is still in evidence, thousands of women are having children, maintaining them outside marriage, and being supported by family and friends to do this without the usual kinds of anxieties. A survey of the Florence Crittenton homes for unwed mothers reveals that they are beginning to experience an increase in the number of women who keep their babies rather than give them up for adoption and that the women who are keeping their children are the non-college-educated group. The supposition or hunch of a number of workers interviewed is that the women are looking to their babies as a means of security which they have not found in their lives to date. Thus, it seems that a motivating factor leading to increased numbers of single-parent families is the need for someone to love and, in turn, to be loved by.

This kind of motivation has a number of implications that expectant mothers should consider prior to accepting the single-parent role as most desirable.

1 What are the implications for the woman herself? What will keeping the child mean in respect to employment, heterosexual relating, and peer support?

2 What are the implications for the child of being labeled, as is the case in many states, illegitimate and being reared in a single-parent family, which, while increasing numerically, still is outside the normative context of society? What impact will questions about his different status and why he has only one parent have on the child's identity formation and personality development?

3 What are the implications in respect to sexual identity formation for

the child? This question is of particular concern if the child is a male being reared by a female and a female being reared without the socializing influence of a male in preparation for educational and community role assimilation. Will the opposite-sex parent modeling result in a tendency, for example, for male offspring to identify with their own sex and become more oriented toward homosexuality or will they become more competent in the areas of emotional expression and non-aggressive relating?

Evidence supported by Dr. Warren Gadpaille, in an article entitled "Biological Fallacies of Women's Lib," suggests that the brain is "programmed" during early embryonic development for masculine or feminine preferences in behavior. According to Gadpaille, the origin of this normal differentiation is the presence or absence of fetal androgens during very early intrauterine life. After the sex chromosomes determine whether ovaries or testes will develop, fetal hormones take over sexual differentiation. The presence or absence of the male hormone androgen not only determines male or female morphology but also organizes the hypothalamus to release sex-specific and sex-appropriate mating and social behavior.[3] This early biological differentiation suggests that males are programmed to be more aggressive and to find satisfaction in such aggressive activities while females are more oriented towards passivity. If this is true, what would be the effect of counter-role conditioning by a single parent oriented toward the opposite type of behavior?

The role of nurses dealing with pregnant women who are considering the future should be twofold. On the one hand they will need to come to grips with their own feelings about the contradictory socialization they have experienced and their feelings about rearing a child in a one-parent family. Secondly, they will need to become competent in reflecting the feelings of the often-confused mother who is attempting to decide on the most desirable course of action. The mother's decision often grows out of her own needs at that point in time, making it difficult for her to project into the future the possible implications of rearing a child in a one-parent family with respect to the impact on the child himself.

BASIC CONSIDERATIONS

As has previously been suggested, a person considering a one-parent family should give thought to her motivation. If it appears to be the need for someone to love and someone to love her in return, the person would be well advised to read Eric Fromm's book *The Art of Loving*. The implications of one-way loving or dependent love, rather than love based on reciprocity and a two-way flow, have been well established in respect to parent-child relating as well as to marital interaction.

Social Stigma

While the unmarried pregnant woman is more accepted today than was the case 50 years ago, the general social response to her situation will be more negative than positive. This, of course, will depend to a large extent on the person's race, ethnicity, or social class. For a goodly number of young blacks and Chicanos the family and peer response to their unmarried pregnant state or single-parent status is one of positive acceptance, primarily because they have proved their femaleness. The adolescent or young teen-ager experiencing pregnancy and childbirth outside marriage often becomes a person of great interest to her same-sex peers, whose questions within their own families have been curtailed in respect to sex, pregnancy, and childbirth. In the middle- and upper-class segments of our population the usual response to an unmarried pregnant female is to speed her away to a home for unwed mothers or to an abortionist with as little fanfare as possible. It is important for nurses to remember the wide range of general responses to the same situation and to consider the person and her specific life situation rather than projecting onto her their own values developed out of their own kinds of class experience.

Working and Parenting

In the United States the general view of the appropriate role of the mother is that of caring for children. For the single-parent mother facing the necessity of providing financially for herself and child there are two major options open to her: (1) obtaining aid to dependent children or some other kind of social welfare assistance, or (2) getting a job. The implication of combining work and parenthood has been for some childrearing authorities that of frustrating the developmental needs of children. Feeling is held that a mother, better than anyone else, can provide the tender loving care necessary for a child to develop a sense of trust, initiative, and accomplishment. Others, who support the development of child day-care centers, communal living, and leaving the work of parenting to professionals, suggest that trust, initiative, and accomplishment can better be fostered through the care of specialists or a group. The single parent should come to terms with the reality of her combined parenting-working roles and deal with her own resulting internal conflicts as well as face the actuality that she will have to rely on others to assist in the child-rearing process.

Sex-role Identification

In the United States we find that sex-role identification is the result of a socialization process wherein males and females are conditioned into their appropriate roles by way of anti-opposite-sex reactions, slogans, and stereotyping. The idea that girls must become girls by not being like boys and vice versa is reflected in the media's description of the American family, parental responses to their children, dating and courtship interchanges, and husband and wife relating. The result of this is general confusion and a good deal of hostility and negativism between the sexes, as well as preparation for homosexual rather than heterosexual relating. Ideally we will arrive at a point someday where the sexes can be made to feel they are complementary rather than conflictual, and role assimilation can take place by way of positive examples rather than negative opposite-sex examples. In the meantime it behooves the person considering a one-parent family to give thought to the implications of rearing a member of the opposite sex without an opposite-sex parental model or to rearing a member of her own sex without the opportunities for reality heterosexual involvement.

Dyadic Relating

One of the realities of the single-parent family is that unless more than one offspring is produced, the parent and child will form a dyad. This means that the two will either be in agreement or at odds without anyone to play the role of mediator. Also, a dyad consisting of only two people will be limited in respect to the number of interaction patterns possible. In a nuclear family consisting of husband, wife, and offspring, psychological and social needs may be met in a variety of ways not possible in a dyadic-pair relationship. When a mother becomes frustrated with the behavior of the child, the father can serve as a release valve by either listening to complaints of the mother or reducing her frustration by shifting her into the wife role and away from that of mother.

Tangible and Emotional Rewards

While most of our status symbols, such as job titles, homes, cars, and paychecks, are tangible and of great importance in enhancing our self-esteem, there are a number of rewards that are emotional. The importance of early childhood stability, consistency, and security is reflected in both the large numbers of people who spend most of their lives in a state of anxiety, fear, or frustration due to early childhood deprivation and in those who are able to deal with diversity and are flexible and mature largely because of having developed a sense of trust in their environment and a feeling of competence in dealing with the world around them. In the one-parent family the task of meeting emotional needs will by necessity fall to a large extent on others. For the working mother locked into our kind of specialized, dehumanized work system, the tendency may well be to use the same kinds of rewards for her child that are provided for herself. Thus, it is of utmost importance that a person considering a one-parent family give thought to the implications of substituting tangible rewards for emotional ones.

SUMMARY

The biases of this author are no doubt reflected in the stress placed on giving thought to implications of taking on the role of a single parent. The orientation of a family life educator and counselor is that of assisting individuals, couples, and families in looking at the reality of their situation, considering the implications of various options, and then supporting them to do the best possible job of human relating, whatever their decision. In the future it will be of great importance that children be desired before they are produced and that we orient ourselves toward providing enrichment experiences and support for families at various stages of the life cycle. The nurse should begin to help women in our society come to view themselves as productive rather than simply reproductive persons. The nurse is in a strategic position to help those women considering one-parent family life provide a positive role model and to assist unmarried women in making a considered decision about rearing a child in a one-parent family.

REFERENCES

1 Golenpaul, Dan (ed.): *Information Please Almanac*, U.S. Bureau of Statistics, Simon & Schuster, New York, 1972, p. 126.
2 Schlesinger, Benjamin: *The One-parent Family*, University of Toronto Press, Toronto, 1969, pp. 113–115.
3 Gadpaille, Warren J.: "Biological Fallacies of Women's Lib," *Hospital Physician*, Medical Economics Inc., subsidiary of Litton Publishing Co., Inc., Oradell, N.J., July 1971, p. 2.

5 | THE COMMUNE

Marna Steinbroner

THE BEGINNINGS

The Driving Force

There are people driven by the inner conviction that life as they live it cannot be all there is. From comfortable homes in White Plains, the ghetto in Atlanta, an apartment with a view of Lake Michigan or the Charles, they surge forward following the urgent need to find, discover, build "something better." That something is the essence of togetherness; coexistence with other humans and with the earth, the water, and the air. It is clear that a technology which pollutes nature and mankind in a megalopolis of humans, each competing for some fast diminishing space, cannot and will not institute any social transformation directed toward slowing mankind's already quickening pace toward extinction.

Communes could not continue to exist without the communard's belief that people who want to change vast social systems must first begin with a change in their own life-style. It is possible that the complex and varied in-

The author gratefully acknowledges the assistance of Ilene Burson in the final preparation of this chapter.

teractions of communal life will enhance individual identity and the potential for interpersonal as well as intrapersonal growth. Communes are the vanguard of an immeasurable social movement addressing itself to the challenge of survival by social transformation. The quest is for that delicate balance between concepts of freedom and togetherness, independence and cooperation, and utopia and realism.

The reader's view of the commune and those who seek to create a life within its scope will depend on his own vision of the future. Is it the desperate fleeing of revolutionary anti-Establishment youth entrenching themselves in preparation for mass revolt or an outpost of new visions, creative energy, and humanistic values? Is it a threat to be guarded against at all cost or an adventure to be explored and investigated with the hope of discovering some intrinsic worth, some hope for social survival?

Historical Perspective

The communal approach to society is not a new phenomenon. Experiments in utopian living have appeared in America as early as the time of the community of Pilgrims. Idealistic inspiration has been the motivating force as groups of like-minded persons withdrew from the masses in search of a more tolerable life-style. In the 1680s these groups were religious sects which sought shelter for their spiritual visions in the American wilderness. During the nineteenth century more than 130 utopian-style communes were established and disbanded. Among those utopian ventures based on religious belief were the Harmonites in Pennsylvania, the Perfectionists and the Shakers in New York, the Zoarites in Ohio, and the Amana Society in Iowa. Several of these religious-based communes survived only because they became business-minded. Two of the most renowned are the Perfectionists of Oneida, New York, and the Amana Society.

Nonreligious communes in the nineteenth century were seeking a change in social order rather than freedom to practice religious beliefs. They identified communal living as the most viable social structure. New Harmony, Indiana, and Brook Farm in West Roxbury, Massachusetts, based themselves on utopian world concepts. Anarchist-socialist communes or "villages" were founded in Ohio, Louisiana, Georgia, and New York.

At the close of the nineteenth century only a few of these experiments continued to exist. Extinction had come because of pressures, both internal and external. Strict rules and celibacy limited the growth and indoctrination of new generations, and rumors of sexual freedoms and perversions moved neighbors to force the groups to disband.

Commune dwellers today share much with history. Their philosophy insists that the communal pattern for society is *the* life-style which all persons will eventually desire. Their commitment is one of intensity, the magnitude of which established society does not comprehend. Their vision is of a superculture shaped to fit the way people really are. As with those earlier utopian-seekers, they are driven by discontent with the present and a fundamental belief that "surely somewhere somehow there is a better way of living—there has to be."[1]

Haight-Ashbury and the Present

The student of social phenomena would trace the present communal movement to the 1960s and the West Coast of America, to the Haight-Ashbury area of San Francisco. The Haight was an older urban neighborhood experiencing the ritual decomposition common to all large cities. A mutation occurred at some point where it would ordinarily have become a black ghetto. Instead there began a slow gathering of postgraduate "beats," aspiring artists and musicians, and mystics. The lack of housing facilities and money for individual rental and the availability of large Victorian houses stimulated the idea of pooling resources and living communally.

By 1967 the Haight had become the Mecca for dissident youth, an experiment in full sense awareness and wholeness. A revelation of self led to a heightened perspective of others. The inhabitants were now dubbed "hippies," and the era of acid rock, body painting, and psychedelic stimulation of sight and hearing was under way. The nation was given its first view of the flower children when 20,000 kids turned out in Golden Gate Park in January 1967 for a "love-in," and the mass media were there to record the event. With the publicity came thousands of young people groping for some place to belong, to be unique, and yet to conform.

This new movement changed the original settlement into a haven for acid heads, runaways, pushers, and bikers. To them the area offered a little of everything: free food, free clothes, a newspaper, a free clinic, free legal services, head shops, and crash pads. The inevitable followed: tourists, the curious, the narcotic agents, and the commercial-minded seller of "hippie momentos."

With this latest invasion the original settlers began to move, in small communal groups, out of the rapidly degenerating Haight-Ashbury district into houses, shacks, and tent communities on the northern California hillsides. They continued to live in a communal atmosphere and turned their work efforts toward building a community and growing their own food. The era of the modern rural commune had begun.

Between 1965 and 1970, 2,000 communal groups were formed. At the outset it was the visceral reaction of disillusioned youth. Now, it is a movement; the creation of a microculture. They reexamined, tested, reevaluated, and revised. They developed smaller, more self-sufficient communities. They worked for harmony with the environment not only in the cultivation of the land, but in the architecture of their building as well. They tried freer forms of family membership and childbearing and rearing. They established home industries of individual craftsmanship. They revived old religions, created new ones, and combined the best of both in a rediscovered awareness of divinity.

Today, one or several communes can be found within reach of every major city in America. Travel long enough and far enough, and the seeker will find *that* commune in which his own ideals and life-style mesh with those of the members already there. If perchance this is not so, he needs only to band with other like-minded people; rent or buy a plot of land, a house, or an apartment; and begin developing a communal family of his own.

PHILOSOPHIES OF COMMUNAL LIVING

Family

Martha's parents and brothers live in a small town in western New York. Charles's parents were divorced, and he had lived with his mother until now. Isaac's wife and daughter were still in an Eastern city. Each member of the commune has in his past some manner of sociological family unit. Yet the most frequent positive response to the commune is, "For the first time I feel I am part of a family." They refer to each other as "the family." Some even have commune names, such as the "Lynch Family" in California and "The Chosen Family" in New Mexico. Thus, the basic philosophy of communal life-style is the establishment of a new family structure with new roles and developmental processes.

For some communes this means having separate sleeping rooms and family dining, recreation, and work programs. Others establish group marriages with sexual partners changing on a scheduled basis or retain monogamous relationships. Some communes practice celibacy. Childrearing varies from single-parent responsibility through biological family units to a separation of children into a special unit apart from parents.

The most constant family activity observed in comparison of communal practices is the togetherness of sharing certain activities, such as group rituals, singing and chanting, drug experiences, religious services, and the observation of festive holidays. Almost without exception, each communal unit has daily family gatherings for prayers, evening songs, or some other activity in which everyone is a participant.

Group and Personal Awareness

The ever-deepening search for self-awareness and self-fulfillment that is common to mankind is the cornerstone of the intimacy and warmth that the commune members are discovering in their extended families. T-group interaction, mutual criticism, or a policy of honesty and uninhibited expression of feeling and gut reactions provide a proving ground for personal growth. It

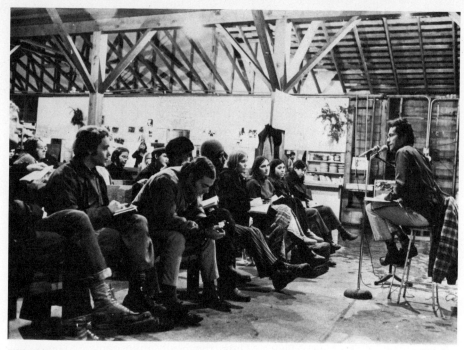

FIGURE 5-1
A devotion to religious study is the central focus of this commune, a colony of the Children of God in Burlington, Wash. The sect has colonies scattered across the United States and Europe sheltering between 2,000 and 3,000 young people. (Courtesy of Wide World Photos)

is a life-style in which all members of the *family* expect honesty and support from other members and receive it. The potential for social change is heightened even if only a few members can consistently meet this standard of openness.

Robert Houriet experienced the directness of this honest approach when he visited High Ridge Farm in Oregon. His recorded conversations, first with Elaine and then with Jean the following morning, illustrate the atmosphere of concerned helping and caring in which criticism is presented.

Later I lay in my sleeping bag, thinking everyone asleep, furtively taking notes on the day's events by flashlight. Lantern in hand, Elaine entered the A-frame. She saw me and smiled knowingly. Removing her layers of raincoats—so many she looked pregnant—she came and sat down beside me. She is a thin twenty-seven-year-old Jewish girl from New York, who graduated in political science from Swarthmore. She has straight, lustrous brown hair which she brushes over her ears, which stick out slightly. Very thick glasses in oval frames help correct her severe myopia. She always wears the same pair of loose, flowered, pajamalike pants. When she chooses to talk to you, her speech is punctuated with anguished gaps to indicate her extremely careful choice of words. "I've noticed . . . from when you first came here . . . that you've held yourself apart from the family."

I was engulfed by tension. She continued, "You introduced yourself rather formally . . . and you said you wanted to be a member of the family. . . ."

"That's right," I said.

"But there's something about you . . . I guess it was tonight that I first realized what it was . . . the way you broke in with that question about Peter . . . it was a question that *intruded*. I saw that you weren't thinking of yourself as a member of the family . . . you were a detached observer in disguise . . . taking notes in your head . . . and secretly at night." She smiled and looked down at my pad. I felt caught.

"Have you ever tried *not* observing . . . just experiencing . . . or do you always remain detached from whatever you're doing?" Man, this chick was what you call laying a trip! And of course all she said was true.

She concluded, "To catch the essence of communal life, you should put your notebook away, and then you may decide it is more important to live it than to write it." I thanked her for revealing my foibles, and we said good night.

(Next morning)

This morning, I tried to start a conversation with Jean as she ground some flour (she baked a dozen loaves and they were eaten in two days), but she didn't respond to my openers. Instead she said, "I agree with everything Elaine told you last night," and paused to let it sink in, all the time continuing to grind, smiling and jiggling her earrings. "What you said during the meeting was with the tone of not caring about Peter or any of us. It was the tone of a ruthless curiosity, digging for a fact to fill out the story. It was your ego speaking."

There was more. She ground away. "I get the feeling when you talk that you are holding back. An aloofness. And that you don't dig the *feeling* of words, only their logical sense. And, you ask too many questions."

Wowwww. I shook my head dumbly and mumbled about having to think over what she said and went off to dig a hole for a fruit tree.[2]

The meaning of these deeply shared experiences in reaching the depths of other human beings cannot be comprehended without participation. It is the life blood of the commune. It is the philosophical rationale for a life-style. It is seen by the communitarian as the hope for mankind; that social growth is the ultimate result of personal awareness. "We've come together in a com-

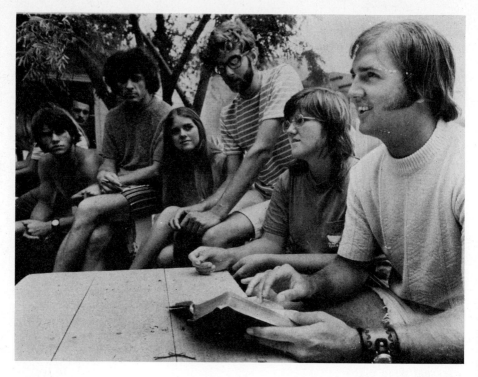

FIGURE 5-2
A scriptural "rap session" is held at a coffeehouse operated as an experiment in Christian evangelism for youths in Virginia Beach, Va. (Courtesy of Wide World Photos)

mune to channel the Truth to one another. Living alone separates you from the richness of life which is a direct result of creating constantly with a group of kindred spirits."[3]

Property and Ownership

The concept of sharing and cooperative venture extends to personal property. Private ownership is, in general, discouraged in most communes. The ideal is for everything to belong to everyone so that everyone treats valuable items, such as tools, with equal care. It is not realistic in view of human nature, past training, and the variation in values placed on material possessions; but sometimes it works. When it does not, there is inevitably strife.

Some communards own the real property in common and run business affairs as a group. More frequently, two or more members actually own the house or the farm, and others pay rent or just live there in exchange for work and companionship or as family members. With a nuclear family group, it does not matter when one parent owns the house; neither does it matter when this occurs in the extended communal family. When problems do develop, the owner may use legal process to change the membership. The family at Bryn Athym in Vermont experienced this when the owner of the property returned one morning with six others he had met on the West Coast. He announced that they were establishing a work-oriented commune and gave the family 30 days' notice to remove themselves or he would call the state police.[4]

Some owner-members, including Chick at Lorien in New Mexico, are content to live in privacy on the land, allowing life to happen as it will, without intervention. Still others in ownership position become the leaders of the commune, as is the case for Kathy and Constantine at Summit House in Cambridge and the original owners at New Buffalo in New Mexico. In the commune the power usually inherent in ownership is controlled, modified, or rejected by the basic philosophy of communal sharing and by the members themselves. Again, each commune is a unique, distinct entity. There is no stereotype.

There are wide variations among communes in the unwritten rules about personal property, private rooms, automobiles, stereos, and their use. When single persons, couples, or biological families have private sleeping units within the commune, they usually retain rights to the furnishings and personal items in their rooms. All items in the communal rooms and all necessary tools for farming, maintenance, and food preparation are owned and used by everyone. Automobiles and motorcycles seem to be the other item of personal property that may be closely guarded by the owners, much to the dismay of other family members. The farm tractor or truck, however, is communally owned.

The basic philosophy of communal living suggests that all property be given to the commune upon admission to be used by anyone who needs it. However, it is evident that few communal families actually adhere completely to this tenet. One exception is that of Twin Oaks in Virginia, a community based on B. F. Skinner's *Walden Two*.

Autonomy and Self-sufficiency

In the American dream each family unit is able to care for its own needs. This autonomy and self-sufficiency is important to communal philosophy. The remarks are similar across the country: "There are no food stamps here." "We are farmers so we can grow our own food." "Even sustenance farming is better than government funds." Books and pamphlets tell how to build a brick house, grow herbs, preserve foods, and make soap, candles, and clothes. The local library usually has a supply of information on other do-it-yourself

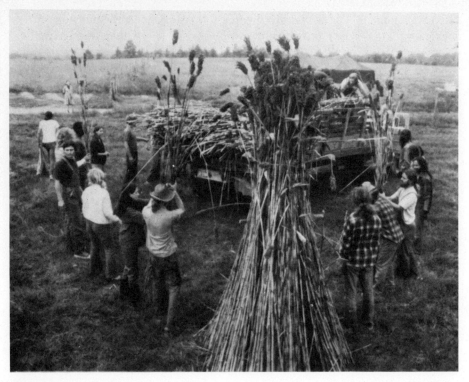

FIGURE 5-3
Members of The Farm near Summertown, Tenn., load sorghum for processing into molasses at a nearby mill. The group of about 400 members came to Tennessee to establish a communal life-style and have been selling molasses to pay for the 1,014-acre farm. (Courtesy of Wide World Photos)

ideas. Local farmers have befriended the members in farming communes, particularly in the New England states. Their knowledge is invaluable to the novice farmer.

The distant goal of self-sufficiency is linked to interdependence with the other communes. The urban communes band together in food co-ops to purchase large quantities of food at lower wholesale prices. Sometimes they contract with nearly agrarian communes; they offer planting and harvesting workers from the city in exchange for fruits, vegetables, and grains from the farm. Handicrafts made at both farm and urban communes may be sold at a co-op store.

Several communes are supported, at least in part, by self-contained home industry. Twin Oaks in Virginia makes hammocks. Messiah's World Crusade operates a natural foods restaurant in San Francisco. Bruderhof communities manufacture community playthings.

Some communes are supported by the outside employment of its members. This is particularly valid in urban settings. The members of Summit House in Cambridge are professional persons who pay a monthly fee for the communal finances. There are members with steady incomes from stock dividends, allowances from parents, and their own savings accounts. These are fairly uncommon, however. More likely, the youths receive some kind of welfare assistance, which frequently serves as a constant irritant to the goals of the commune and may be a cause of much discussion.

MALE AND FEMALE ROLES

Women work in the fields beside the men. A male cooks breakfast for everyone. Women care for the children, sew, and cook. Men work at construction of new buildings. What are the expected male and female roles in a commune? That's just the point; the philosophy is respect for each member and his dream. If Bill wants to cook, he is not degraded by the other men because most likely they cook also.

The household chores are done whenever someone feels right about doing something, by a schedule set up through group consensus, or by chosen work credits. In the agrarian communes the traditional role of women seems to be the one most frequently adopted. Women usually assume the responsibility for child care. They cook, sew, and tend to the housekeeping. In the urban areas the power of "women's liberation" seems to be an influencing factor, and the roles in household chores and childrearing are often equally shared.

The idea of equal regard for role identification is basic to the equality of each human being with every other human being. Understanding of self and of one's individual needs and desires leads to a willingness to accept differences in others. The members of the Hog Farm patterned a structure of rotating leadership on a daily basis including both men and women.

The male in both urban and rural communes may be slightly more inhibited about assuming feminine tasks such as sewing, preserving foods, and caring for children. That hesitancy may be due to the early childhood instillation of distinctly male roles. The men tend toward heavy farm and construction labor. Within the commune setting they are freer to express, experiment with, and experience some of the warmer, more "homey" activities traditionally reserved for women. They express a fuller sense of wholeness because they have transcended the strictly masculine role to that of human being.

What is occurring in the change of role identity is not the development of a unisex, as some suggest, but the discovery that male and female roles in American society are arbitrary and passed on by tradition. They belie the human qualities of toughness tempered with gentleness, strength hidden in warmth, and aggressiveness combined with passivity in the same person. The commune dweller is seeking role identity apart from biological sexual identity.

THE CHILDREN
Childbearing

The most obvious return to the biological, ecological level of living is seen in the almost nationwide communal concept of natural childbirth. Total body-mind awareness, communion with earth and sky, expression of visceral feelings, and the break with technological, plastic, establishment society negates any desire for the anesthetized, sterile, impersonal nature of hospital-centered labor and delivery. The ultimate goal is not merely natural childbirth but natural childbirth at home.

Childbirth is a spiritual, emotional, physiological experience. There is a whole new movement under way to have babies at home attended by husband, children, and those who mean the most to the mother. Dr. Robert Spitzer investigated this trend and found that his previous value systems were being challenged. He writes of the women with whom he spoke:

> They were not kooks, but for the most part were intelligent girls who were not unaware of the medical danger involved. They were willing to take the risk to gain the extreme emotional satisfaction of having their babies at home. To them the advantages of personal growth far outweighted the risk of medical complication. The mothers- and fathers-to-be attended natural childbirth classes and studied the birth process in earnest. [5]

Dr. Spitzer was given the opportunity to participate in a communal birth and found it a joy and spiritual experience not commonly seen in the hospital setting.

> It was extremely moving, a unique peak experience for me as well as the others present. The mother delivered rather than was delivered, and I could see that this kind of family home birth was an outgrowth of a new consciousness, an attempt to regain the shared risks and accomplishments of the reality of frontier life. That was a time rich in rituals when the family built its own shelter, grew its own food, and helped its neighbors. Home birth is a rejection of the prevailing abdication to "experts" of those very activities making for individual and family growth. [5]

The rapid increase of home births is evidence of the viability of the communal movement. The basic tenet of total involvement, so much a part of the communal philosophy, is expressed in the complete sharing of father, mother, and friends in the birth process. The height of such an experience is revealed by Mark in the following description of his participation in the delivery of his son.

Sunshine's still handling all well. I no longer worry about her strength, she's on top of it. I decide to move from her head to her feet with Pat and Barb. Pat notices a bulge in the perineum during contractions. We put scissors, syringe, dental floss and navel clamps into boiling water. Pat shows me perineal massage and how to support the perineum with the palm of my hand to prevent tearing. The bulge continues with each contraction. I start to massage. Sunshine handled the contractions so well, I found it hard to tell exactly when some of them began and ended. Soon with each contraction a little of the baby's head was visible. It's got hair. David was holding a mirror for Sunshine, and Claudia sat nearby. The energy mounted. Soon each contraction brings a little more of the baby's head into view, then slowly it disappears. Now it stays visible between each contraction. I noticed what looked liked a big welt down the baby's head (front to back). To the virgin eye it looked like the umbilical cord. Pat assures me it's only skin forced together, and it's cool. Sunshine starts to push with one foot on Pat's knee, the other on Barb's. I begin to support the perineum which seems very capable of stretching as needed. She pushes. "Far out," "real good," and other such encouragements come from Pat and Barb. It must have been five or six contractions. Each time energy and excitement building, stretching, stretching, pushing, energy, pushing, stretching, then. . . . Like a ball pushed through a bottle neck, the baby's head was in my hand. The head was tightly covered with the caul—remove the caul, my fingernails cut short couldn't dig in, slick as soap on a doorknob. Five hands work fast but gently. Barb gets her finger under the chin and gets ahold of the sac and it tears loose. The face is free.

The face immediately shows expression. Pat sucks a little fluid from the nostrils and throat. It cries. Quickly baby turns sideways as if someone was inside turning it. Another contraction, blam, all red and pink and white-speckled our son was born. Sunshine sits up giggling, and takes him, cord still attached to him and still inside her.

I cry.[6]

An experience of that magnitude will not easily be set aside, no matter what the established health workers suggest. Home birth will be a vital part of the communal scene. Most parents are using some variation of the Lamaze method for childbirth preparation. If a physician is utilized by the parents, he must be one who will allow and even encourage natural childbirth. Pamphlets and magazines and newspaper articles direct communal dwellers to books on the Lamaze methods.

One result of home births is the lack of identity for the child. Not in the sense of personal identity; that is most likely enhanced. For all practical purposes the child is unknown to established authority. As there are no marriage certificates, so there are no birth certificates, no social security numbers, and no draft cards. It is the ultimate in liberation of the child from the numbering systems of society. This practice is not adhered to by all or even the majority at present. The inherent problems are manyfold. In the present society, work, government funds, and scholarships depend upon some identification. To the communard of the future this may be another avenue of social transformation.

Childrearing Practices

Childrearing in most of the communes is an experience shared by the members. Both adults and children seem to thrive in this atmosphere. Each adult has the responsibility and the right to play with, teach, discipline, or just enjoy any of the children at any time. There are many *parents* with many value systems and it seems to be closer to reality.

In contrast, the present American approach is to shape the child's identity and attitudes through the nearly exclusive influence of a single set of adults. It is a very egotistical situation, and the child does not learn to share early in life. Neither do the parents.

Most children live in the same room or unit as their parents. However, each child has a wide variety of adults to interact with during the day. They are shared by many, and an intimacy commonly develops between all of the children and all of the adults. Their primary relationship and loyalty seems to remain with their biological parents.

Some variations are reported. At Olympia, prior to disbanding, each child was free at the beginning of the week to choose an adult to be his official parent that week.[7] The ultimate plans for childrearing at Twin Oaks will be based on the separate units for children suggested by B. F. Skinner in *Walden Two*. At present there are too few children to warrant assigning a person to child care. The children are reared according to behavioral principles. They are placed as an item on the work credit schedule and divided into shifts. The biological parents take one shift and other members sign up to be with the children during the rest of the 24-hour period.[8]

There have been varied problems with the communal approach to childrearing. Some persons find it extremely difficult to allow others a voice and influence in the lives of their own children. Children are sometimes seen as the most private property. At Sunrise they tried communal child care, but soon found there were so many conflicting theories of childrearing that the children once more were given into the total responsibility of their parents. They did interact with a number of other children and adults, however.[9]

The example of High Ridge Farm in Oregon, reported by Robert Houriet, is one which depicts the common concepts motivating members to rear their children as a shared experience. The following are excerpts from that account:

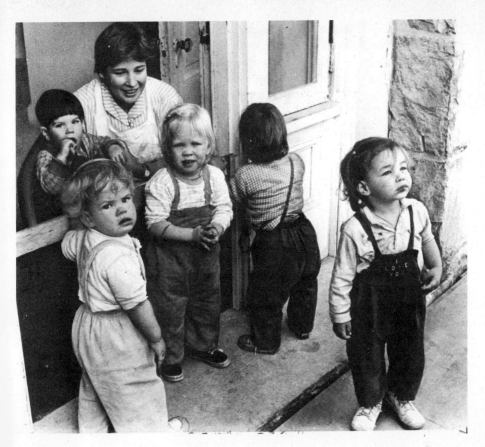

FIGURE 5-4
The sharing of childrearing responsibilities is the rule in some communes. At the Society
of Brothers commune in Norfolk, Conn., one young woman takes care of children while
the families are busy working. (Courtesy of Wide World Photos)

I spent most of the day playing with the children. They had found some
long wooden rods and were engaged in mock swordplay. I watched un-
easily, knowing where it would lead. . . . I let them learn the inevitable
lesson for themselves: Those who play with sticks get hurt with sticks.
Roland got hit hard over the head by Kathy. He retaliated with wild
thrusts. At this point, I intervened, jerked the sticks out of their hands,
laid down a moralistic trip about the difference between playing and
fighting, and diverted their attention to another game. . . . The same
situation could have been handled in a number of ways. Claudia, generally authoritarian, probably would have headed off the swordplay at
the start. Laura might have allowed it to go further than I did, risking

injury. . . . Elaine might have avoided the situation altogether for she avoided the children as much as she avoided everybody; when she did do something with them, it was on her terms, like driving them to the library to see the weekly travelogue film. From time to time, Maureen exploded in violence, usually directed at her own children. . . . Jean was calm and gentle and might have coaxed them into more peaceful play. Altogether, the kids experienced an uneven, inconsistent upbringing by six daddies and five mommies, each of whom could be counted upon to handle the same situation differently. For the kids, the only constant in the communal environment was constant inconsistency. . . . Claudia told me, "I think it's a mistake to bring up kids with the notion that there's a single code of what's good, bad, manly or feminine. The fact is, we're living in a world where all the absolutes have been broken. Each man finds his own path. So to prepare the kids for that, it's better to give them a lot of examples of fathers and mothers who are all different personalities and have different values.[10]

The consistent value at High Ridge Farm and in other communes seems to be honesty with the children as with the adults.

Education for the Children

The goal for education within the communal philosophy is the establishment of communal schools completely apart from the public school system. If the present trend in commune schools is followed, the schools of the future will be open classrooms with each student free to explore and learn as his own interest directs him. It is an effort to retain the natural creativity of childhood and harness it for learning.

The generation of youth now inhabiting communes have found they have much unlearning to do. They spent so many years in the Establishment's educational system that they need a period of *decompression* before they can begin to live communally with satisfaction and success. They want to utilize preventive education with their children. They are determined that each child will be able to find what is most relevant to him and learn to share it with others in an intimate warm relationship.

Most communes do not have enough children to start their own school. Some children now attend the local public schools. Some are tutored at home by one or more of the adults. Generally, school truant officials have not harassed the communes who keep their children home and educate them there. In some of the larger metropolitan areas communes have established cooperative schools. This is true in Cambridge, New York City, Chicago, Los

Angeles, and San Francisco. These are the prototype of the future communal schools.

HELPING THE COMMUNE MEET HEALTH NEEDS
Variables in Providing Care

The earlier segment in this chapter which presented the trend toward home birth introduced the reader to the wary stance the commune takes in relation to established health care facilities. Their experience with poor care, feelings of contamination, embarrassment, and the hospital's tendency to report everything to the police has placed a distinct barrier of mistrust around much of the commune population. The community, on the other hand, frequently views the commune dweller as filthy, disease ridden, drug addicted, and a threat to the health of the area. In fact, it is frequently the sanitation issue that community officials use to disband a local commune when use of drugs or other infractions of the law cannot be used.

Members of the health care professions are becoming leaders in the move to help the commune dweller meet his own needs on his own terms. In many areas the relationships between community and commune have improved to the point of coexistence, if not acceptance. The offer of health care has frequently been followed by involvement of other community volunteers with free legal advice, free farming advice, social service assistance, and offers of part-time employment.

The health needs of the commune member vary to some extent but may include malnutrition, assistance with birth control, hepatitis, venereal disease, and respiratory and psychological problems. They often resist going for care at a hospital or physician's office. Their life-styles and appearance have raised eyebrows and brought lectures and general nonacceptance. If the problem is drug related, they fear being reported to the police. Many cannot afford health care and have no health insurance. Some may be runaways and fear that parents will be contacted. Some have police records and may be fugitives. The usual hospital or clinic admission procedure would bring out most of this judgment-provoking data.

The philosophy and life-style of the commune dweller are the variables which affect any plan for delivery of health care. The objectives of a community health clinic provide for a program designed to offer comprehensive and high quality medical care in a setting that is convenient and acceptable to the recipient. It encourages the development of an interpersonal relationship between staff and patient, involves the residents in the planning and operation of the facility, and is responsive to the individual needs of the target population.[11] To meet both the philosophy of the commune and the objectives of a community-based health program, new methods of health care delivery were established and still others have yet to be explored and instituted.

Public Health Care Facilities

The urban commune is in the ideal setting for its members to utilize free health clinics which were established in several large cities. The clinic is usually staffed by volunteer doctors, nurses, social workers, and laboratory technicians. Admission procedure requires only name, age, and presenting complaint. If the patient decides to use a fictitious name or age, that is accepted. Minimal questions are asked. The atmosphere is non-judgmental. It is the patient with whom the staff's concern lies, not his name, age, or social history except when it has direct bearing on his needs. Such free health clinics have received much publicity, particularly those in California (Haight-Ashbury, San Francisco; Los Angeles; Long Beach) and in Cambridge, Massachusetts.

The newest approach to medical care is the mobile unit. This is a clinic which is also staffed by volunteers. The purpose of the mobile clinics is to take free medical care and counseling to the areas where the target population is most likely to be found. Again the atmosphere is non-judgmental. Frequently a patient tests the staff by requesting help with some minor problem. When he finds that the setting is one in which he can be honest and still be accepted and receive care, he returns to have the more serious problems taken care of.

Many hospital emergency rooms are now staffed by younger doctors and nurses. The red tape has been cut more frequently. Free clinics and some private physicians are referring commune members to the area hospitals where they can find more extensive medical or surgical care without undue hassle.

New Roles for Medical Care

The idea of self-sufficiency is very strong in the commune. When one communal co-op was offered the use of a free medical van their response was, "Leave that for the street kids. Can you teach us about first aid, home delivery, and preventive health maintenance?" The ideal would be a resident health professional—a nurse or doctor who is a member of the commune. In some communes this is a reality.

For the present a more viable plan would be a sort of medical-nursing co-op. It could be volunteers from the community who are trusted by the communards. An exchange program could be planned in which medical professionals from one urban commune provide services to several other communes in exchange for other services.

There are now birth control and abortion counseling centers in many cities. The future may hold the establishment of centers for home delivery staffed by nurse midwives. The need is to help the commune dweller become self-sufficient even in meeting his own health needs either by members who are health professionals or by teaching the commune dwellers how to care for these needs themselves.

THE ESSENCE OF THE COMMUNE

If there is any brief description of the commune or the communal movement today, it might be best said in the words of Robert Houriet as he expressed the only commonality in a comparison of communal roles and life-styles.

> I was eager to find a commune that *was* working out, a group of people who'd been together a year and were happy. . . . Zablocki cautioned me that there was no such beast as a prototypical commune. Each one is a unique attempt to blend economics, art, agriculture, and the spiritual into the natural round of daily life. . . . Every commune wanted to be—and had to be—unique.[12]

REFERENCES

1 Hedgpeth, William, and Dennis Stock: *The Alternative*, Collier-Macmillan, Toronto, 1970, p. 29.
2 Houriet, Robert: *Getting Back Together*, Coward-McCann, New York, 1971, pp. 60–62.
3 Hedgpeth: op. cit., p. 118.
4 Houriet: op. cit., p. 24.
5 "Home Birth," book review in *Ritual*, Science and Behavior Books, Palo Alto, California, 1971, p. 14.
6 Ibid., p. 20.
7 Hedgpeth: op. cit., p. 127.
8 Houriet: op. cit., p. 297.
9 Ibid., p. 9.
10 Ibid., pp. 55–56.
11 Russell, Barbara, and Lynn Lofstrom: "Health Clinic for the Alienated," *American Journal of Nursing*, 71(1):80–83, 1971.
12 Houriet: op. cit., p. 27.

BIBLIOGRAPHY

Brenner, Joseph, "Medical Care without a Hassle," *The New York Times Magazine,* October 11, 1970, p. 30.

Daniels, Ada M., and Alaine Krim: "Helping Adolescents Explore Emotional Issues," *American Journal of Nursing,* 69(7):1482–1485, 1969.

Goldsborough, Judith: "On Becoming Non-judgmental," *American Journal of Nursing,* 70(1):2340–2343, 1970.

Hedgpeth, William, and Dennis Stock: *The Alternative,* Collier-Macmillan, Toronto, 1970.

"Home Birth," book review in *Ritual,* Science and Behavior Books, Palo Alto, California, 1971.

Hommel, Flora: "Natural Childbirth—Nurses in Private Practice as Monitrices," *American Journal of Nursing,* 69(7):1446–1450, 1969.

Houriet, Robert: *Getting Back Together,* Coward-McCann, New York, 1971.

———: "Life and Death of a Commune Called Oz," *The New York Times Magazine,* February 16, 1969, p. 30.

Karmel, Marjorie: *Thank you, Dr. Lamaze,* Lippincott, Philadelphia, 1959.

Lang, Pat: *Home Birth,* Science and Behavior Books, Palo Alto, California, publication in process.

Laurel, Alicia B.: *Living on the Earth,* Vintage Books, Random House, New York, 1971.

"Of Oz and After: Discussion and Letters to the Editor," *The New York Times Magazine,* March 7, 1969, p. 12.

Russell, Barbara, and Lynn Lofstrom: "Health Clinic for the Alienated," *American Journal of Nursing,* 71(1):80–83, 1971.

Sankot, Margaret, and David Smith: "Drug Problems in the Haight-Ashbury," *American Journal of Nursing,* 68(8):1686–1688, 1968.

Smith, David: "Runaways and Their Health Problems in Haight-Ashbury during the Summer of 1967," *American Journal of Public Health,* 59:2046–2050, 1969.

6 | THE EXTENDED FAMILY

Ellen J. Mevis

THE FAMILY

To establish the concept of the extended family, certain generalizations are necessary. The family is composed of individuals who are united by one of several ties: marriage, blood, or adoption. The most fundamental relationship is that of the husband and wife.

A family represents a pattern of group living, and typically members of the family live together in one dwelling area. The number of actual inhabitants can range from a single couple to as many as five generations, including immediate families and relatives. If some members of the family live elsewhere, they still consider it to be their home. Ordinarily the family is culturally, religiously, and functionally oriented, although variations do occur within a single sociocultural complex. In other words, the family household is a group of related individuals living together in a single or joint complex forming a recognizable sociocultural unit.[1]

The related members of this family interact and communicate through the context of their mutually agreed upon social roles which are usually identified in the terms of kinship, such as husband, wife, father, mother, son, daughter, brother, sister, cousin, and so on. Each of these particular roles is established and defined through sociocultural characteristics and expectations.

Within each family unit, roles are interpreted according to traditional or incidental family characteristics. Once established and defined, these roles are continually and powerfully reinforced through the texture of day-to-day experience and events. An established and operative behavioral system provides unity and meaningful direction for the family.[1]

The common culture existing within each individual family is usually derived from exterior sociocultural forces, but in spite of exterior influence, each family maintains its own distinct features. These features evolve through interaction and communication between family members from generation to generation and through which merge general cultural patterns which determine their life style. Other cultural patterns are introduced into the family through intermarriage and incidental interaction and communication with different sociocultural groups. External cultural influences create additional possibilities for development and evolution of the inner culture of any particular family unit.[1]

The "Extended" Family

The "extended" family may be defined as the familial grouping of relatives to form relationships in addition to those normally present in the family situation; the members may inhabit more than one household but will share a common body of domestic, sociocultural, and economic activities.[2] These relationships refer to formations of three or more generations of relatives—grandparents, parents, and their children—allied in a situation involving all as a single family unit. The extended family unit is generally larger than the average American family[2] because of the additional individuals present; therefore, it has a more complex role and organizational structure. When an extended family does not inhabit the same household, it is common to find the separate households in a single locality.

As the result of certain sociocultural, religious, or functional reasons, family units cluster in a particular way. Interdependencies within the extended family are given more emphasis than in the average nuclear family structure. Relationships go beyond and are more complex than those of the nuclear family. The normal biological ties between the members of the extended family are reinforced to a greater extent and relationships tend to be closer and more formalized than one might expect to find in the nuclear family. Therefore, the traditional extended family usually is characterized by being closely knit, inner-directed, and often unfamiliar and unfriendly to those outside its bounds who seem strange or different.

The relationships between members of the extended family, specifically any two members, will be affected to some degree by their sex, marital status, separation in age, and the generation to which they belong.[2] Also significant in the formation of relationships between these members is the factor of whether they have biological or affinal bonds. Each of these factors affects the degree of closeness—between any two members in the family group. In addition to these factors, there often occur particular relationships within a specific extended family group which appear for no apparent reason and are simply the result of some special bond established between the members concerned. An example of this would be the grandfather-granddaughter (or grandson) relationship. Occasionally, when such relationships as these occur, their bond is so strong and influential that it ignores the normal authority patterns and preference associations which exist in such families.

Following this brief introduction to the phenomenon of the extended family is a detailed description of an idealized extended family unit and of some of the significant events which occur in all families (i.e., courtship, marriage, childbearing, education and instruction of children, and old age) for the purpose of demonstrating how such a family unit characteristically reacts to these events.*

The Idealized Extended Family[3]

This extended family unit is composed of a cluster of individual nuclear units who live in their own homes which are usually located near the central and original household inhabited by the grandparents. Among them there is a loosely organized hierarchy of authorities and relationships which are commonly associated with age, actual or potential wealth, and possible utility. This hierarchy often operates as an informal family council through which pressures can be brought to bear on the individual nuclear family units within the larger family structure. Such pressures are utilized to influence members to conform to the family standards and to encourage constant contribution to organized family enterprises and to the welfare and good of all family members.

The integrated extended family circle typically consists of three generations. Members included in this unit range from grandparents, through parents and their children, and as far laterally as uncles and aunts, the resulting first cousins, and often their children. Although it is more common to find these relatives spread into their own nuclear households, the family circle of the grandparents' household—and occasionally that of the parents—is often expanded through the inclusion of aging parents, unmarried sisters or brothers, orphaned cousins, and illegitimate children. The structure of this traditional extended family is organized to handle many of the contingent circumstances and individuals which otherwise must be handled by exterior social and welfare agencies.

---

* *The World of the Family* by Dorothy R. Blitsten has been used as the main reference source for the following discussion of the idealized extended family.

This extended family maintains between its members established and enforced bonds of responsibility and authority. These bonds could be reinforced by actual affection between these same members. As the result of these responsibilities and authorities, inner tensions occasionally occur and are handled within the family unit itself through pressures and influences. During periods of stress, the family's bonds are drawn even closer to present a united front to outsiders.

The extended family represents a closed circle, and undue communication with strangers and outsiders is usually discouraged. It is not common for strangers to be casually introduced into the family circle. The children normally do not bring their playmates and friends from school into the home. While they might certainly have such associations and friendships at school, their most common playmates and companions away from the school are found within their own kin circle. They associate most commonly with their brothers, sisters, cousins, or the offspring of other families with whom they have been in contact for some time. Neither is it common for the working men of the household to regularly bring their colleagues or friends from work into the home, or for neighbors to casually drop in to introduce themselves or for "idle" chat.

Marriage tends to expand the circle of family associations, and there are occasional introductions of long-term friends from either school or work into the family circle, but such occurrences are rare and significant. Thus, the extended family provides its members with a closed, private world of associations which develop into dependable and lasting relationships. For the women and children, the family provides the majority of their entire range of friendships and associations. Such inner-direction adds to the unity and closed nature of the extended family unit. Through it develops a strong feeling of family pride, value, and a sense of obligation to maintain the honor and prestige of the family along with its material and social advantages. These bonds are further strengthened by the concept of the potential contributions which the members can and do make to each other's feelings of personal satisfaction, careers, and possible benefits to the secondary nuclear subunit in assistance in time of crisis, and finally, in terms of likely inheritance. All of these factors contribute in their own way to maintaining the power and strength of the extended family unit.

THE LIFE PROCESS

Courtship

Since preparation for marriage and later integration into the extended family unit is one of the most implicit aspects of the childrearing process, the children from an early age are oriented toward adult life. They are not encouraged or even, in some cases, allowed to become overly involved in adolescent peer group relations or place their own juvenile or adolescent goals ahead of those goals established for them by their elders.

Because of this adult-oriented training and education, by the time the adolescent has reached the age at which courtship and marriage become his primary interests, he is prepared for the demands of married life and the full-time occupation which it will impose.

Generally the young men of the extended family who are of marriageable age postpone their marriage until they have fulfilled their required military training, have entered into an occupation, and have established a means for the support of a family. A variation on this pattern is often manifested in the American Indian and Chicano ethnic groups. Within these groups, which are often characterized by impoverished circumstances, the marriage of the younger members of the family may take place at an earlier age. Occasionally this occurs while they are still in school. Under such circumstances, the male is often expected to drop out of school and go to work to support his new family. The significant factor remains that the male provide capably and immediately for the new wife. This is considered his utmost responsibility to the family and its members.

For the female, marriage alone is assumed to be the fitting and proper career unless the circumstances of her family dictate that she work in order to provide adequately for the family when the male is incapacitated, deceased, or otherwise absent. It is not uncommon for females to discontinue their formal education after they have finished high school or at about age fifteen or sixteen. They are then expected to perfect their skills in such wifely duties as housekeeping, child care, cooking, and sewing. Their training and education in these duties and skills takes place in their home, along with their siblings, under the supervision of their mother or grandmother. By the age of eighteen or nineteen it is assumed that these skills are perfected, and they are then considered to be ready for marriage. At that time they are encouraged by their parents and other relatives to begin actively seeking a lifetime mate.

Through either direct or indirect means, the parents and family influence the choice of the lifetime mate. One of the more subtle means by which this is accomplished is through the inculcation over the years into the child of the family's standards of what is desirable and preferable in a mate of a child of the family. Another means for this is found in the manner in which the extended family limits the range of close associations which its children are allowed to maintain. The associations are restricted to those whom the family would consider to be appropriate mates. A key means by which the parental or grandparental control can be directly asserted is in the fact that they maintain the economic resources and thereby the access to education, career opportunities, and the more desirable living arrangements available to their offspring.

Thus, it is possible for the elders to influence, pressure, or even at times coerce an uncooperative offspring to forego relationships which they consider to be inappropriate or undesirable to the family.

Actual family approval of the mate in a marriage is particularly important. This is so because of the necessity of the chosen mate's fitting into and adapting well to the circumstances of the extended family situation. There is yet another more significant reason why this approval is deemed so necessary. Without such approval the disobedient offspring could—and very likely would—be deprived of the significant practical economic advantages which emanate from the family, ranging from the prestige of membership to the very real—and sometimes sizable—factors of mutual aid and inheritance.

For all these reasons, when the offspring of an extended family arrives at the point of marriage, he is generally well prepared for his new and more responsible circumstances. He realizes that his years of childhood and irresponsibility are behind him, and he is armed with the knowledge of a responsible adult which will increase his distinction and authority within the extended family.

Marriage

Once the marriage partner has been approved and the formal and religious aspects of the marriage have been accomplished, the newlyweds generally attempt to establish themselves in a household separate from, but adjacent to, other members of the husband's family. If this is not practical or possible, they are included quite readily and happily into the household of the parents.

While it is to be expected that some problems will evolve from the newly formed relationships and living arrangement, such strains are effectively reduced because the participants have entered into it with full knowledge and acceptance of its consequences and with highly similar expectations; they have been prepared through their past membership in extended families to deal with such circumstances. With their background and knowledge such a new family relationship has a very high potential for success as compared to the "pioneering" element present in the establishment of completely independent nuclear family life.

Because of the education, training, and orientation of children for adult life present in the extended family, there is a great reduction in importance of the initial period of marriage before parenthood takes place. Since the young couple enter into the marriage with the understanding that the marital relationship is one of interdependence, related closely to their mutual needs, traits, and duties to each other, this usually brief period between marriage and parenthood is a time of preparation for the deeper and more complex marital life which will evolve through parenthood. The emphasis in the extended family is obviously placed on familial continuity, and this concept places a great deal of responsibility and pressure upon the newly wed couple to keep this preparenthood time as short as possible. Because both father-hood and motherhood have an aura of both authority and sacredness, the young couple, as well as all the associated relatives, hope for the onset of the wife's first pregnancy within a very short time after the marriage takes place.

Childrearing

It is a characteristic of the extended family to perpetuate itself and provide for family continuity by encouraging large families. Traditionally, it has only been the period of biological fertility which has acted as a limit on the num-ber of the progeny of the extended family. This tradition has resulted in the fact that while the average number of offspring from a fertile couple has been four or five, it is not unusual to discover six to eight or even more children in nuclear units. Through the social significance attendant upon parenthood in the extended family situation, it becomes personally gratifying to each individual member of the couple—especially the woman—to produce as many children as possible. Consequently, nuclear units in the extended family are much larger, and there are smaller age differences between sib-lings than in the average American nuclear family.

This situation is further helped because within the extended family the burdens of parenthood are significantly reduced through the distribution of both the material and personal costs of childbearing among the family circle, specifically to those either financially or personally capable of sharing the burden. The responsibility of childbearing is reduced for the specific married couple through the structured shared responsibilities and authorities. The relatives are not overly indulgent of the young parents, but they are present and will not shirk any reasonable request for assistance by the young couple if help is needed. The female relatives do help the young mother with her household and child-care duties, and the male relatives can be counted on in times of emergency to provide labor, produce, or financial assistance. There-fore, it is not from lack of personal help that the young nuclear family unit suffers. Because they are not isolated from their relatives, their constant presence and willingness to help create one of the strongest bonds between the nuclear family unit and the main extended family.

The strains developing from the childbearing situation result from the general economic conditions under which the entire family lives. The charac-teristic nature of the extended family to limit both sociocultural and geo-graphic mobility, poor economic conditions, and poor conditions in general tend to significantly influence extended family situations. Occasionally wealth and property are spread throughout the members of some extended families, but it is more often poverty which is commonly shared. This is possibly the most powerful limiting circumstance functional to both the size and maintenance of the nuclear unit of the extended family. As significant and realistic as this factor is, it generally is ignored.

The young mother is expected to keep house well for her husband and children, to live within the financial means which her husband produces, to keep her nuclear family members well fed and clothed, and to teach her children the good manners, respect, and behavior expected of a young member of the family. The father's role is usually somewhat more formally oriented. He is expected to exercise his authority at will over both the wife and children. This does not mean that he normally acts as a dictator and autocrat in the nuclear family situation, but only that the final authority rests in his hands and that he makes those decisions which significantly affect the household. Within this situation, there also lies the powerful, though usually disguised, authority of the mother. Although the authority "officially" rests in the hands of the father, it is often the mother who exerts her influence to direct the course his decision making takes.

Beyond this, the father is affectionate to the children, expecting from them obedience and respect. The child care and household work are considered to be women's tasks, and it is not common for the husband to perform them. The father exercises his authority in the lives of his children by deciding how the child should be reared, what he should be taught, and who his friends should be. Parental approval remains one of the most important and significant factors in the life of the child and operates as a necessary adjunct to the most significant concern for the extended family: family approval.

Although the birth of children creates new strains and pressures upon the relationship of husband and wife, it does not have a harmful effect upon the marriage. The children are definitely an important aspect of the life of the family, but they are never allowed to dominate either the nuclear or the extended family. The family is adult-oriented and not child-centered, as most American families are. The children are trained early to give full precedence and respect to their elders, and this training is additionally reinforced through the child's observation of his parents' behavior in deference to their elders in the extended family relations. The husband and wife relationship is not threatened in the extended family system because the children, though important, are considered to be an integral part of the marital relationship—not a special development from it. Thus, the children are dealt with as a matter of course—they are not spoiled or given a disproportionate amount of pampering or privilege so that they would seem to be actually competing with their parents. There is an important place for the children of the extended family, but that place is maintained only as long as the child demonstrates that he deserves it by his behavior to his elders. Should he exceed that place he is immediately brought to the realization and correction of his mistake by both parental and family action.

EDUCATION AND INSTRUCTION OF CHILDREN

Because in the extended family there are likely to be numerous children and they may be spread over a broad spectrum of ages, there is little distinction made between the initial phases of the childbearing and training process and the later phases of the "launching" of the older children into life. These phases normally are carried on concurrently with several gradations being present in the family at any one time. It is not uncommon to find the situation in which the last child and the first grandchild are approximately the same age. There can be no sharply drawn line between early training and later launching activities except on a purely individual level. The important element in the training and launching of the children is that of providing an expanded series of associations for the child while training him in the significance and importance *to him* of the extended family association. Training and education does not mean in any way the severance of the child from these functions. The direct opposite is, in fact, its intention.

The parental responsibility operative in the extended family continues over a longer period of time than is characteristic of the general American nuclear family. The parental concerns last, in some form or another, throughout the child's entire lifetime. From the training of the child in preparation for his adult life and responsibilities, through his actual marriage and bearing of children, the training and education of those children, their eventual marriage and entering into their occupations, and the concern of the grandparents for their grandchildren, the parental responsibility is much more extensive than might normally be expected. Beyond these considerations the needs of the older generations for care and housing replace the birth and childbearing cycle in such a way as to further extend the parental responsibility. All in all, there is no period to which the parents can look ahead with the intention of having responsibilities out of the way completely, as is characteristic of the nuclear American family. These responsibilities simply continue throughout life in variable forms.

The children are generally indulged while they are young, but this does not continue throughout their childhood. After the child reaches the age of about five or six, a firmer, more extensive discipline is applied. Parental authority is a constantly exercised and respected force in the life of the child of the extended family. The child is taught to respect the authority of the elders of the household. Through this training, by the time the child has reached fifteen or sixteen, he realizes the significance and meaning of his position in relation not only to his own nuclear and extended family, but also within the society in general. He is thus trained to accept the realities of life and understand his position as subordinate until such time as he has obtained adequate prestige or value to the family—and society—to change this subordinate position to a more dominant one.

Early in life the children are given honest and frank appraisals of their own abilities and potentialities. This results from the assumption that not everyone in the family has the same abilities and potentialities, and that if the child realizes this—along with comprehending the extent of his own capabilities—he will concentrate on the development of himself to the fullest extent possible. He is expected to make the best of his natural and inborn capabilities. Any behavior seemingly wasteful or less than that of which he is capable is regarded very negatively and is highly disapproved of by both parents and family elders. The child who is doing his best and attempting to utilize his full capabilities, even though he may be doing less than the other children, is rewarded with the admiration and praise of the family.

The punishment of the children of the extended family rarely reaches the point of physical action. It usually takes the verbal form of "tongue-lashing." The withholding of affection and tenderness is another means through which the elders may punish the misbehaving child. The denial of permission for pleasurable activities of the child is another technique which is effectively used to reprimand and discipline the child. Occasionally the child will actually be held up to the ridicule of others as a means for motivating his proper behavior. Actual physical punishment is generally one of the last resorts which may be applied to discipline and enforce the child's proper behavior.

The daily lives of the children of the extended family are organized and planned out well in advance to conform to the needs and requirements of the extended family situation. Beginning with school, the average day of the child progresses in a well-organized and structured manner. After school come first the required household duties which the child has been assigned and for which he is responsible without fail. These tasks are generally sexually separated: The boys usually perform duties assigned by the father which relate to those duties of the male in the household. The girls aid their mothers and older sisters in a relationship which is much like an apprenticeship to prepare them for the time when they will take over those duties in their own nuclear family unit or offer service to other members of the extended family structure. This clear division of labor between males and females continues from the early period of childhood right on through adulthood and into all aspects of family life.

A primary concern of both the nuclear and extended families with reference to childrearing is in establishing within the child a firm orientation toward the inner circles of the family structure. The child is not allowed any great extent of social initiative or activity outside the extended family circle. This is often carried to the point at which the entrance of the child into school is regarded by the parents as an incursion into their authority and a threat to regulation by the family. In any case, the child is very deeply inculcated with the idea that the family and its demands and requirements have a priority over any outside demands made upon him.

The child is taught a strong competitive spirit which is expressed within the family group in a formalized way. Each of the individual nuclear units of the extended family competes with the others to the desired end of obtaining a larger proportion of the overall resources of the extended family. The gaining of the favor of possible sources of inheritance—from grandparents or unmarried uncles or aunts—is one of the primary objects of this competition. Another area of competitiveness is that of the inner power structure of the family. The power usually rests upon the eldest member of the extended family unit, but there are occasions and incidents in which another member of the family, through wealth, prestige, or special position gained through his own efforts, may be considered as the source of power expressed in the family. Therefore, competition may be a highly effective means for obtaining a base for power within the extended family structure.

As a result of this situation, the child may become adept at the manipulation of certain of his elders quite early in life. Since the favorite grandchild, niece, or nephew has not only garnered for himself an effective ally against parental authority but has also created a closer link between himself and the source of power and possible wealth within the family, the competition for such relationships is often rather keen. The child who does establish such a relationship has also created for himself some degree of equality with the elders in the family and is treated with more deference and tact than he might be otherwise. This applies to treatment from not only family members in general but also his own parents.

These childrearing and launching activities of the extended family have a goal more extensive than the mere preparation of the children for providing for themselves and their children once they become adults. The desired end result of the childrearing and launching process is the development of a family-centered orientation in the child. He is to operate always with the family in mind. He is trained to be a tool of implementation of the family tradition. He is taught that he must apply his powers and efforts to enhance family resources and prestige. By the time the child has completed this educative and training process, his dependence upon the family is an established behavior pattern, and variation from that pattern is unthinkable.

Old Age

Elderly members do not pose the same problem in the extended family as they do in the average nuclear family. There is little reason for an aging member to be anxious over his welfare when he ceases to be self-sufficient. Since respect and deference to elders are taught as the primary aspects of behavior and are reinforced through both training and actual practice, aging members are expected to depend upon the family, and its individual members, more and more as time goes on. The older person is welcomed into the particular nuclear unit which, because of either biological relationship or financial standing, he would most reasonably fit. In this way, the family acts as the social welfare agency in providing for its own members.

Persons of advanced age do not face the problem of being disregarded or losing their prestige and family standing because of their age. In the extended family elders are treated with honor and respect. Usually those who are the oldest have the greatest prestige, if not power as well. The aging male usually works at his occupation as long as he is physically able. Upon his retirement, he may help as much as he can with the normal duties of the male members of the household in which he resides.

For the aging female there are fewer problems in the extended family than may be faced within the nuclear family. They will have gained the confidence and respect of the family members through their past performance as wife and mother. They take great pride in the family which they have engendered and educated into the family tradition. In addition, when the older woman becomes a grandmother she again finds herself in the position of taking a significant role in the childrearing and training process with the children from the new generation.

The care and aid provided for older family members are given as a matter of course and generally without recrimination or resentment. This often entails sacrifice, expecially for those families of low income but it is a duty which must be done—there is little thought of passing the responsibility off onto society in general. The elders do not feel any shame about accepting such aid and care. Since they provided it for their parents, it is expected that their children will do it for them. Any hardship which might derive from this situation is shared by the family on an equitable basis to the extent that it is feasible and possible. Since family unity is the significant factor operative within the extended family unit, this is the only logical means for caring for aging family members.

This idealized description of the extended family is presented to orient the reader to this phenomenon. To further indicate the reality of the extended family in the United States today, two case histories will be presented which are characteristic of this phenomenon. These case histories have been altered somewhat in order to orient them closer to the subject matter for this book. Nevertheless, they represent a true indication of the extended family situation.

THE CHICANO CULTURE

The Mexican-American, or Chicano, population of the United States is basically the result of an intermarriage pattern. Chicanos are the descendants of the early Spanish colonists who invaded the North American continent in the sixteenth century. Their physical characteristics result primarily from the extensive intermarriage which took place between these Spanish explorers and the native Indian populations. Thus, in these Mexican-Americans a situation exists in which European Catholic culture patterns are superimposed upon the already established native culture. The result has been a primarily agrarian, Roman Catholic synthesis. Most of the population inhabits small, independent agricultural communities.[4]

These communities have been characterized throughout most of the past by their isolation.[4] Thus, within these communities there developed a strong internal social organization which had the effect of maintaining past practice over historical change. The two strongest social institutions were the Roman Catholic Church and the family. The leadership in these communities was determined by age and prestige rather than through popular approval or individual characteristics. Leadership emanated from the primary institution involving governmental organization: the family.

The family organizational pattern was of the extended nature. Since the community structure was tightly organized and structured, so was the family life also very formalized and structured. Over the past 400 years there has been little variation in this culture pattern. Today the extended family remains the fundamental organizational pattern for Mexican-American families. Therefore, a closer examination of such families will provide an excellent example of the phenomenon of the extended family which applies to many ethnic groups.

Urban Barrio

The term *barrio* refers to what the Anglo population would call a slum—that is, a generally economically and physically depressed area which is normally inhabited by the more poverty-stricken, primarily Spanish-speaking Chicano families. The barrio is a very tightly woven and somewhat isolated community which is surrounded by the exterior urban population. It is a world which would be difficult for an outsider to penetrate for two reasons: First, because of his unfamiliarity with the conditions and life-style of the barrio, the outsider has no real pre-established terminology or understandings upon which to approach the barrio or its inhabitants. Second, because the outsider is a stranger, he would be regarded with suspicion and mistrust by the inhabitants of the barrio, and he would find it extremely difficult to establish any real contact or communication with the impoverished population there. This mistrust and suspicion which meets any stranger entering the barrio results from not only the characteristic behavior patterns of the poor with regard to strangers, but also from a significant characteristic of the extended family phenomenon which is the organizational pattern for the Chicano families inhabiting the area.

In a certain Colorado barrio environment, there has been recently manifested a strong reassertion of interest in the traditions, music, dances, and folk patterns brought north by the Mexican emigrants whose children now inhabit the barrio. This desire and interest is an expression of minority nationalism through which the Chicano peoples are now attempting to develop a sense of pride and respect for their heritage, which for years has been so denigrated, especially in the southwestern section of the country. One of the primary characteristics of these families which does not need reassertion is that traditional form of family organization which the Chicano family utilizes.

Compadrazgo

While the extended family is the primary pattern upon which Chicano kinship and authority patterns are based, it operates here with an additional aspect. A specific Chicano family unit will offer an excellent example of this. Although this family is relatively small to represent the typical barrio family, it presents a fairly representative illustration of the barrio pattern. In addition to their extended family, the children of the family rely extensively upon the *compadrazgo* system which, in reality, operates as further expansion upon the extended family pattern. The compadrazgo is an old Mexican and Spanish kinship tradition through which each of the children of the family have a set of godparents. The godfather (*padrino*) and godmother (*madrina*) act within the family structure as coparents (*compadres*) and operate in cooperation with the child's real parents to provide additional direction, guidance, and affection for the child. In this sense they actually operate much as the real grandparents of the child might if they were present. The ties of the compadrazgo system are, generally speaking, as strong as blood ties.

In this particular family the "real" family includes the aging grandfather who resides with his son, who functions as the head of the household. The grandfather has had a series of cerebral vascular accidents and is no longer able to function as either a wage earner or source of authority within the family. In addition to the son and his wife, there are three children within the family: The two oldest are both boys and are of grade school age. The youngest, a girl, is six years old. In line with the compadrazgo system, each of these three children has his own set of godparents. These godparents assume certain social, moral, and economic responsibilities toward their godchild and in addition, they function within the social tradition of the barrio by acting as a further link, along with the extended family and kinship systems, to bind together the barrio community in a series of interlocking friendships and responsibility relationships.

The head of the family—that is, the son of the grandfather—has a minimal formal education. He did not graduate from high school because financial difficulties faced by his family at that time forced him to seek employment to provide additional support at the age of sixteen. He has held his present job as a service station attendant for the past 6 years. To gain further funds to support his family he occasionally does odd jobs for two friends of the family who are more affluent and who reside outside the barrio.

The low rents in the barrio section of town have been the prime reason for the father's maintenance of his family in that location. Were it not for this, and given the presence of more money, he would readily move his family to another location in town.

Because he has been able to maintain a fairly dependable work record and income for his family (including his ailing and aging father), the son has obtained his status as head of the household and enjoys the respect of the godparents, neighbors, and relatives for having done so. Although the invalid father provides nothing in the way of sustenance for the family, and little in the way of actual authority, he does receive a great deal of respect and admiration within the nuclear family in which he resides and also among the members of the extended family and godparent system. As the patriarch of the family, his presence is always allowed for whenever it is possible for him to be included, and he is treated with a great deal of deference by everyone in the family. He is admired by all relatives and friends for having been responsible for the rearing, education, and training of his son who behaves in such a responsible and admirable manner toward his father and family. Any man who fathered and trained such a son is due respect and admiration himself within the barrio because such behavior on the part of the son indicates that his father both knew how to raise children properly and succeeded in having done so.

It is not an uncommon practice among Chicano residents of the barrio to "trade" or "loan out" a child to other members of the family, sometimes for as long as a year. The youngest child in the family has been living with a young aunt for 3 months. The aunt has just given birth to her first child, and not only is she happy to have someone in her home to talk to during the day, but she also has a modicum of help available to her. The fact that the young child has been out of the nuclear household has also allowed her mother to take on a part-time job as a clerk at the neighborhood Youth Opportunity Center. The two young boys have also spent time in the household of an uncle but have now reached an age and responsibility at which they are now capable of caring for themselves in addition to performing certain household tasks in the absence of both parents during the day. Thus, it is clear that even the more distant members of the extended family occasionally take a hand in the rearing and caring for the children within its circle and provide aid and support for the parents of any particular nuclear unit.

Wives in Chicano families of the barrio are generally subservient to the wishes of their husbands, except in such cases in which the husband is absent, negligent, or shirks his duties and responsibilities. The mother, however, enjoys the position of being both the religious and moral leader within her own nuclear family unit, for the father's duties tend to be oriented more in the direction of behavioral and disciplinary leadership. Mothers do, however, share the disciplinary tasks of childrearing with the fathers, as is true in the case of this family. The father "lays down the law," and the mother aids him in enforcing it. This is especially true, of course, when the husband is at work and the mother is home.

In this family the father expresses a great deal of affection toward the young daughter. This follows the traditional pattern in which the father is expected to show great affection toward the younger children; this affection gradually changes into a mutually respected distance as the children grow older. Such is the case with the boys of this family.

Motherhood within the Chicano families of the barrio is a much heralded and significant event. This is true especially within the mother's compadrazgo system. Large families are not only traditionally sanctioned, but are also the common occurrence in the barrio. However, in this particular family, the father and mother have expressed the desire to limit the size of their family because of their minimal financial situation. They do intend to have one more child, which will bring the number of children in their family to a total of four, still a large family by Anglo standards.

The mother of this family has related an interesting anecdote concerning the childbirth conditions under which her grandmother gave birth to her children. The grandmother, a first-generation immigrant, delivered her first child in Mexico with the assistance of a midwife, or *parteras* in Spanish. The parteras assisted the pregnant mother prior to actual childbirth with hot teas and oil massages. This had the primarily nonmedicinal effect of relaxing the prospective mother and engaging her affection for the midwife. The whole experience of childbirth with the assistance of the midwife was a satisfying and successful one for the grandmother, and she felt highly confident of the midwife's skills and abilities.

After she had left Mexico and moved to a Southern California city, the grandmother became pregnant again. Little was done until she was about to deliver the second child. At that time the husband set out to find a midwife to assist her. He could not find one, however, in the American city. The couple had neither relatives nor compadres living nearby to help the mother deliver. Finally, the time for actual delivery came, and the mother gave birth with the assistance of the husband only.

Her next child was born in a hospital. The grandmother was very disappointed with her experience in the American hospital. She felt that the doctors and nurses there were cold and uncaring and that the general attitude of those who attended her during the childbirth was impersonal. She complained most of not having been given hot tea or massages. She felt that the American obstetric practices were totally alien to her experience and feelings.

Most of the second- and third-generation descendants of the Mexican grandmother do not express the same feelings of disappointment or resentment toward giving birth in a hospital. In fact, they consider the hospital to be the best place to deliver. Nevertheless, although they are not able to retain the tradition of the midwife (a practice which is illegal in many states today), the Chicano mothers-to-be still retain some of the traditional treatments of the midwife. Some of these are concerned with the diet during pregnancy: They generally avoid eating spicy food (no small effort for Chicano families), chilies, vinegar, and the like. They also traditionally do not eat pork during pregnancy. These dietary prohibitions are based upon their feeling that not eating such foods will aid the new mother in lactation.

In some cities in the Southwest, clinics are in operation to assist pregnant women from the lower socioeconomic areas with both prenatal and postpartum care. In addition, an extensive system of free public health centers has been established within these same sections of the city. These neighborhood health centers are supported by two large health agencies located in the lower-income sectors of the city. These various clinics are funded by local, state, and federal sources and have as one of their major functions the dispensing of medical care, especially prenatal and postnatal care, to their target area residents and other indigent citizens. Thus, not only are medical and maternal care now becoming available to a wider range of citizens than before in these lower-economic areas of town, but these services are of a better quality than they had been before.

The maternity divisions of these neighborhood health centers hold regular clinics for maternal, prenatal, postpartum, and child care instruction throughout the year. By doing so the clinic provides the opportunity for the pregnant woman to see the same physician throughout the period of her pregnancy. In the early stages of pregnancy she is requested to visit the doctor once a month. During the later stages, and according to the doctor's discretion, these visits become more frequent. Also, the pregnant woman is encouraged to attend classes for instruction in adequate hygienic and health practices to ensure the best prenatal and postpartum care for her baby. A significant aspect of this course is intended to explain away the mysteries of urban hospitals and obstetric practices to both the new mother and the mother who will be giving birth in the unfamiliar surroundings of a hospital for the first time.

This aspect of the course also prepares the mother for the possible situation in which the doctor who attends her in the hospital is not the same one who had been treating her at the neighborhood health center. Because of the severe shortages of space and facilities at those hospitals which usually treat patients from the lower-economic areas of town, the postpartum mothers are often discharged within the first 48 hours after delivery, and preparation for this is also necessary. Additional precautions are taken for immediate follow-up care. Usually within 4 hours after she has arrived home with her newborn child, a visiting nurse from the neighborhood health clinic calls upon the mother and child to ensure that everything is proceeding smoothly and is under control. The mother is then encouraged to visit the neighborhood health center if she has any question or worries about either her own or her child's condition.

Special postpartum clinics have been established in the neighborhood health centers in order to provide a more organized approach to postpartum care for both mother and child. At the time of the routine 6-week examination free information about birth control methods, including free paraphernalia, is distributed if the mother so desires. There is no pressure or coercion attached to this part of the routine clinical examination and care, however.

The mother of the family previously discussed gained her motivation and desire to limit the size of her family through this routine part of the neighborhood postpartum clinic. She expressed good feelings about the assistance that she had received in the clinic and hospital in the delivery of her three children. She had several complaints pertaining to her hospital stay, but these were mainly contingent upon the overcrowded nature of the city hospital. During the delivery of her first son she felt that she was being "rushed." She stated that if the clinic doctor were to deliver the baby, a greater feeling of personalized attention would have added to her comfort. She also felt that the hospital doctor was a stranger and was only interested in having her complete the delivery as quickly as possible in order to get on to someone else.

She did wish to impress the interviewer with the fact that she was generally thankful for the action of the neighborhood health center, the visiting nurse, and the hospital. It was her feeling that these services were some of the best provided in the barrio and that they were also of the most direct benefit to the barrio residents, since they place such an importance upon childbearing and children in general.

The Mexican-American outside the Barrio

In an urban setting, where the wage earner has a steady, full-time, dependable job, the extended family continues but in an altered form. This is evident in a larger city where its many levels of job opportunities enable the Chicano family to break away from its reliance on the agrarian pattern and yet remain geographically close enough to permit frequent return visits to the areas of its origin, either New Mexico or old Mexico. Because they so carefully maintain these ties, many of the lower-middle-class Chicano urban families still exhibit many of the characteristics of the extended family.

A family to exemplify this situation might consist of grandmother, father, mother, and six children living together in an older, so-called "changing" neighborhood. Of over 30 families on the block, 85 percent are Anglo, a mixture ranging from WASP Presbyterians and Lutherans to Italian and Irish Roman Catholics. The median age of the heads of the households is about sixty because the majority of the population on the block are retirees and widows. There are not many families with young children in the neighborhood. The older Protestant families on the block tend to regard the Chicano families, about 15 percent of the population there, with disfavor.

Under the heavy Roman Catholic influence present on the block, it is not uncommon to see both Anglo and Chicano neighbors attending the same church services, bingo parties, and other parish activities. There is also a great deal of sharing of garden produce grown in the backyards of these Anglo and Chicano Catholic families. The church has served as a common ground for interest among these families and acts as a unifying influence in this neighborhood—a fact which is also somewhat resented by nearby residents.

Even in this neighborhood where they reside along with retirees who are living in unostentatious comfort, this particular Chicano family occupies the lowest point on the economic and social scale. Their home, which is a large, older house, is rented, and this fact alone sets the family apart from their neighbors, who own their homes. Furthermore, in appearance, the Chicano home falls below the other well-kept properties on the block. Although they are the only family on the block who owns a power lawn mower, the father, who does heavy labor all day, has neither time nor energy to use it often. The job of mowing the lawn is left to the teen-age son, and it is considered one of his responsibilities to the family. He is not as conscientious about this duty, however, as are some of the neighboring retirees who have little else to worry about.

The rather decrepit impression made by the exterior of the Chicano family's home is strengthened by the scantily and poorly furnished interior. A few scattered wall plaques represent the only attempt at interior adornment. In spite of the house's poor overall appearance, it does provide the family with ample living, eating, and sleeping space and is an improvement in housing over their former cramped, dirt-floored New Mexican dwelling.

The grandmother, in her eighties, spends the day sitting on the front porch when the weather permits. Although there are many women on the block who are in the same age group, she makes no attempt to socialize with them in any way. She leaves the house daily to attend mass at the parish church nearby. Occasionally, she spends some time with a married daughter who is more affluent than the son with whom she lives. With her more affluent condition, the daughter has also developed a certain Anglo turn of mind which will not allow her to support her mother or permit her to reside with her for any sustained period of time.

The daughter-in-law with whom she does reside spends the greater part of her day working inside the house cooking and caring for the children and the normal household tasks. She emerges from the house only to hang the laundry or sit for a few minutes with the grandmother. Otherwise, she seldom leaves the house unless accompanied by one of the children or her husband. Her husband expects her to occupy herself fully with the household chores and objects to her spending idle time talking with friends or neighbors. This is a trait quite characteristic of the extended family situation in which the family is formed as a closed unit and none of its members is expected to have undue socialization with outside friends—this also includes friends of the same ethnic origin.

The family's isolated status in a quiet city neighborhood can also be traced to their lower-income status, their minimum concern for the upkeep of the property, and to the fact that Spanish is the language used most freely by the parents and the grandparents. Any attempts the neighbors make to communicate with the father or mother rarely get beyond the "Hello, how are you?" stage. There is, moreover, very little communication with other Spanish-speaking families in the neighborhood. These families tend to be more urbanized, have better jobs, and are property owners rather than renters. Both the men and the women work and attend social activities involving them with groups other than Spanish-American. The younger children, on the other hand, are well known and liked throughout the neighborhood, except for the few neighbors who find them somewhat a trial. Fluent in both Spanish and English, they have many Chicano and Anglo friends.

During pleasant weather the three generations—grandmother, father, mother, and children—gather together on the front porch in the evening. The smaller children occupy themselves with their toys, while the older ones carry on an animated conversation with the adults. Although the teen-age boys in the family go out in the evening with their friends from time to time, the teen-age girls play with the girls across the street but do not go out with them in the evening.

The grandmother apparently plays no functional role in the family in the sense of helping with the housework, cooking, or the rearing of the children. The children seem to enjoy her silent company, but there is a minimum of conversational exchange between them. It is only when her son sits with her in the evening that she becomes animated and converses volubly in Spanish.

Her son, the breadwinner and head of the family, works long hours daily as an unskilled laborer. He rarely does any work around the house or yard but confines himself to keeping the family car in running order. The son takes care of mowing the lawn and cleaning and waxing the car. The girls do their share by vacuuming the interior of the house and washing the windows. Thus, the household and related chores are divided among as many members of the family as are able to perform them. Although there may be occasional altercations, less often a reprimand, over the adequate performance of these duties, they are usually undertaken with less argument and failure than one might expect to find in the average Anglo family.

The father clearly acts as the final authority in both the assignment of these duties and disciplining the children to carry out such duties properly and as requested. He is the clearly recognized head of the family, and in performing this function, he rarely raises his voice or strikes any of the children. From time to time he lays down the law briefly and quietly and very effectively. He is so well established as the authority figure that the children, even the teen-agers, obey without question. He rarely uses any physical methods, such as spanking, to secure the fulfillment of his wishes.

The mother, on the other hand, has to meet the many small crises that plague the normal family from day to day. She can occasionally be heard raising her voice in Spanish. Such scoldings are infrequent and seldom degenerate into nagging. Both mother and children manage to live peacefully with one another but without making any great display of affection. Nevertheless, she gains discipline and accordance with her wishes through the respect and devotion which her children have for her. There is never a serious case of "back talk" or refusal to comply with her wishes; to do so would be to violate the duty expected of a child in the extended family situation. This notion is reinforced by the fact that within the Catholic faith (especially that expressed by the Chicanos) there is a great deal of reverence placed in the person of the mother.

The children are sent to the neighborhood Catholic parish school, but further involvement in parish activities is minimal. Although there are a number of Chicano families in this neighborhood who play an increasingly important part in parish activities, the father of this family confines his activities simply to attendance at church services. He has made no effort to join parish organizations. Neither does the mother join the other Chicano wives in attending the weekly bingo games held at the church. Her social life is very much restricted to home, husband, children, and other close relatives.

Thus, this family provides an example of the tradition of the extended family within the Chicano ethnic group. A similar situation could exist in several other ethnic groups. While many Chicano families who acquire economic and social affluence and security tend to lapse somewhat in the respect and deference given to the original extended family, this has not occurred with the overwhelming number of families. In most of the Chicano families in the Southwest the tradition of the extended family is significant. In fact, it may be said that the extended family is one of the prime factors relevant to understanding the reality of the social and economic condition of the Chicano ethnic group today. Without an understanding of the Chicano extended family, along with all of the relationships and situations which the concept involves, it would be practically impossible to deal with this ethnic group in a realistic manner.

SUMMARY

Generally, it can be assumed that the extended family differs from the nuclear family in that in the extended family the family itself is the basic unit, whereas in the nuclear family the basic unit tends to be the individual. The goals, the survival, and the continuation of the family dominate or supercede the goals of the individual. Moreover, the goals of the family become the goals of every individual within that family. This assumption underlies all family processes, from decision making to childrearing and training. In return, each member is sustained by the family through times of crisis, in fact, throughout his entire life. The extended family differs from the nuclear family also in the fact that the members of an extended family tend to obtain their status from their roles within the family, not from their roles or positions in society. Social roles are sometimes decided by the position or status of the family within the larger community. In dealing with a member of an extended family, then, one is actually dealing with the whole family (the response of the individual member reflects the attitudes of the family).

The very structure and processes of the extended family exist for the sustenance of its members. The family is not only the basic *social* unit, but also the basic unit of education, culture, and moral and ethical training. Sometimes it serves as the only source of medical aid or care. The family is a recognizable unit to which an individual can relate within a larger society.

In many of the societies characterized by extended families, particularly the Chicano and American Indian, there are some basic assumptions about life which differ from those of the predominantly Anglo community. When these assumptions contradict the medical knowledge of the Anglo community, they lead to practices which vary from those prescribed by modern medical science. However fantastic these practices may seem to a medical practitioner, they spring logically from the culture's basic assumptions. In the area of pregnancy and childrearing especially, the assumptions of the Chicano and the American Indian differ extremely from the Anglo point of view.[5]

This summary of an extended family has provided a description of a "classical" extended family. In reality, there are no typical extended families. Many extended families will display some or even most of the traits characteristic of the classic type, but no two will be the same. The families will differ culturally, socially, and economically. Generally, the degree of authority and isolation maintained by the family over the individual will vary at an inverse ratio to that family's socioeconomic status. The families at the bottom of the socioeconomic ladder generally will display more and stronger characteristics of the extended family than those who enjoy more status.

REFERENCES

1 Burger, Ernest W., Harvey J. Locke, and Mary Margaret Thomas: *The Family: From Institution to Companionship*, 3d ed., Crowell, New York, 1966, p. 2.

2 Shanas, Edith, and Gordon F. Streib (eds.): *Social Structure and the Fam-*

ily: Generational Relations, Prentice-Hall, Englewood Cliffs, N.J., 1965, p. 116.

3 Blitsten, Dorothy R.: *The World of the Family*, Random House, New York, 1963, pp. 145–148, 150–156, 158–159.

4 Colorado Commission of Spanish-surnamed Citizens in 1967: *Report to the Colorado General Assembly: The Status of the Spanish-surnamed Citizens in Colorado.*

5 Loughlin, Bernice: "Pregnancy in the Navajo Culture," *Nursing Outlook*, 13(3):55–58, 1965.

BIBLIOGRAPHY

Barnouw, Victor: "Acculturation and Personality among the Wisconsin Chippewa," *American Anthropology*, 52:4, Part 2, 1950.

Blitsten, Dorothy R.: *The World of the Family*, Random House, New York, 1963, pp. 145–148, 150–156, 158–159.

Burger, Ernest W., Harvey J. Locke, and Mary Margaret Thomas: *The Family: From Institution to Companionship*, 3d ed., Crowell, New York, 1966, p. 2.

Burma, John H.: *Spanish Speaking Groups in the United States*, Duke University Press, Durham, 1954.

Cavan, Ruth Shonle: *The American Family*, 3d ed., Crowell, New York, 1966.

———(ed.): *Marriage and Family in the Modern World*, 2d ed., Crowell, New York, 1965.

Christensen, Harold: *Handbook on Marriage and the Family*, Rand McNally, Chicago, 1964.

Clark, Margaret: *Health in the Mexican-American Culture*, University of California Press, Los Angeles, 1970.

Colorado Commission of Spanish-surnamed Citizens in 1967: *Report to the Colorado General Assembly: The Status of Spanish-surnamed Citizens in Colorado.*

The Committee on the Family Group for the Advancement of Psychiatry: *Treatment of Families in Conflict*, Science House, New York, 1970.

Coombs, Madison: *Doorway toward the Light*, U.S. Department of the Interior, Bureau of Indian Affairs, Branch of Education, 1962.

Eggan, Fred: *Social Anthropology of North American Tribes*, University of Chicago Press, Chicago, 1955.

Farber, Bernard (ed.): *Kinship and Family Organization*, Wiley, New York, 1965.

Gamio, Manuel: *The Mexican Immigrant*, Arno Press & The New York Times, New York, 1969.

Gonzalez, Nancie L.: *The Spanish Americans of New Mexico: A Heritage of Pride*, University of New Mexico Press, Albuquerque, 1967.

Heller, Celia S.: *Mexican American Youth: Forgotten Youth at the Cross-roads*, Random House, New York, 1966.

Helm, June (ed.): *Spanish Speaking People in the United States*, American Ethnological Society, University of Washington Press, Seattle, 1968.

Lewis, Oscar: *A Death in the Sanchez Family*, Random House, New York, 1970.

————: *The Children of Sanchez*, Random House, New York, 1961.

————: *Five Families: Mexican Case Studies in the Culture of Poverty*, Basic Books, New York, 1959.

Loughlin, Bernice: "Pregnancy in the Navajo Culture," *Nursing Outlook*, 13(3):55–58, 1965.

Moore, Joan W., and Alfredo Cuellar: *Mexican Americans*, Prentice-Hall, Englewood Cliffs, N.J., 1970.

Opler, Morris E.: *Apache Odyssey: A Journey between Two Worlds*, Holt, New York, 1969.

Parmee, Edward A.: *Formal Education and Culture Change*, University of Arizona Press, Tucson, 1954.

Samora, Julian, and Richard A. Lamanna: *Mexican-American Study Project: Advance Report 8: Mexican Americans in a Midwest Metropolis: A Study of East Chicago*, for Mexican-American Study Project, Division of Research, Graduate School of Business Administration, University of California, Los Angeles, 1967.

Shanas, Edith, and Gordon F. Streib (eds.): *Social Structure and the Family: Generational Relations*, Prentice-Hall, Englewood Cliffs, N.J., 1965, p. 116.

Skolnick, Arlene S., and Jerome H. Skolnick (eds.): *Family in Transition*, Little, Brown, Boston, 1968.

Sussman, Marvin B.: *Sourcebook in Marriage and the Family*, 2d ed., Houghton Mifflin, Boston, 1963.

Underhill, Ruth: *The Northern Paiute Indians of California and Nevada*, United States Department of the Interior, Bureau of Indian Affairs, 1941.

7 | THE NUCLEAR FAMILY

David M. Fulcomer

MATERNITY NURSING AND THE "NORMAL" FAMILY

This chapter will deal with the "normal" nuclear family and its significance to the maternity nursing process. The sociological term "nuclear family" usually refers to the parents and children living within one household. Since much of the reasearch data available is on the middle-class family, that will be the focus in this chapter. However, it is very important that the reader take every opportunity to learn about the many different types of families and to note how the materials presented in this chapter can be used in working with particular types of families.

Special emphasis will also be placed upon the birth of the first child to a married couple and the impact of this birth upon the marital relationship and resulting family relationships. Usually the impact of later children is less severe, though there are exceptions.

What kind of knowledge about nuclear families will be helpful in maternity nursing? How much insight into families can the nurse be expected to know and to use? What are the key concepts, perspectives, and insights that will be especially useful to the nurse? This chapter has been written to help answer these questions.

Families Are Still Popular

Despite all the need for population control and the talk of childless marriages, families are still very important and numerous. Even if reproduction rates continue to decline, all evidence points to millions of families in the future. Although child care centers will increase rapidly and families with alternate life-styles will continue, it is almost certain that the family environment will be extremely important for most adults and children in the future. Therefore, it would seem that families and maternity nursing will be involved to a great degree with each other for as long a time as we dare to predict.

At the end of 1971 almost three-fourths of the population in this country over fourteen years of age was married, and 94 percent of the population lived in families. Americans live in families for the greater portion of their lives. According to the Population Reference Bureau, 2.1 million new families were started in 1968—the highest number since 1946 when the servicemen were returning after World War II. The number of families in the United States now totals more than 50 million.

What Is Happening to Families?

The professional person who works with families needs to be aware of major changes which are occurring in regard to the family. Our society is very complex and is changing rapidly; therefore, any institution within it would undergo significant changes. But it must be kept in mind that not *everything* about the family is changing. Still influential are many traditional concepts, attitudes, and feelings.

The size of families will probably decrease. Women with careers outside the home will undoubtedly increase. In 1966 one-third of all members of the labor force were women; by 1980, at least 60 percent will be women. Working women with children will increase. Already there are approximately 10 million working women with children under the age of eighteen. Almost two out of every five working mothers have children under six years of age.

American families are on the move. Almost half the population five years old and over moved in the 5 years preceding the 1970 census. This mobility will probably increase. Divorce is a big factor and a big problem. More than 500,000 children were involved in a divorce in 1969. Approximately one-fifth of working women are divorced.

Yes, the family is undergoing many significant changes. Probably one of the most important things for the maternity nurse to know is that new parents feel the tremendous pressure of parenthood in our society. This is a definite factor in the reaction of many persons to pregnancy and the coming of children into the marriage relationship. LeMasters speaks of the rate of social change, the conflicting norms, and competing authorities. Parents are being judged by higher standards, by their children, by professionals, and by themselves. The margin for parental error shrinks as the family system becomes smaller. Each child becomes crucial. Each dealing with the child becomes crucial. All this can lead to fear, frustrations, and even guilt, depending upon the parent's expectations of himself or herself as a parent and of his or her mate as a parent.[1]

Parenthood is terribly important to almost all parents, and yet, it is very difficult (although not necessarily undesirable) for most. For many people childrearing and parenthood are more important than marriage as a source of gratification and a sense of self-worth. This is true for many women, and especially for working-class women. Udry says that marriage is a transition to new roles and responsibilities, but under modern American conditions, the adjustment to marriage is not as difficult as the adjustment to parenthood.[2]

Furthermore, parenthood does not "come naturally" to the average wife and husband. It is very demanding. It happens all of a sudden. One has to adjust to it in a much shorter time than either marriage or occupation. And, probably worst of all, less preparation for parenthood is available than for any other major role.[3]

Complicating all this is the terribly romantic approach to marriage and parenthood in our society. For marriage, sufficient preparation is "being in love." For becoming parents, all that is necessary is to want to have one of those wonderful, clean, pretty, smart children! Because having children is highly romanticized in our society, there is a tendency to have a great desire for children but to be unprepared for what they are really like and what it really takes to rear them. Many couples are very poorly prepared for the impact of children on marriage.

This is why many parents experience considerable disenchantment with marriage and parenthood during their first months as parents. Parents usually know little about the nature of children. There is evidence to indicate that the over-romanticizing of parenthood and the lack of preparation for it on the part of most couples is a large factor in causing marital difficulties over the years.

Any help the nurse can give parents in coping with pregnancy and childrearing will have positive results that cannot be measured. Therefore, the nurse should remember the following points:

1 Families are still very important and will continue to be.
2 Size of the family is important.
3 Working mothers will increase in number.
4 Divorce will continue to be a significant factor, with many nuclear families having one or both spouses divorced previously.
5 Parents today feel great pressure, often leading to anxiety and even guilt.
6 Parenthood is of great importance to the sense of self-worth of most parents.

7 Parenthood has to be learned, and learned quickly.

8 The over-romanticizing of children and parenthood affects most couples to some degree.

9 In the United States the average adult is unfamiliar with children. Few have any realistic notions of what effects children will have upon the family.

10 All children and all parents can benefit from an effective and well-handled nursing process.

WHAT IS A FAMILY?

What a family *is* is best seen by the way it functions. What are some of the chief characteristics of the family and the way it operates (structure and function) which the nurse ought to take into account? The following are some important considerations to keep in mind in regard to the couple who are going through pregnancy and childbirth and the early weeks of family life:

1 The myths are out; reality is in. Real people are involved, with all their potentialities for love, hate, and indifference.

2 The family is a special kind of small group. Among other things, it is characterized by:

a Deep, continuing emotional involvement among its members.

b A combination of sexes.

c A combination of ages.

d Strong and intense regulation by society, including society's present confusion over what that regulation should be.

3 Individuals make up the family: therefore, individual needs and tasks are directly and intensely involved.

Each member of the family has his own combination of needs and tasks at any particular moment. Hess and Handel speak of interaction within the nuclear family of husband, wife, and children as a "bounded universe"—a small world of the family's own making—and within this world, the family members work out a dual pattern in which each person maintains his individual separateness, yet remains part of the web of connected relationships. Thus, family life is shaped *within* the participants as well as *between* them.[4]

So, in a very real sense, each person in the family stands at the center of a relationship's context which is peculiar to him. At the same time, since there are other persons in the family, personal uniqueness has to be modified and fit into the necessities of living within the family group.

4 A family is a dynamic, living thing, which is constantly changing as the individual members and outside influences change. Yet, it has a continuity because it is a "bounded universe" of relationships among its members.

Interaction is reciprocal action. Roles played by each family member are related directly to roles played by others in the family. A family is a set of interlocking relationships. Each family works out its own specific ways of coping with the combination of persons and societal forces affecting it.

Henry Bowman describes it this way:

The family is a dynamic institution. It changes in slow, evolutionlike fashion as part of overall cultural change. Each family, too, is dynamic. It changes as the number, ages, needs, and behavior of family members change and as the family as a group adapts itself to fluid circumstances. No matter where the family is found, in whatever area, class, or culture, at whatever period in history, certain broad similarities are to be observed in the stages through which it passes, just as there are broad similarities in the stages through which individuals pass in their development from infancy to old age. . . . [5]

Evelyn Duvall puts it this way:

The family is a unity of interacting persons related by ties of marriage, birth, or adoption, whose central purpose is to create and maintain a common culture which promotes the physical, mental, emotional, and social development of each of its members. Modern families fulfill the promise of this definition through at least six emergent, nontraditional functions: (1) affection between husband and wife, parents and children, and among the generations; (2) personal security and acceptance of each family member for the unique individual he is and for the potential he represents; (3) satisfaction and a sense of purpose; (4) continuity of companionship and association; (5) social placement and socialization; (6) controls and a sense of what is right. [6]

Over two decades ago, Rhoda Bacmeister stated clearly the reciprocity of interaction within a family when she wrote, "This is just human living at close quarters, shifting and frequently illogical, with the love and the flashes of hate, the jolly companionship and the irritations all mixed up. . . ."[7]

In the family, as in all groups, what has gone on before affects what is. Ralph Turner speaks of the sequence of events in the family as a long chain of cause and effect, each link being one episode, and each episode taking some of its unique shape from the sequence of events that preceded it. [8]

This is why the advent of the first child brings a major change in the entire family context. A stranger has been admitted into a close-knit group, and suddenly the balance of the home shifts. Not only has a relationship been added for each older member of the family unit (his relationship with the new baby), but the relationships of all former family members to each other are also changed. In addition to the baby being born, a mother is "born" and a father is "born," and usually there are grandparents being "born" as well as aunts, uncles, and cousins.[9]

VARIATIONS AMONG FAMILIES

Each family situation is always somewhat different from any other. It has its own peculiar combination of circumstances and forces. To be aware of and sensitive to the total configuration and combination of factors in each family is a great asset to the nursing process. To realize that each family has its own particular history influencing it will help the nurse know how to move into that family situation and be more effective in accomplishing nursing goals.

Variation in Form and Structure

Those who criticize our society for being too middle-class, white, and Protestant-centered are correct. Research on families has not escaped this severe limitation. Fortunately, this narrowness is being lessened, but much work remains to be done before we have an accurate overall view and understanding of the many variations among families in our society. The nurse must work within this serious limitation. Yet, the nurse can make use of what knowledge and insight we already have in regard to working with particular types of families.

Minority and nationality groups have distinct cultural patterns within their families. Different socioeconomic classes have distinctive characteristics which influence their families. Families, taken separately, have their own special combinations of ages, sexes, sheer numbers, rituals, and customs. Families differ in the number of kinfolk who have an influence upon them. They differ, too, in major roles their members play *outside* the home which have to be integrated into the life-style of the family within the home. Work roles outside the family are of tremendous importance. Other outside roles can be equally important.

There are significant pieces of research and effective programs for families that help us understand and cope with the variations among families. For example, Tuckman and Regan have made a study of behavioral problems in children as related to family size.[10] The Community Service Society of New York has a project to provide help for very young parents before and after their babies come.[11]

Variation within Families

There are many ways in which each family differs from any other family, even within its own class. These differences can influence significantly how the family functions.

Whether or not parenthood is planned can make a big difference in the relationship between a husband and wife during pregnancy and in their reactions to childbirth and becoming a family. Some professional persons believe that involuntary parenthood is far more tragic than involuntary childlessness, for example.[12]

Motivations for parenthood are powerful factors in how humans cope with the actuality of parenthood. Lantz and Snyder discuss immature and mature motivations. Immature motivations include "holding together a poor relationship," "a means of avoiding loneliness," "a means of realizing unfulfilled goals," and "a means of attaining security." They speak of the mature motivation as viewing the child not as a means to a parental end but as an end in itself.[13]

Some parents—many more than we wish existed—reject their children. Bell points out that some mothers severely reject their children either psychologically or physically and that many American women do not love or want their babies.[14]

The problem of the battered child is not new. But the extent to which it exists in our society is alarming to anyone who knows the facts and who is concerned about human relationships. This problem is evidence that not all mothers and fathers are pleased with the arrival and presence of their babies. We need more facts, and they are hard to get. Various estimates are made, and some authorities believe that at least 9 of every 100,000 children in the United States are victims of violence.[15] No one who works with couples and young children should be unaware of the evidence available and the studies made of the battered child.[16]

Coping with Variations among Families

Nurses need to be aware of the uniqueness of the individual and of the family; yet, it is important to recognize that this uniqueness occurs within a predictable frame of reference. View the individual as unique, but use your knowledge of his age and stage of development to understand better the tasks he may face, the possible reasons for his behavior, and his probable needs. Work with the new parent without typing him as just like other members of his group but use your knowledge of the tasks which he needs to accomplish at this stage of his development as a new parent or as a parent again. It does help to know the family life cycle and the developmental sequences experienced by all families, because this aids in making some predictions about a family's behavior and can open the door to potential problems and needs that are important to a family.[17]

Coping with Personal Feelings about Family Living

Every professional person working with persons and families should be aware of his own values and feelings. What if the nurse does not approve of the way people behave in a family? What should be done about one's own values and feelings? Can they be ignored, or do they have to be faced frankly and honestly? To ignore these feelings is to run the danger of letting them interfere with effectiveness in working with families.

The nurse, like any other human being, is influenced by personal experiences as a family member, past and present. Attitudes, feelings, and expectations regarding family behavior are there. The most professional person in the world has them. The important thing is that the nurse accepts these feelings and learns to cope with them so they do not interfere with understanding, acceptance, and effective work with families. It is not necessary to *like* all family members and all the behavior in a family. Feelings of displeasure, anger, and revulsion are just as normal as positive feelings.

Attitudes, feelings, and expectations regarding family behavior can have a social basis, as well as a personal and familial base. If one has been reared in the middle class, it is almost impossible not to have many middle-class values and biases and the feelings that accompany them. But part of being professional is to know what these are and "allow" for them in the nursing process. In regard to the "naturalness" of biases, one is reminded of the story of the famous Chinese person who, on arriving in the United States, was asked by one of the waiting reporters, "What strikes you as the oddest thing about Americans?" His reply was, "I think it is the peculiar slant of their eyes."

THE NURSE AND THE COUPLE DURING PREGNANCY

Pregnancy is more than most people realize. What happens *during* pregnancy is very important to the nurse, especially because it has so much to do with what happens *after* pregnancy. It is involved in the whole web of relationships husband and wife have with each other, relatives, friends, customs, rituals, expectations of society, and even laws. Pregnancy is definitely an important part of the parenthood experience.

Each Spouse during Pregnancy

Pregnancy, especially the first pregnancy, is quite an experience for both wife and husband. For one thing, each spouse draws upon his or her own experiences, consciously or unconsciously, on how to go about his or her role in pregnancy. It would be very difficult, if not impossible, for anyone to go through pregnancy without some degree of ambivalence. In fact, for most spouses pregnancy is filled with many feelings—anxiety, joy, fear, pride, and self-concern among them. Pregnancy for most couples is a very significant step in further specialization of their relationship. As sex role differentiation decreases in our society, some of this specialization can be eliminated or lessened. But biology itself dictates certain specialization. Whatever new roles arise for each, it is important that each spouse develop feelings of certainty in the importance of these roles and his or her competence in performing them.

The Wife during Pregnancy

Much has been said and written about the woman during pregnancy. Both the physical and emotional dimensions have been explained. It takes a keen mind and diligent work to separate the dependable information from the misleading comments and suggestions. This is one area in which the nurse can be both helpful and supportive. The nurse also can help the wife to understand both what the facts are and the reasons for her feelings. The family background and its influence on the wife at this time can be an important factor. Here is a comment made by a college girl who was making wedding plans:

> Maybe motherhood is not foremost in my plans for marriage, because, frankly, I am a little afraid of it. Mother always emphasized that it was very unpleasant. For several years I believed it was next to the worst thing anyone could go through.[18]

These feelings of fear and anxiety were major problems for this young woman during her first pregnancy. Fortunately, she had contact with a nurse who recognized her feelings and helped her understand and accept them.

The Husband during Pregnancy

As females have suffered so long from sexism, so have males. An aspect of this is the neglect of the husband as an important factor in the pregnancy situation after conception takes place. Generally speaking, he is still ignored as a significant part of the human matrix involved in pregnancy. This carries over into the common tendency to ignore him as a significant parent, except for his financial contribution and "male role image" in parenthood. All members of the family suffer from this.

The ancient ritual of the *couvade* may indicate a long-time and pervasive need for fathers to have their significance noted. In this practice the husband takes to bed, thrashes around, and groans. When the baby is born, friends pay homage to him; after the child's birth, he may go on a strict diet. The details vary from culture to culture, but some anthropologists see this as an attempt by the father to proclaim his importance in parenthood. Others say this ritual is rooted in the man's (husband's) conflicting emotions. It is an interesting custom.

In many respects, the husband's feelings, needs, and problems during pregnancy are not too different from those of his wife, even though this is not usually recognized. Old feelings about pregnancy and childbirth can become important. Mixed feelings, especially shortly after pregnancy is definite, are very common. These feelings are probably reinforced by the popular idea that expectant fathers are lost, afraid, and completely inadequate. One young expectant father wrote:

> Something new was on the horizon. New thoughts and ideas started running through my head. The realization that I was going to be a father was too big to swallow all at once. It's a bit hard for the expectant father to realize exactly what his new title implies. I looked at myself and didn't look any different. The word "father" alone made me think of my own father. The comparison made me wonder if I was old enough to handle the job competently. I still wonder. I am determined to be the best father possible. The truth is, doctors don't seem to realize how many questions arise in the husband's mind.[19]

Dr. David Mace comments on the husband's mixed emotions during pregnancy (he thinks all husbands have them) and the fact that it may be easier to be an expectant mother than to be an expectant father:

> At a time when he is expected to be pleased and loving, and kind and patient, how can he admit to anyone that his real feelings are often surges of fear and resentment?
> In many ways, it's harder to be an expectant father than to be an expectant mother. For the woman, all sorts of exciting things are happening. . . .[20]

The socializing of males is significant. They are conditioned not to express their feelings, especially feelings about personal matters. The need (cultural) for the husband to pretend he knows it all and can cope with it all keeps him from letting others, including his wife, know that he, too, needs reassurance and some helpful information. Many big, powerful males actually feel insecure and inadequate. For many expectant fathers, this may not be a major problem, but the subtle influences of this "trap situation" are probably more far-reaching than is recognized. The nurse who can establish a positive relationship with the expectant father and "sneak in" some pertinent information and reassurance is contributing quite a bit to the pregnancy situation—and the parenthood situation, too. William Genné has written, "The husband who is baffled, bewildered (and, perhaps, belittled) during the nine months of pregnancy will not be able to be a good husband to his wife or a good father to his child."[21]

It is no wonder that in our society many expectant fathers, especially those going through the experience the first time, become increasingly job or work conscious, feeling that now others must depend upon them. Often they think in terms of whether or not they can provide for the needs of their coming children, especially as they think far into the future. (Insurance salesmen are very much aware of this vulnerability of the expectant father.) In times as uncertain as the 1970s, these concerns of the expectant father are multiplied.

Husband-Wife Relationships during Pregnancy

Being pregnant is certainly a matter of emotional and social adjustment for both marriage partners. This leads automatically to necessary readjustments in the husband-wife relationship. A young college man whose wife was pregnant for the first time, has this to say:

> My wife and I had a lot of important changes and adjustments to make to each other and to things in general . . . things like a changed diet and pills for her to take . . . the doctor didn't want her to work as hard. . . . Those weren't the biggest adjustments, though. Right from the start each one of us had a new part to play—a new role—I found out that expectant fathers have to be more considerate of their wives than before. Then, too, it isn't long before they have to assume a few of the household tasks that their wives did before. My wife and I worked out a lot of these adjustments, talking them over at the dinner table. Some of the others didn't get solved that easily. I hope I haven't painted a dark picture, because waiting for the baby so far has been wonderful.[22]

Sexual relationships may have particular significance during pregnancy. This has probably been less of a problem recently, at least among the well-educated, but it still is a common problem for pregnant couples. Women can easily become apprehensive about sexual relations. It is easy for husbands to see this "sexual withdrawal" as something unpleasant connected with pregnancy. Many husbands feel this; few verbalize it. Sometimes the nurse can play a significant part in preventing or lessening this kind of a problem. A "word to the wives" can help if a word to the husbands is not possible. Sometimes both are possible.

Another common problem is for the husband to feel "left out." As one husband expressed it, "I feel like I'm on the outside looking in." And another expectant father expressed it this way: "I feel like the doctor and my wife are in cahoots against me." It certainly is easy for many husbands to feel that their needs are not going to be met (by their wives) in the same way as previously. The facts of the situation tell any husband that he will not continue to be the exclusive interest of his wife—probably never again. Wives often feel the same way. Here, too, the nurse can be of help. In various ways the nurse may help one or both to become less possessive of the other spouse, help one or both to become more able to give up some of the older dependencies upon the spouse, and substitute other things that will make the relationship even more valuable in a personal sense.

Any one or any combination of the following may be important tasks for a couple during the expectancy stage:

1 Acquiring knowledge about and planning for the specifics of pregnancy, childbirth, and parenthood.
2 Realigning roles.
3 Developing new patterns for earning and spending the income.
4 Adapting patterns of sexual relationships to pregnancy.
5 Adapting and reorientating relationships with relatives.
6 Devising housing rearrangements.
7 Adapting and reorientating relationships with friends and the community at large.
8 Learning to communicate even more effectively and positively.

The nurse has many opportunities for helping the couple. This is truly a "teachable moment" for both spouses, especially during the first pregnancy.

MOVING INTO PARENTHOOD

From "romanticized parenthood" to "realistic parenthood" is quite a jump for all too many married couples, especially for the majority who have no real opportunity to learn how to be parents. This is part of the price our society pays for assuming that persons do not need to be taught about human relationships and that even if they did it could not be done.

Most parents, then, have had no "on the job" experience. Regardless of this lack of opportunity to prepare for parenthood, couples are dunked suddenly into responsibility for the care and socialization of the child. Their own childhoods and romantic myths are often predominant, but they are not often very helpful. It is no wonder that so many new parents feel overwhelmed and uncertain. Moving slowly into the new situation would be difficult. The sudden step into this complicated situation is very difficult for many—and very unfair.

Learning to be parents takes time. There is no automatic inborn instinct of parenthood. Children are born knowing how to be children; the skills of parenthood must be learned.[23]

From a Twosome to a Crowd

Ours is a paired society. To function "normally," one is supposed to pair up, especially from adolescence on. Courtship, the wedding, the honeymoon, and early marriage before pregnancy are all great. Then comes pregnancy, and all of a sudden the twosome disappears and one has to operate in a triad—a crowd. Now a third party becomes an involved member of the relationship. Things will never be the same for husband and wife! A classic book on the family states it this way:

> No matter how going a concern a marriage may be, the advent of children causes severe strain between parents. Newborn babies cannot be taken in their stride; they have none. . . . Any orderly, smooth, satisfactory relationship carefully worked out between husband and wife is broken up the very first night the child is home from the hospital. The inability of a child to do anything for itself means that demands are made on parents which create a new relationship between husband and wife. . . . Babies are tyrants.[24]

It is clear, then, that with the arrival of children there is a fundamental shift from a husband-wife relationship to a parental relationship. At least, this is what happens in too many cases. Since couples are usually not prepared for parenthood (and probably have highly romanticized expectations in regard to it), it is often impossible for them to maintain the centrality of the husband-wife relationship while they are rearing a child or children. This is tragic, because a good, healthy marital relationship is desirable for parents and children.

Actually, each time a baby is born, a new learning experience begins for everyone in the family. Being a parent of one child is not like being the parent of two children, and so on. When a child is born, every other child in the family has a new position and a new place in the bounded universe we call the family. Some behavior and some feelings toward others in the family change. A crowd is very different from a twosome! The number of interactions added with the addition of new members is expressed by the following formula, where x represents the number of interpersonal relations and y represents the number of persons:

$$x = \frac{y^2 - y}{2}$$

The following letter written by a very intelligent new mother needs no explanation:

I suppose we had what is common to all first babies the first month—worry. Shall we call the doctor? Why does she cry so? What is *wrong* with the child? It all amounted to mostly nothing, and a bit of colic. It is still difficult to tell the nothing from the colic, but we are classifying symptoms now, and beginning to learn the difference. . . . I doubt that she was nearly as miserable with it as were we. We'd stand over her bed and commiserate with her difficult breathing. I think I drove the doctor almost out of his mind with telephone calls and idiotic questions. . . . Every time we took her to the hospital she fell into a deep sleep, and remained so during all the doctor's examination. The conclusion was that nothing was wrong with her. We began to feel the doctor thought we were unnecessarily picky about the amount of crying she did. . . . Finally the doctor diagnosed colic. To know that nothing is really wrong with her is such a relief that we have relaxed a bit and perhaps in doing so have actually made her colic less serious. . . .

Our daughter, as you can well imagine from experience, has done a thorough job of reorganizing our home, but for the most part things have settled down and some order has come of the chaos of the first few weeks. . . . [25]

Parenthood: Crisis?

In 1957 LeMasters published an article titled, "Parenthood as Crisis."[26] This was a study of middle-class couples which showed that 83 percent of the 46 couples he studied experienced "extensive" or "severe" crisis after the birth of the first child. Several follow-up studies have raised some questions about his instrument and have added other points. It is fair to conclude, however, from the data at hand that the first child in particular introduces some "crisis" conditions to the marital relationship of many couples.

LeMasters found that the mothers reported such things as loss of sleep, chronic tiredness, exhaustion, extensive confinement to the home and resulting curtailment of their social contacts, giving up the satisfactions and the income of outside employment, additional washing and ironing, guilt at not being a "better" mother, long hours, 7-days-a-week schedules, decline in housekeeping standards, and worry over their appearance. Fathers named many of the same things and added decline in sexual response of wife, economic pressure resulting from the wife's retirement plus additional expenditures necessary for the child, interference with social life, worry about a second pregnancy in the future, and general disenchantment with the parental role.

As Udry says, "Marriage is a twosome; three is a crowd. Studies of many kinds of groups have shown that of all human patterns of association, triads are the least stable."[27] A 1967 survey showed that the presence of a child during the first 2 years of marriage doubled the chances of divorce.

This was a Census Bureau survey based on 28,000 households in 701 select counties encompassing every state.[28]

When the chief or only reason for having a baby is based on the romantic conception of parenthood, chances are high that the couple will run into the parenthood-as-crisis situation which LeMasters discusses. The desirability for couples to know what babies are like and what rearing them entails is self-evident if one is concerned about the welfare of the persons involved and the human condition of our society. Parenthood need not be a crisis situation; but, as has been indicated, it can easily be that. Here, again, the nurse can enter the picture and help the couple to cope well with what would otherwise be a very difficult situation.

Shifts in the Husband-Wife Relationship

Regardless of how one may rate or measure the changes caused by the coming of the first baby, there is no doubt that they are profound. Radical changes are caused in the interaction between the married pair. A college student looks back and thinks of herself as a child growing up in the family and her effect upon her parents:

> Children are really peculiar possessions. We arrive at a time when they could be very happy together. They could have more money to spend on each other. They are young. They are happy together. They love each other; and then we come along. They find they have to share their love, work twice as hard, spend half as much time and money on themselves. They get away less. Then they have to begin learning all over again. They have to learn how to play jacks, jump rope, skate, and do all kinds of things they once knew but had forgotten.[29]

Something in this statement indicates that having a child is not all bad. It could be tremendously rewarding, even in the 1970s. A great deal depends upon the preparation the couple have had for this big change in their relationship. Have they developed a really healthy relationship as a couple, with good ability in the skills of handling difference and of communicating? The answer to this question would be very important to the nurse, for it would indicate both how and why husband and wife cope with a new baby. Also, it would help indicate what information is needed and what would be helpful activity on the part of the nurse.

Specific ways in which the husband-wife relationship can be affected by the birth of the baby are discussed in the following paragraphs.

1 No longer can the husband and wife belong *only* to each other. It is possible that one or both may be disturbed that the other has become involved in a new affectional relationship and interpret this as shattering the conception of faithfulness to each other. The romantic approach to marriage in our society makes the closeness and exclusiveness of the couple a symbol of their unity. And this unity is a sacred thing. How romantic and immature are the spouses? This is a very important question.

2 The power relationship and the division of labor can be affected drastically. Blood writes of the revised power structure, division of labor, and personal relationships that are inevitable. He also discusses the loss of mobility, the disruption of routines, the expansion of tasks, and the anxiety about the child's welfare—all of which are common results of the coming of the first child.[30]

3 Each spouse may discover "another" person in his or her marriage partner. Either partner may run into an unexpected syndrome of attitudes, feelings, and behavior that is hard to accept and cope with. The nurse may be able to help them understand what has happened and how to cope with it.

4 A sharp increase in role differentiation and role specialization can occur. (This has been discussed briefly in this chapter in another context.) Preparental relationships are marked by much sharing of roles and activities. Couples vary greatly in how they can cope with this change.

5 Often the sexual relationship has to be adapted to the new family situation. Many husbands are not happy about severe limitations on sexual intercourse for 6 to 8 weeks before the birth of the baby and 6 to 8 weeks after the birth; very few are prepared to adjust well to this. It is common to keep sexual activity limited longer than is necessary. Frequently, the sexual relationship of the marriage never recovers after the birth of the baby. This is not necessary, and it has a very negative effect upon the marital relationship. The wife can be helped by the nurse to understand the husband's needs and what is healthy and possible for the marriage. Too few wives get this kind of help. Sometimes husbands can be aided, too.

6 Both partners may have difficulty in balancing the needs of the child or children with marital and personal satisfactions. Some sound, effective parent education can be of great help at this stage. A primary problem in this stage is to work toward a balance of developmental experiences which will meet the basic needs of *each* family member and of the family unit as a whole. Lack of achieving this is a very common and a very undesirable characteristic of the early parenthood stage.

7 Opportunity for real husband-wife communication may be cut severely. They often no longer have the free time to be with just each other. This is a point at which many marital couples begin to lose the ability to

communicate, and the relationship becomes less and less meaningful to both partners. This is a crucial time for the couple. For many it may be the turning point in their marriage. Here, too, effective parent education would be highly desirable.

8 This may be the point in their married life when the couple stop enjoying each other—a fatal error. The two may start going off in different directions never to really return to each other and the relationship they once cherished. This is a tragedy because it does not have to happen. A young mother in a good marriage writes of some of the things she and her husband had to overcome in order to sustain their own relationship:

> We can't go out so much. We used to ski and travel a lot; and now we have to decide whether to get away from her or take her places. For me now only about 10 to 20 percent of the time is *mine*. I thought that when the baby was born, I would do all sorts of things around the house. But I am very frustrated to discover that there is little time. Then questions come to my mind like: Should I go back to work? When? My husband has been very good with children, but *now* there isn't much that he can do. He tends to feel that Marsha is my kind of baby. At this stage I guess the baby is the mother's.[31]

9 The mother may resent her confinement and her husband's freedom. That this is a common problem is indicated by the many cartoons on this theme. The young infant and child tremendously complicate the wife's role, very often demanding far more time and emotional energy from her than from the husband. (Middle-class fathers participate much more than lower-class fathers in the rearing of their children.) Women tend to become engulfed in the motherhood role.[32]

Here is a letter written by a wife who graduated from college and went into social work until her first child was born. Her husband is a very brilliant young scientist, completely engulfed in his professional roles. This letter was written to a close female friend at 8:00 A.M. [underlining is hers]:

> This has been a hectic year for me, to say the least. I am always tired— too tired to write even the family letters I should! I got pregnant six weeks or so after Susan was born. We bought a house and Dad came to be with us for two months, having disposed of his business.
> I had my hands full—still have. I went to visit my sister for a few days, but when I got home, my help quit. Such a mess to be in. I managed to get Jake started in kindergarten and two babies fed. It's a gay life. I feel as though I've been sexed and babied out for the rest of my days.
> Nothing else to talk about but kids. I don't know what's going on in the outside world. I must close now before the "noisy din" begins. I've

been up since 3:00 A.M. and am about ready to retire again! By spring I'll be a mere shadow of my former self.[33]

Some comment must be made about the working mother having a baby. According to one report, in 1971 there were 3.7 million working mothers with children under five years of age; by 1980 the figure is predicted to be 5.3 million such mothers. And 5 million preschool children have mothers who are employed outside the home.[34]

Another report indicates that in 1968 there were about 10.6 million working mothers with children under the age of eighteen, and 4.1 million with children under the age of six.[35] Still another report indicates that between 1960 and 1970 the number of children under eighteen years of age whose mothers were in the labor force increased from nearly 16 million to nearly 26 million; and almost 6 million of those children in 1970 were under six.

Regardless of what figures and reports one wants to use, it is clear that more and more mothers of young children are in the labor force. There are many ways in which these mothers adapt to the infancy years. The nurse, in working with any family, must be aware of the importance of this type of adaptation.

Kinfolk are important to the young parents. Kinship interaction is different from the "good old days," but it is still a vital part of the young family in many cases. One of the frequent difficulties is that roles of both young and old are not clear. Confusion and even trouble can result. There is another important aspect of the "kinfolk problem" in modern times. Mothering exacts a big price on mothers in a society without the kinship group nearby which is active in helping to take care of the infant on a day-by-day basis. It is significant that modern mothers adapt as well as they do. Nurses should be aware of the type of involvement, if any, of kinfolk in the life of the new family.

Although little helpful research is available, the nurse should be alert to the type of situation that exists when there are older siblings in the family. Older children are prepared in some manner for the arrival of the infant. This preparation may be very inadequate. If so, both children suffer. In the family context siblings are very important to each other. Very little help is given parents in regard to the preparation of older children for the coming of a new baby. This, then, is another neglected area.

It would be safe to draw the following conclusions regarding the "moving into parenthood" stage of the family life cycle:

1 No one is ever completely prepared for parenthood, but the right kind of help can really help.
2 Even if the coming of a baby is a "crisis" in the family, this does not mean it is either good or bad in itself. Properly handled, it is an op-

portunity. Mishandled, it is a disaster. (It is interesting that the Chinese word for "crisis" is composed of two characters. Respectively, they mean "danger" and "opportunity.")

3 Because the evidence is, in part, conflicting, there is no basis for concluding that the coming of children makes a marriage either happier or less happy.

4 How a particular wife or husband reacts to the arrival and presence of a baby depends on many factors.

5 Couples who want their marriage to remain vital and satisfying to them will have to make a deliberate attempt to achieve this. The husband has a major role to play in accomplishing this. (There is no evidence that couples who keep their husband-wife relationship of prime importance have children who are less healthy in any sense. What evidence there is would point in the opposite direction; however, there is little research on this.)

6 The nurse can play a very significant and helpful role in working with families in which there is a young infant. There are many points at which the nurse can move into the relationships in a desirable way. Most parents are open to learning how to cope with their situations.

COMMUNICATION—THE BASIC SKILL

Working with families requires relating to families and family members. Relating positively and effectively requires good communication. This is not easy to accomplish in a society which gives its members little help in learning how to communicate well and, in addition, places many impediments along the way.

Dorothy Lee, the anthropologist, spoke at Iowa State University (June 28, 1962) on "The Human's Potential for Full Existence." She said that people are protesting against the alienation *from* life, saying that we are alienated from ourselves, our own curiosity, our own wonder. The little child, she says, has the motivation, but gradually he loses this. She raised the question, "How can we get people to the point of being themselves, being authentic, being genuine?" She added that we need to learn to relate fully, that the potential for relatedness is infinite, and that "somewhere we have lost our feeling of relatedness."

George A. Buttrick once said, "With all the insistence on intellectual honesty, let us also be emotionally honest." He is correct. We tend to be so anxious to be loved that we are afraid to open ourselves to others for fear of not being loved, thus making it impossible for the other person to know us well enough to truly love us. This basic and tragic fact is discussed thoroughly in an article by Sidney M. Jourard and Ardis Whitman.[36] At various places in his writings, Carl Rogers has spoken of these necessary elements for effective interpersonal communication:

1 A sensitive ability to hear
2 A deep satisfaction in being heard
3 An ability to be more "real," which in turn brings forth more "real-ness" from the other
4 A willingness to receive warmth and care from others, and con-sequently a greater freedom to give love

He often speaks of the necessity of loving the *real* person, hearing what he *really* is saying, and being a *real* person yourself. This, he indicates, makes any relationship more meaningful.

Why this comment on communication? It *is* the necessary skill for relating. The nursing process is basically the matter of relating to other humans. Therefore, nothing is more important than developing the ability to communicate well. No one can communicate perfectly. Everyone has his limitations. But this skill can be developed and improved. Without reasonably good success at it, the nurse can be of little help to young husbands, wives, and their babies. With good communicating ability the nursing process can be of tremendous help to families.

MATERNITY NURSING AND THE NUCLEAR FAMILY

It is fortunate that the nursing profession attracts the kinds of persons who have a deep concern for human development and human relationships. This concern and motivation, plus development of the knowledge and skills necessary, is a combination that will produce a nurse who should relate well to the nuclear family.

As has been indicated, pregnancy, childbirth, and early parenthood are periods in the life of the family when members are open to learning about themselves and how to relate to each other. The maternity nurse is fortunate to be involved with families at a time when they are very "teachable." If the nurse can help the couple move successfully from the relationships developed as a pair, through the process of pregnancy and childbirth, to the realities of parenthood, much will have been accomplished. This is particularly true if the nurse can help the young couple learn to enjoy the rich satisfaction of parenthood and how to practice it for the enhancement of their marriage.

In a society in which feelings are too often unrecognized or belittled, the nurse is in a position to help people understand their feelings and learn how to cope with them. The nurse is not like the census taker in this account:

Census taker: Please give me the number of persons in your household.
Lady: Well, there is Susan, Jackie, Ted. . . .
Census taker: (Interrupting the lady) Thank you, lady, but I don't want their names. I just want their numbers.
Lady: Mister, they ain't got numbers, but they do have names.

If we are to relate effectively with people and teach them, we must regard them as persons, not numbers. This is why it is important that the maternity nurse enjoy encounters with people and families. This is why it is highly desirable that the nurse be aware of and appreciate the ordinary day-by-day joys and sorrows of the young family.

LeMasters and others have warned us against assuming parents to be "guilty" before we even give them a hearing. He reminds us that parents are amateurs, that we should not use professional norms to assess the performance of nonprofessionals. It is indeed important that we learn to relate to people and help people without evaluating them beyond their capabilities.

What is the most important thing a nurse can give to families? It would be very difficult to single out *one* thing. But one is reminded that in her book, *Book of Common Sense Etiquette*, Eleanor Roosevelt wrote that the basis of all good human behavior is kindness. She argued that if you act toward people with genuine kindness, you will never go far wrong.

Pregnancy, childbirth, and early parenthood are indeed short stages in the life of a family, but they are very important "acts" in the play of family living—a drama in which people move in and out frequently. Perhaps Shakespeare described best the dynamic situation the nurse deals with in working with families:

All the world's a stage,
And all the men and women merely players.
They have their exits and their entrances;
And one man in his time plays many parts.

REFERENCES

1 LeMasters, E. E.: *Parents in Modern America*, Dorsey, Homewood, Ill., 1970, pp. 1–16.
2 Udry, J. Richard: *The Social Context of Marriage*, 2d ed., Lippincott, Philadelphia, 1971, p. 437.
3 Rossi, Alice S.: "Transition to Parenthood," *Journal of Marriage and the Family*, 30:26–39, 1968.
4 Hess, Robert D., and Gerald Handel: *Family Worlds: A Psychosocial Approach to Family Life*, University of Chicago Press, Chicago, 1959, p. 19.
5 Bowman, Henry A.: *Marriage for Moderns*, 6th ed., McGraw-Hill, New York, 1970, p. 569.
6 Duvall, Evelyn Millis: *Family Development*, 4th ed., Lippincott, Philadelphia, 1971, p. 5.
7 Bacmeister, Rhoda W.: "Perspective on Parenthood," *Parents Magazine*, September 1951, p. 29.

8 Turner, Ralph H.: *Family Interaction*, Wiley, New York, 1970, p. 20.

9 Fulcomer, David M.: "Becoming Parents," in Ruth Shonle Cavan: *American Marriage: A Way of Life*, Crowell, New York, 1959, p. 418.

10 Tuckman, J., and R. A. Regan: "Size of Family and Behavioral Problems in Children," *Journal of Genetic Psychology*, 111:151–160, December 1967.

11 Progress report in "Briefs," Official Publication of the Maternity Center Association, New York, December 1971, pp. 147–150.

12 Folkman, Jerome D., and Nancy M. K. Clatworthy: *Marriage Has Many Faces*, Merrill, Columbus, Ohio, 1970, p. 188.

13 Lantz, Herman R., and Eloise C. Snyder: *Marriage*, 2d ed., Wiley, New York, 1969, pp. 379–382.

14 Bell, Robert R.: *Marriage and Family Interaction*, 3d ed., Dorsey, Homewood, Ill., 1971, p. 435.

15 UPI story from the International Congress of Pediatrics in Vienna reported in the *Rocky Mountain News*, September 4, 1971, p. 23.

16 Helfer, Ray E., and C. Henry Kempe (eds.): *The Battered Child*, University of Chicago Press, Chicago, 1968; and Kempe, C. Henry, and Ray E. Helfer: *Helping the Battered Child and His Family*, Lippincott, Philadelphia, 1972.

17 Sobol, Evelyn G., and Paulette Robischon: *Family Nursing: A Study Guide*, Mosby, St. Louis, 1970, p. 18.

18 From the personal files of the author.

19 From the personal files of the author.

20 Mace, David R.: "Pregnancy and the Young Husband," *McCalls*, p. 177, April 1963.

21 Genné, William H.: *Husbands and Pregnancy*, Association Press, New York, 1956, p. 15.

22 From the personal files of the author.

23 Fitzpatrick, Elise, Sharon R. Reeder, and Luigi Mastroianni: *Maternity Nursing*, 12th ed., Lippincott, Philadelphia, 1971, pp. 174–176.

24 Levy, John, and Ruth Monroe: *The Happy Family*, Knopf, New York, 1938, p. 243.

25 From the personal files of the author. The last paragraph was written in the same letter by the new father.

26 LeMasters, E. E.: "Parenthood as Crisis," *Marriage and Family Living*, 19:354, 1957.

27 Udry: op. cit., p. 425.

28 Reported in *The Denver Post*, October 11, 1971, p. 27.

29 From the personal files of the author.

30 Blood, Robert O., Jr.: *Marriage*, 2d ed., The Free Press, New York, 1969, pp. 438–444.

31 From the private files of the author.

32 Udry: op. cit., p. 430.

33 From the private files of the author.

34 "Federal Program Silent Revolution . . . Child Development Plans Gather Speed," *The Denver Post*, June 14, 1971, p. 27.

35 Willett, Roslyn: "Do Not Stereotype Woman–An Appeal to Advertisers," *Journal of Home Economics*, 63:549, October 1971.

36 Jourard, Sidney M., and Ardis Whitman: "The Fear That Cheats Us of Love," *Redbook*, 137:83, October 1971.

BIBLIOGRAPHY

Bacmeister, Rhoda W.: "Perspective on Parenthood," *Parents Magazine*, September 1951.

Bell, Robert R.: *Marriage and Family Interaction*, 3d ed., Dorsey, Homewood, Ill., 1971.

Blood, Robert O., Jr.: *Marriage*, 2d ed., The Free Press, New York, 1969.

Bowman, Henry A.: *Marriage for Moderns*, 6th ed., McGraw-Hill, New York, 1970.

"Briefs," Official Publication of the Maternity Center Association, New York, December 1971.

Cavan, Ruth Shonle: *American Marriage: A Way of Life*, Crowell, New York, 1959.

Duvall, Evelyn Millis: *Family Development*, 4th ed., Lippincott, Philadelphia, 1971.

"Federal Program Silent Revolution . . . Child Development Plans Gather Speed," *The Denver Post*, June 14, 1971, p. 27.

Fitzpatrick, Elise, Sharon R. Reeder, and Luigi Mastroianni: *Maternity Nursing*, 12th ed., Lippincott, Philadelphia, 1971, pp. 174–176.

Folkman, Jerome D., and Nancy M. K. Clatworthy: *Marriage Has Many Faces*, Merrill, Columbus, Ohio, 1970.

Fulcomer, David M.: "Becoming Parents," in Ruth Shonle Cavan (ed.): *American Marriage: A Way of Life*, Crowell, New York, 1959, chap. 19, pp. 399–426.

Genné, William H.: *Husbands and Pregnancy*, Association Press, New York, 1956.

Helfer, Ray E., and C. Henry Kempe (eds.): *The Battered Child*, University of Chicago Press, Chicago, 1968.

Hess, Robert D., and Gerald Handel: *Family Worlds: A Psychosocial Approach to Family Life*, University of Chicago Press, Chicago, 1959.

Jourard, Sidney M., and Ardis Whitman: "The Fear That Cheats Us of Love," *Redbook*, 137:83, October 1971.

Kempe, C. Henry, and Ray E. Helfer: *Helping The Battered Child and His Family*, Lippincott, Philadelphia, 1972.

Lantz, Herman R., and Eloise C. Snyder: *Marriage,* 2d ed., Wiley, New York, 1969.

LeMasters, E. E.: *Parents in Modern America,* Dorsey, Homewood, Ill., 1970.

————: "Parenthood as Crisis," *Marriage and Family Living,* 19:354, 1957.

Levy, John, and Ruth Monroe: *The Happy Family,* Knopf, New York, 1938.

Mace, David H.: "Pregnancy and the Young Husband," *McCalls,* p. 162, April 1963.

Rocky Mountain News (UPI story from the International Congress of Pediatrics in Vienna), September 4, 1971.

Rossi, Alice S.: "Transition to Parenthood," *Journal of Marriage and the Family,* 30:26–39, 1968.

Sobol, Evelyn G., and Paulette Robischon: *Family Nursing: A Study Guide,* Mosby, St. Louis, 1970.

Turner, Ralph H.: *Family Interaction,* Wiley, New York, 1970.

Udry, J. Richard: *The Social Context of Marriage,* 2d ed., Lippincott, Philadelphia, 1971.

Willett, Roslyn: "Do Not Stereotype Woman—An Appeal to Advertisers," *Journal of Home Economics,* 63:549, October 1971.

UNIT C
GOALS OF MATERNITY CARE

8 | THE IMPACT OF INDIVIDUAL DIFFERENCES ON MATERNITY CARE

Mildred A. Disbrow and Beverly M. Horn

Individual differences such as age, race, socioeconomic status, cultural background, religion, and education, as well as the geographic areas of residence, have a decided effect on the outcome of maternity care today. The health care delivery system also has a tremendous impact on maternity care. Prior to a discussion of some of these factors, however, it would be advisable to review the current status and trends of maternity care today as reflected in the available statistics.

BIRTH RATES

In the United States, the birth rate has fluctuated over the past three to four decades. The low birth rates of the 1930s plunged to an all-time low of 16.6 per 1,000 population in 1933. This was followed by a gradual increase of births until 1947, when the post-World War II "baby boom" raised the rate to an all-time high of 25.8 per 1,000 population. A slight decrease in births to approximately 25.0 occurred, and this was maintained as a rather stable level for the next 10 years. In 1958 a trend toward a more marked reduction in births began. By 1963 the rate had decreased to 21.7, and by 1967 the rate was 17.8. Finally, in 1968 the rate was 17.5 births per 1,000 population.[1]

TABLE 8-1
BIRTH RATES BY RACE, 1945–1968*

Year	White	Nonwhite	Total population
1968	16.6	24.2	17.5
1965	18.3	27.6	19.4
1960	22.7	32.1	23.7
1955	23.8	34.7	25.0
1950	23.0	33.3	24.1
1945	19.7	26.5	20.4

* Birth rate per 1,000 population.
SOURCE: U.S. Department of Health, Education, and Welfare, Public Health Service, Health Services and Mental Health Administration, National Center for Health Statistics, *Vital Statistics, 1968*, vol. I, Natality, U.S. Government Printing Office, Washington, D.C., 1970.

Racial differences are quite apparent in the birth rate; this can be seen in the data listed in Table 8-1.

When maternity care is under consideration, numbers and rates of births are important. These statistics which are affected by fertility rates are computed by the size and the age groups of women who are in the childbearing years, which are considered to be from fifteen to forty-four years of age. Because of the low birth rates of the 1930s, the fertility rates dropped in the late 1950s and thus affected the birth rate at that time. However, the fertility rate should now increase, since the large number of females born in the early 1950s are now over twenty years old.

MATERNAL MORTALITY

Although dramatically reduced in recent years, maternal mortality rates are still very important. These rates refer to deaths caused by complications of pregnancy, childbirth, and the puerperium. Because of the drastic reduction in rates that have occurred, the basis for computation of the rates has changed. Prior to 1960, the rate was determined on the basis of 10,000 live births; since 1960 it is based on 100,000 live births. The decline in maternal deaths has been consistent, with the 1967 rate at 28.0[2] and the 1968 rate at 24.5.[3] Table 8-2 shows the decline in maternal mortality for selected years.

Although the maternal death rate is low, it should be remembered that the actual number of maternal deaths in 1967 was 987.[4] This large number of deaths should be of serious consequence for those planning maternity care in the future, as almost all causes of maternal deaths today are preventable. Hemorrhage and sepsis should, theoretically, be completely preventable. Toxemia has been reduced markedly in the past, but continued efforts must be aimed at this condition.

The most dramatic reduction in maternal deaths was the decrease in

TABLE 8-2
MATERNAL MORTALITY RATES BY RACE, 1951–1968*

Year	White	Nonwhite	Total population
1968	16.6	63.6	24.5
1967	19.5	69.5	28.0
1965	21.0	83.7	31.6
1960	26.0	97.9	37.1
1955	32.8	130.3	47.0
1951	54.9	201.3	75.0

* Per 100,000 live births.
SOURCES: 1968 statistics from *Statistical Abstracts of the United States*, U.S. Department of Commerce, Bureau of the Census, 1971. Other statistics from U.S. Department of Health, Education, and Welfare, Public Health Service, Health Services and Mental Health Administration, *Vital Statistics, 1967*, vol. II, part A, Mortality.

deaths due to toxemia of pregnancy. For the white population, the ages of thirty to forty-five pose a great hazard in relation to toxemia. The nonwhite population is also affected during these years but has a high rate of deaths due to toxemia at all ages. The total rate of maternal deaths due to toxemia for the white population is 3.3 per 100,000 live births, while the total rate of maternal deaths in the nonwhite population due to toxemia is 15.4.[5]

Hemorrhage is a frequent cause of death and, with the reduction in deaths due to toxemia, has assumed first place as a cause of maternal mortality. The next highest cause of death is sepsis. Frequently, sepsis is indirectly caused from hemorrhage, for the pregnant woman develops infection because of a weakened condition from blood loss. Thus, even in cases of sepsis, hemorrhage may have a major role.

When the causes of maternal mortality are examined more closely, it is evident that they are potentially eradicable, especially in the case of hemorrhage and sepsis. They are causes of morbidity that should never occur today. Therefore, the maternal mortality rates should be reduced significantly in the future. Those concerned with maternal care, especially nurses, should continue to focus on prevention of maternal mortality and morbidity with vigilance.

PERINATAL MORTALITY

Perinatal mortality statistics are also important indices of maternity care. Standards of maternity care have improved, and the rate of maternal deaths is no longer considered to be an adequate index of the quality of maternity care that occurs today. The *WHO Chronicle* indicated that this is appropriate inasmuch as care during pregnancy today tends to be aimed at the fetus, and good fetal care implies good maternity care.[6]

Infant mortality, or the number of deaths in the first year of life per

1,000 live births, is the rate most frequently used in comparing the United States with other countries. At the present time the United States ranks fifteenth among other developed nations.[7] The reduction in infant mortality rates occurred most dramatically from 1920 through 1950.[8] Since then, the decline has been much slower. The discrepancy that exists between the white and nonwhite populations continues. The infant mortality rate among nonwhites in 1968 was 40.8 percent higher than that of whites.[9]

Neonatal mortality, i.e., deaths per 1,000 live births in the first 4 weeks after birth, has declined from a rate of 32.4 in 1935 to 15.4 in 1968. However, in 1968, the neonatal period accounted for 73.2 percent of infant mortality.[10] Implications for research during the neonatal period, as well as concerted effort for improvement of health care during this period should be a high priority for those in the health field.

PERINATAL MORBIDITY

Perinatal morbidity is frequently associated with perinatal mortality as the cause of death. In addition, many infants survive this traumatic period only to be left with serious physiological and neurological deficits. The high incidence of mental retardation, cerebral palsy, and other forms of cerebral dysfunction testify to the grave problems associated with perinatal morbidity. Also, the number of handicapped children born as a result of genetic disturbances, or poor intrauterine environment has continued. Prematurity, the greatest cause of perinatal morbidity, will be discussed in the following section.

Reflection on the preceding array of facts and statements about maternal and infant status today leads to speculation as to what has brought about this situation. Further questions might also be asked, such as What is maintaining the situation currently? What societal changes are occurring that might direct the way to improved care? What is it about being black, being poor, living in an urban area, or being Indian *and* poor *and* living in an urban or reservation setting, that precipitates the discrepancy that exists in the quality of care that is delivered? Who is, in fact, the recipient of maternity care today? What is the "high-risk" population in both maternal and infant categories? Probably the most difficult question to answer is How do the complex variables on all levels—psychosocial, cultural, and physiological—interact? Further, how can health care personnel intervene effectively to promote optimum outcome of pregnancy for the family, based on knowledge of the interaction of these variables?

Much of the research done to determine factors associated with perinatal mortality and morbidity has identified the same factors that are associated with maternal mortality and morbidity. The recurrence in the literature of many of the same factors lends credibility to their importance. Some of the most important are ethnic background, socioeconomic status, reproductive history of the mother, geographic location, age of the mother, the course of pregnancy, and prenatal care.[11, 12]

PREMATURITY

Prematurity has been identified as a major correlate of perinatal mortality. As a single indicator, it is probably the most sensitive index of the interrelationships of individual differences on reproductive outcome. Prematurity can actually encompass both low-gestational-age infants, under 38 weeks' gestation, and low-birth-weight infants. The differences between premature and low-birth-weight infants must be considered when one is searching for causes of morbidity and mortality. Some ethnic groups, the black population for example, have full-term infants of low birth weight.

Premature onset of labor and infants with low birth weight, resulting more frequently in perinatal deaths, recur among certain groups. Hunt has pointed out that because of the frequent association between mortality and social factors, excessive mortality rates may serve to identify neighborhoods and larger areas in the United States that have a high incidence of social handicaps.[13] Peckham has stated that the relationship of a great deal of fetal and infant morbidity and mortality (reflected in premature onset of labor) relates more closely to psychosocial and economic factors than to specific pathologic conditions of pregnancy.[14] A disproportionate number of perinatal casualties occur in certain segments of the population, such as minority groups and particularly the socially deprived. This relationship of sociocultural variables, such as age, race, family, and ecological factors, to the biological factors was also noted by Nesbitt.[15]

Perhaps the most serious reason for consideration of prematurity as reflecting the complexities of the problem of maternity care is the fact that the incidence of prematurity is actually increasing.[16] If prematurity has been the major cause of perinatal mortality and morbidity in the past, its increase is a fearful sign. Gold, in an introduction to Wallace's article, has indicated that even though there has been a 14.2 percent reduction in infant mortality since 1961, the current rate of 21.7 is still high. Prematurity not only continues to be the major cause of infant death but is increasing in incidence.[16] In studying the problem of prematurity, the previous reproductive history of the mother is of major concern. Tompkins has noted three areas that should have priority in obstetric care: adolescent pregnancy, multiparity, and previous history of premature delivery. The mother who has delivered prematurely is very likely to do so again.[17] A previous history of premature delivery, then, signals the presence of a high-risk mother who may deliver a high-risk infant. Shapiro has stated that women who have had one or more premature births have from three to four times the risk of early termination of further pregnancies with low-birth-weight or premature infants than those who have had previous pregnancies ending in mature births.[18]

In addition, Shapiro has pointed out that the risk of fetal death in pregnancies preceded by a fetal death is from two to three times the corresponding rate when only mature live births occurred previously.[18] For maternity care of the future, it is imperative, then, that the past history of the mother in regard to low birth weight, low gestational age, and previous fetal deaths be of major consideration. Wiener, in studying the correlates of low birth weight and low gestational age, used regression analyses with a number of factors and discovered that race and the trimester in which the mother received prenatal care were most significant. Nevertheless, he also stated that those two factors (low birth weight and low gestational age) were not the only causes of maternal and infant difficulties, but that other variables correlated with the mother's race and the trimester in which she received prenatal care.[19] A discussion of some of these factors will follow.

SOCIOECONOMIC STATUS

A factor in the delivery of maternity care which seems to subsume several other factors is that of the socioeconomic status of the mother. Wallace indicated that there was a close relationship between socioeconomic status and infant mortality. She noted that the average infant mortality rates for 1963 for the low-income group (both white and nonwhite) of 17 states was 19 percent higher than the national average.[20] Low birth weight, which in itself can result in morbidity and mortality of the infant, was also associated with low socioeconomic status. Since education is frequently utilized in measuring socioeconomic status, it will be included here.

Education

A number of studies have shown that education is a variable in the outcome of pregnancy. Rosenwaike, in his study, viewed educational attainment of the mother as a major indicator of the parents' socioeconomic status. He found that the incidence of low birth weight was found to vary inversely with the educational level of the mother. This relationship of education to low birth weight was maintained even when he controlled for the mother's age, birth order, source of prenatal care, and timing of prenatal care.[21] Thus, a low level of education of the mother, low economic status of the parents, and the high incidence of low-birth-weight infants were related in his study.

Poverty

Poverty is frequently associated with inferior health, and this is evident in poor maternal and infant health. Bierman, in discussing her experiences in maternity care, has noted that we still know very little regarding the precise relationship between poverty and health and how the various components of low socioeconomic status affect biological functioning and behavior.[22] The inability of the poor to procure health care is well known. Even when care is available, as in urban areas, it may be inaccessible to a majority of the poor. Various studies have been made to determine precisely why health care is not sought by poor mothers, and most frequently lack of transportation and lack of baby-sitting services were the ostensible reasons given. Oscar Lewis has pointed out that profound feelings of apathy, hopelessness, and despair exist among the poor, as they realize that the values of the dominant middle class cannot be realized.[23] Milio proposed and found support for her proposal that the maternity care system, based on values of a middle-class culture, was inaccessible to those who hold an alternate and opposing view of life.[24] An example is the middle-class future time orientation, as opposed to the lower-class present time orientation. Problems associated with the outcome of a pregnancy scheduled to terminate several months ahead are much less important than the problems of today, such as obtaining food.

Further, Strauss has pointed out that the poor are not capable of coping with the complexities of the organizational system of the health care delivery system.[25] Large buildings and impersonalization are in direct conflict with their lack of sophistication in an impersonal situation. Accustomed to dealing on a personal basis, they are confounded by the situation of a large organization. Strauss has indicated that their sense of discomfort in the middle-class world further alienates them from the system devised to bring them health care.[25] Their reliance on personal relationships to achieve their goals cannot be realized, and they withdraw from the health care system as it functions today. Tompkins noted that in most areas of the United States there has been little change in the character and quality of health services delivered to this most vulnerable group, the poor.[26]

ETHNIC BACKGROUND

Another factor, as indicated in the statistics at the beginning of this chapter, closely related to the outcome of maternity care is that of race. Actually, race, culture, and ethnic group are terms which do have precise definitions, but in the literature they are used almost interchangeably. There is controversy regarding the definitions of each term, and the area of overlap in the meanings is significant. Even at the risk of obscuring differences, we have chosen to use these terms to refer to differences in life-style exhibited by a group. It is our feeling that in the pluralistic society (a term which is also controversial) of the United States, the primary differences among racial groups, cultural groups, or ethnic groups appear to exist primarily in the life-styles exhibited by them. To the extent that a difference in life-style indicates a difference in value systems and attitudes, behavior will vary. Thus, if a different life-style exists among groups, there will be different approaches to the problems of health and therefore to maternity care.

The dominant group in the United States whose value system has permeated health care delivery is that of the white middle class. Those with a different sociocultural background have the greatest number of problems in attempting to cope with the system of health care delivery. The poor have a particular problem.

The largest number of the poor in the United States is the nonwhite group. For the most part, included within this group is the black population, the American Indian, the Mexican-American, and the Oriental groups. The various ethnic groups have retained many of the values of their own culture relative to health. The special meanings that childbearing and childrearing have for each group must be considered. The poor results of maternity care in the nonwhite group as witnessed in the statistics cannot be attributed to poverty alone. Each group has special needs that have not yet been met.

Racial and cultural barriers to health care are multiple. The perceptions and belief systems of the nonwhite population regarding the pregnancy area of health care have been shown to vary most from that of the white middle class. Thus, efforts to improve maternity care, based on a value system different from their own, have been significantly unproductive. Maternity care more congruent with the beliefs and life-styles of those for whom it is planned would be more effective.

In 1964, the mortality rate in the nonwhite population was almost twice that of whites in the United States. This fact obscures major differences in the nonwhite population, however, for the highest perinatal mortality rates were in the American Indian and black groups, respectively, whereas the Japanese and Chinese rates were actually lower than those of the white population.[27] Highlighted here, then, is the acute severity of the health problems of both American Indians and blacks. Gold summed up the problem when he discussed the importance of lack of reduction in our infant mortality rate. He expressed great concern over the disparity in statistics and the differential that existed in pregnancy outcome between the white and nonwhite populations.[28]

The American Indian

An ethnic group for whom delivery of maternity care has assumed almost crisis proportions, as viewed from the statistical standpoint, is the American Indian. While the nonwhite population of the United States is approximately 12 percent of the total population, the Indian population is less than 0.3 of 1 percent of the total population and only 2.3 percent of all nonwhites.[29] A definition of the health problem of this group defies those who have attempted it. Determining exactly who is and who is not an Indian is in itself fraught with difficulty, especially in urban areas.

The poor health of the reservation Indian is well documented. A situation of abject poverty exists for most Indians on the reservation. The urban

Indian today is beset by many situations which make him vulnerable to frequent illness and disease, and in the case of pregnancy, a poor maternity risk, resulting in disastrous outcomes. The urban Indian is lost in the shuffle among all minority groups. The studies of urban poor and of minorities are done predominantly with blacks or whites, and the results have been indiscriminately applied to the American Indian. Few studies have been done to determine factors which have precipitated the poor health status of the Indian both on and off the reservation.

The birth rate among Indians is much higher than that in both the white and nonwhite populations. According to Hill and Spector, in 1968 the Indian birth rate of 38.5 live births per 1,000 population was 2.3 times as high as the white birth rate of 16.6, and 1.6 times as high as the nonwhite birth rate of 24.2.[30] Hill and Spector's report also indicated that over the 10-year period from 1958 to 1967 the maternal death rates for Indians averaged about twice that for the United States as a whole.[31] These are just a few of the facts that point to the existence of a very complex health problem.

As previously mentioned, infant mortality rates are recognized as important indices of the quality and quantity of maternal care. The status of the Indian upholds this assertion. In 1967 the infant death rate for infants under one year of age was 32.2 for Indians, 1.6 times as high as the rate for whites. However, the period during which these deaths occurred offers a frightening, if not challenging, situation to the health care worker. Inasmuch as most deliveries of Indians occur in the hospital today, the mortality for the first week of life is the same as that for whites and is lower than that for blacks. In the postneonatal period, Indian rates have been four, five, and six times as large as white rates.[32] A breakdown in continuity of care surely exists. Further, Hill and Spector also noted that in the period 1965 to 1967 more than 16 percent of all Indians who died were under one year of age as compared with 3.8 percent for whites and 10.4 percent for nonwhites.[33] This information should result, it seems, in a mandate for improved maternity care in the future for the American Indian population. This much neglected group surely deserves the immediate attention of health care workers in the area of maternal and child health.

The Black American

The problems associated with maternity care and the black population have been well documented, and this group also remains one of the crucial areas for nursing intervention today. Problems of low birth weight and/or prematurity appear to be almost endemic, statistically, to this specific population. In addition, the probability of plural births, with their coexisting hazards, is $1\frac{2}{3}$ times as frequent for blacks as it is for whites.

In contrast to the American Indian, who is scattered throughout urban areas, the black family in the urban area is even today primarily in the central city. The problems associated with poor housing, poor education, poor recreational facilities, and overcrowding place a great deal of stress on family structure. A breakdown in health is common, and health care is least accessible to this group.

Summary

Racial and ethnic groups in the United States are most frequently members of the aforementioned lower socioeconomic groups, and the complexities of such a combination more frequently than not result in poor health care, and specifically poor maternity care. Thus, in a sense, race and ethnic group is often the crucial variable for the quality of maternity care given, inasmuch as birth into a specific group has placed the mother in a sociocultural milieu with a history of many generations of poverty. Not only American Indians and blacks are included within these groups. The many Spanish-speaking groups, such as Chicanos and Puerto Ricans, and migrant workers, although small in number, have a level of health care that does not begin to meet their needs. Wallach laments the disparity existing between those who have adequate maternity care and those who do not. He pointed out that the need for, and utilization of, professional resources is met most adequately for the white, educated, middle-income expectant mother whose health needs may be least demanding. She has, in most cases, at least an adequate level of health and is in near optimal state for pregnancy. Also, she has the possibility of procuring nutritious foods and paying for professional health care. Those in minority groups, who may be black, Indian, non-English speaking, or low-income mothers with poor nutritional status, get curtailed medical services late, or not at all.[34]

AGE

Age has been considered a rather crucial variable in the outcome of pregnancy. Basic physiological differences exist at various stages during the childbearing years. The adolescent's physiology differs considerably from that of the young mature adult. Also, the immediately premenopausal woman has problems unique to her age group. Besides the physiological considerations, crucial psychosocial variables in the different age groups affect the outcome of maternity care. Utilization of birth control methods, parity, infant mortality and morbidity rates, and maternal complications are just some of the problems that have a direct relationship to the age of the mother.

Adolescence

In women between the ages of fifteen to nineteen a high perinatal mortality rate occurs; this rate declines during the decade of the twenties. During the decades of the thirties and forties there is a rapid increase in the rate of perinatal mortality.[35] As indicated previously, premature labor is one of the most common causes of perinatal mortality, and very young and older mothers are the target groups which have a high incidence of low-gestational-age and/or low-birth-weight infants. Tompkins stated that low-birth-weight and low-gestational-age infants, as determined through reports from maternal and infant care projects, are highest among patients under the age of eighteen and over thirty-five.[36]

The phrase "most vulnerable group" is used repeatedly in the literature to refer to the adolescent who is pregnant. The teen-age mother frequently comes from a low-income group. Although the reproductive outcome for the low-income mother is often poor, it is even more so if she is also a teen-ager. In a study done with a stable low-income rural population in Florida, Held looked at reproductive trends for the years 1967 through 1969. In this geographic area the primigravida formed the bulk of the obstetric population, and teen-agers comprised 75 percent of all primigravidas.[37] His overwhelming conclusion was that teen-agers have to be reached prior to conception.

Tompkins, in a study aimed at reviewing national efforts to reduce perinatal mortality and morbidity, referred to the school age pregnant girl who has the stress of pregnancy imposed during a period of maximal growth and development. He noted that society has a punitive attitude toward a school-age pregnant girl, especially if the pregnancy is out of wedlock, and that rarely can such a girl have the quality and standard of care necessary for a healthy pregnancy.[38] This is a rather sad commentary, not only on society, but also on the status of health care delivery to a most important group in the population. Hunscher and Tompkins also noted in their study the relationship between adolescence and maternal and infant mortality and morbidity. They felt it was a mandate for health care workers to make intensive efforts to improve preventive and remedial care of adolescents who are pregnant.[39]

BIRTH CONTROL

The need to reach the teen-ager prior to the first pregnancy with birth control information has been set as a priority in many of the maternity care programs. Janus, in a study with low-income groups in Washington, D.C., showed that the consistent use of birth control methods varied, depending on marital status and age. Women under twenty years old and those never married practiced birth control the least.[46] Von der Ahe in Los Angeles asked unwed mothers about the use of contraception, and 87 percent denied using it at all.[41] Thus, clearer understanding of the need for and use of contraceptives by adolescents seems to be a priority for maternity care in the future.

NUTRITION

Nutrition has been well documented as a crucial variable in pregnancy. Nutrition and varying degrees of malnutrition should be considered in relation to age but also in relation to pregnancy in general, since it is the single factor most responsible for the outcome of pregnancy. Low-income groups may be in a chronic state of malnutrition. The need of the pregnant woman for an adequate diet during pregnancy is accepted by health care workers. The importance of an adequate state of nutrition prior to the onset of pregnancy is just as crucial. There are many cultural meanings associated with food affecting nutritional status, and ethnic background has a decided influence on nutrition.

Customarily, teen-agers have been known to ignore the rules of good nutrition. Poor eating habits, often associated with food fads, as the macrobiotic diet of today, contribute to increased nutritional deficiency of adolescence. Since the kinds of food eaten by adolescents are frequently high in calories but of poor quality, obesity may occur. This is especially true if pregnancy imposes an alteration in physical activity.

A poor nutritional status at the beginning of pregnancy imposes a severe hazard. If the vital needs of adolescents for normal growth and development are not met, the needs of the developing fetus are severely endangered. Osofsky, reviewing the data relating antenatal nutrition to subsequent infant and child development, pointed out that malnutrition prior to birth can influence subsequent developmental problems.[42] However, the data relative to the effects of malnutrition on the pregnant woman are not as clear. In the case of the adolescent, the additional demands of the developing fetus upon her state of undernutrition may at least predispose her to irreversible conditions of poor health.

Within the philosophy of maternity care today, it is apparent that focus must be placed on the total family. Nutrition has high priority in this relationship, since habits of good nutrition begin in the family context. Concern about the nutritional status for future pregnancies should begin at the time of the child's birth. Hunscher and Tompkins noted that a considerable amount of scientific literature has accumulated, showing the significance of maternal nutrition to the course and outcome of pregnancy. They point out that pregnancy is a unique event, linking past generations, reflecting their health status in current reproductive efficiency.[43]

ROLE MODELS

Another facet of maternity care, with respect to the adolescent, is the imitation of models. For an adolescent, those persons perceived to be most important are considered to be worthy of imitation. This phenomenon is a part of the normal maturation process. Prominent people in sports, politics, and in the entertainment world are frequently used as models.

Many of the models presented to adolescents today deviate considerably from what has been the white, middle-class norms of society. This is especially true with regard to sexual practices and modes of family living. The impermanence of marriage and the questioning of the importance of marriage at all presents the adolescent with a number of "acceptable" alternatives not openly accepted in other times. The conflicts between what parents propose and the currently "acceptable" alternatives impose great stresses upon the adolescent.

Other Age Groups

Although much of the emphasis in this section has been on health care of the adolescent, other age groups have individual differences which affect maternity care greatly. Because adolescence has been relatively neglected, the current focus must be on this group. However, the largest number of babies is born to women twenty to twenty-nine years old.

The highest perinatal mortality occurs in mothers fifteen to nineteen years old. The second most rapid climb is in mothers who are over thirty. The major causes of maternal morbidity and mortality are also quite prevalent in the over-thirty age group. Maternal death rates due to complications of pregnancy, delivery, or the puerperium in the different age groups are the following: thirty to thirty-four years of age, 43.9; thirty-five to thirty-nine years, 72.6; forty to forty-four years, 131.2.[44]

In discussing toxemia of pregnancy, Hendricks notes that in certain women over thirty-five years of age there is a much greater tendency to develop toxemia than in those who are twenty to thirty-four years old.[48] This is especially true when there is an impoverished background and five or more previous pregnancies.[45] Toxemia can also be seen in the younger age groups in the presence of the above conditions but to a lesser degree.

HEALTH CARE DISTRIBUTION

The need for government agencies to become involved in the delivery of adequate maternity care has increased through the years on both the national and local level. Also, a number of voluntary agencies have become involved in the same endeavor. Tompkins has stated that the present situation concerning perinatal mortality and morbidity is untenable and that medical centers, local health departments, and other health professionals must coordinate their work with government efforts.[46] Some examples of efforts of certain groups and their results will be discussed.

Nonprofessionals

Utilization of the indigenous population in an attempt to improve the quality of maternity care has been attempted by many groups. In the District of Columbia, health education aides were used in counseling pregnant women. Success was reflected in a marked reduction in infant mortality and an increase in the number of mothers having prenatal care. Conn's report indicated that the aides moved into the community and encountered problems within the inner-city culture, and this was the precise area that they demonstrated their most valuable asset—familiarity with the life-styles of the women.[47] The aides attempted to deal with whatever stood in the way of the client's getting prenatal care—transportation, baby-sitting, etc.

In 1968, Denver set up a neighborhood health program with decentralization of services. The neighborhood health centers served a population of approximately 20,000. The reported outcomes were favorable, but the report stressed the fact that community involvement was a prerequisite to an effective program.[48]

Morton discussed experiences with a maternity and infant care project in the Los Angeles County Health Department. A multidisciplinary team was used, including the extended role of the nurse in prenatal care. One of the measures to indicate success was the broken appointment rates at the clinic. Prior to the project there were from 30 to 50 percent broken appointments, but after the project was begun these were reduced to 9 to 24 percent. Morton attributed the success of the project to the interdisciplinary teamwork that was involved plus close follow-up of the patients.[49]

In a study conducted by Planned Parenthood, New York City,[50] the use of paraprofessionals to motivate women to return for postpartum checkups was attempted. The paraprofessionals were recruited from the same neighborhood as the patients and had the same sociocultural background. Two comparative studies were done with patients from two hospitals: (1) persons who accepted family planning versus those who did not and (2) women who had failed to keep their postpartum appointments. It was felt that the use of paraprofessionals was very effective, both in getting the mothers back for their postpartum checkups and in helping them to decide on some form of family planning.

In the abovementioned studies, the message that successful delivery of maternity care appears to be dependent on self-involvement of those for whom it is planned comes through loud and clear. Although not specifically noted in these examples, the fact that programs planned by outsiders and executed by outsiders exclusively seem doomed to failure is clearly demonstrated in the literature.

The Free Clinic

A phenomenon of recent years that has had a decisive impact on health care, including maternity care, is the free clinic. In the First National Survey of Free Medical Clinics 1967–1969, Jerome Schwartz noted that the first free clinic was opened in the Haight-Ashbury district in San Francisco in 1967, followed by clinics in Cincinnati, Detroit, Seattle, and Vancouver, Canada which opened that same year. By the beginning of 1971, the total number of clinics was at least 135. A "free clinic" does not necessarily mean that there is no charge but that it is free of eligibility requirements, questions, and "bureaucratic hassle."[51] However, it was noted that free clinic patients have one thing in common: They are without resources to pay for medical care.[52]

This study identified four types of free clinics: neighborhood clinics, street clinics, youth clinics, and sponsored clinics. Not all clinics offered all types of services. Of 59 clinics studied, prenatal and postnatal care was provided by 24 clinics. Street clinics, of which there were 20, included 6 which offered these services, and neighborhood clinics, of which there were 23, included 14 which offered these services. Only 2 of the 9 youth clinics offered prenatal and postnatal care. Lastly, 2 of the 4 sponsored clinics offered these services.

The age groups served by each of the clinics were the following: Neighborhood clinics served families with persons over thirty-five years and children under twelve. Adolescents represented the smallest proportion of patients, and there was also a moderate number of women patients nineteen to twenty-four years of age. The youth clinics had mostly sixteen- to eighteen-year-olds, but also a sizable number of twelve- to fifteen-year-olds. When one considers the previous information regarding age levels, with emphasis on the needs of the teen-ager during pregnancy, the information relative to free clinics poses a problem. Those clinics with the smallest number of adolescents, i.e., neighborhood clinics, offered both prenatal and postpartum care, whereas those who handled the largest number of teen-agers, the street clinics, offered the least. In the street clinic group, only 6 offered these services, with the remaining 14 offering neither prenatal nor postpartum care. One would feel more comfortable about this fact if there was an adequate referral system with follow-up. However, the article on free clinics noted that although many centers made referrals for obstetric care, only four made direct arrangements for delivery and hospitalization.[53]

Home Delivery

An increasingly frequent phenomenon of the childbearing years is that of the desire for a home delivery. Dissatisfaction with maternity care and previous hospitalization has led many disenchanted mothers to request home delivery with subsequent pregnancies. Some of the families of the youth subculture desire an attended, or unattended, delivery at home. The "do-it-yourself" way of thinking has entered into maternity care. The inherent problem in such a situation seems to be a reversal of what has been considered ideal maternity care in our society. Maternity care supervised by professionals, culminating in delivery in a hospital and followed by at least 6 weeks of postpartum care, has been the model. Many facets of this kind of care have been rejected by what is considered to be a significant segment of the population. In the Seattle—King County area the number of home deliveries in 1966 was 32 out of 18,676 or 1.5 per 1,000 births. In 1969, the rate had risen to 2.0 home deliveries per 1,000 births. For the period of January 1, 1971 through September 30, 1971 the number of registered home deliveries had already reached 70.[54] How accurate a picture this is of the total number delivered at home is not known, because there is evidence that some who have delivered at home without medical supervision did not register the births. In addition, the authors are aware of a class of 40 couples in the Seattle area who are currently planning home deliveries with the attendance of a physician or nurse. Apparently, there are many more who do not care to have professional persons in attendance at all.

The implications of such a trend in home deliveries will have to be determined. Rejection of the traditional method of delivery of maternity care has been complete by this group. It would seem that new and unique approaches to maternity care will have to be instituted if this group is to be considered in planning for maternity care of the future.

PRENATAL CARE

In this discussion of individual differences, as they affect maternity care, the concept of prenatal care has only been alluded to. It was not meant to negate its importance. Prenatal care has been shown to have a direct relationship upon the outcome of pregnancy, most likely ensuring a healthy mother and baby. In looking at correlates of low birth weight, Wiener has noted that the trimester in which the mother has obtained prenatal care has been significant.[55]

What factors within the complex of what is called prenatal care are important is not really known. A number of relationships are established, and services are rendered by professionals to the pregnant woman and her husband. Which of these are crucial and which are not remains to be determined by further study. According to Milio, the prenatal care system is structured in a specific way, based on assumptions of middle-class culture.[56] This has proved to be effective for that particular group. The disparity in maternity outcome that exists between middle-class persons and those in the lower class has demonstrated that the traditional prenatal care model is ineffective. Thus, a challenge for health care workers exists; they must be able to meet the needs of the other groups in our society as well as the middle class.

SUMMARY

A great deal can be learned about individual differences that affect maternity care by looking at the statistics of birth rates and of maternal and infant mortality and morbidity rates. The groups having successful maternal and infant outcomes as well as those with less satisfactory consequences can be readily seen. The discrepancies in levels of socioeconomic status, in age, in ethnic background, and in care sought or obtained are evident.

Prematurity, as an example of poor obstetric outcome, is intimately related to all of the factors of individual differences. Inasmuch as prematurity is the major cause of infant mortality, it can be studied in some detail. Further, because in most cases of prematurity there is no demonstrable physiological basis, answers are sought in looking at variations in cultural and social differences.

It is important to recognize that there is a constellational functioning of the many individual differences so that no single one is the controlling factor in the outcome of pregnancy. Poverty is associated with a poor educational background, and both are associated with a poor nutritional background. Minority groups, not members of the middle-class white society, tend to be more frequently in the poverty groups. Place of residence of the poor and of those in minority groups is frequently in an area where health care is inaccessible. Finally, a health care system not responsive to these individual differences can result in the discrepancies we see in maternity care. Thus, we have very fine care, with excellent outcomes for many, while others turn away from the system entirely and inaugurate their own system of maternity care. If health care workers in the area of maternal and infant health can meet the challenge of these special needs, the entire picture of maternal and child care in the future could be altered.

REFERENCES

1 U.S. Department of Health, Education, and Welfare, Public Health Service, National Center for Health Statistics: *Vital Statistics of the United States, 1968*, vol. 1, table 1-1, Natality, Washington, D.C., U.S. Government Printing Office, 1970.

2 ———: *Vital Statistics of the United States, 1967*, vol. II, part A, table 1-16, Mortality, Washington, D.C., U.S. Government Printing Office, 1970.

3 U.S. Department of Commerce, Bureau of the Census: *Statistical Abstracts of the United States*, 92d ed., Washington, D.C., U.S. Government Printing Office, 1971.

4 *Vital Statistics of the United States, 1967*, vol. II, Mortality, table 1-15.

5 Ibid., table 1-16.

6 *WHO Chronicle*, Geneva, Switzerland, June, 1971, pp. 268–269.

7 *Statistical Abstracts of the U.S.*, op. cit.

8 Wallace, Helen M.: "Factors in Mortality and Morbidity," *Clinical Obstetrics and Gynecology*, 13:16, 1970.

9 *Vital Statistics of the United States, 1967*, vol. II, Mortality.

10 Wallace: op. cit., p. 20.

11 Ibid., p. 14.

12 Hunt, Eleanor: "Infant Mortality Trends and Maternal and Infant Care," *Children*, 17:88, 1969.

13 Ibid., p. 89.

14 Peckham, Ben M.: "Optimal Maternal Care," (editorial) *Obstetrics and Gynecology*, 33:864, 1969.

15 Nesbitt, R. E., Jr., and R. H. Aubry: "High-risk Obstetrics. II. Value of Semiobjective Grading System in Identifying the Vulnerable Group," *American Journal of Obstetrics and Gynecology*, 103:974, 1969.

16 Gold, Edwin M.: in Helen M. Wallace, op. cit., p. 11.

17 Tompkins, Winslow T.: "National Efforts to Reduce Perinatal Mortality and Morbidity," *Clinical Obstetrics and Gynecology*, 13:53, 1970.

18 Shapiro, Sam, and Mark Abramowicz: "Pregnancy Outcome Correlates Identified through Medical Record-based Information," *The American Journal of Public Health*, 59:1638, 1969.

19 Wiener, G., and T. Milton: "Demographic Correlates of Low Birth Weight," *American Journal of Epidemiology*, 91:262, 1970.

20 Wallace: op. cit., p. 25.

21 Rosenwaike, Ira: "The Influence of Socioeconomic Status on Incidence of Low Birth Weight," *HSMHA Health Reports*, 86:641, 1971.

22 Bierman, J.: "Some Things Learned," *The American Journal of Public Health*, 59:931, 1969.

23 Lewis, Oscar: "The Culture of Poverty," *Scientific American*, 215:21, 1966.

24 Milio, Nancy: "Values, Social Class and Community Health Services," *Nursing Research*, 16:29, 1967.

25 Strauss, Anselm: "Medical Ghettos," in Anselm Strauss (ed.): *Where Medicine Fails*, Aldine, Chicago, 1970.

26 Tompkins: op. cit., p. 45.

27 Wallace: op. cit., p. 23.

28 Gold, Edwin M.: "Identification of the High-risk Fetus," *Clinical Obstetrics and Gynecology*, 11:1070, 1968.

29 Hill, Charles A., Jr., and Mozart I. Spector: "Natality and Mortality of American Indians Compared with U.S. Whites and Nonwhites," *HSMHA Health Reports*, 86:233, 1971.

30 Ibid., p. 242.

31 Ibid., p. 236.

32 Ibid., p. 238.

33 Ibid., p. 236.
34 Wallach, R., and G. Blinick: "Community Prenatal Care—An Integrated Approach," *American Journal of Obstetrics and Gynecology*, 105:808, 1969.
35 Wallace: op. cit., p. 31.
36 Tompkins: op. cit., p. 53.
37 Held, B., and H. Prystowsky: "Research in the Delivery of Health Care— Changing Reproductive Trends," *American Journal of Obstetrics and Gynecology*, 109:32, 1971.
38 Tompkins: op. cit., p. 48.
39 Hunscher, Helen A., and Winslow T. Tompkins: "The Influence of Maternal Nutrition on the Immediate and Long-term Outcome of Pregnancy," *Clinical Obstetrics and Gynecology*, 13:132, 1970.
40 Janus, Z., and R. Fuentes: "Participation of Low-income Urban Women in a Public Health Birth Control Program," *Public Health Reports*, 85:862, 1970.
41 Von der Ahe, C. B.: "The Unwed Teen-age Mother," *American Journal of Obstetrics and Gynecology*, 15:279, 1969.
42 Osofsky, H. J.: "Antenatal Malnutrition—Its Relationship to Subsequent Infant and Child Development," *American Journal of Obstetrics and Gynecology*, 105:1150, 1969.
43 Hunscher and Tompkins: op. cit., p. 130.
44 *Vital Statistics of the United States, 1967*, vol. II, Mortality, part A.
45 Hendricks, C. H., and W. Brenner: "Toxemia of Pregnancy—Relationship between Fetal Weight, Fetal Survival, and the Maternal State," *American Journal of Obstetrics and Gynecology*, 109:232, 1971.
46 Tompkins: op. cit., p. 56.
47 Conn, R. H.: "Using Health Education Aides in Counseling Pregnant Women," *Public Health Reports*, 84:981, 1968.
48 Cowen, D.: "Denver Neighborhood Health Program," *Public Health Reports*, 84:1030, 1969.
49 Morton, J.: "Experiences with a Maternity and Infant Care (MIC) Project," *American Journal of Obstetrics and Gynecology*, 107:362–368, 1970.
50 Westheimer, R. K., S. H. Cattell, E. Connell, et al.: "Use of Paraprofessionals to Motivate Women to Return for Post Partum Checkup," *Public Health Report*, 85:625, 1970.
51 Schwartz, Jerome L.: "First National Survey of Free Medical Clinics 1967–9," *HSMHA Health Reports*, 86:788, 1971.
52 Ibid., p. 786.
53 Ibid., p. 780.
54 Personal communication with Mr. Harry Dunning, Director of Vital Statistics Section of the Seattle–King County Health Department.
55 Wiener and Milton: op. cit., p. 266.
56 Milio: op. cit.

9 | METHODS OF TEACHING AND COUNSELING

Sylvia J. Bruce and Marilyn A. Chard

FREEDOM TO CHOOSE

What is there about parenthood and prospective parenthood that has created a need for educational programs? Why has this particular period in our history generated such a need to become more knowledgeable? Why did the myth "mother (or father) knows best" break down so completely? This increasing push for education and preparation is by no means confined to affluent and suburban families. Serving the educational interests and needs of parents is fast becoming a professional business. To be sure, it is still one of the weaker aspects of the health care package, and the quality of the educational commitment is frequently secondary to the business enterprise. Nevertheless, the business of educating parents and preparing prospective parents is here to stay, and it must be examined and evaluated carefully and completely.

The effects of the midcentury knowledge explosion and the resulting development of today's technocracy have left no group untouched, including the fabric of family life tradition, belief, and practice. Many forces in today's modern world have influenced family stability, sex roles, kinship relationships, and childbearing practices. The characteristics of our time have cut off many young people from family influences and traditions. There has been a growing awareness of the need to reexamine customs and practices in order to determine purposes and values. Only children used to ask the "why" of things. Fortunately, adults are now beginning to question the purposes of what they do, what they allow done to themselves, and what they have done for themselves.

A flood of unsorted, poorly presented, and ill-digested information has confused both parents and educators. Knowledge will always be used and misused. Helping parents to sort out knowledge and facts will be one of nursing's most critical contributions of the future. The essence of validation of independent practice for nursing will be in the development and advancement of concepts of wellness, prevention, and restoration. Nursing has a choice, and a decision must be made. Our uniqueness, if such it must be, may be in a commitment to concepts of wellness and programs of restoration.

Many prospective parents either are a part of the current movement that is attempting to change the quality and tradition of family life or are already participating in newer forms of social living and child care practices. What was once considered the appropriate domain for maternity nursing practice and expectant parent preparation is now woefully inadequate. Prospective parents are no longer willing to limit their preparation for parenthood only to those needs and understandings which prepare them for the briefest of all their lifetime commitments—pregnancy. Expectant mothers and couples are grappling with such ecological issues as overpopulation and their fear of rearing children in what they view as a substantially polluted world. Knowledge of the so-called freedom experiences manifest in such practices as yoga, hallucinogenic drugs, organic diets, fasts related to social issues, communal living, and transitory coupling is a critical part of the substantive content of today's programs for expectant parents. To continue to limit the scope of programs offered to expectant parents is to ignore the urgency of parental concern and the relevancy of social change and childrearing practices.

One serious caution must be noted, however. Parents and expectant parents should have the freedom to choose the educational program they feel is best suited to them. Making such a choice can be the most difficult and frustrating aspect of the entire pregnancy experience. Generally, educational offerings for parents are not presented or advertised in the most clear and open way. An amazing variety of programs which are offered as preparation for parenthood are actually programs of preparation dealing only with specific aspects of a pregnancy. Education for expectant parents should be broadly based in scope and should include issues beyond the pregnancy cycle itself. If a program is to do less, it should be so advertised. There is no reason why programs for specific pregnancy cycle preparations should not be offered. They are critical to the process, essential to the experience, and are needed by many. They should, however, make no direct or vague claims to being more than they are.

Just what is offered to pregnant women or couples? Some programs are designed specifically to help women cope with the labor process only. Generally, these programs focus on a particular method of self-preparation which may or may not include caretaking and support tasks for the prospective father. Issues related to labor and concerns or questions relevant to pregnancy physiology are also raised but are, for the most part, didactically or prescriptively handled, since they are secondary to the basic purpose of the program. Not only are these programs limited to a specific aspect of a pregnancy experience, but many are limited to just one major approach. Consequently, many expectant women or couples enroll in the course not realizing that only one method will be analyzed and taught. There is nothing wrong in approaching preparation programs in this way *provided* that those who choose to attend are fully apprised of the purposes, goals, and scope of the offering. Perhaps these programs would serve expectant parents more effectively if they were made available to those who have just participated in broader experiences, have had the opportunity to make their preparatory selection from a variety of methods, and are more settled in just how they wish to cope with one specific task—labor.

Another major source of educational offerings for expectant parents could legitimately be referred to as the promotional giveaway programs. The fundamental premise of these programs is that they must sell something—good relations, a specific institution, products, or businesses. The education of prospective parents is blatantly secondary. The qualifications of the nurses conducting these programs may not be a matter of great concern to the sponsors, but they are of critical importance to parents. Given the opportunity, parents or prospective parents will challenge leadership qualifications. Generally, leaders of the promotional giveaway programs are in a safer position if the offerings are geared to imparting facts and dazzling participants. Again, there is nothing fundamentally inappropriate with these offerings *if* the participants know what is being offered as well as what will not be provided.

Promotional giveaways do, however, lay the groundwork for an almost unconscious proclivity to sift out material unrelated to the sponsor and to dwell on facets of content or experience that is of a decided advantage to the supporting business or institution. An example of such a program may be found in the layette section of a large department store. A careful analysis of the content of these offerings would demonstrate an uneven distribution of subject emphasis; more time is expended on bathing supplies, layette items, nursery equipment, and feeding methods than on parental concerns of first trimester issues or preparations and methods of encouraging labor and delivery. Upon completion of a series of lectures or classes the parents are usually given a certificate and a simple case of creams and lotions for the baby. Institutions also provide promotional programs under the guise of preparation for parenthood. The programs are generally shorter, consisting of only two or three sessions during which couples are introduced to the chief-of-staff and the maternity supervisor, attend lectures given by the hospital's nutritionist and chief of pediatrics, and are taken on a tour of the facilities. The main focus of the program is "this is what this hospital can do and has done for you." It is probably only by the sheerest coincidence that these tours usually end just outside the cashier's office.

> Theoretically there is a need for as many kinds of programs as there are expectant parents to attend them. If the purpose of the program is clear and the goals well defined, expectant parents can make intelligent choices regarding the kinds of experiences they feel will be most appropriate for them.[1]

FREEDOM TO LEARN

The traditional expectations of the adult learner involve a situation in which the teacher is the authoritarian communicator of knowledge and the student is a passive receiver of information. Because of past experiences, the student anticipates the ingestion of "pearls of wisdom" which will be regurgitated at a later date as proof to the teacher and to himself that he has learned. Thus, the teacher is seen as the expert authority, the guardian of all available knowledge on a particular subject, and the learner is denied the educational resources within himself and his fellow learners. Yet every adult has a repository of knowledge which he has culled from his experiences. If he can be freed to share his knowledge with his teacher and his fellow learners, then discovery of knowledge will involve a mutual exchange of ideas, beliefs, and experiences. Learning will be side by side rather than face to face. Both teacher and learner will utilize their authority in the educational process.

The independent practitioner in maternity nursing possesses authority because of knowledge of anatomy, physiology, and psychology in relation to the prenatal, intrapartum, and postpartum stages of pregnancy and in relation to menopause. In addition the nurse has sufficient knowledge of human development to provide teaching and counseling experiences for parents regarding offspring of all ages. The parents and prospective parents whom the nurse is teaching and counseling possess authority because of their experiences concerning the physical and psychological changes during the prenatal, intrapartum, and postpartum periods of pregnancy and their experiences as parents of children in various stages of human development. The ability of the independent practitioner in maternity nursing and parents or prospective parents to exercise their freedom to learn will depend upon their exchange of authority. If authority is shared, all participants will be able to assimilate that information which has the most meaning for them.

Principles of Teaching-Learning

Aline Auerbach, a recognized leader in the parent education movement, has identified nine basic assumptions which underlie parent group education and which are based on her experiences over a number of years.[2] The assumptions are as follows:

1. Parents can learn.
2. Parents want to learn.
3. Parents learn best what they are interested in learning.
4. Learning is most significant when the subject matter is closely related to the parents' own immediate experiences.
5. Parents can learn best when they are free to create their own response to a situation.
6. Parent group education is as much an emotional experience as it is an intellectual one.
7. Parents can learn from one another.
8. Parent group education provides the basis for a remaking of experience.
9. Each parent learns in his own way.

The authors have identified five main steps in the teaching process based on their experiences as group leaders. They are as follows:

1. Recruit the group.
2. Develop the agenda.
3. Develop the content.
4. Examine the process.
5. Evaluate the group experience.

Table 9-1 shows the intimate relationship between Auerbach's nine learning principles and the authors' five steps in the teaching process. The fundamental teaching-learning processes can be broadened further and subsequently viewed as methodologies of recruitment, procedure, and process.

RECRUITMENT

The independent practitioner's first step in recruiting a parent group involves identification of philosophy and goals relative to parent education. Nurses should also be aware of their own strengths and limitations as group leaders and as authorities. The nurse then must investigate the various parent education programs which are available in the community. Once this is accomplished either of two things can be done. The nurse can develop a separate program or can serve as a consultant to or a coordinator of existing pro-

TABLE 9-1
THE TEACHING-LEARNING PROCESS

Steps in teaching	Learning principles
1 Recruit the group	1 Parents can learn.
	2 Parents want to learn.
2 Develop the agenda	3 Parents learn best when interested.
	4 Learning is most significant when based on personal experiences.
3 Develop the content	5 Parents can learn best when they are free to respond in their own way.
	6 Parent group education is both an emotional and an intellectual experience.
	7 Parents can learn from one another.
4 Examine the process	8 Parent group education provides the basis for a remaking of experience.
5 Evaluate the experience	9 Each parent learns in his own way.

grams. The latter choice may necessitate suggesting the termination of some programs, the merger of others, or the development of a new program. As a group leader, the independent practitioner must make the choice which is personally as well as professionally acceptable.

Parent education groups are discussion groups based on expectant or actual parent needs. The order and range of topics depend upon group needs. Yet, if it is believed that pertinent material has not been covered, the leader has a responsibility to remind the group of this oversight and to stimulate discussion in the neglected, but important, areas. The group experience "should provide for acquisition of new information as a means of broadening the point of view and enlarging perspectives"[3] based on information culled from the group members.

Because parents can and want to learn, parent group education should be an integral part of prenatal and postpartum nursing care. Independent practitioners in maternity nursing should be familiar with all parent group educational experiences which are available. This information should be discussed with the parents and potential parents with whom the nurse works, thereby affording them the opportunity to choose that group which best meets their needs. Parents can also be recruited into groups through referral. For example, a clinical specialist in maternity nursing may be conducting a prospective parent group in which the topics discussed include the physiology and psychology of pregnancy. Toward the end of the series of eight meetings, a set of prospective parents express their wish to be together during the intrapartum period. The clinical specialist can refer them to an available group experience which will meet their needs. There may be other parents who desire more information regarding their two-year-old. The clinical specialist in maternity nursing can refer them to the clinical specialist in pediatric nursing who will be conducting a series of parent group meetings which will meet this parental need.

Regardless of the work setting (hospital, community clinic, obstetrician's office), the independent practitioner should provide for parent education. The time for conducting meetings and the composition of these groups will be dependent on parents' schedules. For example, prospective fathers may not be free to meet at the same time as prospective mothers. Therefore, there could be two separate groups—one for the men and one for the women. When prospective parents are scheduled for pregnancy assessment appointments and are also attending prospective parent groups, the day for the appointment should coincide with the day of the group meeting and the time for the appointment should be set for one-half hour before or right after the group meeting. The major purpose of parent education is to provide services that are actually needed, at times that are practical, and in combinations that are really helpful (sets of parents, mothers only, fathers only). Regardless of the type of group, the time, and the place, the crucial point is that parents and prospective parents know what the group leader truly plans to provide and in what areas help can be provided for them.

PROCEDURE

Although it has been implied, the authors' premise must be made unmistakably clear: *The teaching-learning interaction or process lends itself best to those situations in which the participants can discuss the topics or issues which are of the most immediate interest or concern to them.* Undoubtedly, there are some leaders who can provide this type of learning situation through methods other than discussion. However, since the more traditional forms of teaching methodologies, such as lectures, panels, symposia, and conferences, are familiar experiences for most, only the discussion process and procedure will be developed in detail.

The discussion procedure involves agenda and content development. At the initial group meeting, the leader first hands out cards to be filled out with certain information, such as name and telephone number. At the same time each group member is given a card with the leader's name and telephone number. The purpose of this exchange is to enable the group members and the group leader to fulfill their obligations to one another. Thus, if the group leader has to change a meeting date, each group member can be telephoned and given the information. By the same token, if a group member is unable to attend a given meeting, he or she can inform the group leader. Missing members do affect group process and procedure. With the mechanism of mutual responsibility established, the leader can inform other group members if a member or members will be absent from individual meetings. If a group leader wishes any additional information, it should be made quite clear why such information is requested and what is to be done with it.

"A first meeting in any group experience is unquestionably a vital one. At this time, the leadership role is explained, and the purpose and function of the group, as well as its limitations, are described."[4] Thus, following the written exchange of information and an explanation of its purpose, it is shared with the group members who the group leader is, why the group leader is there, and the philosophy and goals of parent group education. The participants are then asked to explain who they are and what they hope will be discussed and covered in this discussion series. If their expressed areas of interest and concern are stated broadly, the leader should request more specificity by such questions as, "Can you give me an example?" "Do you have something particular in mind?" Following this "go-around" the leader summarizes the topics raised, grouping the related items under appropriate headings. The leader explains that, as meetings progress, both the leader and the members may add to the agenda. There is no particular sequence in which these topics must be discussed and developed. Thus is the agenda developed and two learning principles are fulfilled: Parents can learn best when they are interested. Learning is most significant when based on personal experiences.

At a recent first meeting of an expectant parent group series, the initial agenda was very superficial, as indicated by the expectant couples who stated the following: "I'm interested in seeing the hospital and delivery room." "I'm interested in care of the baby at home." Since the leader was inexperienced and there were 25 participants in this particular group, the shallowness of the agenda could probably be attributed to the leader's ineptness in working with large discussion groups. However, a more experienced leader would have collected a more meaningful agenda. For example, one expectant father said he was interested in "just what caused it all." The group laughed at this, but the leader never responded to his comment. Yet, had it been said, "I'm not so sure I really understand what you're saying. Can you tell me more?" many pertinent items could have been uncovered, such as, "Why did we become pregnant? It wasn't the right time." "We were practicing the rhythm method of contraception. Why didn't it work?" "I know my wife would know when she is in labor, but what starts labor anyway? The doctor gives you a vague idea of when the baby is expected, but is there anything we can do to start labor? Or does it just happen? Why does it happen?"

By being more sensitive to what seems to be an offhand remark, many issues can be opened, such as the following:

1 Family planning and contraception—techniques, methods, physiology
2 Changing roles from husband and wife to father and mother
3 Unwanted pregnancy—psychological adjustments
4 Becoming parents—responsibilities, fear, worries
5 Harming a pregnancy, i.e., what a couple or mother might do that could start premature labor and result in a deformed infant
6 Physiology of labor—what is true labor, what is false labor?

Not only will the group identify what they want to explore and discuss, but also the leader must assume professional commitment and responsibility to the group in order to help them see the relationship of their general questions and concerns to topics that are specific and pertinent to prospective parents.

Content development involves the identification of a body of knowledge related to the area covered by the group's experience. Content includes a balance between emotional and intellectual material. Its development presupposes the leader's encouragement of open exchange among group members. The first step involves establishing a focus for group discussion; this demands a concentration of attention and the pinpointing of the emotional involvement in the group around a given topic. Therefore, not only is the group better informed, but it is also less fearful and better able to cope with the physical and psychological aspects of the subject matter. The focus helps the members to discuss the same topic and provides a structure which teaches by examples supplied by the members. The group may begin to sense and understand why its members may be concerned about a particular subject.

The group arrives at a focus through a process of clarification—separation of the superficial from the meaningful. The leader picks up the question or request from the group for the purpose of helping the group to become clear about their concerns, feelings, and thoughts around a chosen subject. The leader now carries the responsibility for enabling the group to discuss the topic as productively as possible. The leader must be aware of and sensitive to purposes and readiness for discussion. Input is provided as needed, either to supply information or to correct misinformation when this is not forthcoming from the group. Underscoring and restatement of what individual group members have said and periodic summarization of what has happened up to a given point in the discussion are leadership techniques which help to maintain a productive meeting.

The ultimate goal of any educational parent group discussion is the enhanced ability of the members to cope with present and future demands of parenthood. In the later phases of the group discussion, the members can be enabled to evolve ways of coping which are suitable to them. They can be helped to see the implications of their choices and to face realistically those issues which may not offer a choice. This is content development and in it three learning principles are fulfilled: Parents can learn best when they are free to respond in their own way. Parent group education is both an emotional and an intellectual experience. Parents can learn from one another.

At a fourth meeting of a recent expectant parent group series, the leader collected a small agenda and a topic was selected. The group was told that the leader would prefer to be more specific. Thus, the topic went from "What causes abnormal babies?" to "What can I do to prevent having an abnormal baby?" The original question was academic and general. The second question was more personal and meaningful to the members. This is a step the leader took for the group rather than letting them do it. Had the topic remained

"What causes abnormal babies?" the leader could have turned to the mother who originally raised the question and asked, "What do you have in mind?" The group might have discussed specific diseases and conditions for awhile. The leader then could move in with a restatement of the original question, such as, "Are you perhaps asking if there is anything you can do to prevent or to be sure you won't have an abnormal baby?" The group will usually nod in the affirmative. The leader's next question can be, "What are you doing now that is helping to ensure a good baby?" If there is silence, the leader can say, "Well, let's look at what we've discussed already." The leader will then summarize and have the group select a place to begin. Many issues could have been opened, such as the following:

1 What the parents give to the baby to ensure a healthy start in life
2 What the parents can not control to any predictable degree
3 What the parents, especially the expectant mothers, can do to ensure the best possible outcome

Thus, the focus could have been reached and maintained, and the group could have had a productive discussion through meaningful content development.

As can be seen in the above example, the potential for a productive discussion was there. However, the quality of the learning experience is dependent upon professional competence and social relevancy. The procedures utilized by the leader in discussion groups are merely facilitating devices. They do not take the place of maternity nursing expertise. These same procedures of agenda and content development provide the participants with a more systematic approach to problem solving.

PROCESS

Process involves the utilization of individual behavior as a method of moving the group forward. Therefore, in order to be effective, the group leader should observe and understand individual behavior—words, gestures, silence, facial and bodily expressions, and tone of voice. Individuals possess certain attitudes and predispositions based on previous experience which tend to influence the way in which they interact with each other and with the group leader. Although it may not be possible to fully understand all the meanings of behavior of an individual within the group, the leader must try to see beyond the overt behavior because it has personal significance for the individual who is utilizing it. The leader's key to response to individual behavior is acceptance of the person. Nevertheless, the leader does have a responsibility to intervene when individual behavior is inappropriate and disruptive to the group. The leader seeks to understand through careful listening and maintains focus on the content rather than on the personality.

Once the group has been recruited, its members have expressed their interests and concerns, and a focus has been found, the leader should utilize process to enhance the group experience. In order to pave the way, it might be helpful to set aside time either at the beginning or at the end of the first two or three sessions to discuss the process of forming a group. Thus, members can be prepared for initial feelings of disappointment. They may have expected to take notes while the leader talked. Once in the group they discover that they are expected to be active participants. This is difficult to do with a group of strangers. People (participants and leader) have to get to know one another before they can take risks. Before the group is really formed, some people may elect to leave and new members may arrive. It usually takes three meetings before the group becomes "permanent" and cohesive.

The group leader should identify process very subtly to the group; this can be done when the group process is *not* working because members are directing all their questions to the leader and not using each other, or when they are "doing their own thing" and not listening to each other. At such times the leader might say, "We don't seem to be working as a group. Let's slow down." Or "What's the matter with everyone tonight? No matter what we agree to discuss, it just falls apart." A summary of what has occurred up to that point may then help the group to refocus.

Remember the father who wondered "just what caused it all"? The response of the group to this was just laughter. The leader could have seen this group laughter as a cue. Was it anxious laughter? Was it hilarious laughter? Did it mean that other group members also had questions or concerns about how such things happen? The leader must be sensitive to group as well as individual behavior in order to provide a productive meeting. The leader's use of behavior and content will determine the participants' freedom to share their authority with one another and to try new behaviors. Not only should group members feel free to explore and analyze a situation presented within a group, but they also should be able to apply this learning in their daily lives.

Evaluation of the group experience is provided when both leader and parents discover for themselves what they have learned and ascertain how they could have learned more. It is important that the leader realize that each person learns in his own way and at his own rate. Members should be encouraged to do this and to come to their own decisions. Because this experience is one which is freely chosen by the participants, the leader should not demand a verbal or written evaluation. Rather, this should be anticipated, on a behavioral level. Toward the end of the series, group members may exhibit their unwillingness to leave by congregating at the end of a session "just to talk." An expectant mother may deliver before the last session but attend this last session with her newborn. Some members may just say, "Thank you. This really helped."

The leader can enhance personal learning by keeping records of each session in a series. Through careful examination of these records, the leader can ascertain what has been done that was helpful to the group or that hindered the group process. The leader can also realize the clues that were missed and the quality of content which was discussed, analyzed, and utilized by the participants.

In parent group education, the leader teaches procedure to the parents through agenda and content development. Process is used to facilitate the group's learning. Through process, the last two learning principles are realized: Parent group education provides the basis for a remaking of experience. Each parent learns in his own way.

Through the exploration of recruitment, procedure, and process, the relationship between the nine learning principles and the steps in teaching have been established. Yet this chapter is concerned not only with teaching but also with counseling. Is counseling different from teaching? Is it inherent in teaching? Are the terms counseling and teaching synonymous? Herein lies a dilemma.

The Dilemma of Teaching-Counseling

Some may see teaching as mechanical fact-giving and counseling more personal and feeling-oriented. This does not mean that they cannot be afforded simultaneously in a teaching situation. Others believe that counseling is something which is beyond the scope of teaching. The authors use the terms interchangeably. Teaching is not effective unless it deals with feelings. Emotions such as fear, hate, and anxiety can inhibit learning, while love, openness, and trust can enhance learning. The feelings dealt with during the teaching-counseling process are based on the present. Delving into the unconscious would be therapy. The independent practitioner in maternity nursing, when working with parents and prospective parents, is interested in how parents perceive facts and how they deal with them as applied to the present. This practitioner is not equipped to handle psychological problems, which are the realm of the clinical specialist in psychiatric nursing.

Much of this chapter has been directed toward parent group education. This does not preclude the efficacy of teaching-counseling on an individual basis. There may be times when problems cannot be handled appropriately in the group. Although feelings have relevancy to the individual and to group members, one participant's feelings are not always relevant to the entire group. They may be too personal and thus embarrassing to other group members. The leader should be sensitive to this group feeling, intervene, and arrange to see the participant personally.

Individual teaching-counseling can also be provided by the independent practitioner in maternity nursing in practice settings (hospital, community health center, obstetrician's office). Problems which are of immediate concern to the parents and prospective parents should be handled as they arise rather than being deferred to the parent group meeting time. *The same teaching-learning principles of group settings apply in these situations.* The great difference lies in the fact that the nurse and the parent must give more of themselves because they are the only two involved as opposed to a group of nine to twelve couples.

Parents will have freedom to learn when they are aware of the educational opportunities which are available to them as parents and prospective parents. This knowledge presupposes their right to choose from a variety of parent group education experiences when the philosophies and goals of each program have been interpreted to them. Then they can choose that program which will meet their educational needs. Their freedom to learn will be enhanced when group leaders acknowledge parents' authority and supplement it with their own.

FREEDOM TO TEACH

Parents who are free to learn need nurses who are free to teach. As simplistic as this statement appears to be, it in no way ensures an easy implementation. Classes, courses, tours, and demonstrations traditionally offered to expectant parents by maternity nurses have not been widely known as free experiences for either the nurse or the participants. The content or focus of a majority of these classes and courses generally has been instructive in approach and physiomedical in scope. Nursing theories, science, and practice have been abysmally absent. Nursing knowledge and skills are certainly not unknown to maternity nurses. The freedom to use these knowledges, unfortunately, is a little used freedom. Just why this is so is a point of historical interest but is not germane to the decision to change. If change is wanted, change can occur. Why it has not occurred can become a preoccupying exercise of little academic merit.

Professionalism Revisited

The maternity *nursing* role as it is practiced today can best be described as static and passive. Maternity nursing practice is a mere reflection of the larger issue—professional obsolescence. Whether nursing ever *was* or now *is* a profession is a moot question. What it *will* become is an issue of urgent concern. Other professions have defined their parameters of practice, stated their goals, and developed the content of their role while simultaneously implementing their service. But nurses have practiced their role as defined by others and are only now beginning to evolve their own definition of what nursing care should be.

Today's practitioners must have the integrity required to allow changes to occur that will ensure the rebirth of their profession as a legitimate form of practice and service. Nursing, however, and maternity nurses are no exception, must earn the right to professionalism and independent practice. This can only occur when present-day practitioners can recognize and value the strength and integrity that is realized through standards, knowledge, research, and scholarship. When nursing *practices* are carefully examined they leave much to be desired, for the art and science of nursing is remarkably absent. When nursing *thought* is evaluated the tragedy rests in the omission of implementation. Although obviously overdue, it is not too late to legitimize thoughts, ideas, and intuitions.

Parents have a right to learn, and nurses have a right to teach, but only if they first accept the responsibility to learn. The freedom to teach assumes there is a willingness to learn.

Self Reexamined

Self-development is a professional responsibility of the independent practitioner in maternity nursing. In order to develop, one must have something on which to build. Hopefully, the independent practitioner has a broad background in the liberal arts, including anthropology, psychology, sociology, history, literature, and human development. Today, an historical sense of nursing seems to be sadly lacking. How many independent practitioners can determine whether history has changed nursing or nursing has changed history? How has history affected nursing? Upon what must independent practitioners build in order to change their self-image and earn the freedom to teach parents and prospective parents?

When anthropology, psychology, sociology, literature, and theories of human development are taught from an historical perspective, the learner begins to acquire a sense of history. In teaching parents, the nurse who has experienced this approach will be able to identify practices and values held by some parents who seem to belong to a different era. The nurse can begin to understand why these values and practices are important to work colleagues.

In order to understand and deal with the social issues of today the independent practitioner must have an understanding of our technocracy and how it developed historically, with the impact of two world wars, the philosophy of pragmatism, and the explosion of knowledge in the fields of technology, medicine, and psychology. How many independent practitioners can understand the reasons why the counter culture has emerged and delved into the area of psychedelic experiences? Where have members of this culture seen value placed? They have seen value placed on the authority of scientific knowledge which espouses the development of the intellect and ignores the psyche. Thus, they perceive human relationships as lacking in love and understanding.

Suppose an expectant mother who had taken LSD came to a community health center. She had read that fetal chromosomal abnormalities can be determined through analysis of amniotic fluid. Upon her request an amniocentesis was performed. Examination of the amniotic fluid showed no abnormalities. Although the expectant mother has been assured that the fetus has no known chromosomal defects, she is still fearful and expresses her anxiety to the clinical specialist in maternity nursing who works out of the community health center. If the clinical specialist places nursing values on the authority of scientific knowledge, the expectant mother will be referred to the test results. If the clinical specialist believes in the authority of the psyche as well as the intellect, not only will the test results be used as assurance, but the expectant mother will be helped to explore her feelings. Until the reasons for her feelings are understood, the expectant mother may be unable to believe that the fetus is doing well. Thus *care* has been demonstrated by the clinical specialist.

Professional nurses have a responsibility to themselves and to their clients to come to grips with today's social issues. The quality of parent teaching and freedom to teach will be limited if they do not face these issues. The parents' freedom to learn will be inhibited through their lack of knowledge. Without a firm background in the liberal arts and in *nursing,* how can nurses help parents to find relationships between knowledge and feelings in order to reshape their own learning? How can they teach legislators what nursing is? And how can parameters of practice be defined so that a nurse practice act congruent with the professional concepts for nursing practice can be legislated and enacted? These nurses must reexamine themselves as professionals, enhance their strengths, and acknowledge their limitations by building upon what is already known, identifying what needs to be known, and accepting the responsibility to learn it. Only then will the nurse have the background to merit the freedom to teach.

FREEDOM TO DEVELOP

Education for parent development and expectant parent preparation should be viewed as a parental right. The quality of programs offered to parents and prospective parents should be no less than the quality of educational experiences provided for children and young adults. In this respect the development of new programs and the consultation provided to existing ones should be the responsibility of institutions involved in the teaching-learning interaction. To do less would be to undermine the fundamental assumption that a democratic system of government works best when its members are informed, are free of unrealistic concerns, and are operating in a state of wellness.

The University and the Community

Colleges and universities have long been under attack for what has been perceived as an insensitivity to the social and educational needs of the communities in which they are located. All too few communities view institutions of higher education as integral and necessary components of an efficient and productive human condition. One is more likely to hear them described, and this is particularly true of highly congested urban areas, as institutional forms that take the services, facilities, and resources of the community but remain uncommitted to the realities, issues, and ills of human need. Without question, there are variations of both forms of practice. There is no valid reason, however, why universities should continue to remain patently unresponsive to the country's largest and most neglected group—parents. Parenthood is the only occupation for which there is no systematic mode of preparation and no continuing education programs for parental development. Is there any reason why universities and colleges should not develop these programs and courses for parents?

Certainly it is a justifiable expectation to look to and depend upon the universities for the development of a wide variety of learning resources and materials. If the premise that schools of nursing should produce general family health practitioners at the baccalaureate level and specialist practitioners through programs at the graduate level is accepted and operative, then the need for providing practitioner experiences commensurate with societal needs will be of critical concern to the faculties of nursing. There is no doubt of the benefits of mutuality when schools of nursing provide educational programs for parents and these same programs provide teaching-learning sources for students and faculty. Services for parents and expectant parents should be ongoing and continuous even though there will be times when these experiences are needed more by parents than by students and faculties. Such services should not be provided just for those periods when students need particular learning experiences.

Parents and the Video World

A variety of teaching-learning devices and approaches can be developed and utilized to enrich and vitalize programs and services offered to parents. Video tapes can be developed around particular developmental tasks of children, can focus on certain common but troublesome family interactions, or could follow a parent discussion series. These tapes could be used by nurses from outside the university who are leading discussion groups either for their own continuing education or to facilitate the process and development of their groups. Parents who wish to direct their own learnings also should have access to these video tapes. There is no reason why parents and expectant parents should not be able to use university facilities to meet their own needs in learning how to cope with or manage their children or their pregnancy.

The Right to Develop

Parents have a right to learn the roles they must assume in helping their families to grow and develop, and universities have an obligation and social commitment to be sensitive and responsive to meeting the fundamental purpose of their being. Maternal–child health services must begin to accept the continuing education of parents as a service of equal importance to the education of nurses and physicians in the field of maternal–child health care.

REFERENCES

1 Bruce, Sylvia J.: "Do Prenatal Educational Programs Really Prepare for Parenthood?" *Hospital Topics,* November 1965, p. 104.
2 Auerbach, Aline B.: *Parents Learn through Discussion,* Wiley, New York, 1968, pp. 23–28.
3 Bruce, op. cit., p. 105.
4 Bruce, Sylvia J.: "What Mothers of 6- to 10-Year-Olds Want To Know," *Nursing Outlook,* 12:40, September 1964.

PART II

PLANNING THE FAMILY: CHILDBEARING AND CHILDREARING

People throughout the world are becoming increasingly aware of and concerned about the steadily rising population and the inherent effect this rise will have on the quality of life and the delicate balance of nature. Man continues to study diligently for answers to the question of how a level of population can be maintained through reproduction that will not exploit the environment.

We live in our environment, and our biopsychosocial lives are molded by our environment. A healthy environment provides conditions that nurture the development of choice human characteristics. Ideally, each person should contemplate these factors before adding another human life to the already heavily populated milieu.

A recognized basic human right entitles individuals to exercise their choice regarding spacing of children and limitation of family size. However, contraception is only one of several important components of planning a family. Other components include infertility and conception problems, legal and illegal abortion, genetic counseling, and the psychosocial and cultural considerations inherent in these components.

Many thousands of couples each year find with deep disappointment that they seem to be unable to have the baby they want so very much. Roughly 15 percent of all couples experience difficulty in producing a child. This is frustrating for these people who try in vain to have a child. They become anxious and upset, and the partners often blame each other for their inability to reproduce. The study of infertility is another component of family planning. Just as research has defined effective ways to limit reproduction, it also has provided a body of knowledge about ways to stimulate reproduction.

Some women, for various reasons, find it impossible to allow pregnancy to continue. These women seek either a legal or illegal abortion. However, very often the woman who seeks a legal abortion is confronted with a maze of legal, medical, and religious obstacles. Abortion is a complicated situation in which many variables need to be considered. Nonetheless, it is one more aspect of family planning with which nurses are confronted.

Genetic counseling is usually sought by couples with a familial history of birth defects or by those who have produced a defective child. Rapid developments in the study of genetics over the past few years have added genetic counseling as one more vitally important component of family planning.

The psychosocial cultural factors implicit in planning a family were spoken of by Sigmund Freud many years ago. Yet it is only recently that health professionals have begun to concentrate their attention on these factors. Education, income, society, and religion, to name a few, certainly influence a couple's ability and efforts to plan a family. However, it is an interplay of *many* different psychosocial cultural factors in each human being's life that dictate what family planning means to an individual.

Contraception is an equally important component of family planning. Nurses often are involved in helping clients to choose a method of contraception. The choice of method must be made by the client after the necessary details on each method have been shared with them. Therefore, it is basic to nursing education that nurses be oriented to all aspects and methods of contraception.

Planning a family necessitates anticipatory and preventive delivery of health care by professionals. In their roles as counselors, case finders, and educators nurses can assess those clients who need or are interested in family planning. Nurses can inform these clients of the services available, provide information about the services, and help them seek the actual care. Nurses can then act as liaisons between physician and client by interpreting and explaining the medical regimen for family planning as well as by delivering follow-through nursing care. An evaluation by nurses of the effectiveness of nursing intervention with clients in planning a family is essential.

10 | ECOLOGICAL FACTORS IN FAMILY PLANNING

Joan Carvell and Fred Carvell

Ecology refers to the study of the relationships between organisms and between organisms and their environment. Until recently most people concentrated on the biological aspects of ecology without giving much consideration to the human and sociological considerations that deal with the spacing of people and institutions and their interdependency. The discussion in this chapter will emphasize these aspects of ecology rather than the biological.

The concept of ecology involves a complex network of dependency among living things. Many of the interrelationships go unnoticed by man until the delicate balance of nature is disturbed. Some ecologists have attempted to explain the network of natural interdependency through the use of a multilayered pyramid. At the base of this pyramid lies the earth and sea, which support all life. The next layer consists of all forms of plant life which support insects and smaller forms of animal life. The remaining layers of the pyramid are composed of various members of the animal kingdom. Ultimately, man sees himself at the apex of the pyramid. It may be argued that this topmost position of man is more correctly attributable to his ego than to his animal superiority; however, it is difficult to find another living thing that has done more to exploit the environment or endanger the existence of living things in each layer of the pyramid.

Although the pyramid is a simple representation of a very complex network of relationships, it serves to illustrate several important points. First, each layer of the pyramid supplies the food and resources for the layers above it. In turn, each layer is dependent upon the layers below it for survival. Second, ecological balance is maintained as long as each layer reproduces in sufficient numbers to ensure its continuance while supplying the needs of the layers above it, resulting in a system of complex interdependencies.

The critical question for the survival of all living things, including man, is how to maintain a level of population through reproduction that will not overtax the supportive environment. Nothing is more germane to man's survival than the birth and death rates; yet these two factors alone are not the primary determinants of his standard of living. A sound and healthy environment for man implies much more than maintenance of ecological equilibrium, the conservation of natural resources, and the control of the biological layers that occupy the pyramid beneath him.

Man not only survives and functions in his environment, he is shaped by it—psychologically, physically, and socially. To be healthy, the environment and standard of living sought by man must therefore provide conditions that favor the development of desirable human characteristics. Each set of parents *should* consider this factor before making the decision to add another human life to the existing stock of mankind. However, it may be unrealistic to expect man to suddenly become concerned about such a broad topic as ecology when he has little understanding of the factors that affect the social and psychological environment in his own family.

Man can take three philosophical approaches when considering his impact on the environment.

First, he can believe that the ultimate control of the earth lies outside man. Therefore, he is justified in neither worrying about its problems nor taking action to prevent catastrophe.

Second, he can believe that the destiny of man and the earth lies in his own hands. Thus, man should plan even his own subsequent evolutionary process so that the best kind (and number) of man in the best kind of world results.

Third, he can believe that he cannot and perhaps should not control his entire destiny, and yet by virtue of his rational nature, he will always act to control significant portions of his future.[1]

If man is to act in accordance with the third philosophical approach and make the attempt to control his own population growth, he should begin by understanding the importance of his relationship to other elements in the ecological system. To do this requires new insights and knowledge. This chapter begins with a general explanation of what environmental education is about and why it is important in helping to attain such insights. Other topics relate to various aspects of population growth and the impact such growth has on resource utilization, urbanization, pollution, and living standards.

Each potential set of parents should consciously make the decision whether or not to have children. Those who make no decision may end up reproducing by default. Obviously, not all potential parents will attempt to engage in the thought-provoking mental process that leads to making either a positive or negative decision. However, those who do decide to curb their own reproductive process will also have to make the decision on the appropriate means to be used for taking such action. The means should be appropriate for them and in accordance with their own values and beliefs.

Other chapters in this book deal more specifically with methods of birth control. This chapter, hopefully, provides information that can be used as the framework within which the decision to control population can be made by individuals more intelligently and with greater understanding.

WHY ENVIRONMENTAL EDUCATION?

For more than a decade man has shown an increasing awareness of the changing ecological balance and the role he has played in it. Ecology has become a *cause célèbre* for crusades and conferences both at local and international levels. State and federal legislation has been affected, advertising campaigns launched, and ecology-related fads in organic foods, natural cosmetics, clothing, and posters have become prevalent. Life-styles based on *a return to nature* have had widespread appeal among those who have joined rural communes.

There are variations in the levels of concern and understanding among those who are advocates of conservation and other environmental programs. The viewpoint of the scientist, industrialist, land developer, physician, student, farmer, or politician is colored by his spectrum of experience. In short, each person's perspective of ecology is influenced by his own understanding and ideals and his vested interests in either protecting or exploiting natural resources.

Despite the increased publicity on ecology, understanding of the interdependence and interrelationships among living things and their environment is more apparent than real among the majority of people. Yet the course of man's future lies in his comprehension of the consequences of his exploitation of nature. The allocation of natural resources and the resulting changes in the environment will vary according to man's priority of demands from the earth. Until priorities change, man seems destined to continue to pollute his environment, overpopulate, and create environmental problems that endanger his life-style and health.

The urban dweller is confronted by environmental problems resulting from overcrowding, rats, roaches, poor solid waste and sewage disposal, air pollution, and environmental blight. The rural dweller faces the consequences of ruinous strip-mining practices and timber harvesting, excessive or inappropriate use of agricultural chemicals, and the encroachment of the overflow of urban population. It is little wonder that the urban dweller trapped in the squalid living conditions of the ghetto does not share the same degree of concern over the purity of mountain streams that the rural dweller or Sierra Club conservationist may voice. Yet, inhabitants of both environments ultimately must face the consequence of air, water, and surface pollution.

Not only do the urban and rural environmental problems impose visual and aesthetic distractions, they pose genuine health hazards and have long-range consequences which affect the survival of both animal and plant life. An important implication of the widespread and growing concern man is showing toward the environment is his increasing awareness that should an ecological disaster occur, it will not differentiate between nations as political units, races, ideologies, ages, or geographic locations. Thus, the importance of ecological awareness affords a point of view not limited to the narrow approach that often accompanies temporary solutions framed by economics, politics, or singular nationalistic interests.

The ecological balance has never been static, but with the recognition of the threat to the human environment, concern and steps toward action are emerging. The individual in this complex world who wants only to understand the problems of his immediate locale or whose perspective is limited to his own technical field (and this would include nursing) is, at the least, a hindrance to society and more likely a threat to the environment.

Today man possesses much of the scientific and technological knowledge necessary to solve many environmental problems. However, decisions regarding man's use of his environment are seldom based solely on scientific knowledge. Human decisions are affected by emotion, custom, oversight, economic feasibility, political expediency, social desirability, or religious belief. Certainly individual human decisions regarding planned parenthood are influenced by the same factors.

It is difficult to make wise decisions about the environment without an understanding of economics, history, political science, sociology, psychology, the humanities, and the physical and natural sciences. This calls for a new approach to education which will provide an ecological perspective for all aspects of learning. The need for such an approach was the force behind the passage of the Environmental Education Act of 1970. This act was an outgrowth of a national commitment to a search for enlightened life-styles and provides a working definition of environmental education.

Environmental education is an integrated process which deals with man's interrelationship with his natural and man-made surroundings, including the relationship of population growth, pollution, resource allocation and depletion, conservation technology, and urban and rural planning to the total human environment. Environmental education is a study of the factors influencing ecosystems, mental and physical growth, living and working conditions, decaying cities, and population pressures. Environmental education is intended to promote among citizens the awareness and understanding of the environment, our relationship to it, and the concern and responsible action necessary to assure our survival and to improve the quality of life.[2]

Under the broad, general definition adopted by Congress in the Environmental Education Act of 1970, population growth becomes a key element in understanding the interrelationship of man, his environment, and the quality of life he enjoys. This relationship is germane to the medical profession of which nursing is a part and, more specifically, to the role of planned parenthood which is discussed in this part of the book. The following sections of this chapter deal with the magnitude of population growth and the factors that contribute to continued growth.

POPULATION GROWTH

The term *population explosion* has been used by demographers to describe the rate of increase in the world's population during the past several decades. The use of the term implies that a problem exists—overpopulation. This perception is reinforced by the news media and reports from such agencies as the United Nations indicating that nearly two-thirds of the existing population live at the edge of survival with malnutrition or starvation. These reports indicate that in certain parts of the world there are more people than can be supported by existing food supplies and necessary health services. According to reports from the Food and Agriculture Organization of the United Nations, food production is failing to keep pace with rising population growth in many sectors of the world. This means there will be little relief unless a better balance can be struck between people and food production.[3]

The United Nations *Demographic Yearbook* reports that the world population, which exceeded 3.6 billion in 1970, is expected to reach 4.5 billion by 1980 and 6.5 billion by the year 2000. Some demographers project even higher world population levels by 2000. Although there is no statistical evidence to indicate precisely how many people the earth can support, it can be assumed that earth, having finite and exhaustible resources, cannot indefinitely support such increases in population.

Concern about implications of the population explosion might best be understood by reviewing the past record of population growth. The world's population did not reach 1 billion until 1850. In 1925, 75 years later, it reached 2 billion; it only took 37 years to reach 3 billion by 1962. World population is expected to expand by another billion, reaching 4 billion by 1977. This latest 1 billion increment is expected to take just 15 years.

Population growth is the result of a sequence of industrial, medical, and agricultural revolutions that began nearly 200 years ago in England. Until then, the doubling time for the world's population took about 1,500 years. Even a cursory review shows that once world population reached 1 billion, it only took 75 years to double the first time. To double the second time (from 2 to 4 billion) it will take about 52 years. Thus, it is easy to see that the term population explosion is no misnomer.

An average person has approximately 38 million pulses per year. Nearly two infants will be born for each of these pulses. At present the world population expands by 70 million persons each year. This means that, in theory, every 6 to 7 weeks the world population increases sufficiently to populate the world's largest city, Tokyo—that is, roughly 9 million persons.

In addition to the problems posed by the absolute increase in population, further complications accrue as a result of the extraordinarily uneven growth rates around the world. In the industrialized and technologically advanced nations, those mainly of Europe, the Soviet Union, North America, Oceania, and Japan, the annual rate of increase is relatively low—about 2 percent. However, in other locations where nations are still in the early stages of technological development—namely, Asia, Africa, and Latin America—the yearly rate of increase is rapid, often twice the rate of the more developed nations. At the current rate of increase, by the year 2000 the developing nations will add more than five times as many people to the world as the more advanced nations.

Factors of Population Growth

Thus far, the discussion has centered on population growth. Two factors have contributed to this growth: natality (birth) rates and mortality rates. Although birth rates have played a role in population growth during the past 25 years, there is little question that the reduction of mortality rates has become the dominant factor for increasing populations.

Approximately half the population in the world today has been born since 1945. Improved medical care has resulted in a substantial reduction in infant mortality rates, allowing a greater number of infants to survive than ever before. At the same time that a higher portion of infants live to the age of procreation, improved health services and technology have helped to extend the life expectancy of persons born prior to 1945. The extension of life expectancy for adults is the reason people under the age of twenty-five do not constitute an even higher portion of the total population. For example, in the United States the life expectancy of a person advanced from thirty-three to seventy years (more than doubled) between the time the Pilgrims first settled New England and 1970.

Although the recent emphasis on youth in the United States has given the illusion that the average age of the population is getting younger, actually the opposite is true. In 1970 the median age in the United States was

25.9 years. In 1910 it was only 24.1 years. The net result of more people living longer has been that the average age of the population has risen, even though more youths under the age of twenty-five are alive today than ever before.

The large portion of youths approaching or at childbearing age has major implications for world population. In the underdeveloped and emerging nations roughly 40 percent of the population is under fifteen years old compared with 25 to 32 percent in the more advanced nations of Europe and North America.[4]

Because birth rates are related generally to the number of women of childbearing age (ages fifteen to forty-four) in a given locale, the avalanche of youth in emerging countries is an ominous sign for future population growth in such areas as Latin America, South Asia, and Africa. In these areas the birth rate is often 40 per 1,000 persons, nearly double that of the more advanced nations. Thus, high birth rates are already occurring in the countries with the largest potential childbearing population yet to come.

When high birth rates are combined with lowered mortality rates, it is not difficult to understand that even if birth rates were reduced to the replacement level (i.e., limited to two children) population would continue to expand. It is estimated that it would take nearly 60 years, or almost a lifetime, before the world's population would stop growing.[5]

POPULATION GROWTH AND USE OF NATURAL RESOURCES

The quality of life for man is irrevocably tied to the quantity of people and the level of their material demands for goods and services. As the population increases, assuming that a given standard of living is to be maintained, increases in resource utilization must also occur. In simple terms, production must keep up with the requirements of the population. In the United States most citizens have high levels of expectation regarding these requirements. Although, as a nation, we are the world's greatest producer, we are also one of the world's most avid consumers. Robert and Leona Rienow illustrate this point:

> Every 8 seconds a new American is born. He is a disarming little thing, but he begins to scream loudly in a voice that can be heard for 70 years. He is screaming for 56,000,000 gallons of water, 21,000 gallons of gasoline, 10,150 pounds of meat, 28,000 pounds of milk and cream, 9,000 pounds of wheat. . . .[6]

The same child will also scream for school buildings, clothes, housing, automobiles, paper, plastic, steel, electric power, and other materials and services that he considers his share. His share, when combined with the shares of all other Americans, constitutes about half the total material production of the world.

The expectations of Americans continue to grow. It is estimated that in 1880 each American used roughly 50 tons of raw materials per year to sustain his standard of living. By the mid-1960s the amount of raw materials had grown to 300 tons per year. Based on an average life span of seventy years, each American is supported by 21,000 tons of raw materials which are not replaceable within many lifetimes.

Aside from the depletion of natural resources—i.e., iron, oil, coal, wood —to provide material goods for our expanding population, these raw materials are the basis for supplying the energy we require to supply electricity and heat for our homes, run our factories, and provide our transportation. It is estimated that the standard of living we currently enjoy in the United States uses 150,000 calories per person each day. Three thousand or less of these calories are required for physical nourishment; the remaining calories are used for production, transportation, and running laborsaving appliances.

Modern life-styles in industrialized nations are supported by raw materials used at a rate never before known to man. The rapid utilization of materials and energy has been brought about because man's material needs and wants have accelerated. The technology of production has kept pace with the demand to convert increasing quantities of raw materials into more usable or desirable forms—automobiles, washing machines, housing, highways, television sets. Technology has helped man apply scientific knowledge in such fields as medicine, aerospace, communications, and production. At the same time that technology has extended man's power over nature, it has contributed to the pollution of our air, water, and landscape which detracts from the habitability of the environment. Often other living things that are part of the ecological system pay the price of man's unbridled application of technology. Insects and plant life die because of indiscriminate use of chemicals. Living things in rivers, lakes, and even the oceans are unwittingly diminished or altered because of industrial and human wastes that are deliberately or unthinkingly pumped into waterways.

URBANIZATION

Mass production has provided the material goods for the populations who live in technologically backward countries as well as those who live in industrialized nations. Both beneficial and nonbeneficial effects have resulted from the mass production processes man has developed. Industrialization creates jobs, and thus the people can work to earn the means to acquire the material goods that are produced. Industrialization also has accelerated the increasing concentration of populations in urban centers around the world. Not only have nations grown in population, but cities with their suburban areas are getting larger. Less than 15 years ago the world had only 29 cities which had

1 million residents. Now there are 133 such cities. Not only are big cities getting larger and more numerous, but middle-sized cities are increasing in number. According to the United Nations *Demographic Yearbook*, in 1970 the world had 1,784 cities with more than 100,000 people residing in each one. This was a 20 percent increase in the number of such cities over the previous decade. Now more than one-third of the world's population lives in urban areas—quite a transition from the days when the farm was the primary living and production unit of society.

Throughout the world people have been moving from rural areas to more densely populated urban areas. In the United States alone, two-thirds of the population live on one-fiftieth of the land area in and around urban centers. With the current population trends indicating that we will number nearly 300 million by the year 2000, accommodations for the increase of 100 million people will mean crowding them into existing cities or building the equivalent of a new city with a population of 250,000 every 40 days for the next 30 years—35 more Los Angeleses, or 250 Newark, New Jerseys.

POLLUTION

The impact of an urbanized concentration of man in all areas of the world has resulted in a concentration of waste—solid, liquid, and gaseous—that has increased per capita along with the growing per capita use of materials and energy, intensifying pollution problems. The types, sources, and amounts of wastes increase with population growth, industry, and use of technology and natural resources. Many types of wastes are expected to increase even more rapidly than population.[7] Unless dramatic changes are made in the existing production processes and energy utilization patterns of man, increases in consumption will continue to mean compounded increases in pollution. The paradox of man's behavior lies in his efforts to raise his material standard of living which has inevitably resulted in the destruction of pure water, clean air, plant and animal life, and ruination of the landscape that contribute to his well-being, health, and aesthetic pleasure.

Since man has conceptualized the planet earth as a self-contained space ship, he has also been faced with the reality that he can no longer dispose of his garbage merely by dumping it over his backyard fence. This is true whether he is seeking to dispose of aluminum cans or radioactive waste materials.

LIVING SPACE FOR MAN

In addition to the rising pollution problems resulting from the interaction of population growth, industrialization, urbanization, and increased consumption patterns, other factors have become significant in assessing the quality of life man enjoys—population density and the living space each person has at his disposal which may result in crowding. Although these two space factors are interrelated, they are not the same thing.

Population Density

Population density refers to the number of people per designated area and is most frequently calculated on the basis of a square mile. This gross index is an indication of the amount of land that is available in a given country to support each individual living in it. It indicates how much land is available to grow food, provide recreational space, erect homes, and accommodate other human uses.

The figures in Table 10-1 indicate the approximate populations, density, and land area for 12 selected countries. It will become apparent that population density varies among nations without regard to their global location or stage of technological development. For example, in the most populous nation in the world, China, the density is less than in some highly industrialized nations in Europe (West Germany, United Kingdom, France). Yet China's density is considerably higher than any country in North America (United States, Mexico, Canada). Comparison of population densities provides a gross basis for determining how much land is available for population expansion, but it does not provide any indication of how rich in mineral deposits the land is, nor does it tell about the topography which might make the land uninhabitable. These factors are important in determining the usability of the land.

In general, it can be said that countries with the most fertile soil, abundant water, moderate climates, and bountiful natural resources attract and support the highest number of people. This may be reflected in population density; however, population density alone does not indicate the standard of living of the population. Other factors, such as the status of technology, affect living standards more than the land-people ratio.

Crowding

Social scientists have turned increasing attention toward other factors of man-space relationships. In the face of burgeoning cities with crowded living conditions, a number of studies have been conducted to determine the effects of limited space on behavior. Citing evidence gained from observing the behavior of rats placed in overcrowded conditions, Edward T. Hall has attempted to project the effects of crowding on human behavior. Hall's analysis leads to the conclusion that the stress produced from overcrowdedness contributes to a sense of disorganization and ultimate breakdown of normal social relations among people. The term "behavioral sink" was used to designate the gross distortions of behavior among the rat population that was subjected to excessive crowding. Delinquency, sexual deviations, violence,

TABLE 10-1
POPULATION SIZE AND DENSITY FOR SELECTED COUNTRIES

Country	Approximate population (in millions)	Density per square mile	Area in square miles (in thousands)
China (Mainland)	730.0	197.8	3,690.5
India	524.0	415.3	1,261.5
Soviet Union	237.8	27.5	8,647.2
United States	202.0	**55.7**	3,614.3
Japan	101.0	708.0	142.8
West Germany	58.0	606.1	95.7
United Kingdom	55.3	586.9	94.2
France	50.3	238.3	211.2
Mexico	47.3	62.1	761.4
South Korea	30.5	801.6	38.0
Argentina	23.6	22.0	1,071.9
Canada	20.8	5.4	3,850.8

SOURCE: Compiled from the United Nations Statistical Office, 1968.

and crimes along with other symptoms of behavioral breakdowns such as drug addiction, mental illness, nervous tension, and other physical and psychological disorders are often attributed to the overcrowded and squalid conditions found in inner cities and ghettos, where as many as a quarter of a million human beings are crowded into a few square miles, as they are in Harlem.

Hall sums up his conclusion regarding overcrowding in cities with this statement:

The implosion of the world population into cities everywhere is creating a series of destructive behavioral sinks more lethal than the hydrogen bomb. Man is faced with a chain reaction and practically no knowledge of the structure of the cultural atoms producing it. If what is known about animals when they are crowded or moved to an unfamiliar biotope is at all relevant to mankind, we are now facing some terrible consequences in our urban sinks. Studies of ethology and comparative proxemics should alert us to the dangers ahead as our rural populations pour into urban centers. The adjustment of these people is not just economic but involves an *entire way of life.*[8]

Not all social scientists agree that overcrowding has the effects of which Hall warns. Opponents of Hall's theory say that crowding seems to have little effect on juvenile delinquency or mental illness. As evidence, they refer to the fact that New York City, which is the most densely populated city in the United States, has a lower crime rate than many other cities. More important, within New York City, areas with the highest densities do not necessarily have the highest crime rates. However, even those who do not agree that population density is a causative factor in social breakdown do find that lack of sufficient space in the home is associated with more crime, mental illness, and probably other forms of social disorientation.

Living space is related to status and economics not only in amount but also in quality. The high-status and upper-income individual has better space and more of it. Most attempts to equalize the situation on a limited scale seem to fail because persons with higher incomes also have greater mobility and will move to places where more space is available and where their prerogatives will be recognized.[9] It is not surprising that people will avoid juvenile delinquency, congestion, and air and noise pollution if they can. Thus, the last two decades have seen a mass migration of families from the city to the suburbs. This move has been largely among the middle-income and higher-income population who have abandoned the core city and left behind concentrated populations of the elderly, nonwhite, and low-income families. Although the blighted living conditions of the inner city may have been reason enough to escape, the suburb, in many cases, was no utopia. Lack of architectural imagination, conformity, poor construction, and social isolation were often the price for families who sought to own their homes on a 50 ft × 100 ft treeless lot. The move of many families to suburban developments only postponed rather than eliminated the declining social and living conditions.

POPULATION AND LIVING STANDARDS

Before discussing the implications of family planning as it affects the individuals involved, it might be useful to summarize a few generalizations about population and its impact on standards of living.

1 With the present status of technology and social organization among nations, there is little possibility of raising the material standard of living for the vast majority of people living in underdeveloped nations to the level enjoyed by those living in developed nations. As the population in the underdeveloped countries multiplies, the likelihood of raising its standard of living to western levels becomes even more remote.

2 There is a strong probability that the standard of living enjoyed by the developed nations will have to be modified, if not lowered, as more people in underdeveloped nations acquire and demand more material goods and as pollution becomes an increasing barrier to existing production methods.

3 The production processes and consumption patterns of modern man are creating pollution problems at a faster rate than he has been able or willing to solve. Therefore, even if population growth were not a

factor, man will have to improve his efforts to clean up the environment if he wishes to improve the living conditions of the millions of people who reside in urban centers.

4 The population base of the world is accelerating at an increasing pace with each generation. Although there is no known optimal long-range population level, given a finite set of resources to support and feed the population, growth cannot continue indefinitely. Therefore, man individually and collectively will ultimately have to face population control or a substantially reduced standard of living.

It has already been established that the efforts of the medical and health fields have resulted in lower mortality rates among all age groups. Therefore, reducing the birth rate will not, by itself, solve the population-related environmental problems faced by man. However, one cannot forego or eliminate the long-range consequences for man if birth rates are not reduced. The question is: How should the reduction be brought about?

REDUCTION OF BIRTH RATES

Many demographers have observed that certain conditions tend to reduce birth rates. Rapid economic development and rising manufacturing and industrial production accompanied by increasing urbanization and limited living space have resulted in a relative disadvantage for large families. The downward trend in birth rates in the United States strongly indicates that there has been a voluntary reduction in birth rates. This self-imposed reduction was noted five or more years before contraceptive pills became widely available or the intrauterine device (IUD) widely used. During the past decade birth rates in seven European countries have dropped below the replacement level. A half dozen other European countries are rapidly reaching the zero population growth (ZPG) level. Although the migration of workers between countries may distort the growth rate of some countries, taken as a whole, birth rates in both Eastern and Western Europe have shown an absolute decline.

In a number of other countries, most notably Sweden and Japan, declines in birth rates are attributed to legalized abortion rather than contraception. Sterilization by vasectomy of the male and tubectomy of the female has been used and promoted in a number of developing nations. India, for example, reported that 4 million males have been vasectomized during the past few years. However, it is also reported that sterilization among males in India has shown a decline in popularity despite measures to promote it. At the same time, sterilization procedures are gaining popularity in the United States. Although not as popular as oral contraceptives, used by an estimated 8 million persons in 1970, or the condom, employed by another 5 million, sterilization was obtained by an estimated 1 million Americans last year.

In 1965, more women than men requested the operation, but in 1970, 75 percent of the requests were from males. The Association for Voluntary Sterilization reports that the most frequent requests came from middle-aged fathers of three children. Another trend appears to be the rising number of calls for sterilization from younger people and from people with no children.[10]

Reduced birth rates have also been attributed to a number of changes in social patterns and institutions. It is claimed that postponement of marriage until a later age has helped reduce birth rates in Mainland China. It is noteworthy that the number of marriages in the United States has shown a declining trend during the early 1970s. What the long-range effects of postponed marriages or reduction in the number of marriages will be on birth rates is yet to be measured; however, if the pattern of the past decade continues, the developed nations will see a substantial reduction in average family size by 1980. Presently in the United States the average completed family size includes 2.7 children; by 1980 it is expected to drop to 2.4 children.

Barriers to Population Control

Proponents of ZPG have launched a strong campaign against reproduction. Neutral observers could easily conclude that if antipopulation groups have their way man would soon become an endangered species. Although there are signs, most notably in more developed nations, that reduced birth rates can and will be attained, there are many widespread factors that militate against sustained reduction in birth rates. Paul R. Ehrlich discussed one of the deep-rooted barriers to birth control in his book on population growth:

> Billions of years of evolution have given us all a powerful will to live. Intervening in the birth rate goes against our evolutionary values. During all those centuries of our evolutionary past, the individuals who had the most children passed on their genetic endowment in greater quantities than those who reproduced less. Their genes dominate our heredity today. All our biological urges are for more reproduction, and they are all too often reinforced by our culture. In brief, death control goes with the grain, birth control against it.[11]

In addition to cultural habits, other social and political forces oppose the practice of birth control or abortion. For example, some nations promote the theory that a larger population will contribute to their own political, economic, or military power. Some nations have and do reward marriage and childbirth with acclaim or actual financial benefits.

Although many nations do not overtly reward childbirth or large families, there is still a strong cultural belief that growth is good. It may make little difference as to the type of growth—gross national product, number of cars produced, tons of steel, sales volume, or population—as long as the current figures show increases over previous ones. Cities take pride in their population increases between censuses. Nations look to their increased numbers for military strength and a larger labor supply. As long as a culture treats quantitative increases as having intrinsic value, there will be little substantial action to make anything smaller. This will be true whether one is dealing with population or the number of automobiles produced. Thus, population will tend to increase in such a culture because of the implicit sanction given to growth.

For some people a major barrier to birth control is direct religious opposition, most notably the Roman Catholic Church. On numerous occasions Pope Paul VI has expressed the attitude of the church toward artificial birth control.

> Instead of increasing the supply of bread on the dining table of the hunger-ridden world, as modern techniques of production can do today, some are thinking in terms of diminishing, by illicit means, the number of those who eat with them. This is unworthy of civilization.[12]

Opposition to "illicit means" of birth control will undoubtedly delay the reduction of birth rates in underdeveloped nations where a large portion of the population is Roman Catholic. Time will tell whether the Roman Catholic Church will change its position about birth control or whether developing nations in the sphere of its influence can gain a foothold on economic progress so that reduced birth rates will occur as they did prior to widespread use of contraceptive technology in the advanced nations.

If all political and religious sources of resistance to contraception were eliminated, the long-range effectiveness of birth control methods in many underdeveloped nations would still depend upon the development and implementation of inexpensive, less burdensome methods than presently exist. In many countries the level of illiteracy is a hindrance to widespread distribution of information and medical advice on family planning and birth control. Pills that must be taken daily will no doubt have to be replaced by methods that may last for longer periods of time if contraception is to become truly workable for many women who are confused about present methods. Perhaps the future lies with the development of a safe temporary male sterilization technique.

THE DECISION TO PLAN A FAMILY

Although proponents of ZPG often give the doctrinaire impression that *no* family should have more than two children (i.e., replacement of the parents), most groups encouraging family planning emphasize that it is a means for *spacing* children as well as regulating their number. Most parents when considering family planning are not concerned with futuristic abstractions or global population forecasts. They are more directly concerned with their own physical ability and psychological willingness to incur the added responsibility for rearing a child.

This poses questions that each family must be prepared to answer. After careful consideration some couples may decide that despite cultural pressures they will remain childless. Others may find that despite the publicity of ZPG they want to have more than two children. In either case family planning has stressed the right of parents to have the number of children they want, not the right of society (church, government, and so on) to have the number of children it needs. When the majority of parents want children, population will continue to increase. Thus, many population and environmental experts agree that the effectiveness of a self-limiting population is dubious when the decision to procreate remains with the discretion of the parents. Yet the idea that anyone else should share in the decision is regarded by many as an extreme danger to personal freedom.

Although the self-limiting population concept may prove inadequate over the long run, there is little chance that it can succeed if man remains unaware of the human and environmental consequences of overpopulation and the role each individual plays in creating such a condition.

REFERENCES

1 Carvell, Fred, and Max Tadlock: *It's Not Too Late*, Glencoe Press, Beverly Hills, Calif., 1971, pp. xix-xx.

2 Environmental Education Studies Staff: excerpts from the *Environmental Education Act, 1970*, Office of Education, U.S. Department of Health, Education, and Welfare, 1970.

3 Brody, Samuel: "Facts, Fables, and Fallacies on Feeding the World Population," in Paul Shepard and Daniel McKinley (eds.), *The Subversive Science*, Houghton Mifflin, Boston, 1969, p. 74.

4 Kormondy, Edward J.: *Concepts of Ecology*, Prentice-Hall, Englewood Cliffs, N.J., 1969, p. 83.

5 For further discussion on the impact of limited birth rates on the population of specific countries in the world see *The Two-child Family and Population Growth; An International View*, compiled by the U.S. Bureau of the Census, Superintendent of Documents, U.S. Government Printing Office, Washington, D.C., 1970.

6 Rienow, Robert, and Leona Train Rienow: *Moment in the Sun*, Ballantine Books, New York, 1967, p. 3.

7 Lamson, Robert W.: "The Future of Man's Environment," *The Science Teacher*, vol. 36, no. 1, January 1969.

8 Hall, Edward T.: *The Hidden Dimension*, Doubleday, Garden City, N.Y., 1966, p. 155.

9 Sommer, Robert: "Planning *Not Place* for Nobody," *Saturday Review*, April 5, 1969, p. 69.

10 Tuthill, Sue: "Today's Health News," *Today's Health*, October 1971, p. 8.

11 Ehrlich, Paul R.: *The Population Bomb*, Ballantine Books, New York, 1968, p. 34.

12 Excerpts from Pope Paul VI, *Christmas Message to the World*, 1963.

11 | INFERTILITY

Elizabeth M. Edmands

Family planning in its broadest sense encompasses the desire on the part of the couple to determine whether or not they will have children, how many, and at what intervals they will conceive. Currently the emphasis is on curbing a rapidly expanding population in the United States and abroad. However, this situation has little meaning for most couples who are having difficulty in producing at least one child of their own. *Infertility* is a relative term implying inability to have children as readily as most couples do. The terms sterility and infertility are commonly used interchangeably, but *sterility* actually represents the incapacity to conceive.

Nursing has been involved for many years in the education, counseling, and care of persons who seek assistance for the problem of infertility. New knowledge and techniques of diagnostic and therapeutic procedures have had a profound effect on the nature and extent of nursing responsibilities in this area. They call for all the sensitivity, compassion, and understanding the nurse can give, for they involve not only intimate relationships between the couple, but also a need for confidence and trust in the professional staff.

HISTORICAL PERSPECTIVE

Man may not have realized the relationship between coitus and pregnancy until he was well along in his intellectual development. However, we do have evidence that barrenness was recognized over 4,000 years ago (Egyptian medical papyri), and there are numerous references to it in the Old Testament. In the fifth century B.C. Hippocrates developed theories about woman's inability to conceive and wrote of his prescribed remedies. Soranus, a Greek physician in the second century, wrote a number of books on gynecology. His writings indicate that he recognized the relation of emotional factors and good physical health to conception.

It was not until the year 1677 that Leeuwenhoek and his German medical student, Ham, while examining human semen, saw what they called animalcules through a simple microscope. There were spermatozoa. It was also in the seventeenth century that de Graaf described the ovarian follicle, but not until 1827 did von Baer see the first ovum.[1]

Numerous were the contributions of many medical scientists to the development of knowledge both before and after these critical discoveries. Names such as Rubin (tubal insufflation), Knaus-Ogino (fertile-infertile period), and Klinefelter (chromosomal abnormalities) are prominent today. These men and others did their work in the twentieth century. Less than 100 years ago, experts were writing that the best time to achieve pregnancy was just before and after the menstrual period. They even hypothesized that male children were conceived premenstrually and females postmenstrually. Therefore, it is evident that scientific diagnostic procedures and treatment of infertility are modern accomplishments, based on concepts that had their origin in antiquity but their critical refinements only in this century.

There have been few religious prohibitions to the procedures involved in the study of infertility. A notable exception is the objection of the Roman Catholic Church and strict Orthodox Jews to masturbation, withdrawal, or use of the condom to obtain semen samples for the study of the male factor.

INCIDENCE AND CAUSES

Fifteen percent of all couples will experience difficulty in producing a child. They are either infertile or sterile. The drive to reproduce is nearly universal, and failure to do so is regarded as a major tragedy in some cultures and some families. Fortunately for the infertile couple, the same search for an effective way to limit reproduction has provided insight into ways to stimulate it.

Infertility is found in all nations and all races. It occurs in all economic groups and social classes. However, there is a difference in its etiology depending on some of these factors. For example, in the United States in the lower-economic group, pelvic inflammatory disease and postabortal sepsis contribute to a high incidence of tubal closure. Behrman and Kistner state, "An overall review of recent literature dealing with the major causes of infertility reveals a gradient of this order: cervical factor, 20 percent; tubal factor, 30 to 35 percent; male factor, 30 to 35 percent; hormonal factor, 15 percent. Among private patients the cervical factor is much lower and the hormonal factor much higher."[2]

Four factors that contribute generally to a normal couple's ability to conceive are (1) the age of the female partner, (2) the age of the male partner, (3) the frequency of intercourse, and (4) the length of exposure. The peak of fertility in the female is reached at about twenty-four years of age. There is a gradual decline until about age thirty, then the decline becomes more rapid. It is a rare exception for pregnancy to occur after the female is fifty years of age. The male peak is also reached at twenty-four to twenty-five years. The decline is also gradual, but there are reported cases of male fertility remaining as late as eighty to ninety years of age.

It is estimated that a frequency of sexual intercourse averaging four times per week is most likely to produce conception in a 6-month period. Depending on all other factors, average couples not using contraception will conceive at the rate of 25 percent the first month, 65 percent in 6 months, 80 percent in a year, and 90 percent in 18 months.[3]

Infertility often has multiple causes. There are male and female factors and those that relate to the couple as a unit. For each partner these factors can be grouped as general, developmental, endocrine, and genital disease. For the couple as a unit, there are the factors of sexual knowledge and adjustment, immunologic incompatibility, and minor factors which might not be significant in one partner, but in combination produce a subfertile threshold.[4]

In spite of the fact that infertility management has made considerable progress, there will remain from 5 to 10 percent of all couples for whom no medical reason for their barrenness can be determined.[5]

DIAGNOSTIC APPROACH AND THERAPY

The Couple

Although it is usually the female partner who first seeks medical assistance for infertility, it is considered unwise to subject her to more than the most simple diagnostic procedures unless the male partner also agrees to an evaluation. The couple is entitled to a full explanation of the tests and procedures involved and the reasons why they are done. An overall plan is made in progressive steps, and testing usually continues until critical defects are found, pregnancy occurs, or the plan is completed. The length of time required is usually estimated from 6 to 18 months. The couple should fully understand what is expected of them, for their consistant cooperation is essential to the study. They will also want to know something about costs. These estimates will obviously vary according to the findings, but they should know that complex diagnostic evaluation or corrective surgical procedures requiring hospitalization will increase the costs of the investigation.

The decision of a couple to seek help with an infertility problem is frequently therapeutic in itself. Some physicians and infertility clinics report conception occurring before tests have been made or soon after—sometimes before any treatment is possible. It may be that there is improvement in psychological outlook, followed by release of tension when the couple realizes that their problem is not unique or that they have transferred their burden to someone who is skilled in helping them.[6]

The basic premise of fertility has been described in a booklet published by the American Fertility Society.[7] The following clear, concise statements describe quite simply what processes must take place in order for pregnancy to occur:

1 Male:
The husband must produce a sufficient number of normal, motile spermatozoa which have access through patent pathways to be discharged on ejaculation from the urethra.

2 Male and Female:
These spermatozoa must be deposited in the female in such a way that they reach and penetrate the cervical secretion, and ascend through the uterus to the tube at the time in the cycle appropriate for fertilization of the ovum.

3 Female:
The wife must produce a normal fertilizable ovum which must enter the fallopian tube within a period of a few hours, and become fertilized. The resulting conceptus must move into the uterus and implant in an adequately developed endometrium, and there undergo normal development.

In some women who have no other demonstrable cause for infertility, sperm-immobilizing or sperm-agglutinating antibodies have been found in the blood plasma. When the male partner uses a condom only and the woman does not use any vaginal lubricants, her titer of circulating antibodies tends to fall in time. These findings suggest that some women make antibodies to their male partner's sperm, and some become pregnant after the antibody titer falls.[8]

Couples need to realize that infertility problems may be complex, often involving psychosocial factors as well as physical impairments. Some couples will be extremely embarrassed because of the necessity to reveal aspects of the personal life which they have considered private. Infertility diagnosis and treatment can be a threatening experience for any couple. It can also be a time when wise counseling and skillful interpretation of findings can promote understanding and empathy between the couple regardless of the outcome of the investigation.

The Male Partner

Usually the male partner is referred to a urologist for diagnosis and evaluation. Only recently have some gynecologists included the actual examination and treatment of the male. In either case, close cooperation and coordination of testing and reporting are essential.

HISTORY

A complete history is of primary importance. This will include medical, social, sexual, and occupational factors. Medical factors of vital importance are past and present illnesses, especially mumps, orchitis, venereal diseases, and surgical procedures. Social habits to be noted include excessive smoking, alcoholism, and fatigue. Sexual aspects such as use of precoital lubricants, premature ejaculation, impotence, and coital positioning may all have significance. Occupational exposure to radioactive substances, gasoline and carbon monoxide fumes, excessive heat, or certain metals may be etiological factors. Prolonged excessive heat to the genital area may affect spermatogenesis.

EXAMINATION

Physical examination will include special emphasis on observation of secondary male characteristics, endocrinopathy, presence of congenital abnormalities such as undescended or atrophic testicles, hypospadias, cryptorchism, and absence of vas deferens.

LABORATORY STUDIES

Laboratory studies include those of basic routine evaluation appropriate for age or any presenting symptoms of pain or disfunction. Nearly all clinicians include tests for thyroid function and, if indicated, may add other endocrine studies. A complete semen analysis is usually done. Authorities differ on the number of specimens required, but if the first is abnormal, usually a minimum of three, collected at intervals of 2 to 4 weeks, are sufficient. A period of continence corresponding to the usual frequency of intercourse is recommended prior to obtaining the specimen. The specimen is obtained by masturbation or coitus interruptus and collected in a clean, dry, glass jar. It should be transported to the doctor's office as soon as possible and no later than 2 hours after collection.[9]

Factors and standards (not absolute) for examination of the seminal fluid are as follows:

1 Liquefaction: complete within 10 to 30 minutes
2 Volume: 2.5 to 5 cc
3 Motility: proportion forward moving related to time of ejaculation
4 Count: minimum normal 40 million per cc or a total count of 125 million per ejaculate
5 Morphology: normal sperm heads in 80 percent of count[10]

TREATMENT

In general, treatment of male infertility has been discouraging. Correction of underlying conditions affecting general health can be instigated. Elimination of external factors such as heat, radiation, or exposure to certain fumes and metals may be beneficial. Habits of excessive smoking, drinking, and fatigue can be curtailed. Surgical treatment of congenital abnormalities and obstructions may be possible. Coitus at regular intervals of approximately every 2 or 3 days will encourage sperm motility without appreciably decreasing sperm count. All these measures increase the probability of conception and certainly are in no way harmful. Frequently reassurance, instruction in coital techniques, and emphasis on timing of intercourse in relation to ovulation are helpful to the male partner who is subfertile but not sterile.

The Female Partner

Often the female partner who is having difficulty in achieving a pregnancy prefers to consult her own source of medical care first. This procedure is advisable for if there is any chronic medical condition or known abnormality, this information can be communicated on referral to the physician or infertility clinic. However, few general practitioners are equipped to do a complex study, and unless there is an obvious minor correctable condition, most generalists will not delay referral to a specialist. Infertility studies are ideally conducted by a team of specialists, such as gynecologists, endocrinologists, psychiatrists, and marriage counselors with consultation from others, depending on the nature of preliminary findings.

HISTORY

The history required of the female is even more detailed than that of the male partner. In addition to medical, surgical, and social factors, a complete menstrual history including onset, frequency, duration, pain, and amount of flow should be recorded. It is important to know about use of contraceptives —kind, duration and cessation of use, and side effects, if any. Coital frequency and timing in relation to ovulation must be explored. Other factors include vaginal and pelvic infections, abdominal and pelvic surgery, and use of intravaginal lubricants and douches.[11] If a previous pregnancy has been achieved, full details on the course and outcome are essentials. During history taking it is possible to obtain some estimate of the patient's attitudes toward coitus, marital relationships, and the degree of anxiety in relation to her failure to conceive.

If no previous evaluation of the time of ovulation has been made, the patient is instructed to keep a basal body temperature (BBT) chart. During the monthly cycle, women who ovulate have biphasic curves. As ovulation takes place within a 24- to 72-hour period of the temperature change, the woman who has uterine bleeding but is not ovulating does not have this biphasic pattern.[12]

EXAMINATION

A complete physical examination is performed, during which time observation is made of the general body contour, the relation of weight to height, breast development, and evidence of a female pattern of hair distribution. A thorough pelvic examination includes evaluation of any abnormality or infection. Specifically in relation to the patient's ability to conceive, the examiner evaluates the hymen, clitoris, cervical os, and the size and position of the uterus and also looks for evidence of tumors, malformations, or endometriosis.

LABORATORY STUDIES

Laboratory procedures begin with basic routine urinalysis, serological examination for syphilis, blood count, sedimentation rate, and chest x ray. Tests for thyroid function and a Papanicolaou smear are always done. If any purulent secretion is noted on vaginal examination, it should be stained and cultured for gonococci.[13] Some examiners also do a hanging drop slide for *Candida (Monilia)* and *Trichomonas*, especially when there is a complaint of dyspareunia. If there is a history of irregular menses, amenorrhea, hirsutism, acne, or excessive weight gain, basic endocrine studies are also done.

Three important diagnostic tests that can be done in the physician's office or on an outpatient basis are discussed in the following paragraphs:

The Sims-Hühner test is a postcoital examination of cervical mucus. It is done at the time of ovulation and from 1 to 12 hours after coitus. The purpose of the test is to determine sperm survival and motility. Also, the characteristics of the cervical mucus can be determined. Normally at ovulation it forms a thin, continuous thread when pulled apart (spinnbarkeit) and when dried on a slide takes on a fernlike pattern called aborization. Both of these phenomena disappear during the progesterone phase following ovulation.

The endometrial biopsy is performed to test for ovulation. The optimal time is the sixth to eighth day after the shift in BBT, or if this is obscure, at the first day of menstruation. It is then possible to determine whether uterine bleeding is anovulatory. If the biopsy shows abnormal tissue, it should be followed by curettage to be sure there is no malignancy.

Tubal insufflation is also known as the Rubin test. It is diagnostic but may also be therapeutic. The best time to perform the test is 3 to 4 days after menstruation. It is preceded by a pelvic examination to rule out any evidence of infection, which would be a contraindication. With the patient in the lithotomy position, carbon dioxide is introduced into the fallopian tubes, through the cervix and uterus. Pressure readings under normal conditions show a rise and fall. Also significant is the pain in the shoulder experienced by the woman with tubal patency. Tests should be repeated if pregnancy does not occur after a normal test or if there is evidence of obstruction.

As a result of these tests, other examinations may be indicated. *Hysterosalpingography* enables the examiner to investigate tubal patency by visualizing the tubes through fluoroscopic or x-ray examination. *Culdoscopy* is done as a hospital procedure, usually under spinal anesthesia. By injecting methylene blue into the cervix with the culdoscope in place, further visualization of the tubes is feasible. *Laparoscopy* is being done more frequently as instruments have been perfected. Some examiners believe this is preferable to culdoscopy because, if indicated, corrective procedures can be carried out immediately after the examination.[14]

TREATMENT

The defects found on examination of the female are more likely to be amenable to treatment than those of the male. However, the degree of severity, the type of defect found, and the relationship of multiple defects are critical factors in the probability that their correction will enable pregnancy to occur.

Estrogen deficiency may be treated with small doses of this hormone over a period of several months. Other endocrine defects may be more difficult to assess and treat in relation to infertility because of their complexity and interrelatedness. Anovulation is often successfully treated with drugs like clomiphene or human menopausal gonadotrophin. Removal of any vaginal or uterine obstruction to the flow of seminal fluid may require only a simple surgical procedure. Gradual dilation of a closed cervix and treatment of cervical inflammation with antibiotics have been used, but it is questionable how specific such measures are in improving the patient's fertility. Pelvic endometriosis may be treated both by surgery and by suppression with progestagens. Disease and obstruction of the oviducts are the commonest organic cause of infertility in women, and the treatment is usually plastic surgical repair.

The purpose of the complete diagnostic study is to uncover all contributing causes for infertility. Return of fertility is usually the result of a change of threshold, rather than the discovery and correction of a single blocking factor. Successful outcome in the study of infertility can be measured by the discovery of a cause or by an exhaustive study which determines no known medical impediment. Psychosomatic factors may impinge on the ultimate achievement of pregnancy in either of these groups. However, the supportive measures provided by skilled counseling have been known to be effective to the couple's resolution of their problem. This may be their ability to produce a child or successful adaptation to childlessness or adoption.

Alternatives

ADOPTION

For the couple found to be permanently sterile or even for the couple for whom no medical cause for infertility can be found, adoption may fulfill their desire to become parents. The physician usually is not equipped to make judgments or provide the complex guidance that prospective adopting parents need to determine if this course of action is advisable for them. It is his responsibility to see that those who desire to pursue adoption are referred to a responsible counselor or agency.

Not all couples who are unable to have children of their own can provide the care and nurturing needed by adopted children. Some couples who seek diagnostic help are motivated by a desire to know whether they are fertile or infertile so they can decide about continued use of contraceptives. Still others consider their infertility as evidence of something abnormal. They do not desire a child, but only reassurance of their normalcy.[15]

It is not as easy today to adopt a baby of the desired sex as it was a few years ago. Availability of contraception and abortion are decreasing the number of women who carry an unwanted pregnancy to term. However, older children, those of mixed race, and those with physical and mental deficiencies are still available and just as much in need of love and support. Wise counseling can often make such an adoption a satisfactory and fulfilling experience for the parents and the child.

There are few, if any, well-documented studies on the incidence of conception after adoption. Two studies, one of which was reported by Hanson and Rock[16] in 1950, and the other by Tyler, Bonapart, and Grant[17] in 1960, found very small percentages of adopting couples who later achieved pregnancy. Evaluation of couples who did conceive suggests that they may not have received an exhaustive infertility work-up or may have been among the 10 percent who spontaneously achieve pregnancy with or without adoption when no medical cause can be found. The reason that it is such a common belief that pregnancy follows adoption may be due to the drama involved or the optimistic expectations generated by this achievement when all the facts are not known.

ARTIFICIAL INSEMINATION

There are two types of artificial insemination possible today. They are known as AIH (artificial insemination by husband) and AID (artificial insemination by donor).

For those couples in whom no medical pathology can be found and yet pregnancy does not occur, the physician may suggest that a semen specimen from the husband (AIH) be introduced by syringe into the vagina at the mouth of the cervix. This is a simple procedure which is timed to coincide with the ovulation period. Usually three inseminations are carried out each cycle over a period of three months or until pregnancy is achieved.[18]

When it has been proved by exhaustive study that the male is azoospermic but the female is capable of producing a child, the couple may want to consider artificial insemination by a donor (AID). Although this is a medically sound procedure, it may have legal complications in some states. Further discussion of technique, medical and legal aspects, and social implications may be found in specialized texts dealing more extensively with this subject.

NURSING INVOLVEMENT
Case-finding, Counseling, and Referral

A nurse living or working in a community will need to be sensitive to local attitudes toward women's roles, motherhood, parenthood, and the meaning of children. Since the desire for children is nearly universal, no matter what motivates that desire, it is fairly certain that most married couples expect to produce a child within 3 or 4 years.

In many situations, whether at work or as a neighbor in the community, a friendly, approachable nurse may be the first person to learn that a woman or a couple are doubtful about their ability to conceive. Others, however, will be reluctant to initiate a query because of embarrassment or lack of knowledge that anything can be done. Perhaps the first manifestations may be marital stress or physical and emotional symptoms.

How can these couples who need help be approached? There is a time for subtle suggestion, and there is a time for the direct approach. When nurses must talk about any delicate or serious problem, they try to find a time when privacy can be assured, when the subject can be introduced naturally into a conversation, and when the recipients of their messages are most likely to understand. When the subject is infertility, they may expect that this emotionally charged topic can bring forth denial, resentment, blame toward anyone but self, and frequently profound grief. One woman described her reaction: "I've been frantic to talk about this to someone. I'm glad you brought it up, but now I feel exposed."[19] Mixed reactions are common, but when handled by a skillful, compassionate interviewer, there is usually relief and gratitude.

Perhaps one of the most important things for the nurse to know is that any couple who desire a child and have cohabited normally for a year without using contraceptives are entitled to a full infertility evaluation. If either partner is over thirty-five years of age, they should be referred for medical help after 6 unsuccessful months.[20]

Public health nurses working in their districts are frequently approached by a mother-in-law, a relative, or a neighbor to ask what can be done. This situation can involve sensitive and complex relationships. Two actions are possible. Preferably, nurses can suggest that the woman or couple be referred to them for discussion and information. If this seems unlikely to happen, then necessary knowledge and means of referral to competent resources should be given.

It is not always the couple who has never reproduced that needs counsel; it may be the couple with one child who is experiencing problems with a second conception. Age and the interval since last delivery are critical factors. Those couples who have been using contraceptives and stop because they desire a pregnancy should be counseled regarding expectations and medical intervention if they are not successful. The interval will depend on age and the type of contraceptive used.

Counseling in infertility requires that the nurse be knowledgeable about human reproductive anatomy and physiology, sexual practices such as frequency and timing of intercourse, likelihood of conception for age and length of coital exposure, procedures involved in male and female fertility investigations, and available resources for referral. The nurse also must be able to gauge the amount of information that can be absorbed by the particular individual or couple at a given time. The first objective may be simply to establish a comfortable relationship that will invite discussion.

Procedures in counseling will vary with the situation. A formal or informal history is often the opening wedge to ascertain the direction for further exploration. If the counseling is in response to a query, a base line of the couple's knowledge needs to be established before the counselor can proceed.

Even today there are married couples with an abysmal lack of knowledge of how conception takes place. Many do not understand when ovulation occurs or that it is of short duration. Old wives' tales and superstitions abound, not only in the poorly educated, but in some who give an outward appearance of sophistication. Perhaps it is in this basic teaching that nurses can make a unique contribution. Women who have doubts or apprehension about intimate, personal female problems are far more likely to seek out another woman, and particularly a nurse, whom they believe has the answers. The male nurse also has a unique contribution to make in relation to the male sex partner. Answers to some of these questions may be all that is needed by some couples in order to achieve a pregnancy.

Referral procedures will vary with the circumstances within which the case-finding and counseling take place. It is obvious that those who have a private physician should be referred to this source first. If there is an infertility clinic within the community, medical referral may be required. If so, a medical clinic or private physician may be the actual referring agent. However, the nurse should be knowledgeable about resources within the community, state, or region and about costs, eligibility, and the number of visits usually required for a basic evaluation. This information can be helpful to the couple seeking advice and may enable the nurse to work in partnership with the physician to provide a supporting referral team.

Care and Support

After the couple have been referred to a diagnostic resource, they may still need the interest and encouragement that can be provided by the referring nurse. Inquiry regarding progress and further clarification of the reasons for procedures may provide the stimulus to continue the diagnostic process. The public health nurse is often in a position to give such continuity of care.

The nurse working in an infertility clinic or with the physician who is carrying out the procedures has a critical role to perform. The female nurse will relate closely to the woman, and the male nurse can be helpful to the man. A dignified yet friendly approach, an unhurried manner, patience, and understanding are qualities that can make the nurse an invaluable member of the examining team.

Although procedures may have been explained innumerable times, the patients in their anxiety often have questions about these procedures or want reassurance that a test is really needed. Nurses learned long ago that patients frequently wish to appear self-confident, knowledgeable, and unafraid before their physician but will express their concerns and ask for interpretation of information from the nurse. This pattern should not be discouraged, nor the fact belittled, for each profession has its own role in relation to the patient.

Some of the procedures may be painful, unpleasant, tedious, and require repetition. A nurse who can explain the procedure and inform the patients what is expected of them will not only make the procedure more endurable, but may actually encourage the relaxation that is essential for the test or treatment to be properly done. During the gynecological examinations, the female patient appreciates a kind, sympathetic nurse by her side who can anticipate her needs or ease her discomforts.

Nurses must be aware that both partners are under stress and that it will increase as procedures become more complex. For the patient and the staff, each test holds the expectation that it will reveal what is wrong. While waiting for the results of these tests, hopes may soar that a remediable defect will be found. It is one of the few situations in which the determination of medical normalcy is not always a welcome diagnosis.

Coordination with Other Disciplines

Throughout the nurse's contact with the patient or couple, more information will be received. Some of it will have little pertinence to the evaluation, but some may be highly significant. A nurse who is alert and sensitive to subtle clues and has the judgment to decide their relevance is a great asset.

Opportunities for communication and coordination of activities with other disciplines occur under a variety of circumstances. Prior to referral nurses may need to discuss their plans with the local physician or a social worker. At the time of referral, their knowledge of the situation relayed by telephone or written report may give focus to an immediate problem or to a complex, involved background. The nurse in the infertility clinic or specialist's office will work closely with other members of the team. Communication with others, such as the physician, the marriage counselor, the social worker, or the psychologist, will take place during routine procedures as well as at case conferences.

Nurses engaged in multiphasic screening may be the first to detect unrecognized or subconscious infertility among apparently normal persons. In counseling patients who are getting contraceptives or abortion, a nurse must be aware of their interrelatedness to infertility. When appropriate, such information should be given to the couple. In areas of the country where health manpower is scarce, physicians may not be able to give as high a priority to infertility as to lifesaving measures. It may be that a well-informed nurse can provide the counseling, referral, and guidance that is needed in many of these circumstances.

REFERENCES

1 Guttmacher, A. F.: "Past Attitudes Especially toward Female Infertility," in C. A. Joel, *Fertility Disturbances in Men and Women*, S. Karger, Basel, Switzerland, 1971, pp. 317–326.
2 Behrman, S. J., and R. W. Kistner: "A Rational Approach to the Evaluation of Infertility," in *Progress in Infertility*, Little, Brown, Boston, 1968, p. 1.
3 Ibid., p. 3.

4 Ibid., p. 6.

5 Ibid., p. 3.

6 Ward, Mildred W.: "One Thousand Pregnancies in Infertility Cases," *International Journal of Fertility*, 10:7, 1965.

7 *How to Organize a Basic Study of the Infertile Couple*, The American Infertility Society, Birmingham, 1970.

8 Personal communication from Dr. Robert W. Noyes.

9 *How to Organize a Basic Study of the Infertile Couple*, op. cit., p. 11.

10 Ibid., pp. 11–12.

11 Behrman and Kistner: op. cit., p. 10.

12 Iorio, Josephine: "Infertility and Sterility," in Josephine Iorio (ed.), *Principles of Obstetrics and Gynecology for Nurses*, 2d ed., Mosby, St. Louis, 1971, p. 360.

13 Behrman and Kistner: op. cit., p. 12.

14 Ibid., pp. 13–17.

15 Iorio: op. cit., p. 355.

16 Hanson, F. N., and J. Rock: "The Effect of Adoption on Fertility and Other Reproductive Functions," *American Journal of Obstetrics and Gynecology*, 59:311, 1950.

17 Tyler, E. T., J. Bonapart, and J. Grant: "Occurrence of Pregnancy Following Adoption," *Fertility and Sterility*, 11:581, 1960.

18 Guttmacher, A.: *Birth Control and Love*, Macmillan, New York, Bantam edition, p. 233.

19 Personal communication.

20 Guttmacher: *Birth Control and Love*, p. 203.

BIBLIOGRAPHY

Behrman, S. J.: "Management of Infertility," *American Journal of Nursing*, 66:552–555, 1966.

————: "The Complete Fertility Work-up," *Hospital Practice*, October, 1966, p. 50.

Cavanaugh, John A.: "Rhythm of Sexual Desire in Women," *Medical Aspects of Human Sexuality*, 3:29, 34, 35, 39, 1969.

Dillon, Harriet B.: "The Woman Patient," *Nursing Clinics of North America*, 3:195–203, 1968.

Kaufman, Sherwin A.: *A New Hope for the Childless Couple*, Simon and Schuster, New York, 1970.

————: "Impact of Infertility on the Marital Sexual Relationship," *Fertility and Sterility*, 20:380, 1969.

————: "Male and Female Infertility: In an Age of Population Explosion, Why a Child Isn't Born," *Medical Insights*, 3:14–21, 1971.

————: "Physical Clues to Sexual Maladjustment in Women," *Medical Aspects of Human Sexuality*, 4:38, 1970.

Kleegan, Sophia J., and Sherwin A. Kaufman: *Infertility in Women*, Davis, New York, 1966.

McCulley, Lee B.: "Health Counseling of Women," *Nursing Clinics of North America*, 3:263–273, 1968.

Novak, E., and Seegar G. Jones: *Novak's Textbook of Gynecology*, 7th ed., Williams & Wilkins, Baltimore, 1965.

Westin, Bjorn, and Nils Wisvist (eds.): *Fertility and Sterility: Proceedings of the Fifth World Congress*, Excerpta Medica Foundation, New York, 1967.

12 | ABORTION

Sandra L. Berry

Nurses have been caring for women having therapeutic abortions for years. Today, many nurses are caring for women having legally induced abortions. What is the difference between legally induced abortion and therapeutic abortion? Historically, therapeutic abortion has referred to those which were done on the basis of poor health of the mother and were usually recommended by several physicians. In some states women, or women and their husbands, now have the opportunity to decide if they want to continue a pregnancy, and after consulting a physician, they may be eligible for an abortion. The indications for legally induced abortions vary, depending on the individual state law; however, the major reason is an unwanted pregnancy. These indications may include mental or physical health, probable fetal deformity, rape or incest, or social problems; in some instances, request by the pregnant woman is the only indication necessary. The two terms, therapeutic and legally induced, have become synonymous in medical usage. Abortion, as used throughout this chapter, refers to legally induced abortions performed under the auspices of the new state laws.

As laws change and abortion becomes socially acceptable, nurses throughout the United States will be caring for women who elect to undergo these procedures. Therefore, it is the nurses' responsibility to be aware of the facts regarding abortions and the effects on the women having them as well as the effects on the nurses who are giving care.

HISTORICAL PERSPECTIVE

Even the earliest written records give evidence that physicians and scholars have had something to say about abortion. Some were concerned about the ability of a family or a state to care for a large number of children. Others sought a means to select for survival only those who were physically and mentally sound. Still others were interested in finding a safe way for a woman to rid herself of a pregnancy that was poorly timed or sired by the wrong male.

Apparently, in these ancient times abortion brought forth few feelings of condemnation, for the custom was universally practiced. Often the failure to dislodge a fetus or the birth of an unwanted child resulted in the practice of infanticide, the exposure of an infant to harsh elements and lack of care or feeding.

In the royal archives of China about 3000 B.C., the first description of an abortive technique was recorded. In 1550 B.C. the Egyptian papyri also recorded abortion methods. The Greek philosopher Aristotle recommended that abortion take place "before life and sense have begun," especially for those who have "an aversion to exposure of offspring."[1]

Early Greek, Roman, and Egyptian writings contained many descriptions of methods, ranging from herbs to foreign objects inserted in the vagina to produce irritation of the uterus. Few advocated surgery, although some gynecological instruments had already been developed. Although Hippocrates is credited with stating opposition to abortion in his famous oath, recent scholars have questioned whether the antiabortion section may not have been written by his disciples, the Pythagoreans, who believed that the soul was present from the moment of conception.[2]

It is over the issue of *when life begins* that most legal, moral, and religious controversies have taken place throughout the centuries. Some writers express the view that even now "we seem no nearer agreement than the Greeks."[3] Aristotle claimed that the soul entered the body 40 days after conception for the male and 80 days for the female. Plato, at about the same time, was arguing that life begins at birth. At the other extreme, the Stoics maintained that the soul was infused at puberty.[4] It is evident that individual philosophers and scientists had many different opinions, and also that these opinions influenced how society dealt with this issue in relation to abortion at different periods of time.

The early Judean and Christian teaching about the value of an individual life had the strongest influence on the moral issue. "In actuality, previous to 1803, abortion appears to have been largely regarded as a church offense and was punishable only by religious penalties. The first English Abortion Statute, the law of 1830, made abortion a crime."[5] No one knows for certain what combination of circumstances motivated the passage of this law at this time. Possibly widespread disease, infanticide, poverty, and high death rates were providing little enticement for couples to attempt to raise large numbers of children, and the government decided to intercede.

In 1821, Connecticut became the first state to pass an abortion law. Throughout the remainder of the nineteenth century various states gradually developed their own laws. A number of factors influenced the adoption of these laws. Prior to these statutes, abortion was done chiefly by barbers, who also did minor surgery and bloodletting to cure various ailments. Gold was discovered in 1849, and the Civil War lasted from 1861 to 1865. The need to settle the West was hindered by the loss of life from war casualties and by the increased demand for abortion due to wartime pregnancies. This demand brought unskilled, unscrupulous amateurs into the abortion business, and as a result, the maternal mortality rate soared. Legislators sought some way to stem the practice and to increase the birth rate so they made abortion a criminal offense. It is pertinent to note that in the impetus for enactment in most states, neither ethics nor religion played a major part.[6] However, the latter part of the century was also the Victorian era, noted for adherence to Puritanical concepts of sin. The pregnant unmarried girl had to be punished and was not allowed to conceal evidence of her wrongdoing. Abortion would have removed this evidence.[7] So the laws on the books were made more stringent by revision and by stronger attempts at enforcement.

In spite of the fact that there was no national law and each state had enacted its own legislation, there were few changes during the first half of the twentieth century. By midcentury, evidence accumulated that demand for abortion had reached a figure equal to a substantial proportion of live births. In the face of this demand only a small percentage were done by physicians in hospital settings, and illegal abortion has flourished.[8] Only in the last two decades has there been an attempt to inform the public of the horrors that take place in the clandestine, degrading, unclean places of most illegal abortionists. Lader states, "Untrained and often thoroughly incompetent abortionists are surely the most terrifying product of the underworld which feeds on the abortion system."[9]

ABORTION REFORM

"The first decisive move for reform in either Britain or the United States originated in 1938 in the solitary courage of an eminent London surgeon, Aleck Bourne."[10] A fourteen-year-old girl had been raped by soldiers, and Bourne decided to perform an abortion and then notify the police. This test case made medical history and his acquittal provided the first liberalized guidelines for practicing physicians.

Four European countries—Sweden, Denmark, Norway, and Iceland—pioneered in abortion reform to produce laws that allowed for liberalization

TABLE 12-1
MAJOR CATEGORIES OF ABORTION LAWS IN THE UNITED STATES,
JANUARY 1, 1971

Major categories of state abortion laws	*States having similar abortion laws*
I Abortion allowed only when necessary to preserve the life of the pregnant woman.	Arizona, Connecticut, Florida, Idaho, Illinois, Indiana, Iowa,* Kentucky, Louisiana,† Maine, Michigan, Minnesota, Missouri, Montana, Nebraska, Nevada, New Hampshire, North Dakota, Ohio, Oklahoma, Rhode Island, South Dakota, Tennessee, Utah, Vermont, West Virginia, Wyoming
II Indications for legal abortion include threats to the pregnant woman's life and forcible rape.	Mississippi
III "Unlawful" or "unjustifiable" abortions are prohibited.	Massachusetts, New Jersey, Pennsylvania
IV Abortions allowed when continuation of the pregnancy threatens the woman's life or health.	Alabama
V American Law Institute Model Abortion Law: "A licensed physician is justified in terminating a pregnancy if he believes that there is substantial risk that continuance of the pregnancy would gravely impair the physical or mental health of the mother or that the child would be born with grave physical or mental defect, or that the pregnancy resulted from rape, incest or other felonious intercourse."	Arkansas, California (does not include fetal deformity), Colorado, Delaware, Kansas, Maryland (does not include incest), New Mexico, North Carolina, South Carolina, Virginia
VI Abortion law based on the May 1968 recommendations of the American College of Obstetricians and Gynecologists allows abortion when the pregnancy resulted from felonious intercourse, and when there is risk that continuance of the pregnancy would impair the physical or mental health of the mother: "In determining whether or not there is substantial risk (to the woman's physical or mental health), account may be taken of the mother's total environment, actual or reasonably foreseeable."	Oregon
VII No legal restriction on reasons for which an abortion may be obtained prior to viability of the fetus.	Alaska, Hawaii, New York, Washington

VIII	Legal restrictions on reasons for which an abortion may be obtained were invalidated by court decisions.	District of Columbia, Georgia, Texas, Wisconsin‡

* *State v. Dunklebarger*, the Iowa statute which is couched in terms of saving the life of the woman, has been interpreted to suggest that preservation of health is sufficient. 221 N.W. 592 (Iowa, 1928)

† Although the Louisiana abortion statute does not contain an expressed exception to the "crime of abortion," the Louisiana Medical Practice Act authorizes the Medical Board to suspend or institute court proceedings to revoke a doctor's certificate to practice medicine in the state when the doctor has procured or aided or abetted in the procuring of an abortion "unless done for the relief of a woman whose life appears imperiled after due consultation with another licensed physician." La. Rev. Stat. Ann. 37:1261.

‡ The abortion laws of several other states have been ruled unconstitutional by lower state trial courts; however, these decisions are binding only in the jurisdiction in which the decision was rendered.

SOURCE: From table 21, U. S. Department of Health, Education, and Welfare, Public Health Service, "Abortion Surveillance Report—Legal Abortions, United States Annual Summary, 1970," *Center for Disease Control: Family Planning Evaluation*, p. 39.

for "humanitarian" needs. Howerver, none of these countries has approached the marked permissiveness found in Japan or other Eastern European countries. In spite of this movement for reform, abortion is still prohibited except for medical emergencies in nearly two-thirds of the world.[11]

As of 1971, one of the countries in which abortion was still restricted was the United States. The American Law Institute in 1962 developed a model code which has been used as a basis for most of the reform legislation to date. In 1967, Colorado was the first state to adopt new legislation, and within the next 4 years, 16 other states passed modifications of their original laws.[12] Four of these states—Alaska, Hawaii, New York, and Washington—have been the most liberal. Their reform calls for no restrictions for the nonviable fetus and provides for "abortion on demand" or arrangements that can be made between the patient and her physician.

ATTITUDES OF MAJOR RELIGIONS

In the United States, attitudes toward abortion and consequently abortion reform are influenced by the positions of its three major religions, Roman Catholicism, Judaism, and Protestantism. In other parts of the world where one religion predominates in a country, the position closely adheres to the accepted attitude of that specific faith. Neither Buddhist nor Hindu theology contains any scriptural prohibitions against early abortion. Islam prescribes to the belief that life begins after 150 days, and Shinto holds that life begins at birth. Therefore, the debate over abortion as a moral or ethical issue rarely occurs for them.

The Roman Catholic Church has taken a firm position on abortion. Since 1869 when the church abolished the 40- and 80-day theories of animation, it has strictly prohibited abortion when termination of pregnancy is the prime motive for the operation. Only when there is underlying pathology for which an operative procedure is required and the termination is a natural by-product is it tolerated.[13] The church has been strong in its opposition to abortion reform, calling it an outrage against humanity. It deals harshly (by immediate excommunication) with those Catholics who deliberately procure an abortion or help someone to do so.

The Jewish theologians have been more flexible in their interpretation of when life begins. Although there is some disagreement among them, generally they consider the moment of ensoulment as belonging to those "secrets of God." They usually consider the fetus as part of the mother until it is born.[14] In this interpretation there is no conflict with their legal and ethical standards in relation to aborting a pregnancy. The Jewish position has been handed down by great rabbis and teachers through the centuries.[15] There may be some rejection of modern interpretation by Orthodox Jews, but in general, the emphasis has been on protecting the life of the mother.

The Protestant position can hardly be said to be uniform. There is wide range of belief of many religious tenets, which hold to positions of extreme conservatism and equally unrestricted liberalism. However, the National Council of Churches of Christ in 1961 issued a statement stressing the sanctity of potential life and condemning abortion as a method of birth control *but* approving hospital abortion "when the life or health of the mother is at stake." The General Assembly of the United Presbyterian Church issued a similar statement on policy in 1962. Prior to this in 1958, the Lambeth Conference which included representatives of the American Protestant Episcopal Church, as well as those of the Anglican Communion, also declared that abortion is allowed "at the dictate of strict and undeniable medical necessity."[16] Other denominations during the decade of 1960 through 1970 have brought the issue to their assemblies with the result that a number of them have issued statements equally free in their interpretation.

In many communities Protestant clergy and Jewish rabbis have formed Abortion Counseling Services. Their primary purpose is to provide guidance to qualified medical care as a deterrant to the use of the illegal abortionists. Some of these services also include provision for guidance to the woman or couple who wish to continue with the pregnancy but need medical or financial assistance.

HEALTH AND SOCIAL ASPECTS

Medical Contraindications

The issue of abortion is surrounded by multiple aspects of health and social concern. During the past decade the pace of attitudinal and technological changes has accelerated the need for legislative action. All of these changes are highly significant to the concepts and practice of nursing.

Medical indications for abortion as a lifesaving measure have decreased, and the focus has changed to concern for the health of the pregnant woman and the risk of a defective child. However, conditions such as hypertension, cardiac disorders, cancer of the breast or cervix, kidney disease, and psychiatric illness are still indications for medical intervention, depending on their severity. In some of the psychiatric indications such as severe psychoneurosis, previous postpartum psychosis, schizophrenia or neurological disease, mental deficiency and situational reactions, the decision to perform an abortion must be considered in relation to its effect on the woman's future mental health.[17]

The major studies involving the degree of psychological sequelae in women having legally induced abortions have been done in Sweden. These few studies show that the stronger the indication for abortion the greater the risk of unfavorable psychological sequelae. Approximately 25 percent of the women expressed mild to serious self-reproaches on follow-up 22 to 30 months later.[18]

The Osofskys studied psychological reactions to abortion in New York City in 1970.[19] They interviewed approximately 400 patients immediately after the procedure with the following results:

60 percent happy	15 percent unhappy
66 percent no guilt	6 percent guilt
78 percent relieved	9 percent angry

There were no significant negative sequelae. Positive attitudes of staff made for significant acceptance of the procedure.

More psychological studies of the effect of abortions are needed. Presently, research is being conducted on the psychological motivation of women requesting abortion, psychological sequelae as a result of abortion, and other ramifications. This is being explored in the United States and abroad.[20]

Threat of Deformity of the Child

Each year in the United States between 80,000 and 160,000 defective children are born.[21] In states in which reasons for abortion are reported, less than 1 percent have been performed on the indication of potential fetal abnormality.[22] Rubella during the first trimester, massive exposure to x rays, history of previous genetic defects, and the consumption of teratogenic drugs, prescribed or self-administered, are a threat of deformity to a fetus.

Two procedures are used to detect fetal deformities. Amniocentesis is a means of detecting a small percentage by microscopic examination of fetal cells. It is limited in use because of possible complications, such as infection or initiation of labor. When there is probable exposure to German measles, a positive rubella blood titer indicates the disease did occur. Most abnormalities will not be detected until birth or years after.

Age of the Mother

The age of the mother is an important consideration in determining the degree of pregnancy risk. Pregnancy before the age of sixteen and after forty is generally considered to involve increased risks of complications.

Rape or Incest

It has been calculated that there are approximately 800 rape-induced pregnancies in the United States per year.[23] It is often difficult for the woman who has been the victim of rape or incest to obtain an abortion. There may be complicated legal requirements of proof as well as state restrictions. Some women have abortions done under the guise of a psychiatric condition due to the emotional trauma of forcible rape.

Social or Family Problems

Social issues such as poverty, marital stress, unwanted pregnancy, and excess number of children do not elicit the same acute emotional impact as do issues such as rape or incest. However, these issues are the major reasons women seek abortion, both legal or illegal. Reports from the few studies, surveys, and lay literature concerning attitudes of nurses, physicians, and laymen reflect prevailing opposition to abortion for social reasons.[24-30] The controversy over legislation for abortion on request is another clue to the interest of society in the protection of the embryo.

INCIDENCE

Legal and Illegal Abortion

Nurses should be aware of the extent of society's demand for abortion. As abortion laws are being liberalized, the demands for abortion are coming from several sources: (1) women seeking therapeutic abortions, (2) women having criminal abortions, and (3) women with unwanted pregnancies who are not seeking abortions.[31] The demand for abortion increases dramatically following legal change.

Before any of the states changed their laws, the estimated number of therapeutic abortions performed annually in the United States was about 8,000.[31] Estimates on the number of illegal abortions per year in the United States were between 200,000 and 1,200,000.[31] In 1970 a total of 180,119 abortions were reported to the Center for Disease Control from 19 states, 13 hospitals, and the District of Columbia.[32]

Variables

In 1958 in a book she edited, Mary Calderone reported on a onetime Baltimore abortionist, Dr. Timanus, who told of having performed 5,210 abortions in a 20-year period. Of these abortions, the majority of women (84 percent) were between twenty-one and forty years old; 53 percent were married, and 35 percent were single. Of these patients, 3,149 had no children while 2,061 had one to five children; more than one-third of the women (35 percent) were between twenty-one and twenty-five years old, 24 percent were between twenty-six and thirty years old, and 25 percent were between thirty-one and forty years of age.[33]

The late Dr. Kinsey published a study of a sample of 8,000 white females with a pregnancy total of 6,300. Among all women in the sample ever married, 22 percent had abortions in marriage by the age of forty-five. Among all the single white females who had coitus, 20 percent had abortions.[34]

The foregoing statistics were from yesterday, before liberalization of laws began. Between January 1, 1967, and December 31, 1970, 16 states had passed new abortion laws.[35] Unfortunately, reporting systems are not in effect in each state. Based on the information that is available from selected states, it is possible to describe demographic characteristics of the population of women who have received legal abortions.

AGE

The age distribution of women who have had legal abortions (Table 12-2) shows the largest number of abortions (59.4 percent) were obtained by women between the ages of fifteen and twenty-four years. Unmarried women

TABLE 12-2
INDUCED ABORTION BY AGE IN SELECTED STATES, 1970*

Age groups	Number of abortions	Percent of total
Under 15	505	0.7
15–19	18,155	23.7
20–24	27,404	35.7
25–29	13,772	17.9
30–34	8,497	11.1
35–39	5,737	7.5
Over 40	2,294	3.0
Unknown	395	0.5
Total	76,759	100.0†

* Alaska, Colorado, Delaware, Georgia, Hawaii, New York City, Upstate New York, Oregon, and South Carolina.
† Note that the total is actually 100.1 because of rounding off of percentages. This applies to other tables in this chapter.
SOURCE: U.S. Department of Health, Education and Welfare, Public Health Service, "Abortion Surveillance Report—Legal Abortions, United States Annual Summary, 1970," *Center for Disease Control: Family Planning Evaluation*, p. 14.

under the ages of eighteen or twenty-one years, depending on state laws as to when a woman is of age, still have the disadvantage of required parental permission in most states and, as a result, are forced to carry unwanted pregnancies to term.

MARITAL STATUS

Table 12-3 shows that two-thirds of the women who received abortions were not married at the time of their abortions. The classification of unmarried women includes those who have never married and those who are separated, widowed, or divorced.

TABLE 12-3
INDUCED ABORTION BY MARITAL STATUS IN SELECTED STATES, 1970*

Marital status	Number of abortions	Percent of total
Married	10,344	33.4
Unmarried	20,647	66.6
Total	30,991	100.0

* Alaska, Delaware, Georgia, Maryland, Upstate New York, Oregon, and South Carolina.
SOURCE: U.S. Department of Health, Education and Welfare, Public Health Service, "Abortion Surveillance Report—Legal Abortions, United States Annual Summary, 1970," *Center for Disease Control: Family Planning Evaluation*, p. 17.

PARITY

Approximately one-half of the women (49.2 percent) who had abortions in the small number of reporting states had no living children (Table 12-4).

TABLE 12-4
INDUCED ABORTION BY PARITY IN SELECTED STATES, 1970*

Number of living children	Number of abortions	Percent of total
0	741	49.2
1	188	12.5
2	210	14.0
3	179	11.9
4	102	6.8
5	75	5.0
Unknown	10	0.7
Total	1,505	100.0

* Alaska, Georgia, and South Carolina.
SOURCE: U.S. Department of Health, Education and Welfare, Public Health Service, "Abortion Surveillance Report—Legal Abortions, United States Annual Summary, 1970," *Center for Disease Control; Family Planning Evaluation*, p. 20.

GESTATION

Most women have abortions performed in the 9th through 12th weeks of gestation. There is a fairly wide variation among these states as to when abortions are performed. Two-thirds were performed before the end of the 12th week of gestation and 97.5 percent by the end of the 20th week (Table 12-5).

TABLE 12-5
INDUCED ABORTION BY GESTATION IN SELECTED STATES, 1970*

Weeks of gestation at time of abortion	Number of abortions	Percent of total
Less than 9	2,768	19.4
9–12	6,712	47.1
13–16	2,220	15.6
17–20	2,187	15.4
21–25	255	1.8
More than 25	17	0.1
Unknown	85	0.6
Total	14,244	100.0

* Georgia, Hawaii, Maryland, Oregon, and South Carolina.
SOURCE: U.S. Department of Health, Education and Welfare, Public Health Service, "Abortion Surveillance Report—Legal Abortions, United States Annual Summary, 1970," *Center for Disease Control: Family Planning Evaluation*, p. 22.

INDICATIONS

The first four indications for abortion shown in Table 12-6 are the legal indications for abortion in states where the American Law Institute Model was

TABLE 12-6
INDICATIONS FOR INDUCED ABORTION IN SELECTED STATES, 1970*

Indication	Number of abortions	Percent of total
Mental health	15,103	76.6
Physical health	813	4.1
Risk of deformity to fetus	223	1.1
Rape or incest	173	0.9
Other	477	2.4
Unknown	2,933	14.9
Total	19,722	100.0

* Alaska, Colorado, Delaware, Georgia, Hawaii, Maryland, North Carolina, Oregon, South Carolina, and Virginia.
SOURCE: U.S. Department of Health, Education and Welfare, Public Health Service, "Abortion Surveillance Report—Legal Abortions, United States Annual Summary, 1970," *Center for Disease Control: Family Planning Evaluation*, p. 21.

adopted. The stated reason for most abortions listed under "other" was "unwanted pregnancy." Slightly more than 75 percent of these abortions were performed for mental health indications.

METHODS

Since most abortions were performed by the 12th week of gestation, the majority of women had a dilatation and curettage (D&C) or evacuation (D&E) procedure (Table 12-7). It appears that women are better educated concerning the safety of having abortions early in their pregnancies.

TABLE 12-7
PROCEDURES USED FOR INDUCED ABORTION IN SELECTED STATES, 1970*

Procedure	Number of abortions	Percentage of total
D&C	26,201	34.8
D&E	30,687	40.8
Saline induction	12,615	16.8
Hysterotomy	1,307	1.7
Hysterectomy	536	0.7
Other	74	0.1
Unknown	3,768	5.0
Total	75,188	100.0

* Alaska, Georgia, Hawaii, Maryland, Upstate New York, New York City, Oregon, and South Carolina.
SOURCE: U.S. Department of Health, Education and Welfare, Public Health Service, "Abortion Surveillance Report—Legal Abortions, United States Annual Summary, 1970," *Center for Disease Control: Family Planning Evaluation*, p. 24.

PROCEDURES
Abortion Resources

A woman who is faced with the possibility of an unwanted, unplanned pregnancy usually needs counseling and referral services. In large metropolitan areas there are agencies which provide pregnancy testing as a part of their counseling services. In smaller cities and rural areas it is more difficult to obtain this kind of help. However, in some areas, pregnancy testing is now being offered through the resources of health departments, outpatient facilities, neighborhood clinics, and doctors' offices. Frequently in these settings, nurses are called upon to counsel and refer.

When the test is positive for pregnancy, a woman must make her next decision—what to do about it. She needs basic information about medical, legal, and financial aspects of abortion and about the alternatives that are open to her. If she is considering abortion, she needs to know that her decision cannot be postponed indefinitely because of the developing fetus.

Today, regardless of where a woman is in the United States, she does have access to an abortion referral group or agency.[36] Local resources will vary according to availability and the legal status of abortion in a particular state. Such resources might be a private physician, a hospital, a Planned Parenthood affiliate, a clergy consultation service, or a health or social service department. If assistance cannot be found locally or in the state, national groups such as the Abortion Reform Association, the Association for the Study of Abortion, the National Association for Repeal of Abortion Laws, the National Clergy Consultation Services, and the headquarters of Planned Parenthood—World Population may be of assistance.

If a woman wishes to explore the services available to her if she should decide against abortion, local agencies such as social service, health departments, or private physicians may be equipped to help her carry the pregnancy to term. Several new national organizations such as Birthright, Birthchoice, and others with similar titles have recently been developed. They state that their chief purpose is to provide a pregnant woman with the opportunity to make a choice.

Review Committees

In the majority of states, the laws in general prohibit abortion except in situations of rather severe physical disease. In order to conform to these laws, hospitals have set up review committees consisting of several physicians of various specialties to deal with the requests for therapeutic abortion. Most hospitals have set limits on the number of abortions they will perform in a reporting period. With this degree of rigidity, it may be extremely difficult for women in need to be considered candidates.

Medical, Psychological, and Social History

In any abortion case, the need for a complete history consisting of social, psychological, and medical aspects cannot be overly stressed. Various professionals may be involved, including nurses, social workers, and physicians. In some instances, different aspects of the history may be taken by several persons, thus breaking the continuity of care. If it is possible, within the system, for a counselor or nurse to follow the patient throughout her entire abortion experience, this will assist in the patient's self-acceptance and a more positive approach toward the entire procedure.

In many instances, there is a general format (record system) which can be used as a guide. If nurses take the initial history, they should individualize their questions to the patient and be attuned to important cues given by the patient which need further investigation. During this time, rapport can be established with the patient which may reveal important details that should be passed on to the physician to be utilized when he takes a medical history or performs the physical examination. Many histories can bring forth information which will assist the nurses in caring for the patient throughout her abortion experience, including follow-up in the community.

If the patient is having her abortion for psychiatric reasons, there may be only a summary or a statement by the psychiatrist to the effect that this is the basis for the abortion. In these instances it is of great importance for nurses to be able to utilize the information obtained in the social history and counseling sessions to help them accept this patient and as a basis for beginning nursing care.

Methods by Length of Gestation

The commonly used methods of legally inducing abortion are (1) dilatation and curettage; (2) dilatation and evacuation (suction method); (3) saline induction; and (4) hysterotomy. There is research being done with prostaglandins, which are fatty acids normally produced by the human body. This procedure is being used experimentally in place of saline induction in some medical centers. At this time, we are mainly concerned with the four commonly used methods and the variations on these procedures.

DILATATION AND CURETTAGE; DILATATION AND EVACUATION

Up to the 12th or 14th week of gestation, abortion is usually performed by either dilatation and curettage or dilatation and evacuation. Either of these procedures may be done in a hospital, a clinic, or an abortorium. Wherever the procedure takes place, the room is set up similar to an operating room. The patient is given a preoperative medication and either a regional or inhalation anesthetic. The cervix is gradually dilated until a curette or suction tube can be inserted. If curettage is used, the uterus is scraped clean with the curette. If suction is used, a rubber, glass, or plastic tube is inserted into the dilated cervix, and the uterine contents are evacuated.

SALINE INDUCTION

If the pregnancy is past 14 weeks of gestation, saline induction can be done. This procedure is usually done in a hospital clinic or treatment room, and the patient will remain hospitalized until the abortive process is complete and she has stabilized. Local anesthesia of the abdominal wall is used. A 4- to 6-inch 18 or 20 gauge needle is inserted through the abdominal and uterine walls until the amniotic sac is entered. Amniotic fluid is withdrawn in an amount approximating the volume of saline to be used. Approximately 200 cc of hypertonic saline solution is then administered by drip through an intravenous infusion set or by syringe through the needle into the amniotic sac. Following the injection, the patient must await the onset of "labor." Usually between 12 and 36 hours, the patient will begin experiencing uterine cramping which continues at increasing intensities until the fetus is aborted.

HYSTEROTOMY

Hysterotomy is a surgical procedure performed after the 15th week of gestation. A small incision is made transabdominally, through the uterine wall. The contents of the uterus are then removed. This method is sometimes referred to as a "mini cesarean section." Usually the procedure is accompanied by tubal ligation.

Complications

Complications due to abortion vary according to the method used and the age, health status, and psychological well-being of the patient. In general, the longer the gestation, the more likely are the chances for complications (Table 12-8). According to Dr. C. Hendricks's report on pregnancy termination,[37] the following range of percentages were reported from those states with new laws:

Dilatation and curettage	0 – 8.2
Dilatation and evacuation	0.5– 1.2
Saline induction	4.0–12.6
Hysterotomy	9.3–24.8

In some of the states with liberalized abortion laws, maternal mortality has lessened, the number of admissions to hospitals because of incomplete abortions has decreased, the premature and infant death rates dropped, and the rate of illegitimate births also decreased.[38]

TABLE 12-8
REPORTED COMPLICATIONS OF INDUCED ABORTION, BY METHOD

Complications	D&C	D&E	Saline induction	Hysterotomy
Incomplete abortion	+	+	+	−
Postabortal bleeding	+	+	+	+
Postabortal infection	+	+	+	+
Perforation	+	+	−	−
Cervical lacerations	+	+	−	−
Hypernatremia	−	−	+	−
Hypofibrinogenemia	−	−	+	−

CODE: + Complications which apply to method
      − Complications which do not apply to method
SOURCE: Charles H. Hendricks, "Pregnancy Termination: The Impact of New Laws," *The Journal of Reproductive Medicine*, 6:60–70, 1971.

Contraception

One of the effects of liberalized abortion laws in general has been the availability of information to many women about methods, or more effective methods, of contraception and sexuality. Women now seeking abortions are from all socioeconomic levels; thus, for the first time all women have a more equal opportunity to decide the number of children they want.

Recidivism

Since data are only available over a 2- or 3-year span, it is very difficult to identify the characteristics of women who have had repeated abortions. There are, at this time, no reports of studies on the incidence of recidivism available in the United States. A study is currently ongoing in New York City by Daily and Pakter.[38] Rovinsky, Chief of Obstetrics, Elmhurst Hospital, New York City, has been looking at this problem both psychologically and socially. From his experience, the young teen-ager does not appear to be a repeater. Women that are repeating seem to have poor ego development in that they do not use or are inconsistent users of contraceptives, thus exposing themselves to the risk of repeated abortion.[38] Dr. Lebensohn (psychiatrist, Washington, D.C.) believes that these women are in need of psychiatric care but do not recognize their problems and are not interested in treatment.[38]

Women who are now having abortions are being counseled during the abortion experience concerning contraception, and many are asking for help to go on contraception immediately following the process. Perhaps this will help decrease the number of repeated abortions until we have some results from ongoing studies which may help to identify the repeater.

PSYCHOLOGICAL AND EMOTIONAL ASPECTS FOR THE PATIENT (OR FAMILY)

Decision Making

In spite of the fact that the issue of abortion is more freely discussed today than in the past, there is no universal opinion of its justification or acceptance. Pro-groups are strong in advocating that it should be a decision between a woman and her doctor. Anti-groups proclaim loudly that it is murder and cannot be sanctioned under any circumstances. Opinion polls indicate that most people have their own concepts of when it is right and when it is wrong. Yet, many say they are confused and don't know what they believe.

Against this background, it is understandable that persons who are confronted with an unwanted pregnancy are ambivalent in making their own decision. Professional people and all those in counseling roles need to be aware of the potential factors that may impinge on the decision-making process. Generally, the husband or the sexual partner is not directly involved in the counseling sessions. Yet, he may be the one on whom the ultimate decision rests.

The woman carrying an unwanted conceptus has some very personal concerns, both physical and psychological. For example, she may question whether she is really destroying a life, or whether the procedure will be more painful or distressing than a full-term delivery. She may wonder what other people will think of her, particularly her family and nursing staff. She may have concerns about expense or the people in whom she has put her trust. Fear of the unknown cannot be completely eliminated by the best of counselors, but it can be diminished by skillful interviewing and emotional support.

Institutionalization

During the patient's institutionalization, whether it be an outpatient or inpatient procedure, she should be treated as a person who has many feelings that need continuous attention. Everything that the patient having an abortion encounters should be carefully explained. Many of the patients expect to be rejected and disapproved of by nursing personnel and physicians.

After undergoing the abortion procedure, the patient does not expect a visible reward. She has experienced a procedure which, when finished, brings her a feeling of relief: It is over!

Psychological Sequelae

What about a few hours or a few days later when she is at home and a feeling of depression suddenly appears? How accountable does she feel now for the decision that she made? Is this guilt she now feels? Whom can she go to? What if she does not feel any guilt or contempt for what she has done? Dr. Margolis has reported on a follow-up study and corroborated his data with four other studies in the United States. He concluded that abortion is "often helpful to the life situation adjustment of these patients. The legal, social, and medical sanction for interruption of pregnancy results in minimizing untoward guilt and depressive reactions, leaving the majority of women a sense of rightness of their pregnancy terminations, now culturally approved."[39]

NURSING CARE

Counseling and Interviewing

The woman wanting an abortion comes to the hospital or abortorium either with no previous counseling or with comprehensive counseling by someone who has prepared her very adequately for the procedure she is about to experience. It is very important for the nurse who initially interviews the woman to find out what she has already been told and to restate anything that has been misunderstood or not synthesized. A follow-through with the same information by the nurse can help the patient to feel more relaxed and able to concentrate on the deluge of information that is to befall her, regardless of the method she is to undergo. The patient may appear to have no knowledge of what will occur even though she has been counseled by someone before admission. This patient may be experiencing some ambivalence in her decision, or a low frustration level, and needs reassurance and support to be able to follow through with her decision.

The nurse is in a unique position as the one person to whom the patient may communicate with the most freedom, if she is given the opportunity. Communication by the patient may be an expression of positive or negative feelings. Regardless of what the patient's expression may be (hostile, fearful, angry, flippant), the nurse can assist her by being aware of why she is reacting in such a manner and encouraging her to express her feelings. Every patient will not verbalize to the same extent. Those who hesitate to express their feelings may respond to nonverbal cues such as touch or the frequent presence of a caring, accepting nurse.

Care during Procedures

The setting the patient enters is dependent upon gestation and procedure and will be a major factor in the amount of nursing time she receives. If the patient comes into a hospital, clinic, or abortorium for a D&C or D&E, these procedures are completed, the patient is observed for several hours, and then she is released if there are no complications. If the patient is hospitalized for a saline induction or hysterotomy, she will be in contact with nurses from 2 to 6 days. These procedural differences thus bring up variations in nursing care.

Depending on the situation, the patient may or may not have been in this clinic before for her counseling and laboratory work-up. This may include a pregnancy test, urinalysis, complete blood count, serology, gonococcus smear, Rh type (Rh negative women may be given RhoGam after abortion), and a Pap test. The patients will see a nurse for an interview and, if indicated, a social worker. The doctor will examine the patient and schedule her for the procedure. In some instances, the patient returns at another time, and in other cases, the procedure is done that day.

Regardless of the particular routine of the clinic, there are reported experiences from nurses and patients which can serve as a basis for nursing care. One very important aspect of abortion is the nurse's ability to exhibit a relaxed and comfortable atmosphere. The more frank and direct the nurse can be, the more the patient will feel free to interact, whether on an individual or group basis. In many instances, the woman is accompanied by her boy friend or husband. He should be encouraged to sit in on the counseling sessions (individual or group) if the patient concurs. If the patient is to be hospitalized for a saline abortion, then the sexual partner should feel free to be with the patient whenever he is able. In the case of some adolescents, a parent or both parents may accompany the girl. After the nurse has interviewed the girl alone, together they should decide on the amount of time her parents will spend with her during the procedure.

DILATATION AND CURETTAGE OR DILATATION AND EVACUATION

A woman having a D&C or D&E should be told what she can expect throughout the entire procedure. After receiving the preoperative medication, the patient will be taken to the procedure room and given an anesthetic. Upon awakening, the patient may experience abdominal discomfort similar to menstrual cramps. Most patients will have an intravenous infusion running which was started preoperatively for induction of anesthesia or as a prophylactic measure. This will be discontinued in a short period of time. The nurse will check the patient for excessive bleeding and vital signs frequently during the first postoperative hour. In most cases, the patient can be ambulated with assistance in an hour. If the patient complains of feeling weak or tired, she should be reassured that this is not unusual and may persist for as long as a week. The patient may be given Methergine in 0.2-mg tablets which could cause her to have more severe cramping than she has been experiencing. An analgesic may be given every 4 hours as needed.

If the patients are in a clinic or abortorium, they may be in a lounge where they may talk with each other during the recovery time. Many programs have either a group meeting to go over postoperative instructions and answer questions, or individual consultation with a nurse before discharge. Most women are still feeling too many effects of medication and the procedure to retain this information. A printed sheet for future use is of great value.

SALINE INDUCTION

After the patient has been interviewed and adequately counseled concerning saline induction, she may be admitted immediately or go home to return at a later time. Depending on the hospital, the procedure may be done on an inpatient or outpatient basis. In some places, an enema is given to lessen the pressure at the time of the abortion. The abdomen may be shaved and the patient is asked to void just prior to the injection to make the level of the bladder as low as possible. The nurse may find that the patient asks some very disturbing questions while the doctor is injecting the saline. These questions need to be faced by both patient and nurse as honestly as possible.

The patients are not given any medication or anesthetic (except local anesthetic at the injection site) so that they will be able to report any sensations related to possible side effects of the procedure. Intravascular injection would produce heat sensation, dry mouth, tinnitus, tachycardia, or severe headache. A small amount of the saline solution is injected; if none of these symptoms occur within 1 minute after injection, the remaining saline is infused. Generally, patients do not experience pain during the procedure except at the beginning when the needle penetrates the peritoneum. Vital signs are checked every 15 minutes until stable and usually stabilize rapidly. The patient is then allowed activities and food as desired.

Fetal movement generally decreases soon after saline injection, and fetal death has been documented within 1 hour.[40] With the infusion of such a hypertonic solution into the amniotic sac, all surrounding tissue is dehydrated. However, the exact reason for fetal death or the induction of uterine contractions is unknown.[40]

There is a latency period from the time the patient receives the injection until she experiences labor. The patient may complain of an intense thirst for a few hours after injection, and she should be encouraged to drink as much as she desires. During this time, she may become quite talkative or uncommunicative. Of all times during the whole abortive process, this appears to be the time that is most stressful. If there are several patients undergoing the same procedure, one may find they group together and support each other to the exclusion, at times, of the nursing staff and family or friends. If the patients are talkative with the nurse, they should be encouraged to ventilate their feelings. Often while these patients are awaiting labor, members of the hospital staff will walk into their rooms several times during each shift to ask, "Is anything happening?" Soon the patient begins to wonder if there is something wrong because nothing is occurring.

Once the patient begins experiencing contractions, this crisis situation begins to have an ending. This labor period is one of negative expectation due to the end result. Regardless of this, the patient needs physical and psychological support throughout this laboring process. Medication for pain may be given if needed to provide relief and rest. A clear liquid diet should be provided to supply some caloric intake. Once the patient has partially dilated, she is kept in bed until she aborts.

The patient should be instructed to call the nurse when she feels rectal pressure. During the abortive process, the nurse may deliver the fetus and placenta. If the placenta is not expelled immediately, the cord should be clamped and cut and the fetus removed. The placenta generally separates on its own or with the Crede expression (slight pull on the cord along with fundal massage). After two hours, if the placenta still remains attached, surgical removal may be necessary. The placenta must be checked to ascertain whether or not fragments have been retained.

Following complete abortion, the patient may be given Deladumone or started on an oral regimen of Tace or stilbestrol to prevent breast engorgement. The patient usually expresses feelings of relief. After she is bathed and offered something to drink, she will probably be exhausted and fall asleep. If there are no complications, she will be discharged usually within 4 to 6 hours.

HYSTEROTOMY

The patient experiencing a hysterotomy usually has two areas of concern, one being the abortion, the other the loss of capability to reproduce. Abortion combined with sterilization indicates that the patient has come to a decision concerning family size. When this patient enters the hospital, she is usually treated by the staff very much like any patient having abdominal surgery, often with complete disregard for the pregnancy or approaching abortion. This is reflected in the fact that this patient, generally, is not given the emotional support she needs as an abortion patient. Just being given a chance to express her feelings might assist in her recovery. What she does receive is routine postoperative physical care such as instructions on turning, coughing, and deep breathing which do not meet her psychological or emotional needs. She usually remains in the hospital for about 5 days.

Referral

Referral following the abortion can be very detrimental to the patient if she has not been consulted in this decision. Many patients are fearful of the knowledge of the abortion getting back to their homes. Many have had the abortion done away from home and do not want public health, mental health, or private physicians knowing about their decision. In other instances, the patient was initially referred for abortion by these same agencies or physicians and the follow-through assists the patient in continuing care back in her own community.

Follow-up Care

It is of great importance that all women going home after having an abortion be aware of possible complications. Vaginal bleeding will continue for 1 to 3 weeks, but if it becomes heavier than a menstrual period, or if the patient passes large clots with the bleeding, she should consult her physician. She should also see him for fever over $100.6°F$, severe persistent pain, or burning on urination. The first menses usually occurs 2 to 8 weeks after the abortion and may differ from that which the patient has previously experienced. The menses may be heavier or less in quantity and may be either of a longer or shorter duration.

If lactation begins, it is usually mild and lasts less than 48 hours if the breasts are not stimulated. Using a tight brassiere, or binding the breasts and using an ice bag will ease the discomfort until the engorgement decreases.

Normal physical activity can be resumed as rapidly as desired. Increased fatigue is often noted for a few days. Showers and washing hair can be done immediately, but tub baths or swimming should be avoided for at least 1 week or for as long as the physician orders.

Return appointments are made for 2 to 4 weeks after the abortion. It is of utmost importance for the patient to have this examination to ensure that the reproductive organs have returned to the prepregnancy state. Although most physicians suggest that patients abstain from sexual intercourse until after their return appointment, most patients resume sexual activity when they, the patients, desire.

Family Planning

At some time during the abortion experience, the nurse should introduce the subject of family planning if the patient has not already requested information. In some instances in which the patients are having D&C's or D&E's, they have given permission for an IUD (intrauterine device) to be inserted while they are still under anesthesia. If this service is available, it is of importance to include family planning in the preabortion counseling.

During the time the patient is making her decision for abortion is not when she would be motivated toward thinking about a method of birth control. Once the decision is reached, then she is ready to pursue the outcome— abortion. After the abortion, the patient is discharged within a few hours, and at this time she is emotionally drained. The next possible contact with the patient is 2 to 4 weeks later, *if* she returns for her postabortion examination. This may be too late! Probably the optimum time to approach the subject of contraception is when the woman has been settled into her hospital room after admission to the hospital.

Counseling on contraception is of importance to these women who are or have been faced with the reality of an unwanted pregnancy. The nurse may find several opportunities which will be psychologically right for discussion of contraception with these patients.

PSYCHOLOGICAL AND EMOTIONAL ASPECTS FOR THE NURSE

Since 1967, when Colorado and North Carolina liberalized their abortion laws, nurses have been expected to be part of the medical team providing care to patients having abortions. However, there were no considerations taken as to the psychological reactions that might occur in the nursing personnel working with these abortion cases.

In 1970 *RN* polled 500 of their subscribers (*RN* panel) concerning the attitudes of nurses toward abortion and patients who have abortions.[41] The majority of nurses were opposed to abortion on demand, but 93 percent could accept having abortions for some reasons. The reasons given for abortion were rape, fetal defect, and physical impairment of the mother. Abortion for psychological reasons was not an acceptable indication. The greatest opposition toward abortion for out-of-wedlock pregnancies came from the younger nurses.

Medical personnel in Colorado reported having problems in accepting the care of patients having abortions under the new laws.[42] Some personnel refused to take part in abortions, particularly those done for psychiatric reasons when the need for the procedure was not completely obvious. Inservice training and reeducation helped to alleviate some of the difficulties which occurred.

Dr. John McDermott, Jr., presented a paper on the unexpected crisis in patient care in Hawaii when their abortion law was repealed.[43] Within one month after the change, hospitals began to ask for mental health consultation because of psychological reactions of the nursing staff. The reactions were of varying intensities among the staff, depending on the procedure involved. The description was of a kind of "combat fatigue" which resulted from an increased work load and emotional stress. Part of the problem here, as with other medical institutions performing abortions, was that the nurses were not well prepared for the new procedures nor for the new kinds of patients they were to encounter. Most nurses who select maternity nursing as their occupational role think in terms of bringing life into the world, not taking it away. Consequently, it was quite evident from the negative reaction which was encountered that nurses were unprepared for this shift in role.

The nurses' persistent identification with the fetus seemed based on their inability to identify with the abortion patients themselves. Nurses were horrified at women who talked about the fetus as though it had no human characteristics, while they, the nurses, placed very definite humanizing characteristics on the fetus. The young girl patients on the service aroused anger in the nurses, who felt that they were playing games with sex. Ambivalent feelings were expressed over women becoming pregnant in spite of excellent contraceptive methods being available.

Small group sessions were utilized with these nurses, first allowing for ventilation of feelings and then looking at general patient dynamics.

Because of continuing problems evolving from attitudes of health personnel toward abortion, the Center for Disease Control interviewed health care providers in 16 states in an effort to find out how they felt about abortion in late 1970 and in 1971. They found that religion was an obvious, but not the most important, personal factor. The most important factor was the person's general feeling about social change: "Those who identify on some level with the forces of change are quite likely to view legal abortion as an improvement in society's way of handling unwanted pregnancy, while those who see societal change as the cause of problems fear legalized abortion as one more in a series of steps down the road to moral decay."[44]

They found that the attitudes of the nursing staff directly affected the morale of the patients. When the nurses expected their patients to feel some remorse over the abortion, the patients did feel guilty and sad. On the other hand, if the nurses communicated to patients that they were not sick, but had a solvable problem, they seemed to feel much better after the procedure and the nurses felt good, too.

The abortion situation is a complicated one with many variables to be considered as we prepare student nurses to care for patients having abortions. Working with such patients and having understanding staff members and instructors who are available for verbalization of feelings will assist the student in caring for another patient in need.

REFERENCES

1 Lader, Lawrence: *Abortion*, Bobbs-Merrill, Indianapolis, 1966, p. 75.
2 Ibid., p. 76.
3 Knutson, Andie L.: "When Does a Human Life Begin? Viewpoints of Public Health Professionals," *American Journal of Public Health*, 57:2163–2177, 1967.
4 Ibid., p. 2163.
5 Guttmacher, Alan: "Abortion Yesterday, Today, and Tomorrow," in A. Guttmacher (ed.), *The Case for Legalized Abortion Now*, Diablo Press, Berkeley, 1967, p. 4.
6 Personal communication from Arthur Jones and Elizabeth M. Edmands.
7 Lader: op. cit., p. 89.
8 Lebensohn, Zigmond: "The Right to Abortion" in "Abortion and the Law," *Res Ipsa Loquitar*, 23:15, 1970.
9 Lader: op. cit., p. 64.
10 Ibid., p. 103.
11 Westoff, Leslie A., and Charles Westoff: *From Now to Zero*, Little, Brown, Boston, 1971, p. 137.
12 Ibid., p. 138.
13 Guttmacher, Alan: *Birth Control and Love*, Bantam Books, published by arrangement with Macmillan, New York, 1970.
14 Westoff and Westoff: op. cit., p. 129.
15 Lader: op. cit., p. 98.
16 Ibid., p. 99.
17 Ryan, Joseph A.: "Liberalized Abortion Laws—Immoral and Dangerous," *Medical Opinion and Review*, pp. 104–105, February 1966.

18 Ekblad, Martin: "Induced Abortion on Psychiatric Grounds: A Follow-up of 479 Women," *Acta Psychiatrica et Neurologica Scandinavica*, Supplementum 99, p. 170, 1955.

19 Osofsky, J. D., and J. H. Osofsky: "The Psychological Reactions of Patients to Legalized Abortion," paper presented at American Orthopsychiatric Association Meeting, March 1971.

20 David, Henry P.: "Abortion: Public Health Concerns and Needed Psychosocial Research," *American Journal of Public Health*, 61:513–514, 1971.

21 Hardin, Garrett: "Abortion—or Compulsory Pregnancy?" in Garrett Hardin (ed.), *Population, Evolution, and Birth Control*, Freeman, San Francisco, 1969, p. 295.

22 Kahn, James B., Judith P. Bourne, John D. Asher, and Carl W. Tyler, Jr.: "Surveillance of Abortions in Hospitals in the United States, 1970," *HSMHA Health Reports*, 86:426, 1971.

23 Hardin: op. cit., p. 294.

24 Westoff, Charles F., Emily C. Mors, and Norman B. Ryders: "The Structure of Attitudes toward Abortion," *Milbank Memorial Fund Quarterly*, 47:33, 1969.

25 Rossi, Alice S.: "Abortion Laws and Their Victims," *Trans-Action*, 3:8, 1966.

26 Vincent, Clark E., C. Allen Haney, and Carl M. Cochrane: "Abortion Attitudes of Poverty-level Blacks," *Seminars in Psychiatry*, 2:311, 1970.

27 Frye, Bobbie S.: "Attitudes toward Abortion of a Selected Group of Nurses," unpublished master's thesis, University of North Carolina, 1971, pp. 17–21.

28 "What Nurses Think about Abortion," *RN*, 33:40–43, 1970.

29 Sherwin, Lawrence, and Edmund W. Overstreet: "Therapeutic Abortion," *California Medicine*, 105:337–339, 1966.

30 Peck, Arthur: "Therapeutic Abortion: Patients, Doctors, and Society," *American Journal of Psychiatry*, 125:109–115, 1968.

31 Tyler, Carl W., Jr., and Jan Schneider: "The Logistics of Abortion Services in the Absence of Restrictive Criminal Legislation in the United States," *American Journal of Public Health*, 61:490, 1971.

32 U.S. Department of Health, Education and Welfare, Public Health Service: "Abortion Surveillance Report—Legal Abortions, United States Annual Summary, 1970," *Center for Disease Control: Family Planning Evaluation*, pp. 3–5.

33 Calderone, Mary S.: *Abortion in the United States*, Harper, New York, 1958, pp. 60–61.

34 Ibid., pp. 50–55.

35 U.S. Department of Health, Education and Welfare, Public Health Service, "Abortion Surveillance Report," p. 3.

36 Ebon, Martin (ed.): *Every Woman's Guide to Abortion*, Pocket Books, New York, 1971, pp. 119–147.

37 Hendricks, Charles H.: "Pregnancy Termination: The Impact of New Laws," *The Journal of Reproductive Medicine,* 6:60–70, 1971.

38 Harting, Donald, and Helen J. Hunter: "Abortion Techniques and Services: A Review and Critique," *American Journal of Public Health,* 61:2101–2102, 1971.

39 Margolis, Alan J., et al.: "Therapeutic Abortion Follow-up Study," *American Journal of Obstetrics and Gynecology,* 110:246, 1971.

40 Cronenwett, Linda R., and Janice M. Choyce: "Saline Abortion," *American Journal of Nursing,* 71:1754, 1971.

41 "What Nurses Think about Abortion," *RN,* 33:40–43, 1970.

42 Thompson, Horace, David L. Cowen, and Betty Berris: "Therapeutic Abortion: A Two-year Experience in One Hospital," *Journal of the American Medical Association,* 213:995, 1970.

43 McDermott, John F., Jr., and Walter F. Char: "Abortion Repeal in Hawaii: An Unexpected Crisis in Patient Care," paper presented at the 48th annual meeting of the American Orthopsychiatric Association, Washington, D.C., March 23, 1971.

44 Report by Judith Bourne presented at the Conference on Abortion Techniques and Services, New York City, June 3–5, 1971.

BIBLIOGRAPHY

Bennett, Elizabeth: "Abortion," *Nursing Clinics of North America,* 3:243–251, 1968.

Branson, Helen: "Nurses Talk about Abortion," *American Journal of Nursing,* 72:106–109, 1972.

Cronenwett, Linda R., and Janice M. Choyce: "Saline Abortion," *American Journal of Nursing,* 71:1754–1757, 1971.

Felton, Geraldine, and Roy Smith: "Administrative Guidelines for an Abortion Service," *American Journal of Nursing,* 72:108–109, 1972.

Fronseca, Jeanne D.: "Induced Abortion: Nursing Attitudes and Action," *American Journal of Nursing,* 68:1022–1027, 1968.

Goldman, Alice: "Learning Abortion Care," *Nursing Outlook,* 19:350–352, 1971.

Keller, Christa, and Pamela Copeland,: "Counseling the Abortion Patient Is More Than Talk," *American Journal of Nursing,* 82:102–106, 1972.

Malo-Juvera, Dolores: "Preparing Students for Abortion Care," *Nursing Outlook,* 19:347–349, 1971.

"Personal Experience at a Legal Abortion Center," *American Journal of Nursing,* 72:110–112, 1972.

University of Colorado, School of Nursing, Workshop on Family Planning: "Abortion," *American Journal of Nursing,* 70:1919–1925, 1970.

13 | GENETIC COUNSELING

Janet M. Stewart

The ultimate goal of every pregnancy is to produce an individual who is anatomically perfect, intellectually normal, and functionally capable of an independent and productive life. Most pregnancies culminate in such an individual, but in a certain percentage—small, but significant—something goes wrong. A child is born with a congenital anomaly which may be immediately obvious or which may not become apparent until later on in childhood or even in adult life. He may be mentally retarded, or his behavior or emotional stability may be such that he is not capable of functioning independently in society. In some instances the cause for such a problem is known; in others, it cannot be determined. In the minds of the parents, however, many questions are raised: "Will this happen again? Can it be prevented? What are my chances of having a normal baby next time?" Genetic counseling is an attempt to answer these questions. Genetic factors are of major importance in some abnormalities, in others they are a contributing factor, and in a third group their role is negligible. We as medical personnel may know into which group a certain abnormality falls; but parents rarely do, and they usually imagine the worst.

The incidence of congenital abnormalities is estimated to be 3 to 5 percent of all births with an even higher occurrence if an individual is followed into adult life. This incidence is fairly constant, but the significance of these defects is increasing. Perinatal mortality due to prematurity and infection is decreasing. Improved nursery and surgical techniques are allowing children to survive who previously would have died. These children are now living reminders of the pain, expense, and frustration of rearing a handicapped child. Parents, in their increasing sophistication, are seeking to learn the genetic implications of the defect in their particular family.

CHROMOSOMES AND CHROMOSOMAL DEFECTS

All hereditary material, in the form of deoxyribonucleic acid (DNA), is carried as genes on the chromosomes. All somatic cells in the human body contain 46 chromosomes (diploid number), or 23 pairs of chromosomes; one member of each pair is maternal in origin, the other paternal. Twenty-two of these pairs are known as autosomes; the remaining two chromosomes are called the sex chromosomes, two X chromosomes consituting a female (46, XX) and one X and one Y a male (46, XY). These somatic cells divide by a process called mitosis.

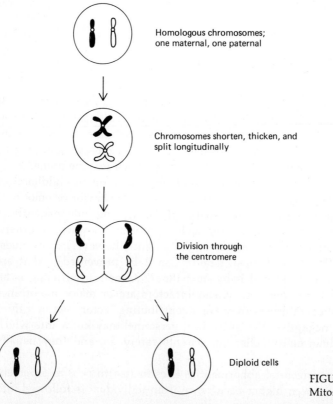

Homologous chromosomes; one maternal, one paternal

Chromosomes shorten, thicken, and split longitudinally

Division through the centromere

Diploid cells

FIGURE 13-1
Mitosis.

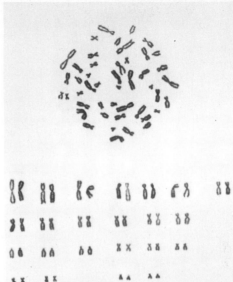

FIGURE 13-2
Normal female karyotype.

Each chromosome becomes shortened and thickened and splits longitudinally into two chromatids joined at a point called the centromere. This is the form in which most chromosomes are pictured. They are then aligned on a central spindle and split longitudinally through the centromere, thus separating the two chromatids which then migrate to opposite ends of the cell. Cleavage occurs to produce two genetically similar cells.

In the germ cells of the body, a unique process known as meiosis occurs. The chromosomes again shorten and thicken and split into two chromatids joined at the centromere. Homologous pairs are arranged together, and at this time material may be exchanged between the paired chromosomes (crossing over). The paired chromosomes then separate (disjunction) and move to opposite poles, forming two cells with 23 chromosomes each (haploid number). Each cell contains either an X or a Y. This is then followed by a mitotic division in which there is a longitudinal split at the centromere and migration of the chromatids to opposite poles. In this manner ova and sperm are formed, each with 23 chromosomes. At the time of fertilization, one ovum and one sperm unite to form a cell with the full diploid chromosomal constitution, and from this cell the fetus develops.

Chromosomes are most commonly studied in lymphocytes. Phytohemagglutinin is added to peripheral blood to stimulate mitosis and agglutinate erythrocytes. After 3 days, the cells are arrested in mitosis by the addition of colchicine to the culture medium. At this stage the chromosomes have split into chromatids and are readily visible under high magnification. The photographic record of the chromosomal constitution of a cell is called a karyotype.

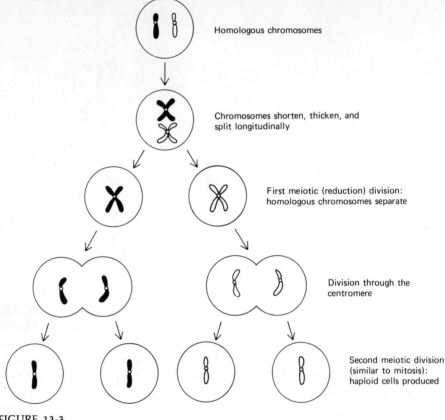

Homologous chromosomes

Chromosomes shorten, thicken, and split longitudinally

First meiotic (reduction) division: homologous chromosomes separate

Division through the centromere

Second meiotic division (similar to mitosis): haploid cells produced

FIGURE 13-3
Meiosis.

Abnormalities may occur during meiotic or mitotic division, producing an individual with a chromosomal defect. These abnormalities may involve one of the autosomes or the sex chromosomes and consist of too much or too little chromosomal material. Approximately 1 in every 150 live-born infants will have a chromosomal defect; half of these will involve the autosomes and half the sex chromosomes. As high as 25 to 50 percent of spontaneous abortions will also have a chromosomal aberration.

Autosomal Defects

The most common autosomal defect is known as Down's syndrome, or mongolism. The affected individual has an extra number 21 chromosome for a total of 47, trisomy 21. During meiosis, the two paired 21 chromosomes fail to separate (nondisjunction), and two dissimilar cells are formed, one with 24 chromosomes and one with 22. The latter cell is nonviable and dies. The

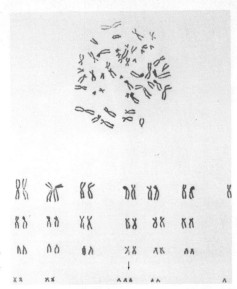

FIGURE 13-4
Karyotype of a male with trisomy 21, or
Down's syndrome. Extra 21 chromosome
indicated by arrow.

former cell then unites with a haploid gamete and the result is an individual
with 47, XX (or XY), 21⁺ karyotype. The clinical features of Down's syndrome are well known and are listed in Table 13-1. Most children with
Down's syndrome are born to mothers over thirty-five years of age. At the
time of the birth of a female child all ova are in the early stages of meiosis.
They remain dormant until the time of ovulation, as long as 35 years later.
It is believed that these older ova are more prone to nondisjunction.

    Down's syndrome can occur in two other cytogenetic forms. An occa-
sional child with Down's syndrome will have only 46 chromosomes. This includes one large abnormal chromosome which consists of the translocation of
the extra 21 to another chromosome, usually a number 14. One of the parents, usually the mother, may have a balanced translocation, that is, 45
chromosomes including the translocation. Although the number of chromosomes is deficient, the amount of chromosomal or genetic material is essentially normal and the translocation carrier is clinically a normal individual.

TABLE 13-1
CLINICAL FEATURES OF DOWN'S SYNDROME

Small head	Short, broad neck
Slanting palpebral fissures	Congenital heart disease
Epicanthic folds	Short broad hands
Speckling of the iris	Transverse palmar creases
Low-set, simply formed ears	Curved fifth finger
Protrusion of the tongue	Hypotonia
High palate	Mental retardation

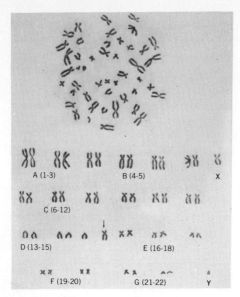

FIGURE 13-5
Translocation Down's syndrome with abnormal chromosome shown by arrow.

She is, however, at an increased risk for having subsequent children with Down's syndrome. Translocation Down's syndrome is more common in younger mothers, but the most common type of Down's syndrome born to a young mother is still the standard trisomy 21. Clinically, the child with a translocation type of Down's syndrome is indistinguishable from the child with the more common form.

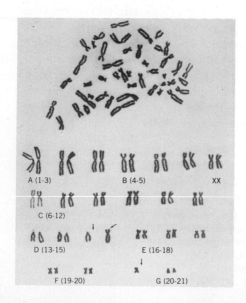

FIGURE 13-6
Balanced translocation carrier for Down's syndrome. Vertical arrows indicate missing D and G chromosomes; oblique arrow points to D/G translocation chromosome.

Occasionally an individual will have a mixed population of cells, some normal and some with an extra 21. This is known as mosaicism and is due to nondisjunction at a later stage of cell division. The clinical features and intellectual potential of these individuals vary with the proportion of abnormal cells.

Infants have also been born with trisomy 13 and trisomy 18 but have many severe abnormalities and rarely live beyond a few months of age (Table 13-2). Translocations are fairly common in trisomy 13.

The total absence of an autosome is felt to be incompatible with life, although a few exceptions have been reported. Partial deletions of the short arm (p−) or the long arm (q−) of various chromosomes have been described and, in a few instances, seem to comprise specific syndromes. A deletion of the short arm of chromosome 5 results in severe mental retardation and a catlike cry in infancy, the cri du chat syndrome.

A deletion of the long arm of chromosome 18 may be associated with maxillary hypoplasia, stenotic ear canals, and a conductive hearing loss. Material may be lost from both the long and the short arms of a certain chromosome, and during cell division, these two arms may become adherent, forming a ring. These individuals clinically resemble the picture seen with a single deletion.

Sex Chromosome Defects

Unlike the loss of autosomal material, an individual may lose one of the sex chromosomes with surprisingly little effect. The 45, Y zygote is not viable, but the 45, X individual (Turner's syndrome) has a female appearance or phenotype with the abnormalities listed in Table 13-3. She also has streak ovaries, develops few secondary sex characteristics, and is usually infertile. She is often of normal intelligence but may have perceptual difficulties. It is

TABLE 13-2
CLINICAL FEATURES OF TRISOMY 13 AND TRISOMY 18

Trisomy 13	Trisomy 18
Arhinencephaly	Low birth weight
Microphthalmia/anophthalmia	Low-set, malformed ears
Facial clefts	Prominent occiput
Polydactyly	Micrognathia
Scalp defects/hemangiomata	Short sternum
Congenital heart disease	Overlapping fingers
Severe retardation	Flexion contractures
	Spasticity
	Congenital heart disease
	Genitourinary anomalies
	Severe retardation

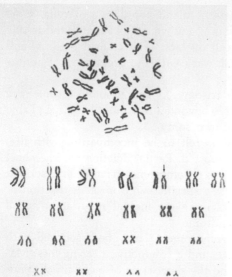

FIGURE 13-7
The cri du chat syndrome. Arrow shows deletion of short arms of chromosome number 5.

usually not known if the lost chromosome is of maternal or paternal origin, and, indeed, this probably varies.

The presence of the Y chromosome is essential for the early development of a male phenotype, but it actually carries few, if any, known genes. At first glance it would appear that the normal female has a double dose of the genetic material carried on the X chromosome. The work of Barr and others,

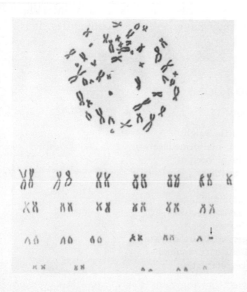

FIGURE 13-8
Karyotype of a male with a ring 18 chromosome indicated by arrow.

TABLE 13-3
CLINICAL FEATURES OF TURNER'S SYNDROME

Short stature	Hyperconvex and/or deep-set nails
Lymphedema	Excessive nevi
Low hairline	Renal anomalies
Webbed neck	Broad chest
Cubitus valgus	Wide-spaced, hypoplastic nipples

however, has shown that females have a darkly staining body found adjacent to the nuclear membrane in nondividing cells, a body not found in the normal male. It has been postulated that this Barr body represents one of the X chromosomes which is randomly inactivated early in fetal development. Thus, the genetically active material on the X chromosome is equal in males and in females. This is known as the Lyon hypothesis.

A female may have a 47, XXX constitution and have two Barr bodies, representing two of the three X chromosomes that have been inactivated. While it has been felt in the past that these individuals are retarded and infertile, more recent evidence indicates that many may be normal. A male with a 47, XXY chromosomal picture may have testicular atrophy and sterility. This is known as Klinefelter's syndrome.

Recent attention has been focused on the 47, XYY karyotype and its possible association with tall stature and aggressive or criminal behavior. This association has not been proven. Individuals with more X chromosomes (48, XXXX or 48, XXXY) usually have more severe physical abnormalities and mental retardation.

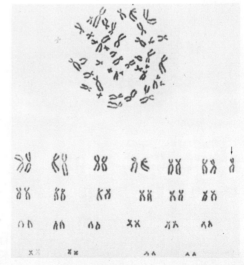

FIGURE 13-9
Turner's syndrome: 45, X.

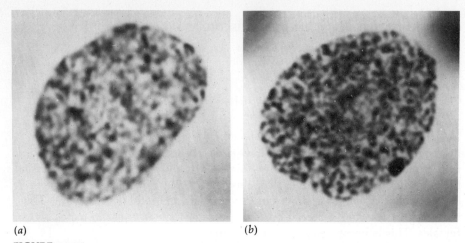

(a) (b)

FIGURE 13-10
(a) Normal male cell, no Barr body. (b) Normal female cell, single Barr body.

PATTERNS OF INHERITANCE

The chromosomal defects that have been discussed are grossly obvious in a standard karyotype. Defects involving single genes, however, are much more discrete and invisible by any currently used technique. The determination of the hereditary nature of an abnormality is done in two ways: (1) by the careful study of an individual family, and (2) by a study of the inheritance pattern of that particular defect as previously reported in the literature.

Genes occur in pairs and are located on homologous chromosomes. One

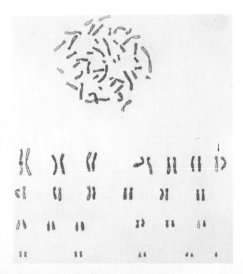

FIGURE 13-11
Klinefelter's syndrome: 47, XXY.

is maternal in origin and the other paternal. If the two genes have the same effect, the individual is said to be homozygous; if the effect is different, he is said to be heterozygous. The expression of each gene depends upon its inter-action with other genes and with the environment.

Genetic defects can be inherited in three well-known ways and in a fourth less well understood but commonly occurring manner.

Autosomal Dominant

A condition or trait is said to be dominantly inherited if it is manifest in the heterozygous state. This is a vertical type of inheritance with an affected in-dividual having a 50 percent chance of passing the gene on to each of his off-spring. An unaffected individual, in most cases, does not carry the abnormal gene, and all of his offspring will be normal.

Case 1. A. G. (Figure 13-12, III-1) is a five-year-old boy with bilateral cataracts and a left club foot noted at birth. The club foot has been cor-rected by casting, and his development has been normal. The cataracts are small and do not interfere with vision. His mother (Figure 13-12, II-1) has bilateral cataracts and colobomata, as does a maternal aunt (II-2). A maternal uncle also has cataracts (II-3) and has one son with cataracts and aniridia (III-2), a daughter with cataracts and colobomata (III-3), and a second daughter with cataracts and aniridia (III-4). The maternal grandmother (I-1) also has cataracts and colobomata. All other family members are normal. The affected family members carry a dom-inantly inherited gene for eye abnormalities, variously expressed as cata-racts, colobomata, and aniridia.

Dominantly inherited traits have several distinguishing characteristics. They are usually milder, since the gene is passed on by the affected individ-ual who is able to reproduce. Occasionally, the onset of symptoms does not occur until after the reproductive years, e.g., Huntington's chorea. There is much variation in the clinical manifestations of a dominant gene as shown in Case 1. This is known as variation in expressivity. A few individuals are severely affected, while those at the other end of the spectrum may be so mildly affected that they have no obvious clinical manifestations of the gene. If this occurs, a gene is said to have decreased penetrance. Often, however, if sought, some mild and clinically insignificant finding is present which identi-fies the abnormal gene.

On occasion a dominant trait will seem to appear *de novo*. An affected child will be born to normal parents with a negative family history. In this case, a spontaneous gene mutation has occurred. The parents of such a child are not at an increased risk for future pregnancies, although the affected in-dividual himself would have a 50 percent chance of passing the trait on to his offspring. Many dominantly inherited traits have a high mutation rate, and

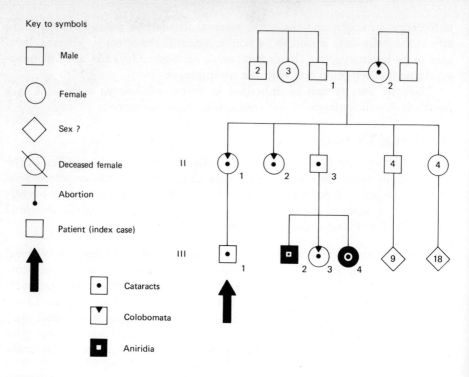

Key to symbols

☐ Male

◯ Female

◇ Sex ?

⊘ Deceased female

Abortion

☐ Patient (index case)

⊡ Cataracts

⊡ Colobomata

■ Aniridia

FIGURE 13-12
Case 1: Pedigree illustrating autosomal dominant inheritance.

indeed, some of the more severe conditions seem most often to be new mutations, e.g., Apert's syndrome, or acrocephalosyndactyly.

Autosomal Recessive

A condition is said to be recessively inherited if it is manifest only when the individual is homozygous for the defective gene. This is a horizontal type of inheritance with the carrier parents often being asymptomatic and having a 25 percent chance of producing an affected child. One-half of their children will be carriers like themselves, and 25 percent will be genetically normal. In many cases, recessive conditions are more severe as the abnormality is passed on by the asymptomatic carrier and the affected person need not reproduce. If a particular recessive condition is rare, there is an increased incidence of consanguinity in the parents. Conversely, if parents are related, there is an increased chance that an abnormality in a child is recessive in nature.

Case 2. M. W. (Figure 13-13, II-10) is a fourteen-and-a-half-year-old girl with a profound bilateral sensorineural hearing loss first suspected at one year of age. She wears a hearing aid and has attended schools for the hearing handicapped. M. has two older sisters, ages thirty-one and thirty-two (Figure 13-13, II-4 and 5), who also have profound hearing losses and goiters. They have been diagnosed as having Pendred's syndrome, an autosomal recessive condition characterized by hearing loss and a goiter which appears in adolescence. Both sisters have children with normal hearing. M. has no thyroid enlargement to date. Both parents have normal hearing, and there is no other family history of deafness.

The distinction between dominant and recessive inheritance is not strictly true. If our tools are sophisticated enough, an abnormality can be detected in the "normal" carrier parents. Galactosemia is a defect due to the deficiency of the enzyme galactose-1-P uridyl transferase. The homozygous individual has little or no detectable enzyme. The carrier has an enzyme level that is roughly 50 percent normal. Although clinically asymptomatic, he is not biochemically normal, and the gene does manifest itself in the heterozygous state.

Sex-linked

If the gene for a particular trait or abnormality is located on the X chromosome, the condition is said to be inherited in an X-linked, or sex-linked, manner. The condition is X-linked recessive if it is manifest only in the male who is hemizygous, that is, the abnormal gene on the single X chromosome is genetically unopposed. The female who has a normal gene on one X chromosome and an abnormal gene on the other is a carrier and usually asympto-

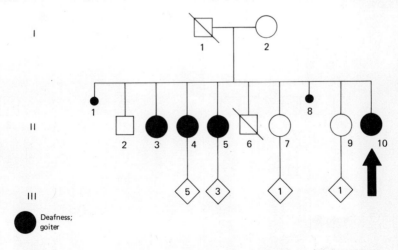

FIGURE 13-13
Case 2: Pedigree showing autosomal recessive inheritance.

matic. In reality, because of the random inactivation of the X chromosome, the female carrier may have varying degrees of symptomatology. This is an oblique kind of inheritance. The carrier female passes the gene on to 50 percent of her sons, who then manifest the abnormality, and 50 percent of her daughters, who are also carriers. An affected male has all normal sons and all carrier daughters. The cardinal feature of an X-linked trait is the lack of male-to-male transmission, since the male may only pass on his Y chromosome to his sons.

Case 3. T. N. (Figure 13-14, IV-2) is a twelve-month-old boy with an athetoid form of cerebral palsy diagnosed at ten months of age. Laboratory studies including serum uric acid and ceruloplasmin are normal. He has an older normal brother. A maternal first cousin (Figure 13-14, IV-4), an uncle (III-3), a second cousin (IV-6), and two first cousins of the mother (III-5, 6), are all males who have a similar type of cerebral

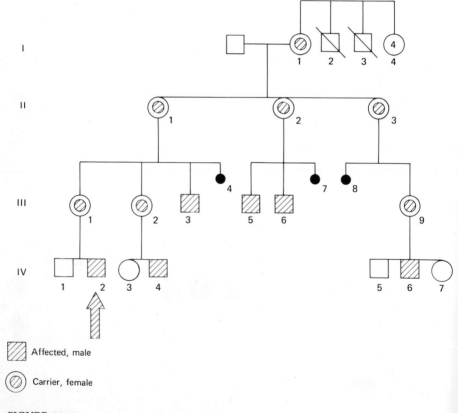

FIGURE 13-14
Case 3: Pedigree demonstrating X-linked recessive inheritance.

palsy and associated mental retardation. This is a rare X-linked form of cerebral palsy. The carriers (I-1; II-1, 2, 3; III-1, 2, 9) are clinically normal.

More rarely, an X-linked trait may be dominantly inherited, e.g., vitamin D resistant rickets. In this case, heterozygous females are also affected but less severely than the hemizygous male. Again, there is no male-to-male transmission.

Polygenic

Many of the more common congenital abnormalities, such as cleft lip, cleft palate, spina bifida, and pyloric stenosis, are not inherited in one of the manners described above, and yet these defects often cluster in families. It has been postulated that multiple genes contribute to these defects and that each individual has a threshold above which the abnormality will be manifest. This is known as polygenic inheritance. The more severe the defect, the more predisposing genes present. The less commonly affected sex requires more predisposing genes to demonstrate the abnormality. Unlike single gene defects, the recurrence risk varies with the number of affected persons in the family. Practically, the principles of polygenic inheritance are often applied in genetic counseling situations. Normal parents who have one child with a cleft lip and cleft palate have a 4 percent recurrence risk figure for future pregnancies. If one of the parents is also affected, the risk increases to 17 percent. With normal parents and two affected children the risk is about 9 percent.

INBORN ERRORS OF METABOLISM

Metabolic errors are disorders of protein, often characterized by abnormal or missing enzymes which interfere with the metabolism of certain endogenous or exogenous substances. A few of these abnormalities are dominantly inherited (Type II hyperlipoproteinemia), some are X-linked (Hunter's syndrome), but most are autosomal recessive disorders. Most metabolic errors are rare, but they assume an importance out of proportion to their frequency. There are several reasons for this. First, they are often associated with mental retardation; second, if detected early, many of the metabolic errors can be treated and the retardation thus prevented; and third, an increasing number of these conditions can be diagnosed early in pregnancy (see following paragraphs). Three inborn errors of metabolism will be considered here briefly.

Phenylketonuria (PKU)

PKU is one of the best known of the metabolic errors. It was first described in 1934 by Følling, and in 1953 Jervis identified the missing enzyme as phenylalanine hydroxylase. Affected persons are unable to convert phenylalanine to tyrosine, resulting in an accumulation of phenylalanine and certain metabolic by-products. Infants with PKU are usually normal at birth but within the first few months of life they show progressive developmental delay, often with eczema and seizures. Untreated, most phenylketonurics are severely retarded. Dietary treatment was first attempted in the mid-1950s and, with some modifications, is the therapy used today. After the diagnosis has been confirmed, the infant is put on a diet restricted in phenylalanine. Since this is one of the essential amino acids, certain amounts are necessary to ensure normal growth. In essence, this is a diet with little protein which is supplemented by a commercial milk substitute containing low levels of phenylalanine. Results of early dietary treatment have been encouraging; mental retardation is either prevented or markedly ameliorated. It is apparent, however, that for dietary restriction to be effective, it must be started within the first few months of life. For this reason, several screening methods have been developed, and in many states PKU screening of the newborn has been made compulsory by law.

The incidence of PKU ranges from 1:15,000 to 1:20,000, and it comprises 1 percent of the population in an institution for the mentally retarded. It is an autosomal recessive condition and carriers are identified by a phenylalanine loading test with measurement of phenylalanine levels and the phenylalanine:tyrosine ratio. Although this test is helpful, there may be overlap with normal, and carriers cannot always be identified with certainty. Unfortunately, the missing enzyme, phenylalanine hydroxylase, has only been found in the liver, making the measurement of exact enzyme levels an impractical method for the diagnosis of the disease or the identification of carriers. At this time, PKU cannot be diagnosed in utero.

Many questions remain unanswered about this abnormality. The exact cause of the mental retardation is not understood. There are some individuals with the disease who have a normal or near normal IQ. No consistent metabolic differences have been identified in these individuals. The exact level at which the serum phenylalanine should be maintained during treatment has not been determined, nor has the age at which the diet can be discontinued. It would seem that most brain growth has been completed by the age of five or six years and that the diet can be safely discontinued at this time. It is also known that mothers with PKU give birth to a very high percentage of children with mental retardation and microcephaly. Since most of the treated individuals will now marry and reproduce, some type of maternal treatment during pregnancy must be devised which will ensure enough phenylalanine to allow normal fetal growth but not so much as to cause retardation.

Maple Syrup Urine Disease (MSUD)

MSUD is a much less common metabolic error in which there is an accumulation of the branched chain amino acids leucine, isoleucine, and valine. This is felt to be secondary to the absence or depression of the decarboxylase enzyme or enzymes. Clinically, these infants are also normal at birth but by one week of age, they develop poor feeding, vomiting, lethargy, hypertonicity, and seizures along with a characteristic odor to the urine suggestive of maple syrup. Untreated, most infants die shortly after birth; survival is associated with severe retardation. Treatment is similar to PKU. An artificial diet is used which contains restricted amounts of leucine, isoleucine, and valine. Again, early treatment seems to be effective in preventing mental retardation, but the diet is more difficult to maintain with frequent fluctuations associated with infection. Dietary treatment may be necessary throughout life. This, too, is an autosomal recessive condition. Carriers can be identified and an intrauterine diagnosis can be made in the first trimester of pregnancy.

Galactosemia

A third metabolic error, galactosemia, is due to a deficiency of the enzyme galactose-1-phosphate uridyl transferase, resulting in an inability to convert galactose-1-phosphate to glucose-1-phosphate. These infants develop failure to thrive, vomiting, diarrhea, and signs of liver disease shortly after milk is introduced into the diet. Untreated, many go on to develop cataracts and mental retardation. Therapy consists of the elimination of galactose from the diet by using commercial milk substitutes which are galactose-free. Dietary treatment has been quite effective. A second, less common form of galactosemia is due to a deficiency of the enzyme galactokinase. Affected persons may have cataracts but seem to be spared the liver disease and the mental retardation. Both forms of galactosemia are autosomal recessive. Enzyme levels can be determined in fibroblasts and leukocytes, and heterozygotes have 50 percent of the expected normal enzyme value. An intrauterine diagnosis can be made by measuring the enzyme level in fetal fibroblasts.

There are many other inborn errors of metabolism. Although rare, these conditions must be considered in children with early deterioration or mental retardation, particularly if the family history indicates other similarly affected persons or if there is consanguinity. The potential for prevention of the secondary complications of these errors makes early diagnosis imperative.

GENETIC COUNSELING

Most frequently, genetic counseling is given to parents who have had one abnormal child. It should also be offered to siblings of such an individual and to the affected person himself when he approaches marriage and parenthood. Less commonly, more distant relatives may seek genetic counseling, or related individuals who are contemplating marriage may want genetic advice.

The genetic evaluation and counseling may be done effectively in many places by a variety of persons, and there are advantages to having the counseling done by a person familiar with the family. It is absolutely imperative, however, that the diagnosis be correct. The less common dominantly inherited form of cleft lip and cleft palate must be differentiated from the usual polygenic type. The child with multiple abnormalities who fits into a previously described recessively inherited syndrome must be identified. For this reason, referral to a genetic center is often advisable.

The actual steps involved in genetic counseling vary with the complexity of the problem, but often the process is simpler and less expensive then expected. A careful history is always taken, and it should include any environmental factors in the pregnancy which might explain the abnormality. The family history is taken in pedigree form and is as extensive as possible. It is often necessary to obtain medical records or photographs of relatives who may have a similar abnormality. A careful physical examination is made of not only the affected individual (the propositus or proband) but often of other family members as well. The detailed history, including a pedigree, and the careful physical examination are the hallmarks of a good genetic evaluation. The amount of laboratory work required prior to genetic counseling varies considerably. Some of the tests which may be done on the proband and other family members are listed in Table 13-4. It is not necessary to do a karyotype prior to genetic counseling unless a chromosomal defect is suspected.

When the evaluation has been completed and the diagnosis made, the parents then return for the actual counseling session. Both parents are required to attend, and the counseling is done in an unhurried and relaxed atmosphere. They are given the final diagnosis and the risk figures for future pregnancies. In most centers, actual advice about future children is not given, but rather an attempt is made to give parents the factual knowledge necessary to make a wise decision. This not only includes the recurrence risk figures but also the significance of the diagnosis and the prognosis for the child. Parents who have not yet lived with a child with cystic fibrosis will not comprehend the severity of the disease. When possible, an attempt is made to minimize guilt; however, in situations in which one parent is obviously the carrier of the gene causing the defect, it is often better to acknowledge the guilt and help the parent deal with it. In many instances one counseling session is not enough. Parents may hear nothing beyond the word "Down's syn-

TABLE 13-4
SOME LABORATORY TESTS DONE ON PROBAND AND FAMILY

Viral titers	Carrier tests
Viral cultures	X rays
Dermatoglyphics	Other blood tests appropriate
Buccal smear	for suspected disorder
Karyotype	

drome." Additional sessions may be necessary to review the information given, answer questions, and clear up misconceptions. A nurse or social worker may be the key figure in these follow-up meetings. If parents decide against future children and seek advice about contraception or adoption, appropriate information can be given at this time. There is good evidence that parents who seek genetic advice will usually make appropriate and expected decisions about future children.

THE ROLE OF THE NURSE

When an imperfect child is born, the parents often see many physicians, and the child may be immediately transferred to a medical center many miles away. Their most frequent and consistent early contact may be with the maternity nurse. It is important, therefore, that this nurse recognize the need and indications for genetic counseling. After the initial shock, the parents will have many questions and will need to talk with someone who is comfortable discussing their child. They need to be encouraged to voice their many questions. "What is the significance of my child's defect? What caused it? Is it hereditary?" Although the nurse may be unable to answer many of these questions, the parents can be guided to appropriate resources, such as genetic counseling clinics, after discussion with the pediatrician, obstetrician, or family practitioner.

Prior to discharge, the nurse, with the approval of the attending physician, should make the arrangements either to follow the family personally or to refer them to a community health nurse. The importance of this long-term, continuing contact with the family cannot be overemphasized, and through it the nurse can play an important role in the genetic counseling process.

Before Counseling

The nurse can help the family contact a genetic counseling clinic and should arrange transportation if necessary. The family can be prepared for their appointment by discussing what will be done and by collecting information on family members who have similar medical problems. The family can also be helped to formulate their questions and their apprehension can be eased.

During Counseling

It is most desirable that the nurse attend the counseling session with the family. The role of liaison between the family and the genetic counseling clinic will be much more effectively filled if the nurse has talked with the counselor and has heard directly the information given to the family.

After Counseling

It is at this point that the nurse becomes one of the most important figures in the counseling process. By virtue of training and background and close contact with the family, the nurse is the ideal person to follow through on genetic counseling. To do this there must be a good understanding of the basic principles of genetics as described above. The nurse can answer questions and elaborate upon information given to the family. If the questions are too complex or if the family's basic understanding of the information is poor, a return appointment to the clinic can be arranged. As parents make decisions about future pregnancies, the nurse can discuss contraceptives and make referrals to family planning clinics or adoption agencies.

In the majority of cases, after the genetic counseling has been completed, the parents must learn to live with their handicapped child. The nurse now becomes a major source of support for the family by answering questions about prognosis; by helping with daily problems of feeding, development, etc.; and by referrals to appropriate places for medical care and educational planning. Intimate knowledge of community resources makes the nurse one of the most important contacts for the family.

The "luxury" of genetic counseling has traditionally been confined to the middle and upper classes. These people have been verbal enough to ask their questions, and their physician, often an old friend, has been able either to answer them or to find the answers. The same questions exist in the minds of parents of all classes, but those of a lower socioeconomic group or those with a language barrier may have difficulty expressing them. Traditions inherent in their culture may discourage such questioning or may supply erroneous answers. Medical care is often fragmented and sporadic, and families may never see the same physician frequently enough to raise more than the very urgent questions about immediate problems. The community health nurse is in a unique position and knows people of all classes and all ethnic backgrounds. Such a person is often the only consistent contact many people have with the professional community. It is important, therefore, that the nurse recognize those families who need, but who are unlikely to get, genetic counseling and discuss the issue with them, arranging for referral. It is important that the family wants this information, as this motivation is essential for the genetic counseling to be effective. If there is a language barrier, the nurse should either function as or provide an interpreter for the counseling session.

It is obvious that the nurse, both in the hospital and in the community, is of vital importance in genetic counseling. A nurse makes the referrals and answers the questions which arise after the counseling and is the single most important person in the expansion of genetic counseling to people of all classes. A sound background in genetics is essential to fill this role effectively. Such a background will be increasingly important in the future.

ADVANCES IN GENETIC COUNSELING

The field of genetics is old, antedating even the work of Gregor Mendel in the 1860s; yet, it is also very new. It was in 1956 that man's chromosomes were first accurately counted and in 1959 that LeJeune described the first chromosomal abnormality—the trisomy 21 associated with Down's syndrome. Progress has been rapid in the past 15 years, and many of the new techniques are of practical significance for all involved in genetic counseling. Since 1963, amniotic fluid has been aspirated from the uterus late in pregnancy to predict the involvement of an infant with an Rh incompatibility. More recently, amniotic fluid has been aspirated from the uterus earlier in pregnancy (12 to 16 weeks) to diagnose a variety of chromosomal and metabolic disorders. This fluid contains cells from the fetal skin and the amnion, which is also fetal in origin. These cells can be cultured, the chromosomes examined, and the sex of the fetus determined. Various enzyme assays can also be done and an ever-increasing group of metabolic defects can be diagnosed early enough to terminate the pregnancy if the parents so desire and if an abortion on genetic grounds is legal in that particular state. Table 13-5 is a partial list of abnormalities which can be diagnosed in utero. This list is *not* complete and is growing daily. When a specific question arises, a genetic center should be contacted. Early amniocentesis is a new technique, and the long-term implications are not known. Evidence to date, however, would indicate that it is a safe procedure. In most genetic centers, amniocentesis is currently being recommended in the following situations:

1 Previous child with a chromosomal defect.
2 Either parent a balanced translocation carrier.
3 Both parents carriers for a diagnosable metabolic defect.
4 Mother a carrier for an X-linked disorder. A potentially affected male could be aborted and a female carried to term.
5 Mother over forty years of age. This is a controversial indication, but since the risk of delivering an infant with a chromosomal abnormality increases markedly with age, many consider it a valid reason for amniocentesis.

The nurse should be familiar with the indications for amniocentesis and should discuss this with appropriate families.

TABLE 13-5
SOME ABNORMALITIES WHICH CAN BE DIAGNOSED IN UTERO

Chromosomal disorders
Metabolic disorders

Tay-Sachs disease	Maple syrup urine disease
Niemann-Pick disease	Glycogen storage disease
Hurler's syndrome	Galactosemia
Hunter's syndrome	Lesch-Nyhan syndrome

For many years, a simple technique has been available to screen for X chromosome abnormalities. Cells scraped from the buccal mucosa or cells from the amnion could be stained and the Barr bodies counted. Within the last 5 years a new fluorescent stain has been developed, and it has been demonstrated that the Y chromosome, even in the interphase or nondividing cell, can be identified as a brightly staining body. Buccal, amnion, or umbilical cord cells can now be stained by this new technique, and an effective tool has been developed to screen for abnormalities of the Y chromosome. This same fluorescent staining technique has enabled individual chromosomes to be identified. Each chromosome has a striking and unique pattern of alternating bright and dark bands, enabling it to be specifically identified. Minor deletions or additions and more subtle chromosomal abnormalities can thus be detected and studied.

There has been considerable progress in the development of new genetic techniques. There must be similar progress in the expansion of genetic counseling, increasing its availability to all those in need. The role of the community nurse in genetic counseling has been described. The nurse can also fill an expanded role in a genetic counseling center and can be trained to take the pedigree, print and interpret dermatoglyphics, examine family members for certain specific abnormalities, and do much of the initial evaluation under the supervision of a physician who would assist in making the diagnosis. The

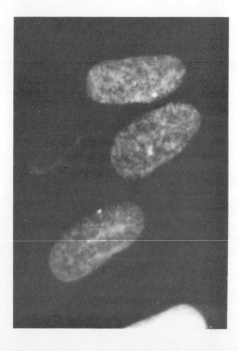

FIGURE 13-15
Fluorescent Y body in interphase or resting cell; this indicates the presence of a single Y chromosome.
(*Reproduced by permission of Journal of Pediatrics, 79:305, 1971.*)

nurse could then participate in or even do the genetic counseling and follow through with the family as has been described.

The nurse may also play an expanded role in the community itself. By spending a period of time in training at a genetic center, a nurse can be taught the techniques of a genetic evaluation and can then return to a job in the community, the schools, the state health department, etc. In appropriate situations, the nurse could begin an evaluation, discuss the findings with a physician from the genetic center, and go with the family for an abbreviated counseling session during which the diagnosis would be confirmed and the specific risk figures discussed. Further interpretation and discussion could be done by the specially trained nurse after the family has returned home. The expanded role of the nurse in genetic counseling is new, but it is feasible today and potentially very rewarding.

Some of the most exciting medical advances today are being made in the field of genetics. A maternity nurse or a community health nurse with basic genetic knowledge or with expanded skills can be in the center of this new and exciting activity.

BIBLIOGRAPHY

Bearn, A. G.: "Cell Culture in Inherited Disease—With Some Notes on Genetic Heterogeneity," *New England Journal of Medicine*, 286:764–767, 1972.

Bergsma, D. (ed.): "Intrauterine Diagnosis," *Birth Defects: Original Article Series*, vol. 7, no. 5, April 1971.

Carr, D. H.: "Chromosomal Abnormalities in Clinical Medicine," in A. G. Steinberg and A. G. Bearn (eds.), *Progress in Medical Genetics*, vol. 6, Grune & Stratton, New York, 1969, pp. 1–61.

Carter, C. O.: *An ABC of Medical Genetics*, Little, Brown, Boston, 1969.

———, J. A. F. Roberts, K. A. Evans, and A. R. Buck: "Genetic Clinic: A Follow-up," *Lancet*, 1:281–285,1971.

Eller, E., W. Frankenburg, M. Puck, and A. Robinson: "Prognosis in Newborn Infants with X-Chromosomal Abnormalities," *Pediatrics*, 47:681–688, 1971.

Gordon, H.: "Genetic Counseling," *Journal of the American Medical Association*, 217:1215–1225, 1971.

Greensher, A., R. Gersh, D. Peakman, and A. Robinson: "Screening of Newborn Infants for Abnormalities of the Y Chromosome," *Journal of Pediatrics*, 79:305–306, 1971.

Hecht, F., H. E. Wyandt, and R. W. Erbe: "Revolutionary Cytogenetics," *New England Journal of Medicine*, 285:1482–1484, 1971.

Lynch, H. T., G. M. Mulcahy, and A. J. Krush: "Genetic Counseling and the

Physician," *Journal of the American Medical Association*, 211:647–651, 1970.

McKusick, V. A.: *Human Genetics*, 2d ed., Prentice-Hall, Englewood Cliffs, N.J., 1969.

Milunsky, A., J. W. Littlefield, J. N. Kanfer, E. H. Kolodny, V. E. Shih, and L. Atkins: "Prenatal Genetic Diagnosis," *New England Journal of Medicine*, 283:1370–1381, 1441–1447, 1498–1504, 1970.

Nadler, H. L., and A. B. Gerbie: "Role of Amniocentesis in the Intrauterine Detection of Genetic Disorders," *New England Journal of Medicine*, 282:596–599, 1970.

Reisman, L. E., and A. P. Matheny: *Genetics and Counseling in Medical Practice*, Mosby, St. Louis, 1969.

Robinson, A.: "Clinical Genetics," in E. S. Taylor, *Beck's Obstetrical Practice*, 8th ed., Williams & Wilkins, Baltimore, 1966, pp. 621–640.

Smith, D. W.: *Recognizable Patterns of Human Malformation*, Saunders, Philadelphia, 1970.

Stanbury, J. B., J. B. Wyngaarden, and D. S. Fredrickson: *The Metabolic Basis of Inherited Disease*, 3d ed., McGraw-Hill, New York, 1972.

Stevenson, A. C., B. C. C. Davison, and M. W. Oakes: *Genetic Counselling*, Lippincott, Philadelphia, 1970.

14 | PSYCHOSOCIAL AND CULTURAL FACTORS IN FAMILY PLANNING

Miriam T. Manisoff

The decision by any individual couple to delay or limit childbearing is based on a most complex interaction of social and economic conditions and pressures, cultural norms, conscious and unconscious motivational factors, and emotional attitudes toward childbearing. With the introduction of highly effective, coitus-independent methods of conception control, many of the former barriers to effective contraception were removed. Indeed, many of the so-called motivational problems were eliminated, as is attested to by the studies on the increasing use of contraception. What we are seeing now is a convergence of values and a pattern of fertility control behavior approaching universality. By 1965, 90 percent of all white married couples had used or expected to use some means of contraception. In 1965 87 percent of couples wanted four children or less, and low-income couples wanted the same number of children as those of higher incomes. Nonwhites wanted slightly fewer children than whites.[1]

INCREASING ACCEPTANCE OF FAMILY PLANNING

Pohlman enumerates many factors now operating to bring about greater parental choice in conception.[2] Newer, more effective, more acceptable methods have been developed. There is greater professional and scientific acceptance and commitment as well as public interest in contraception, and a number of social trends now favor individual choice. These trends in family life include a shift from the "institutional" to the "companionship" family in which children may be a liability, even though they are desired; the change from having children as a duty to having "wanted" children; the altered parental roles with the woman working and the husband helping to rear children; and a willingness to plan and interfere with "nature."

The United States is moving toward a universally favorable attitude of acceptance of family planning among all American women, whether urban or rural, white or nonwhite, rich or poor, Catholic or non-Catholic. Among the factors which may be contributing to this norm of acceptance are the increasing number of working women, the greater number of two-income families required by our high standard of living, and increased urbanization which makes the large family an economic liability rather than an asset and imposes additional penalties for large families in difficulties in obtaining adequate housing. The effect of the women's liberation movement may also be a factor.

CAUSES OF UNWANTED FERTILITY

Why, then, in the face of this norm of acceptance, is there an estimated unwanted fertility rate each year in this country of 20 percent of total births— 32 percent among the poor and near poor and 15 percent among the nonpoor? For the nonpoor, some of this percentage can be accounted for by the fallibility of current methodology. Only the oral contraceptives are almost 100 percent effective, but they require constant and repeated use and have side effects. Improvement in reducing unwanted fertility for the nonpoor group can probably be achieved through improved technology in methods, more widespread education, and the provision for back-up abortions in cases of contraceptive failure. For the low-income couples, there is a need for a catch-up program to provide services which will give them the same degree of access to modern contraceptive methods which is available to the nonpoor.

Regardless of income, there is one group for whom services are relatively unavailable—the sexually active teen-ager. The Executive Board of the American College of Obstetricians and Gynecologists at its meeting in May 1971 pointed out that the "never-married, never-pregnant, sex-involved female has not yet been reached with effective contraception." It recommended that "the unmarried female of any age should have access to the most effective methods of contraception," and urged the removal of legal barriers which restrict the physician's freedom to provide services for minors. The American Medical Association, the American Academy of Pediatrics, and the American Academy of Family Physicians have now endorsed the recommendation that teen-age girls who are likely to conceive should have access to medical consultation, contraceptive advice, and methods consistent with their needs. Since 1969, numerous states have enacted statutes broadening the rights of minors to give effective consent for contraception. Sociologist Phillips Cutwright concludes from a cross-national analysis that illegitimacy in the United States can only be reduced by making effective medical contraception services available, accessible, and well advertised to all without restriction as to age, marital status, or previous pregnancy and backed up by abortion on request.[3] Out-of-wedlock births occur in all age brackets within the childbearing years.

Although most United States couples have used or plan to use contraception, there appears to be a divergence in the methods typically used by various socioeconomic groups. Couples in the higher socioeconomic levels (who can afford private medical care) tend to use more reliable, medically supervised methods of birth control, while low-income couples (who have less access to such care) depend more on the less reliable, nonmedical methods available from drug stores. The medically indigent, in addition to achieving less success in determining completed family size, also have more "timing failures" than the well-to-do. From 1960 to 1965 the annual fertility rate among the poor and near poor was 153 births per 1,000 women aged fifteen to forty-four, compared with a rate of 98 per 1,000 among the nonpoor. Nearly half of the children growing up in poverty in 1966 were members of families with five or more children under the age of eighteen in spite of the expressed preference of low-income parents for families of two to four children. More than one-fourth of all families with four or more children in 1966 were living in poverty, and four out of ten were either poor or near poor, based on Social Security Administration definitions. The higher fertility found among the poor cannot alone account for the growth in American population, since this group makes up only one-fourth of our population. The significance of unwanted high fertility among the poor lies in the additional burdens it imposes on the poor themselves.

The disparity between poor and nonpoor effective contraception is related to accessibility—financial and otherwise—of services. Wherever free or low-cost family planning services have been offered at convenient locations under conditions of respect, dignity, and free choice, unusually high patient acceptance has been found. However, while the network of government services is expanding, there still exists a tremendous gap between need and availability. In 1969 a little more than 1 million of the 5 million medically indigent estimated to need subsidized services were being served through all available public and private family planning programs. It is estimated that the comparable 1970 patient load will approximate 1.4 to 1.6 million, or 30 percent of fertile, low-income women in need. About seven out of ten were still lacking effective access.

VOLUNTARY NATURE OF FAMILY PLANNING

In the United States today there is no official national policy of population control. Couples who practice family planning do so to achieve personal objectives, based on their own goals and not as part of a government population policy. Our governmental family planning program is designed to help people achieve their own desires as to family size and spacing, based on individual voluntary decisions.

All the major religions now agree that family planning is an obligation of responsible parenthood. Pope Paul's encyclical of 1968 continued the approval of the rhythm method only.

Through the Department of Health, Education and Welfare, the government defined its policy with regard to population and family planning in 1966 in terms of improving the health of the people, strengthening the integrity of the family, and provision of freedom of choice to parents to determine the spacing of children and the size of their families. The Commission on Population Growth and the American Future was established by Congress in 1970. Its *Interim Report* in 1971 identified population growth as an intensifier or multiplier of problems—environmental, economic, political, and social—which impair the quality of life in this country.[4] In 1972 the commission will recommend whether a national policy is desirable and, if so, what the policy should be. The Family Planning Services and Population Research Act was passed by Congress in December 1970, authorizing for the first time substantial amounts of public monies ($382,000,000 over 3 years, 1971 to 1973) to underwrite contraceptive services and to sponsor research for new and improved methods.

PSYCHOSOCIAL FACTORS IN FAMILY PLANNING

The reasons couples use or fail to use contraception, in addition to the factor of availability, stem from many emotional and social needs. In contemporary society, parenthood is considered the norm. Social pressure is felt by those remaining deliberately childless. Among the poor, even more than among the nonpoor, social scientists hold, parenthood brings a sense of status and a sense of personal adequacy. And, of course, among rich and poor, the birth of wanted children is a joyful event.

Many cultural values and concepts emphasize the importance of childbearing. Parenthood may be used to "prove" an individual's femininity or masculinity, virility or potency. Some parents may continue to conceive in the attempt to have a child of each sex; others in the belief that children will hold a fragile marriage together. Some religious beliefs hold that children are an expression of God's will or punishment, not to be changed by human decision. Conception and pregnancy are interpreted by psychologists as a possible way to show independence from parents, or as payment or punishment for having sex. Couples may feel that good parents should have as many children as they can afford. Bearing children may be used to compensate for a husband's neglect; to express the husband's conscious or unconscious hostility by repeatedly making his wife pregnant; to obtain increased attention from a spouse; to relieve boredom; to provide a creative outlet in an otherwise uncreative life; or to prove male dominance or female importance. Parents may believe that large families are better for the children or may want to give their child a sibling. The child may be viewed as an extension of oneself or a way of reliving one's life vicariously.

Motivations for the use of contraception are often expressed in terms of economics. The financial costs of rearing children are high. It may cost as much as $40,000 to rear and educate a child through college. Psychosocial reasons often operate on the subconscious level and are less likely to be acknowledged because they may appear selfish. Childbearing and rearing can interfere with a mother's social life, career, and physical appearance. It subtracts time from enjoyment and self-development. It may represent a sacrifice of husband-wife relationships and impair intimacy, romance, and sexual relations. The shift in attention from spouse to child may evoke jealousy in the husband or wife. However, these psychological "costs" of children may, by some parents, be seen as rewards rather than penalties if, psychologically, they have a strong need for punishment. Ignorance and fear of contraceptive methods may also be factors in their nonuse, but such barriers are usually most amenable to correction through education.

Motivation and Contraception

The stronger the desire to avoid conception, the more effective contraceptive practice is likely to become. Parents approaching or achieving desired family size tend to use more effective methods and to use them more skillfully and consistently. They take fewer chances and achieve a lower rate of unwanted conceptions.

The acceptability of specific methods also affects contraceptive use. In the days when the diaphragm was almost the only female method available, patient motivation was considered to be a great problem, and much attention was focused on improving it. With the introduction of methods which did not involve vaginal manipulation—repugnant to many women because of its possible association with masturbation—patient motivation was found to be much less of a barrier. Since the most effective methods—the pills and the IUD—have troublesome and possibly frightening side effects, it is most important to prepare patients in advance for possible difficulties, so as to reduce anxiety and to enable them to cope.

According to Dr. Hans Lehfeldt unwanted pregnancy may be due to conflicting motivation.[5] Some couples fail to use contraception consistently and regularly because they are ambivalent about pregnancy and willfully expose themselves to possible failure by misuse of the method or "forgetting" to take their pills. They alternate between contraception and exposure and may need psychological help to elicit and clarify their ambivalence so that they can either practice effective contraception or become happy parents.

Couples may also harbor fears related to the use of contraception that they will lose their capacity for sexual enjoyment or ability to give sexual pleasure. Men may feel that it will lead to extramarital activity by the wife or that inability to impregnate her will lessen his status in the eyes of his sociocultural group. Among minority groups, there may be beliefs that the motivation for offering contraception is racist in origin and that family planning programs are designed to keep them a minority, rather than to help them. Women who, because of poor sexual adjustment, have used fear of pregnancy to avoid coitus may be unable to use a method which would eliminate that excuse.

Dr. Robert E. Gould has identified reasons people often give for having children—reasons which are not uniformly valid for child or parents:[6]

1 Our parents want grandchildren.
2 We can afford it.
3 I want to be somebody.
4 I need to be needed.
5 A baby will give me something to do.
6 It will help our marriage.
7 It's the only way to prove you're a man.
8 We don't want to be different.
9 I want him to have the things I never had.
10 A child is my only claim to immortality.
11 A baby will keep a woman in her place.
12 Children are a blessing.
13 Children are a gift of destiny or chance.
14 Children ensure security for parents in their old age.
15 Many sons are needed to ensure continuation of the family name.
16 Children are useful and can help parents in the home and at work.
17 Additional children are no problem.

Since family planning encompasses assistance in achieving desired family size through spacing and limiting pregnancies as well as through help in cases of infertility, we need to consider some of the psychosocial factors which may exist among those denied a child.

Psychosocial Factors in Infertility

Unwanted infertility, or involuntary childlessness, is a problem for about 15 to 20 percent of married couples in the United States.[7] It has been a concern of people since ancient times: The Ebers papyrus describe a test for female fertility, and a Greek text attributed to Hippocrates mentions, incorrectly, that a woman is most fertile immediately after menstruation. The desire for children, stemming from basic human desires and reinforced by societal pressures for parenthood, can produce in those who are involuntarily childless feelings of guilt, frustration, and inadequacy as males or females.

The effects and role of psychological and emotional factors in infertility are most complex. Although a number of writers agree that such factors exist, they also indicate that it is difficult to identify them or to document them scientifically.[7-10] For example, indirect clinical evidence exists, based on repeated findings, that a small percentage of women with sterility problems become pregnant soon after registering for infertility therapy and before any medical treatment has been instituted, or after adopting a child. The occurrence of pseudocyesis in a woman anxious to become pregnant is also cited as an example that psychological factors are operating in infertile women. The reciprocal nature of psychological factors and infertility is pointed out by Drs. Buxton and Southam.[10] Psychological conflicts about pregnancy and marriage also affect fertility.

Inability to conceive affects the psychological condition and state of mind of both males and females. Social pressures on couples to reproduce can produce tension within the individual who finds herself barren and may put her on the defensive. This in turn produces feelings of guilt and inadequacy which can further affect her fertility. Very often tension arises between husband and wife; each blames the other for the infertility.

Many theories have been advanced to account for the effect of emotional factors in achieving pregnancy. Dr. James A. Peterson indicates that inadequate emotional integrations operate (1) by directly affecting endocrine or tubal functions, (2) by inhibiting sexual adjustment essential to conception, or (3) by interfering with the development of sympathetic understanding between marital partners needed for cooperation in achieving parenthood and in child nurture.[9]

The relationship of sexual response and sexual adjustment to fertility is implicated in Dr. Peterson's findings of a "low order of sexual adjustment" in many cases of infertility. The emotional disturbances which influence success or failure of infertility programs, he explains, must be dealt with through exploration of:

1 The *meaning* of sterility for the patient in her social setting, along with attempts to ventilate and minimize guilt or self-demeaning reactions

2 The degree of adjustment of the couple's marriage and ways of dealing with possible marital conflicts

3 The degree of sexual adjustment and any frigidity or impotence which may interfere with impregnation

4 The degree of emotional disturbance in the husband and wife to de-

termine to what extent neurotic conflict may be interfering with medical therapy

SERVICE-RELATED FACTORS IN FAMILY PLANNING

Nurses working in public health family planning programs among the medically indigent should be concerned with clinic-related factors. While many studies have surveyed factors of family planning knowledge, attitudes, and practice among patients, few have addressed themselves to relating the purveyor's knowledge, attitudes, and practices to patient needs. It is possible that the most difficult obstacles may exist not in the patient, but in the professionals responsible for making services available.

Nurses in family planning clinics should keep in mind that family planning is an elective service; the patient is not propelled by acute pain or disease. Patients can easily be deterred from attendance if they find demeaning, unsympathetic attitudes among staff, lack of privacy, or long waiting periods. Other practical issues which may affect acceptance are cost, inconvenient clinic hours, distance which the patient must travel to reach the clinic, availability of public transportation and baby-sitters, and the variety of methods from which patients may choose, together with full information as to their use.

NEGATIVE STAFF ATTITUDES

Concepts of the Goals of Family Planning

Other problem areas may involve staff. The basic concept of the doctor or nurse as to the goals of family planning may be negative. Some consider family planning as a means to control population (with the frequent implication that particular groups should be singled out). It is important to distinquish between family planning, as a voluntary individual decision, and population control, a societal issue. If the nurse's approach to patients is based on the concept of population control, it is likely to boomerang, and the service may be rejected by the patient. The statement, "Nobody should have more than two children" as an introduction of family planning to a couple has proved a disaster. The nurse who critically says, "*How many* children did you say you have?" is conveying to the patient personal family planning goals—not necessarily the patient's. The primary goal of family planning is to reduce the gap between desired and achieved family size. There are also important secondary objectives, including (1) improving the physical, emotional, and economic health of the family; (2) fostering happier, more fulfilling sex relationships for parents; (3) giving parents the freedom to decide the number and spacing of children; and (4) reducing abortion and illegitimacy.

Attitudes toward the Poor

Some nurses hold negative, punitive, or demeaning concepts about the poor. These may be expressed in such phrases as "They're too dumb, too lazy, too uninterested to use family planning." "People who have had fun should pay for it." "If they don't accept family planning, they're just stupid." "They can't support what they have now, why should they be allowed to have more." "Why should we use tax money to support promiscuity?" "They don't care how many they have." Most of the time these statements are not true. More important, these attitudes can be serious obstacles to patient education and acceptance. While the phrases may vary, contempt or disrespect in word, tone, or facial expression of nurses or other staff members will predictably evoke unfavorable patient reaction. The family planning staff should be selected for positive attitudes to family planning because basic attitudinal changes take time, training, and effort, and for some, change may not be desirable or possible. Those without tolerance should be reassigned to other, less sensitive services. To underline the importance of these attitudes, a study by William Darity showed that almost 90 percent of patients interviewed cited "kind treatment" as the characteristic they most liked about a health department family planning program.[11]

Concepts of Self

Into our functioning as professionals we bring our concepts of self, both positive and negative. The negative may easily interfere with adequate functioning in family planning. For example, nurses may feel they do not know enough to discuss family planning properly with patients. Young unmarried nurses may feel they cannot discuss family planning at all. Outmoded beliefs that this teaching invades patient privacy still persist. Nurses may harbor fears that patients will be offended; they may feel that "It's none of my business." "Why should I force my attitude on someone else?" "I feel too uncomfortable talking about this." These attitudes can prevent the nurse from offering information which the patient has a right to know. Identifying this sense of inadequacy in staff can lead to its early resolution. Role playing has been found an effective antidote. So has the assignment of a neophyte with an experienced family planning educator.

Attitudes toward Sexuality

Negative concepts of sexuality may exist in both patients and staff and may make effective education more difficult. Such attitudes may be conscious or unconscious, and essentially they consist of the idea that sex is sinful and pregnancy is an appropriate punishment for it. Reflections of this are the attitudes that unmarried girls should not be told about birth control, that family planning promotes promiscuity, or that patients with many children are oversexed.

Service Providers and Service Consumers

Another source of difficulty may lie in the whole relationship of service providers vis-à-vis service consumers. Often reflected in the styles used with patients is the underlying assumption that the providers know—ipso facto—what is best for the patient. Professional education and experience do prepare nurses to assess a problem from an objective viewpoint. But nurses can learn much about the "hard knocks" and existential know-how on which patients base their views.

CONSUMER ATTITUDES

Effects of Previous Experience

Patients' views of family planning services are influenced by their previous experience with public medical care facilities. Since family planning is so intricately connected to such emotional areas as sex and reproduction, staff in these services must use particular tact in dealing with patients who may already be hostile to care provided from such "charity" agencies. Every staff member, professional or nonprofessional, will need to be trained to be respectful of patient feelings and sensitivities. Regulations set by the administration will need to be flexible enough to take into account the life circumstances and attitudes of patients.

Attitudes among the Poor

Consider for a moment the implications of the fact that public health programs of family planning are directed at low-income groups. Among these groups there are a number of incentives for the use of family planning. These include the fact that no one wants pregnancy at all times, the desire for sex without danger of conception, the influence of peer attitudes, and economic and health reasons. Realistically, there also exist among low-income groups some explicit barriers to the use of family planning. What has been called the "powerlessness syndrome" can be a very real thing. This may be expressed as "the odds are against you anyway, so live for today, take a chance, and what will be, will be." To be offered power against births without power in any other sphere may not be enough for some. The dominance of the male in sex relations among this group, with the woman dependent on the man for companionship, sex, attention, and groceries, may also be a problem, particularly if the man equates his virility with impregnating a woman.

Among this low-income group there may also exist a dislike and mistrust of medical personnel and facilities, since the obvious power of doctors and nurses may serve to emphasize the patient's own lack of power.

Lack of Consumer Participation

Among the poor and minority groups in particular, family planning programs have come under criticism for the lack of involvement of the consumer in planning, policy-making, and decision. It is increasingly important that consumer participation be considered in an area such as family planning so that services will be responsive to and representative of those for whom they are intended.

CONSIDERATION FOR THE NURSE

In the development of a personal working philosophy and role, nurses are reaching for a better understanding of some of the obstacles which may exist in the patient, in the services, and in themselves. We can perhaps emphasize the need for nurses to see and place the patient's needs above their own and to respond to those needs, even if talking about sex or birth control makes the nurse uncomfortable at first. If this is an area of patient need, the professional responds with help for that need. Linked to this is the ability to observe and understand the scene from the patient's point of view, for nurses must be able to put themselves in the patient's seat, as a recipient of service. For example, students or staff nurses in clinics can "shadow" a patient through a clinic, wait with her, hear the instructions and questions she gets, note the time she spends waiting, observe where and how she is directed and the times she gets lost, and find out how she feels about her experience.

In trying to help patients who forget or confuse their instructions or who say they want to use family planning but never get around to attending the clinic, nurses can try to develop understanding of their own feelings. By considering the effects of the patient's environment and experiences, nurses can achieve a better comprehension of why patients act or react as they do, and minimize their own feelings of anger and impatience. The nurse can attempt a more open approach to methods of patient education and to search for more realistic teaching which involves the patient in the process. Nurses can encourage greater patient participation in clinic administration, possibly through use of neighborhood advisory committees.

Nurses must have faith in their patients' ability to grow, improve, and learn. They should try to be nonjudgmental, to refrain from imposing their attitudes, standards, and ways of life on families with different cultural or economic orientation. If possible, they should learn to understand and operate within the patient's cultural framework—to meet patients at their own level and proceed from there. Above all, in their relationships they should try to create an atmosphere of mutual respect and understanding by encouraging patients to feel a sense of freedom in choosing—or refusing—a family planning method.

Nurses need to consider both initial and continuing inservice education, through cooperative efforts for all staff members in contact with patients—clerks, receptionists, aides, etc. Attempts should be made to provide continuity of service, such as bringing together hospital and clinic nurses. There are hospital family planning programs in which a patient is begun on a method with no provision or follow-through to see that she continues that method at a community facility when the hospital clinic is not convenient. Improved interagency communication is another goal for achieving better service. Nurses, nurse educators, and students need opportunities—in small groups—to discuss and evaluate their feelings about sex and sexuality so that they can develop ability and comfort in talking with patients about matters related to family planning and sexuality.

HEALTH CONCERNS IN FAMILY PLANNING

A concern for maternal and infant health is integral to the interest in and provision of family planning services. Perhaps of greatest concern are those who are socially and economically deprived and with whom high-risk conditions are most commonly associated. Among the factors which are implicated in increased risk to mother or child are parental age (under eighteen and over forty), birth interval (less than 15 months between pregnancies), and a history of premature births, infant deaths, abortion, obstetrical complications, diabetes, cardiovascular disease, or venereal disease.[12]

Studies have repeatedly shown the relationship of infant mortality and other adverse pregnancy results to high parity and short intervals between births. Such relationships are intensified among poor women with repeated pregnancies in rapid succession whose health is already impaired by inadequate nutrition and living conditions and poor medical care. Nowhere in the health field is poverty as directly implicated in the cost of human well-being and life.

Maternal and infant mortality and morbidity rates increase when the interval between children is less than two years. Among births which occur at less than 15-month intervals, the infant mortality rate is four times the natural rate. The premature birth rates among babies born less than 12 months apart occur at double the rate for those born at 24-month intervals. After the fourth child the risk of fetal and neonatal death increases. Studies have also substantiated the fact that perinatal mortality increases with the age and parity of the mother. The unmarried mother and her infant are at significantly greater risk from mortality, premature births, and pregnancy complications. A definite correlation has been found between multiparity and obstetric diseases and gynecological complications. Multiparity also has an aggravating effect on many other diseases, such as cardiovascular disease, cancer, epilepsy, hypertension, and rheumatic heart disease. Women who have had five children have about three times the chance of developing diabetes as nulliparous women. Since poor women are more likely to suffer from malnutrition, anemia, chronic vascular disease, tuberculosis, and toxemia, it is important that pregnancy be postponed in women with such conditions until they can be treated, for the protection of mother and child.

In assessing the need for family planning guidance, the nurse can utilize her knowledge of the patient's and the family's medical and social history. While all women in the childbearing years can be considered as potential family planning patients, the following are particular indicators for offering information:

1 The mother has just had a pregnancy.
2 The last two pregnancies were less than 18 months apart.
3 The mother appears physically or emotionally depleted.
4 The mother, father, or other family members have a history of physical or emotional disability.
5 The mother is under eighteen or over forty years old.
6 The family already has four children.
7 There is a history of premature births, obstetric complications, tuberculosis, or heart disease.
8 The mother is unable to cope with her existing children.
9 There is marital conflict related to the birth of unwanted children.
10 There is a seriously handicapped child requiring much care.
11 There are one or more out-of-wedlock children.
12 The mother is working or plans to work.
13 A sexually active teen-ager is present in the home.
14 The family is having difficulty in maintaining economic independence or is already receiving public assistance.
15 There is evidence that any of the children in the family are abused or battered.

Although nurses, as health educators, are rightly concerned with the knowledge, attitudes, and values of their patients regarding family planning, it is interesting that one professional health educator considers such factors often not sufficient as causal factors in the adoption of preventive health behavior, such as family planning. Lawrence Green has found that individuals often have the appropriate beliefs and attitudes and adequate knowledge to produce a recommended behavior, and yet it does not materialize.[13] Conversely, the expected preventive health practice is seen in those without such knowledge and attitudes or they may be acquired following the behavior. Green suggests that social pressure and social support may be more important than knowledge and that influence in matters of health tends to come from informal social sources close to the individual. The use of indigenous para-professional workers with whom patients can identify can be a valuable way to increase patient utilization of family planning services. The "satisfied patient" herself is, of course, an excellent source of such influence and in many family planning clinics, the primary source of new patients.

Psychosocial factors in family planning are only recently being given the attention of psychiatrists and social scientists. Yet, as early as 1898 Sigmund Freud wrote[14]

> Theoretically it would be one of the greatest triumphs of mankind, one of the most tangible liberations upon the bondage of nature to which we are subject, were it possible to raise the responsible act of procreation to the level of a voluntary and intentional act, and to free it from the entanglement with an indispensable satisfaction of natural desire.

REFERENCES

1 Westoff, Charles, and Norman Ryder: "United States: Methods of Fertility Control, 1965," *Studies in Family Planning*, no. 17, February 1967.
2 Pohlman, E. J.: *The Psychology of Birth Planning*, Schenkman, Cambridge, Mass., 1969.
3 Cutwright, Phillips: "Illegitimacy: Myths, Causes and Cures," *Family Planning Perspectives*, January 1971.
4 Commission on Population Growth and the American Future: *Interim Report*, U.S. Government Printing Office, Washington, D.C., March 16, 1971.
5 Lehfeldt, Hans: "Psychology of Contraceptive Failure," *Medical Aspects of Human Sexuality*, May 1971.
6 Gould, Robert E.: "The Wrong Reasons to Have Children," *New York Times Magazine*, June 1970.
7 Guttmacher, A. F., W. Best, and F. Jaffe: *Birth Control and Love*, Macmillan, New York, 1969, pp. 235–245.
8 Van de Velde, T. H.: *Fertility and Sterility in Marriage*, Heinemann, London, 1931, p. 167.
9 Peterson, James A.: "Emotional Factors in Infertility," in Edward T. Tyler (ed.), *Sterility*, McGraw-Hill, New York, 1961, pp. 282–299.
10 Buxton, C. Lee, and Anna L. Southam: *Human Infertility*, Harper, New York, 1958, pp. 203–216.
11 Darity, William: "Continuing/Discontinuing Users of Oral Contraceptives," in A. Sobrero and S. Lewit (eds.), *Advances in Planned Parenthood*, Schenkman, Cambridge, Mass., 1965.
12 Manisoff, Miriam: *Family Planning: A Teaching Guide for Nurses*, Planned Parenthood—World Population, New York, 1971, pp. 13–23.

13 Green, Lawrence N.: "Status Identity and Preventive Health Behavior," *Pacific Health Education Report*, School of Public Health, University of California, Berkeley, 1970.

14 Freud, Sigmund: "Sexuality in the Aetiology of the Neuroses," collected papers, vol. I, Hogarth, London, 1949 (quoted in Lee Rainwater, *And the Poor Get Children*, Quadrangle, Chicago, 1960).

BIBLIOGRAPHY

Berelson, Bernard: "Beyond Family Planning," *Studies in Family Planning*, Population Council, February 1969.

Bumpass, Larry, and Charles F. Westoff: "The Perfect Contraceptive Population," *Science*, September 1970.

Commission on Population Growth and the American Future: *Interim Report*, U.S. Government Printing Office, Washington, D.C., March 16, 1971.

Darity, William: "Continuing/Discontinuing Users of Oral Contraceptives," in A. Sobrero and S. Lewit (eds.), *Advances in Planned Parenthood*, Schenkman, Cambridge, Mass., 1965.

Green, Lawrence N.: "Status Identity and Preventive Health Behavior," *Pacific Health Education Report*, School of Public Health, University of California, Berkeley, 1970.

Gould, Robert E.: "The Wrong Reasons to Have Children," *New York Times Magazine*, June 1970.

International Planned Parenthood Federation, "Relations between Family Size and Maternal and Child Health," London, July 1970.

Kessler, A., and S. Kessler: "Health Aspects of Family Planning," in E. Diczfalusy and U. Borell (eds.), *Control of Human Fertility*, Wiley, New York, 1971.

Lehfeldt, Hans: "Psychology of Contraceptive Failure," *Medical Aspects of Human Sexuality*, May 1971.

Lidz, Ruth W.: "Emotional Factors in the Success of Contraception," *Fertility and Sterility*, vol. 20, no. 5, September–October 1969.

Manisoff, Miriam: *Family Planning: A Teaching Guide for Nurses*, Planned Parenthood—World Population, New York, 1971.

———: "Counseling for Family Planning," *American Journal of Nursing*, vol. 66, no. 12, December 1966.

———: *Family Planning Training for Social Service*, Planned Parenthood—World Population, New York, 1970.

Maxwell, Joseph W., and James E. Montgomery: "Societal Pressure toward Early Parenthood," *The Family Coordinator*, October 1969.

Planned Parenthood—World Population: "Family Planning Services in the United States: A National Review 1968," *Family Planning Perspectives*, October 1969.

Pohlman, E. J.: *The Psychology of Birth Planning*, Schenkman, Cambridge, Mass., 1969.

Public Family Planning Clinics: "Proceedings of Conference," G. D. Searle & Co., Chicago, September 1966.

Rainwater, Lee: *And the Poor Get Children*, Quadrangle, Chicago, 1960.

————: *Family Design*, Aldine, Chicago, 1965.

Wallach, Edward E., and Celso-Ramon Garcia: "Psychodynamic Aspect of Oral Contraception," *Journal of American Medical Association*, vol. 203, no. 11, March 1968.

Westoff, Charles, and Norman Ryder: "United States: Methods of Fertility Control, 1965." *Studies in Family Planning*, no. 17, February 1967.

Wyatt, Frederick: "Clinical Notes on the Motives of Reproduction," *Journal of Social Issues*, vol. 23, no. 4, October 1967.

15 | METHODS OF CONCEPTION CONTROL

Miriam T. Manisoff

All current as well as experimental methods of family planning are based on the principle of "intervention," that is, the interposing of barriers to or the interruption of the complicated series of physiological events in humans which constitute the process of conception. The ideal method would be completely safe, reversible, inexpensive, free of all side effects, simple to obtain and use, 100 percent effective, and not related to the time of coitus. Although we have approached some of these ideal standards, no single method meets all these criteria. Research to develop new and improved methods is a vital need if we are to achieve the ideal. Methods now in use can be categorized as those which require medical services (pelvic examination, prescription, or surgery) and those which the patient can obtain and use without medical supervision.

HELPING PATIENTS TO CHOOSE

In guiding couples to a choice of a method, it is important to ascertain which one will be most acceptable to them, since consistency of use is a critical factor in effectiveness. A method may be considered highly effective theoretically, but if the couple finds it unpleasant, distasteful, or difficult to use, it is unlikely they will use it consistently, if at all. This, of course, implies that they be given enough detail about each method so that they may make an informed initial choice and so that they be made aware of the availability of alternative methods; in this way they may later choose another method if the first choice is found to be unsatisfactory.

Consideration should always be given to the acceptability of the method to the male partner, since his opposition can be a serious barrier to effective use. Therefore, both factors of acceptability and effectiveness need to be considered, the aim being to select the most effective method which will be used consistently.

ORAL CONTRACEPTIVES

Oral contraceptives contain synthetic forms of the hormones progesterone and estrogen, either in combined form or in sequence. The dosages and types of hormones in the pills vary among the 15 to 20 brands now on the market, and the schedules for taking them also vary. The older brands are 20-day pill regimens in which the patient starts taking the pill on the fifth day of the menstrual cycle, counting the day that menses begin as day one and taking one pill a day for 20 days. She then stops taking the pills, waits for her next menstrual cycle, and repeats the procedure. The patient should be cautioned not to skip any days. She should be instructed to take the pill at approximately the same time each day and never to wait more than 7 days for the next menstrual period. If her period has not started by the seventh day, she should begin the next cycle of pills that day. If menses do not appear by the seventh day following the second pill cycle, she should report this to the physician. If the patient forgets to take her daily pill, she is to take it as soon as she remembers, even if this means taking two the next day. If she neglects her pill for 2 days in a row, she should be advised to continue the daily schedule, but to use an additional contraceptive (such as foam or the condom) for the remainder of the cycle. Patients should also understand that they are protected from pregnancy at all times, even on those days when they are waiting for their next period. The protection starts with the first series of pills if they are begun within the first 7 days of the menstrual cycle. Patients who decide to discontinue the pills in favor of another method should be informed that their next menstrual period may be delayed for up to 3 weeks and in some cases longer. Cessation of pill-taking at any point prior to completion of the full cycle of pills will result in withdrawal bleeding. Guidance to patients, therefore, should include mention that it is advisable to complete a pill series in its entirety before discontinuing oral contraception.

Oral contraceptives are also available in the more convenient 21-day regimens in which the patient takes a pill each day for 3 weeks continuously, then suspends for 1 week and resumes for the next 3 weeks—the so-called "3 weeks on, 1 week off" method. The menstrual period usually occurs during the 7 days off the pill, but patients must restart the pill after 7 days whether or not menses have occurred. In another variation, the pills are in a 28-day package and the patient takes the pills continuously and in sequence. The final seven pills are placebos. All the varieties described above consist of hormonal combinations.

Sequential pills are packaged so that patients take 15 or 16 consecutive pills containing only estrogen, followed by five pills containing both estrogen and progesterone. The sequential pills were designed to simulate the natural hormone events more closely than the combination pills, but they have a somewhat lower effectiveness rate.

Mode of Action

The primary action of the oral contraceptives is the suppression of ovulation through the inhibition of the follicle-stimulating hormone by estrogen, similar to its mechanism in pregnancy. The progestin contributes to the contraceptive effect by causing the cervical mucus to become thick and less penetrable to sperm. The pill also alters endometrial development so that it is out of phase for implantation. It may interfere with tubal transport of the ovum.

The effectiveness of combination oral contraceptives is considered virtually 100 percent in preventing pregnancy *provided* that they are taken as directed. This proviso emphasizes the importance of patient instruction and checking for patient understanding. The nurse, using language appropriate to the level of the patient's comprehension and education, plays an important role in ensuring proper use.

Side Effects

Side effects similiar to those of early pregnancy are experienced by some women due to the pregnancy-like hormonal status produced by the pills. These side effects can be slight or serious. They include nausea, dizziness, bloating, tenderness, headache, weight gain, and breakthrough bleeding. The symptoms usually disappear within the next two to four cycles, but if they persist, a shift to another preparation may be necessary. If side effects persist with various preparations, discontinuance of the medication and provision of a different method may be necessary.

Since the pills may suppress lactation, it is usually advised that they not be used for new mothers who plan to nurse their babies until the milk supply is well established.

Other side effects, which are considered desirable, are a decrease in the menstrual flow; reduction of dysmenorrhea, premenstrual tension, and vaginal discharge; improvement in acne conditions; and regulation of the menstrual cycle. In rare instances, patients report increases in libido and feelings of euphoria, perhaps induced by the release from worry about unwanted pregnancy. A few patients have also reported depression and reduction of libido.

Less common side effects also include an increase in skin pigmentation (chloasma), which clears when the medication is discontinued, and an increase in acne or hirsutism. Vaginal infections may be more common. In women who have menstrual irregularities before starting the pills, amenorrhea may persist after discontinuing them. Pre-existing uterine fibroid tumors may enlarge occasionally when the oral contraceptives are used.

The most severe side effect which has been noted is thrombophlebitis. There is an increased risk of morbidity and mortality from pulmonary embolism or cerebral thrombosis among patients using the pill, higher in women over thirty-five years old than in younger women, and a history of thromboembolic disease is a contraindication to their use. Since pregnancy carries a six to ten times higher risk of thrombophlebitis and embolism than does the use of the pills, their use in patients without such history is considered justified by most physicians.

Other contraindications to the use of oral contraceptives are a history of breast or uterine cancer, serious liver disease, or undiagnosed vaginal bleeding. Use with medical caution is indicated in migraine, uterine fibroids, heart or kidney disease, asthma, high blood pressure, diabetes, and epilepsy. No causal relationship has been found between the oral contraceptives and any type of malignancy.

It is apparent that careful and continuing medical supervision is required for the use of this method. A careful history, pelvic and breast examination, blood pressure determination, urinalysis for glucose and protein, and a Pap smear should be completed before the initiation of pill therapy. Patients should be educated as to the necessity for periodic medical examinations and reporting of untoward symptoms.

The Food and Drug Administration now stipulates that all pill manufacturers include with their product a standard information flyer cautioning patients about possible side effects and suggesting that they ask their doctor for a booklet with further information. Physicians prescribing the pills must be able to provide patients with this pamphlet, which has been prepared by the American Medical Association.

Acceptability

The oral contraceptives appear to be the most acceptable of all methods which can be used by women, being chosen by about 75 percent of patients seen in Planned Parenthood clinics. It is estimated that 15 to 20 million women are using these pills throughout the world. However, in the United States, about 32 percent have discontinued use of the pills by the end of 1 year, and 47 percent by 2 years, usually because of the side effects encountered.

INTRAUTERINE DEVICES

Intrauterine devices, often referred to as IUDs, are small plastic or metal forms to which a "tail" of nylon threads is usually attached. Some different types of IUDs are shown in Figure 15-1. There is a wide variety of shapes and sizes available. The device is inserted through the vagina and the cervical canal into the uterine cavity. IUDs are usually inserted via a straw-shaped inserter with a plunger. The device is pulled into a straight line as it is loaded into the inserter, and can be easily introduced without dilating the cervix. The insertion of a Lippes loop is shown in Figure 15-2. The inserter is then disengaged and withdrawn from the vagina. The nylon threads extend into the vagina and are used to check on the presence of the device in the uterus. The disengagement of the inserter and the extension of the tail into the vagina are shown in Figure 15-3. The doctor can remove the device by pulling the threads. Those devices which cannot be opened for such extension (the so-called "closed" devices) require their own individual inserters. The devices regain their original shape after placement in the uterus and can be left in place for an indefinite time.

All devices must be inserted under sterile conditions, usually by a physician, although nurse-midwives and nurses trained to do the procedure increasingly perform this function under medical supervision. The doctor uses sterile gloves, and the device and inserter are sterilized before use. Cold sterilization is used for the plastic devices and inserters, and presterilized packs of them are now available. A complete pelvic examination and Pap smear are done prior to insertion to rule out contraindicating pelvic disease. The physician passes a uterine sound to ascertain the direction and tightness of the uterine canal. He may use a tenaculum to stabilize the cervix during the insertion. The preferred time for insertion is during the last few days of the menstrual period, since this usually rules out an existing pregnancy. The device is also easier to insert at this time, and the slight bleeding which usually follows

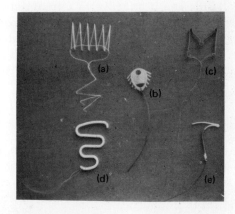

FIGURE 15-1
Five types of IUD's. (*a*) Majzlin spring device; (*b*) Dalkon shield; (*c*) "M" device; (*d*) Lippes loop; (*e*) "seven" device.

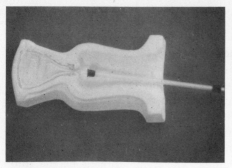

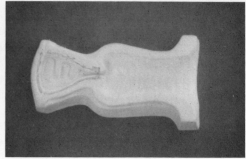

FIGURE 15-2
Insertion of a Lippes loop.

FIGURE 15-3
The Lippes loop inserter has been withdrawn, leaving the "tail" extending into the vagina.

insertion is less alarming to the patient, since she can consider it as part of her menses. Insertion can also be made immediately after delivery or abortion or at the time of the postpartum visit.

Mode of Action

The exact way in which the IUD works to prevent pregnancy in humans has not as yet been determined. It was originally thought to increase tubal motility and speed ovum transport. Thus, the egg, if fertilized, would be too immature for nidation on reaching the uterus. However, this theory has not been substantiated. It is now believed that the IUD, like the pill, may have more than one effect on the reproductive chain of events. One possibility is that the presence of a foreign body in the uterus produces a spermicidal or blastocidal substance. Another theory is that the IUD's presence causes an increase in macrophages in the uterine cavity and that their increased numbers are hostile and destructive to a fertilized ovum. Another mechanism which may be operating is an alteration in the normal endometrial phase needed for the reception of a fertilized ovum. The latest research development in the method is a device in the shape of a T, which has a thin copper wire wrapped around the leg of the T. The wire releases copper ions which appear to be spermicidal or antinidative.

Effectiveness

The IUDs, while less effective than the oral contraceptives in preventing pregnancy, are still among the most effective methods available. Approximately 20 to 30 percent of women either expel the device involuntarily or have it removed because of side effects. Among those who retain the device, there is a failure rate of about 2 percent of women per year during the first year of use, but this rate declines in later years. Older multiparous women retain the device better than nulliparous women. If pregnancy occurs with the device in place, the IUD usually does not need to be removed, since it does not interfere with the pregnancy.

Side Effects

The most common side effects are bleeding following insertion and heavier menstrual periods for some months after insertion. If the bleeding is severe and continues, the device may need to be removed. Cramping or pelvic pain is also common and may be severe enough to warrant removal. Involuntary expulsion of the device, particularly at the time of menstruation, may occur. It may be reinserted and will usually be retained in about half of such cases. Patients should be instructed to check with their finger for the presence of the nylon threads in the vagina about once a week and always after their period. If they cannot feel the threads, they may have expelled the device without noticing it and should be instructed to return to the doctor and to use an alternative method until they have been reexamined. Although the threads are discernible to the patient's examining finger, it is rare for the partner to be aware of them during intercourse. Patients should be told that they may experience the side effects noted above and that if the side effects are severe, to report them to the doctor.

Among the more serious side effects of IUD insertion are possible occurrence of exacerbation of pelvic inflammatory disease (PID) and uterine perforation after insertion. PID can usually be treated without removal of the device. Perforations may occur, but they are rare, and are usually symptomless in the case of open devices. This may require removal of the device, especially if it is of the "closed" type. There is no evidence that the IUD causes cancer of the uterus or endometrium.

The contraindications to the insertion of an IUD are pregnancy or suspected pregnancy, the presence of acute or subacute pelvic inflammatory disease, and a history of infected abortion or postpartum endometritis during the previous 6 weeks. In patients with menometrorrhagia or a class III Pap smear, insertions should not be made until proper investigation has been completed.

Acceptability

IUDs have been found highly acceptable to clinic patients, judging by the rates of continuation observed. About 80 percent were found to be still using this method after 1 year and 70 percent after the second year. Continuation rates for private patients are not available. Among the possible reasons advanced for this high acceptability are the facts that the IUD, once inserted, requires little, if any, further action or decision by the patient; it is coitus-independent and therefore aesthetically preferable; its cost or upkeep is low; and it is easily removed and completely reversible.

The nurse is often expected to explain this method and to answer the questions of the patient who will have or has had an IUD inserted. It is reassuring for the patient to be shown the device and to be instructed as to how and where it will be inserted, using a model or diagram. She can see that the device is not likely to be lost inside her, and she should be informed as to what the possible side effects are so that she will not be unduly alarmed if they occur. She can also be told that the IUD will not interfere with sex relations, the use of tampons, or the douche. Most women will also want to know how reliable the IUD is in preventing pregnancy, and it is important that they be aware that the IUD is not 100 percent effective.

DIAPHRAGM WITH JELLY OR CREAM

The diaphragm is a shallow cup of soft rubber with a flexible metal rubber-covered rim, approximately 2 to 4 inches in diameter. It is designed to fit snugly in the upper vagina between the symphysis pubis and the posterior fornix, covering the cervix. There are also some special diaphragms in other shapes for women with very relaxed vaginal tissues or other anatomical difficulties who cannot be fitted with a standard diaphragm. Diaphragms come in various sizes, measured in millimeters (50 to 105 mm), and each patient must be individually measured and fitted by a physician or trained nurse to ensure proper coverage. The thimble-shaped cervical cap, made of rubber or plastic, is designed to fit snugly over the cervix. This device, however, is not used very frequently in the United States.

The diaphragm is always used with contraceptive jelly or cream spread on it. A diaphragm and tube of cream are shown in Figure 15-4. In addition to careful fitting, this method requires that patients understand female anat-

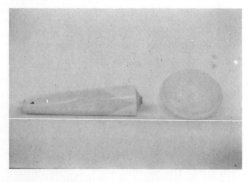

FIGURE 15-4
Diaphragm and contraceptive cream.

omy, how the diaphragm works, and how to insert the diaphragm properly. They will also need to be given the opportunity to practice insertion and checking for correct diaphragm placement. Patients should be instructed that the size may need to be changed after the birth of a child or pelvic surgery or if there is a considerable loss or gain of weight (10 pounds or more).

Mode of Action

The diaphragm acts as a mechanical barrier to the entry of sperm into the cervix, as shown in Figure 15-5. The primary function of the diaphragm, however, is to hold the spermicidal jelly or cream in contact with the cervix. This fact should always be emphasized in instructing patients.

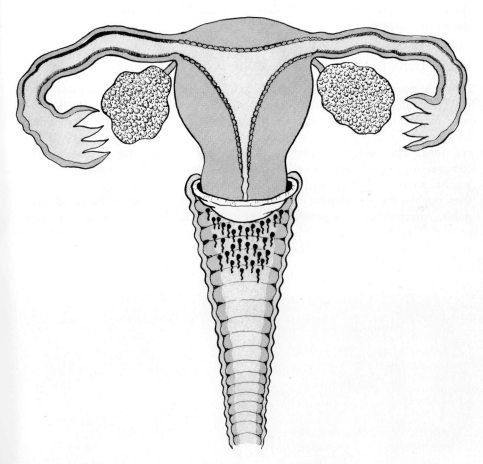

FIGURE 15-5
Entry of sperm into the cervix is prevented by use of the diaphragm.
(*Drawing by Mary McGovern.*)

Effectiveness

The theoretical effectiveness of the properly fitted, correctly used diaphragm with jelly or cream is high, with a failure rate as low as three pregnancies per 100 women per year. However, it is a fairly complicated method and requires consistent and repeated use, involving some degree of vaginal self-manipulation—distasteful to many women—and preplanning in relation to coitus; therefore, its actual use and effectiveness is much lower than in theory, with 10 to 15 pregnancies per 100 women per year. It also requires the availability of privacy and sustained motivation on the part of the woman, which may be in short supply for many patients in the lower socio-economic groups. It has no medical side effects. About 5 percent of patients in Planned Parenthood clinics now choose this method. Prior to the advent of the pills and the IUD, it was probably the most used method for women in the United States.

Instructions to the Patient

Probably no other method requires as much careful and usually time-consuming instruction for the patient. Two visits are usually needed before the patient may use the diaphragm for protection. On the first visit she is examined by the physician, a Pap smear is taken, and the proper size diaphragm is ascertained. The patient is then asked to insert the diaphragm herself, first compressing the rim between the thumb and forefinger and passing it into the vagina, aiming it in the direction of her coccyx, as shown in Figure 15-6. She then pushes the rim nearest the front of her body up behind the symphysis pubis. Alternatively, the patient may attach the diaphragm to an inserter and push this as deeply as possible into the vagina, give it a half turn to release the diaphragm, and remove the inserter. The patient then checks to see if the

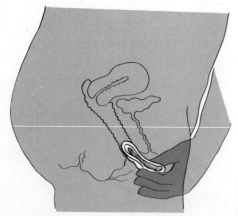

FIGURE 15-6
Insertion of a diaphragm.
(*Drawing by Mary McGovern.*)

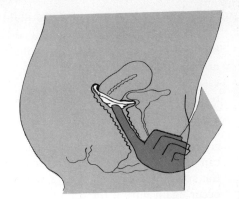

FIGURE 15-7
The woman uses her longest finger to check for proper positioning of the diaphragm.
(*Drawing by Mary McGovern.*)

cervix is covered by the rubber dome of the diaphragm by inserting her longest finger into her vagina and feeling for the rounded knob of the cervix. This procedure is demonstrated in Figure 15-7. It is advisable to have the patient feel her cervix before and after insertion so that she can distinguish the covering of the rubber. She can be told that the cervix will feel like the tip of her nose.

It is most helpful for the patient to be shown a model of the pelvic organs, into which a diaphragm can be inserted, so that she will better visualize what she is doing. The patient is usually given a "practice" diaphragm to take home with her before actually relying on the method for protection. She is instructed to return in a week, having inserted the diaphragm at home, so that her positioning of the diaphragm can be checked again after she has had the opportunity to practice insertion and removal. She may insert the diaphragm in a squatting or lying-down position, or standing up with one foot raised and resting on a chair or toilet seat. Removal of the diaphragm is done by hooking a finger around the rim nearest the front of her body and pulling. The patient should also understand that when using the diaphragm for contraception, it *must always* be coated thinly with about a teaspoonful of contraceptive jelly or cream. The diaphragm may be inserted with the dome up or down, if both sides have jelly or cream on them. After removal, the diaphragm is to be washed with mild soap and water, patted dry with a towel, lightly powdered with unmedicated talcum or cornstarch, and replaced in a container or safe place. The patient does not need to douche in connection with this method, but she may do so if she wishes to after removing the diaphragm.

At the return visit, when the patient is again examined, the doctor can see if she has properly placed the diaphragm. He may also at this time change the size originally given her, since some patients are tense on the first visit and more relaxed on the return visit, when a larger size fits better.

Patients should also be encouraged to adopt the habit of inserting the diaphragm before retiring every night as part of their usual routine, whether they expect to have intercourse or not. This reduces the likelihood—and bother—of having to get up and insert it during the night. If intercourse does not take place, the diaphragm will simply be removed in the morning. In any case, the patient should be told to be sure to insert the diaphragm before intercourse, regardless of when it takes place. If intercourse occurs more than 2 hours after the diaphragm has been inserted, additional jelly or cream should be inserted with an applicator before sex relations. Following intercourse, the diaphragm must not be removed for *at least 6 hours,* although it can remain in place longer. The 6-hour interval is necessary to ensure that the sperm deposited in the vagina will all be inactive or dead. If sex relations occur again during the 6 hours, the patient should insert more cream or jelly and leave the diaphragm in place for 6 hours following the last coitus.

The patient should understand that she may urinate or defecate while she is wearing the diaphragm. If her menses should start during that time, the diaphragm will not interfere. She should also examine the diaphragm from time to time to check for holes or tears, particularly around the rim, by holding it up to a strong light. The patient often needs reassurance that the diaphragm cannot get lost inside her. She can readily see this if the nurse can show her the pelvic model and point out the absence of any passageway large enough for the diaphragm to go through from the vagina into the interior of her body.

Patients should be told to return once a year to see the physician or sooner if she has any problems with the method. Young women who are just beginning regular intercourse should return in about 3 months to have the size rechecked. Patients should also know where they can obtain additional supplies of the cream or jelly as they need them and should be cautioned against using any other lubricant, such as petroleum jelly, as a substitute, since these may cause the rubber to deteriorate and are not spermicidal.

STERILIZATION

Voluntary elective sterilization of either male or female is a medically accepted means of conception control which is legal in all states. It differs from other methods of contraception in that it involves a surgical, usually irreversible procedure. It is the most reliable way to avoid unwanted pregnancy.

Voluntary sterilization should be actively considered for those couples who have achieved a family of desired size, particularly in cases in which there are serious medical contraindications to another pregnancy or in which other temporary contraceptive methods have been found to be unacceptable. Patients interested in this method should be fully informed as to its nature and consequence, since male sterilization is considered reversible in only 20 to 40 percent of cases. There is no way of predetermining this for specific individuals. However, newer techniques are improving the chances of reversibility. The recent development of sperm banks, in which the frozen sperm of a man who plans to have a vasectomy can be deposited and kept indefinitely for future use, may make male sterilization more acceptable.

Doctors feel that both man and wife should be emotionally mature and sure of their determination not to have any more children. They should also have a clear understanding of the permanence of the procedure. Doctors may expect both husband and wife to give written consent. Since these procedures do not involve removal of any glands or organs, normal potency and functioning of the hormonal system are not affected.

In women, there are a number of procedures, involving tubal ligation or partial or total salpingectomy, which may be used. These usually involve an abdominal incision so that the tubes may be ligated, and a portion excised or the two cut ends cauterized. Female sterilization can also be done vaginally (culdoscopy) or through a very small abdominal incision using a laparoscope. Sterilization in women is preferably done in the immediate postpartum period, since at this time the tubes are more readily accessible. Hysterectomy is also sometimes used as a sterilizing procedure, but unless there is uterine pathology, it is hard to justify its use in place of the more conservative sterilization procedures which have lower mortality rates.

For the male, the procedure, vasectomy, involves merely the closing of the vas deferens which carries the sperm. An incision of ½ to ¾ inch is made in each side of the scrotum so that the tubes can be lifted out, cut, and tied off, thus blocking the passage of sperm. The testicles continue to form sperm which are then absorbed in the body. Usually, this minor operation is performed in the doctor's office under local anesthesia.

After sterilization, the male will still have orgasm and ejaculate, although the semen contains no sperm. The quantity of the ejaculate does not diminish noticeably after a vasectomy, since the secretion of the testes which contains the sperm constitutes only about one-tenth of the amount of ejaculated semen.

Vasectomy does not produce sterility immediately, since mature sperm remain in the vas deferens and accessory glands beyond the area of ligation. Men who have been sterilized should be cautioned to continue contraceptive use until their semen can be reexamined by the physician about 8 weeks or following 10 ejaculations after the operation to ensure that it is sperm-free.

Although voluntary male sterilization has been widely used in India, its acceptance in this country appeared relatively low until recently (an estimated 100,000 Americans yearly). Through education and understanding of the fact that vasectomy does not castrate a man or "change his nature" but simply removes his ability to impregnate a woman, it is becoming an increasingly popular method of permanent contraception. Public acceptance, combined with greater availability of the procedure from physicians and clinics, has resulted in a startling increase. In 1970, according to the Association for Voluntary Sterilization (*A.V.S. News*, Summer 1971), a study showed that approximately 750,000 vasectomies were performed and that probably 3 million living Americans of childbearing age have now obtained sterilization.

THE RHYTHM METHOD

The rhythm method is the only birth control method (besides total abstinence) which is officially approved by the Roman Catholic Church. It is also referred to as "safe period," "periodic continence," or "temporary abstinence."

This method is based on the fact that a woman is fertile only around the time of ovulation and that if she abstains from intercourse during that time, she is unlikely to conceive. Usually a woman ovulates once during each menstrual cycle. The ovum has an active life of 12 to 24 hours during which it can be fertilized. Sperm cells, once within the uterus, are viable for about 72 hours during which they can fertilize the ovum. Thus, there is a minimum total of 96 hours (4 days) during each menstrual cycle when conception is possible. To these 4 days an additional margin of several days is added to allow for variation in the exact day of ovulation.

To calculate the safe period by the calender method, the woman should have a written record of the date of onset of her last 12 menstrual periods. From this record, the number of days in each of these menstrual cycles is listed, counting from the first day bleeding began to the day before the onset of bleeding of the next menstrual period. From this list, the longest cycle and the shortest cycle are selected. The number 18 is subtracted from the number of days in the shortest cycle to give the first day of the fertile or unsafe period, and the number 11 is subtracted from the number of days in the longest cycle to give the last day of the fertile period. Thus, if a woman had cycles ranging from 25 to 31 days, she would abstain from intercourse from the seventh day of her current menstrual cycle (25 − 18 = 7) until the twentieth day of her cycle (31 − 11 = 20). The woman will need to continue her written record of menstrual periods so that the calculation is always based on the 12 most recent menstrual cycles.

The accuracy of the safe period method can be improved by charting the woman's basal body temperature. This is based on the fact that the basal temperature (taken immediately on awakening and before any activity whatsoever) of a woman is more or less constant during the first part of the menstrual cycle until the day of ovulation. At that time it drops slightly and then rises to a level somewhat higher (usually five-tenths to seven-tenths of a degree) than it has been and remains at the higher level for the balance of the cycle. If there is no cold or infection to account for this elevation, the woman can consider herself beyond the fertile period when the elevation has persisted for 3 days. Special basal temperature charts are available from Planned Parenthood—World Population for recording the temperature curves, and special basal thermometers may be used.

The effectiveness of this method can be considered satisfactory for highly motivated, carefully selected women with fairly regular cycles, who have the intelligence and self-discipline, as well as a cooperative marital partner, to understand and practice it correctly and rigorously. It also costs nothing. However, many couples find it impossible to have "sex by the calender" instead of by inclination. The use of the rhythm method has also been implicated in studies that indicate it may predispose to fetal abnormalities or abnormal gestation because when accidental pregnancies occurred the ovum or sperm involved were more likely to be "past their prime."

Most couples who, because of religious convictions, prefer to use this method will need assistance and considerable support from the doctor or nurse. It is contraindicated in women for whom a pregnancy poses a serious medical danger.

CONDOMS

The condom, a rubber or synthetic rubber sheath, is the most widely used device for contraception in this country and in many other parts of the world. It is also the oldest device and one of the few under male control. It is highly effective, particularly when used in conjunction with the insertion of contraceptive vaginal jelly or cream by the woman. The spermicide provides protection in case the condom should break or slip during intercourse.

The condom ranks almost with the diaphragm in effectiveness, having an accidental pregnancy rate of about 3 percent. The popularity of the condom is no doubt due to the fact that it is relatively inexpensive, simple to use, and readily available without a doctor's prescription. It carries the additional advantage of protecting against venereal disease and is also used clinically in the treatment of vaginal moniliàsis and trichomoniasis to prevent reinfestation by the male. Condoms are particularly appropriate for use when intercourse is not taking place frequently and regularly, as among unmarried young couples, and when there are contraindications or difficulties in using other methods.

Its disadvantages include the fact that the sexual act must be interrupted to apply the condom to the erect penis, and many couples find that it dulls sensation. The latter fact, however, may be an advantage in cases of premature ejaculation.

Condoms are made with plain ends or with a teat tip, prelubricated or dry. To use the condom correctly, care should be taken in unrolling it over the erect penis to see that no air is left in the condom's tip or, if it has a plain end, that it is not drawn too tightly over the end of the penis, since the air may cause it to burst or may cause an overflow of semen from the open end. After orgasm, the penis must be withdrawn before the erection disappears. The upper rim of the condom must be held firmly during withdrawal so that it does not slip off into the vagina.

VAGINAL FOAMS, JELLIES, AND CREAMS

These preparations contain spermicidal chemicals and materials which immobilize sperm and form a film over the cervix to deter sperm from entering. They are inserted deep into the vagina with a plastic applicator which has been filled from a container. Insertion must take place within an hour before each coitus. If intercourse is repeated, or if more than an hour has elapsed since insertion, another full applicator of the preparation should be inserted. Douching is not necessary, but if used, it *must be delayed until 6 hours* after the last intercourse, since the protection of these materials may be washed away before the sperm are dead or inactive.

Foams are considered somewhat more effective than jellies or creams and are also less likely to be messy or drippy. These methods are rated less effective than the diaphragm or condom. Like the condom, they are readily available without prescription, relatively inexpensive and simple to use, and are especially useful as an alternative or temporary method (e.g., when a woman has forgotten to take her pills for 2 days) or for women who are having infrequent intercourse.

VAGINAL FOAMING TABLETS, SUPPOSITORIES, AND SPONGES

These methods are not as widely used in the United States as other vaginal methods and are ranked among the least reliable. Their main advantage is their simplicity, availability, and low cost. The foaming tablets are moistened with water or saliva to start their foaming action and are inserted no more than 1 hour before intercourse.

The woman must wait at least 5 minutes after insertion to allow the foam to be generated. Vaginal suppositories do not need moistening, but require a brief time—about 10 minutes—after insertion to allow them to melt and disperse in the vagina. The vaginal sponge is used by moistening with a spermicidal liquid and squeezing it to produce a foam. The sponge is inserted deep into the vagina and left in place until 6 hours after intercourse. No douching should be used with these methods until 6 hours after coitus.

WITHDRAWAL (COITUS INTERRUPTUS)

This is an ancient technique which requires the male to interrupt coitus by removing his penis from the woman's vagina prior to orgasm so that the ejaculate is deposited well away from the vagina or external genitals. It requires no devices or chemicals and is available under all circumstances at no cost.

Estimates as to its effectiveness vary, since this depends on the ability of the individual male to judge and control his time of orgasm. Studies indicate that it may rank with the diaphragm and condom for effectiveness, but many men lack the control necessary for its successful use. Many couples consider the interruption psychologically disturbing, and anxiety about whether withdrawal will take place in time can also be a deterrent to satisfactory sexual intercourse. For couples who have found this method acceptable and reliable, there is no need to urge a change to another method. It can also be useful as an emergency method when other means are unavailable.

UNRELIABLE METHODS

The postcoital douche is a very ineffective method of contraception, despite its fairly wide use, since the sperm enter the cervical canal within seconds after ejaculation, from where they cannot be flushed by douching. Its main value, since it reduces the number of sperm still within the vagina, is in an emergency, such as after the breaking or slipping of the condom.

It is possible that prolonged lactation may delay pregnancy for up to 10 months by delaying the return of ovulation, but in the United States it is not considered a reliable or useful method.

RESEARCH METHODS

Possible sites and means of intervention in the reproductive chain of events are being studied in the effort to develop new and more effective means of contraception. Such experimental methods are, of course, not available for general use. Among those of great interest today are the continuous progestins and the prostaglandins. It has been found that daily doses of small amounts of synthetic progestins, which do not suppress ovulation, produce a cervical mucus which is thick and hostile to sperm, and also produce an out-of-phase endometrium in which the ovum cannot implant. The progestins can be administered by mouth or by long-acting injection or subcutaneous capsules which release the daily dose required.

Prostaglandins are fatty acids, originally isolated from a number of body tissues and now synthesized, which can stimulate the myometrium to terminate pregnancy, or the tubal musculature to hasten egg transport sufficiently to prevent fertilization. They may also produce corpus luteum degeneration and prevent or interrupt nidation.

Morning-after pills, using large doses of estrogens from 3 to 5 days immediately after unprotected coitus, have been found almost completely effective in preventing pregnancy. This technique, however, can be considered only as a backup emergency measure because of the high estrogen dose involved and the accompanying nausea and vomiting.

Reversible male sterilization through the use of metal valves which can be turned on or off, removable clamps, or plastic plugs placed within the vasa deferentia is also being studied.

BIBLIOGRAPHY

Davis, Hugh J., and John Lesinski: "Mechanism of Action of Intrauterine Contraceptives in Women," *Obstetrics and Gynecology*, vol. 36, no. 3, September 1970.

Guttmacher, Alan F., W. Best, and F. S. Jaffe: *Birth Control and Love*, Macmillan, New York, 1969.

Harkavy, Oscar, and John Maier: "Research in Reproductive Biology and Contraceptive Technology: Present Status and Needs for the Future," *Family Planning Perspectives*, vol. 2, no. 3, June 1970.

Hartman, C. G.: *Science and the Safe Period*, Williams & Wilkins, Baltimore, 1962.

Karim, S. M. M., and G. M. Filshie: "Use of Prostaglandin E2 for Therapeutic Abortion," *British Medical Journal*, no. 5716, July 25, 1970.

Manisoff, Miriam: *Family Planning, A Teaching Guide for Nurses*, 2d ed., Planned Parenthood—World Population, New York, 1971.

Neubardt, Selig: *A Concept of Contraception*, Trident Press, New York, 1967.

Peel, J., and M. Potts: *Contraceptive Practice*, Cambridge, New York, 1969.

Segal, Sheldon J., and Christopher Tietze: "Contraceptive Technology: Current and Prospective Methods," *Reports on Population/Family Planning*, Population Council, no. 1, October 1969.

Wood, H. Curtis, Jr.: *Sex without Babies*. Whitmore, Philadelphia, 1967.

PART III

CHILDBEARING AND THE NURSING PROCESS

Childbearing is one of the most significant and personal experiences in the life of a couple. It is viewed by most families as being a planned and happy event in their lives. Producing a healthy baby is the natural anticipation of expectant families, and no couple expects to experience complications during pregnancy or in childbirth. In order to assure the necessary care to promote a healthy experience, prevent complications in the expectant mother or developing fetus, provide as normal a delivery as possible, have a healthy baby, and give the appropriate teaching and counseling to the family in infant care and development, every expectant couple must receive the highest quality of maternity care provided by knowledgeable, expert, caring, and supportive health practitioners.

Since maternity nurses are being offered and are accepting more responsibility in the management and supportive components of total family care during pregnancy and childbirth, it is imperative that they also be accountable for their actions. Thus, the nurse needs to continually evaluate her understanding and utilization of current scientific knowledge and the nursing process as they relate to the expectant woman and her family. Some questions the nurse might ask herself are: How current is the knowledge that I use in my nursing practice? Do I truly believe that the biopsychosocial needs of the woman are the basis for nursing actions? In my nursing practice, am I incorporating the steps of perceiving, assessing, planning, implementing, and evaluating so that others can recognize, understand, and participate appropriately in the nursing actions? Does every expectant or new mother with whom I interact understand through my relationships and actions that I am interested in her and her family as individuals? Do my actions and expressions reflect a knowledgeable and harmonious working relationship with other health team members?

Today's maternity nurse must be an excellent listener, teacher, and counselor and an expert practitioner, and she must be able to perform these roles in such a way that the expectant or delivered woman and her family perceive that the nurse is truly interested in and concerned about them.

Regardless of the setting in which the nurse first meets the expectant woman—the clinic, the doctor's office, or the home—it is essential that the nurse's approach be personally focused. How the nurse initiates the nursing process will determine the cohesiveness of the relationship and the effectiveness of the nursing care.

The physiological and emotional changes that occur in the woman during pregnancy are fairly well understood by most nurses. Helping the expectant mother and family gain the same understanding is a necessary and valuable preparation for childbirth and their parental roles. Understanding what the pregnant woman experiences will also help them understand fetal development and how each influences the other. Expectant parents frequently want information about travel, recreation, and sexual activity, and they are particularly interested in knowing if certain activities cause any harm to the mother or the developing baby.

The importance of good nutrition during pregnancy has been recognized for a long time but unfortunately has not always been included as an essential component of nursing care. How to assist families in improving their eating habits is not always easy. Knowing about and believing in the importance of good nutrition, the nurse has many opportunities to strengthen and support the health of women and families through sound nutrition education.

Preparation for childbirth is an accepted and expected service in maternity care. There are many methods of teaching just as there are a variety of different ways individuals prefer to learn. Some couples express an interest in group discussions while others prefer to listen to a stimulating lecture. Others wish to talk individually with the nurse or other health professional. Still others prefer to read a book. Regardless of the method, couples are expressing the need and desire to know more about pregnancy and childbirth, and the authors of the following chapters have identified and described several effective methods of preparation for childbirth utilized by the maternity nurse today.

Just as the nurse needs to be knowledgeable about the many physiological and emotional changes that occur during pregnancy, the nurse is also expected to have a comprehensive understanding of the stages of labor and the reactions and responses of the laboring woman to these various stages. The authors clearly discuss the needs of the woman and her family during labor and provide helpful approaches for the nurse to use in her management and supportive care during this critical time.

Very often the expectant woman will express the desire to have the nurse who has assisted her in pregnancy be with her and her family during childbirth. When relationships have been meaningful, it is difficult to go through the process of establishing new ones, especially when sufficient time to do this is not always available. A woman approaching labor has no control over when it will start. Women in labor express the need to have someone with them to assist, comfort, and support them. Many want their husbands with them, and when they wish to be together, this should be arranged. Both husband and wife should be given the information, support, and assistance they want and need during this memorable experience.

Continuity of care is essential throughout pregnancy and childbirth. Because the maternity nurse who cared for the family during pregnancy is not always able to assist during labor and delivery, it is imperative that the nurse in labor know the maternity care given during pregnancy. Only when the unique needs of each woman and family are known by all health personnel involved in the plan of care can there be continuity and consistency in implementing the plan. It is also important for the nurse who cares for the mother and family in childbirth to inform the nurse of the special needs of the family after delivery. How the nurse implements this continuity of care is dependent upon the needs identified by her and by the family.

Scientific research in maternity care is continually being investigated. The authors have incorporated many of the current findings in research to assist the nurse in her own learning so that she can be more knowledgeable, confident, and effective in implementing the nursing process.

UNIT A

MANAGEMENT AND SUPPORTIVE CARE DURING PREGNANCY

16 | INITIATING THE NURSING PROCESS

Rosie L. Acton

Antepartal care, or management and supportive care given during pregnancy, has maternal and fetal safety and health as its goals. In recent years these goals have expanded to encompass supporting an informed rewarding life experience for a family. Emphasis is on the informed, participating family. With this has come increased counseling and teaching in prenatal settings plus more written material on parenthood with the expectant parents in mind. The management and supportive care given during pregnancy differs in relation to many social, cultural, ethnic, and financial circumstances. The differences are also reflected in the nature of the professional delivering the service.

Financial circumstances—namely, poverty—limit the number of families who seek antepartal care. Efforts are being made to make services available. With the emphasis on health as a right, perhaps more mothers will seek antepartal care, and the risks of childbearing for the poor may be reduced. Sweden, a country where antepartal services are available to everyone, has the lowest infant mortality rate in the world.[1] With Sweden's infant mortality rate at 12 to 13 per 100,000 for several years, the United States remains at 21 to 25 per 100,000. In the United States in 1969 the infant mortality rate was 21.6 per 100,000.[2]

PROFESSIONAL ROLES WITHIN THE HEALTH SYSTEM

The nurse, physician, midwife, and other specialized personnel collaborate to provide the services required by the family. The nurse acts as the patient advocate, teacher, and counselor concerned with the total experience of the patient. The midwife or physician is the diagnostician, process facilitator, and technical specialist. The physician differs from the midwife in his ability to also diagnose and treat medical complications of pregnancy. These roles are not necessarily clearly defined and much overlap is usually the case. Nurses, doctors, and midwives have many similar skills. The following factors may influence who provides what services to patients:

1 The strength or weakness of a particular skill makes a difference in how the professional performs. Nurses have technical and interpersonal skills. If interested in technical performance, the nurse may act mainly as a technical assistant to the physician. When the nurse values interpersonal and teaching skills, more time is spent counseling, supporting, and teaching patients.

2 Circumstances may often dictate the practice of a nurse. If the nurse works in a prenatal facility that serves 100 women a day, individual teaching and counseling may be difficult. One would expect group sessions in this setting and perhaps use of skilled volunteers from the community with whom the nurse would work very closely.

3 The patient's prior conceptions of nurses influence the early nurse-patient interactions. If patients have not had previous experience with nurses as counselors and teachers, the nurse will need to be articulate in interpreting and establishing the role with patients. This role is often supported by physicians with the referral of the patient to the nurse for information. In return the nurse keeps the physician informed of the patient's response; this helps nurture the colleague response to patient needs.

4 The availability of other professionals influences how the nurse works with families. Small rural communities have limited numbers of allied health personnel, such as dietitians and social workers. In large clinic-type organizations, there are often social workers and dietitians available to meet the needs of patients in such areas as placement of babies of unwed mothers or specific dietary problems. Some facilities, when able, use these resources in teaching sessions with pregnant women and their families. Usually they have a minimum of time available, and they see only those patients with the greatest need. This emphasizes the need for nurses to make accurate patient assessments and to refer those who require other professional services.

5 If there is a physician shortage in the community, nurses may perform differently. The minimal number of physicians to provide care to

patients emphasizes the need for collaborative effort and the use of the most appropriate person for services the patient needs. This points toward the probable use of nurses and midwives to provide more antepartal care to women with apparently normal pregnancies. We may see nurses working with families to facilitate self-monitoring and also as the primary health worker for the family. This would support a trend toward family care, not merely maternity care.

6 The nurse's stronger preparation in interpersonal skills influences the health services available to patients. This preparation makes the nurse the best prepared person to work with families as they deal with the very real life changes of enlarging a family. The interpersonal support of coping mechanisms and teaching is best done by nursing and should be the assumed role of nursing.

The patient will seek the person she feels will meet her present perceived needs and proceed on a trial-and-error basis. This is especially true in regard to information. Often the patient may not know where to find the most appropriate source of information. The nurse needs to be skilled in watching for cues. Establishing relationships with reception personnel so that they will refer patients who seem hesitant or uncertain is one step. Emphasizing this part of nursing practice when talking with physicians will increase the opportunity for nurses and physicians to collaborate in regard to patient needs. Nurses must keep physicians informed so that they know how to work with us. Nursing must follow through by keeping accurate, concise, clear records so others may also work with the nurse in delivering service to patients.

Patients come to health facilities with various perceptions or stereotypes of physicians and nurses. We can determine what these are and perform that way or ignore them and "do our own thing." We can try to understand their expectations and attempt to interpret what services we can offer. Studies have shown that patients are willing to use nurses as counselors rather than physicians if nurses can meet their needs.[3] Edith Anderson speaks of programs in which the maternity nurse may manage the normal pregnancy of a mother after the initial medical assessment.[4] These trends will mean more and more responsibility in nursing and emphasize the need for skill in establishing long-term relationships with patients. The nurse will need interpersonal communication skills to interpret the nursing role to patients and knowledge and judgment to perform it.

ANTEPARTAL RECORD

A woman calls an office or clinic to make an appointment when she thinks she is pregnant. She is asked some questions by a receptionist, and an appointment is made for a pregnancy test. When the results of the pregnancy

FIGURE 16-1
EXAMPLE OF AN ANTEPARTAL OR OBSTETRIC RECORD

	DATE

PATIENT'S NAME: LAST   FIRST   INITIAL   AGE

MAIDEN NAME   BIRTH DATE   RACE   RELIGION   OCCUPATION

ADDRESS   PHONE   MARITAL STATUS
M-S-W-D-SEP   EDUCATION

HUSBAND   AGE   OCCUPATION   HEIGHT   WEIGHT

MEDICAL HISTORY

FAMILY MEDICAL HISTORY: (Tuberculosis, Hypertension, Heart, Diabetes, Neurology Epilepsy, Allergies, Multiple Births, Congenital Anomalies)

MEDICAL HISTORY	POS		POS
Nephritis		Psychological disorders	
Heart disease		Epilepsy	
Hypertension		Drug sensitivity	
Rheumatic fever		Allergies	
Tuberculosis		Blood dyscrasias	
Venereal disease		Blood transfusions	
Gynecologic disease		Operations, accidents	
Iso-immunization		German measles	
Diabetes		Virus infections	
Thyroid disfunction		X rays	
Phlebitis varicosities		Smoking	

COMMENTS:

MENSTRUAL HISTORY

Onset Age	Interval	Duration	Amount
LMP	PMP	Normal?	EDC

PREVIOUS PREGNANCIES

No.	Date	Place of confine-ment	Duration of gestation	Duration of labor	Type of delivery	Born A/D	Sex	Weight	Complications Maternal	Child
1										
2										
3										
4										
5										
6										
7										

Summary, number
of pregnancies

	Full term	Premature	Abortions Stillborn	Children now alive	Multiple births

FIGURE 16-1 (Continued)

PRESENT PREGNANCY

Nausea	_____	Edema	_____
Vomiting	_____	Abdominal pain	_____
Indigestion	_____	Urinary complaints	_____
Constipation	_____	Bleeding	_____
Headache	_____	Breast changes	_____
Dizziness		Fatigue	_____
Visual disturbance	_____	Weight gain	_____

COMMENTS:

PHYSICAL EXAM: T   P   R   BP   WT   WT before LMP

EENT	Abdomen
Fundi	Height of fundus
Teeth	Breasts
Thyroid	Nipples
Heart	Tumors
Lungs	Fetal heart
Extremities	Presentation or
Varicosities	position
Edema	Pelvic exam
Skin	
Nodes	

COMMENTS:

Bony pelvis _____

Diag: Conj.   cm   Trans. diam. outlet   cm   Shape sacrum

Arch   Coccyx   SS. notch

Ischial spines   P. sag

Inlet	Midpelvis	Outlet	Prognosis for delivery
__Adequate	__Adequate	__Adequate	
__Borderline	__Borderline	__Borderline	
__Contracted	__Contracted	__Contracted	

LABORATORY EXAMINATIONS: Blood Type and Rh_____Hgb_____
Urinalysis: Albumin _____ Sugar _____ Microscopic _____
Pap smear: Date _____ Results _____
G. C. culture: Date _____ Results _____

FIGURE 16-1 (Continued)

PRENATAL RECORD

EDC	Parity		Nonpregnant weight

Date of visit	
Week of gestation	
Blood pressure	
Weight	
Headache	
Dizziness	
Nausea Vomiting	
Edema	
Urine tr. sym.	
Bleeding	
Height of fundus (cm)	
Presentation and position	
Station	
Fetal motion	
Fetal heart rate	
Est. fetal weight	
	Urine protein	
L	Urine sugar	
A	Antibody titer	
B	Hemoglobin	
Next visit	
M.D. initials	

SPECIAL INFORMATION

Type of delivery planned   Sensitivities

Anesthesia planned   Nutritional status

Hospital   Breast-feeding planned?

                                                          Physician's Signature _____

FIGURE 16-1 (Continued)

PROGRESS NOTES AND/OR CONSULTATIONS

Date:

Postpartum exam
Time: post delivery _____ Complications _____

T _____ P _____ BP _____ WT _____

Breasts and nipples _____

Abdomen _____

Perineum _____ Vagina _____

Uterus: Position _____ Size _____

Cervix _____ Adnexa _____

Rectal _____

Cytology _____

Infant's condition _____

Remarks _____

Recommendations _____

Referrals _____

Date _____

Physician's Signature _____

test are positive, an appointment is set for the woman to see the nurse an
the physician.

When the woman arrives at the institution, an admission clerk or
secretary gathers initial data and sets up the chart. This gives the nurse an
physician some basic information prior to seeing the patient.

In a clinic that uses nurses as assessors of patient needs, the nurse an
patient meet, and the nurse puts the patient at ease and conducts an initi
interview. From this an assessment of the patient is written, and a plan c
care is entered in the chart. This antepartal record with its nursing asses
ment and plan of care will facilitate the patient's pregnancy experience an
coordinate the work of the various people the patient will contact during he
pregnancy. The record is updated at each prenatal visit. It will be sent to th
hospital labor and delivery areas when the patient is admitted to have he
baby. Her experience will be recorded as she goes through labor and deliver
and is admitted to the postpartum unit. It will also be used by physicians an
nurses to provide care while she is in the hospital and to plan for her car
when she goes home. The information may generate a referral to a publ
health nurse. The public health nurse uses it for the home visit and returr
it to the clinic where it is used for the first postpartum visit. By this time
tells the entire story of her pregnancy, labor and delivery, postpartum reco\
ery, and home adjustment. At the first postpartum appointment, 5 or 6 week
after delivery, an evaluation is then made of her experience and family plar
ning services are offered.

In some institutions the antenatal record is a combined medical and nurs
ing record. In others, the records are separate with some overlapping of ir
formation and are cross-used by the two professionals. A separate nursin
record form can be sent out to the public health nurse to use when making
home visit (see Figure 16-2). This probably could not be done if it were
combined record. There are advantages to both types of records. In man
institutions the record must stay on the premises. It is the record of the pa
tient, but the institution is responsible for its safety. Nursing records such a
those shown in Figure 16-2 can be mailed because they were originally de
signed for this purpose.

THE NURSING ASSESSMENT TOOLS

From the time of the initial patient visit, the nurse makes observations an
seeks information to formulate a plan of care. The assessment draws on th
nurse's knowledge, skill, experience, and judgment. Often part of this proces
is unconscious. As in any first meeting, trains of thought quickly take shape
The purpose of a nursing assessment is to clearly direct the effort put fort
and to make it conscious and purposeful.

NURSING INFORMATION RECORD

E.D.C._____

Date of 1st Clinic Visit:_____

Phone:_____

Patient:_____ Age:_____
Occupation:_____
Future Plans:_____
Husband:_____ Age:_____
Occupation:_____

Family:_____
_____
_____
_____
_____
_____
_____
_____

Concerns of the Patient:_____
_____
_____
_____
_____
_____
_____
_____
_____

Problems observed by Staff:_____
_____
_____
_____
_____
_____
_____

Knowledge and Attitudes Concerning Labor and Delivery:___
_____
_____
_____
_____
_____

Infant Care:_____
_____
_____
_____
_____
_____
_____
_____
_____
_____
_____

FIGURE 16-2

The nursing information record. This record is used at the University of Minnesota Hospitals to record the nursing assessment and the plan of care. It travels from the clinic to the labor rooms, to the postpartum unit, to the public health nurse, and back to the clinic. This circle movement provides continuity throughout the childbearing experience.

Date of Interview and Tour of Obstetrical Area:_____

General Observations:

   1. Appearance:

   2. Behavior During Interview:

   3. How Patient Communicates:

Previous Hospitalizations:_____
Reason(s) for Hospitalization:_____

Comments:_____

Hospital Discharge Notes:_____

Family Planning:_____

FIGURE 16-2 (Continued)

The assessment is a picture of the important data about a patient. The data the nurse requires is that which indicates the kind, quantity, and extent of service the patient needs. Most assessment plans contain broad categories of information which then are individualized for each patient. The information may be gathered by an interview, by asking the patient to fill out a questionnaire, or through both. Because of the personal patient information involved in maternity nursing, an interview is more appropriate and helpful.

This initial assessment or picture of the patient's situation is the baseline tool of the nursing process. The nurse validates the picture obtained with the patient and develops a plan of action. The assessment will be altered as the patient situation changes. This is a nonstatic matrix which changes with the living process.

Assuming there is consensus that the nursing process is data gathering, validation, interpretation, validation, plan of action, implementation, and evaluation, the assessment represents the first four steps in this process. The shift to the plan of action and its implementation is often not sharply demarcated. It often involves giving information or teaching which evolves from the initial assessment interview. The nursing process in this type of patient relationship is like a form that flows, expands, and contracts to varying degrees in a changing pattern. An illustration of this pattern follows.

At the initial interview the nurse noted that the patient seemed anxious and tense when the appointment with the physician was explained (data gathering). This cue was investigated by asking if the woman was nervous and if she had had a pelvic exam before (validation and interpretation). The patient's reply was negative regarding the pelvic exam, and she replied that she was nervous (validation). The nurse offered to stay with the patient and explained ways she could relax (plan of action). The patient sighed with relief and said that would be helpful (validation). The nurse evaluated the plan of action by observation of the patient during the examination, by noting her relaxed body and manner after the examination, and by listening to her statement that "it won't be as difficult next time" (implementation and evaluation).

This experience, the action taken, and the response of the patient now become part of the assessment or picture of the patient. It indicates other areas the nurse should pursue. If this woman has never had a pelvic examination before, how much gynecological health care has she had? What is her knowledge of sexuality? Thus, each situation leads into another, and the nursing process is further modified and reconsidered. This was only one area involved in the first interview; there were other areas in which this same process occurred and which directed the information the patient received and influenced how the interaction would go at her next clinic appointment.

Categories of Information in an Assessment

The categories of information are described as follows:

1 What is the patient like? This would include age, marital status, occupation, ethnic group, size, appearance, and personality.
2 What are her resources? Level of intelligence, close family and friends, energy level, and apparent ability to cope with change or stress might be included in this area.
3 What are her goals and values? This might include body image, whether the baby is a planned pregnancy, if she is working and if her job is important to her, and noting her life-style.
4 How much knowledge or experience does she have? This would include whether this is the first baby, the existence of younger brothers and sisters, if she has cared for small babies, and whether she has read any books for prospective parents or attended expectant parent classes.
5 What are her expectations and concerns? A difficult and uncomfortable pregnancy, the change of life patterns with this addition to the family, and worry about labor and delivery should be noted.
6 Does she have any problems which may influence the course of the pregnancy? Examples might be existing diabetes or heart disease. She may be having financial problems, or she may be overweight. This might be an unwanted pregnancy, or she might be unmarried.

From this information a plan of nursing care and a patient record is established which facilitates work with the family. This record is used to plan teaching and the use of community resources and as a base to anticipate problems the family might encounter during the course of the pregnancy.

Interviewing

There are three basic purposes of the interview:

1 To gather information
2 To disseminate information
3 To establish a relationship

Some nurses use the initial interview as a time to focus on gathering patient information to be used as base-line data. This is often combined with giving information regarding the services of the agency. The third goal is an assumed goal by most nurses, and it is often expected to occur naturally. All three goals are sought in an interview, but all require different emphasis at different times, both during the interview and during pregnancy.

PERSPECTIVES OF INTERVIEWING

In a new interpersonal situation, people have the need to maintain self-esteem. This is done by feeling out the values within the situation. This is intensified in situations that will extend over a given time. When prospective parents come to a health facility they are very interested in what the people are like and how they will be treated. If the nurse is able to demonstrate caring, respect, and value of people, this will enhance the service rendered. This sets the whole atmosphere of the interview situation. If the nurse is concerned with what patients think of nursing knowledge and tries to impress them, difficulty may arise. Trying to impress patients may be perceived as patronizing. The probable result is that the patient only tolerates the nurse. The goal is a relationship of honest caring and give-and-take.

PERSONAL OR OBJECTIVE INTERVIEWING

An interview may be a personal or impersonal experience—personal if a reciprocal relationship is established, impersonal if it is merely a question and answer session. Assuming that a personal experience is desirable for maternity patients, the nurse needs to understand what is happening in the interview situation and why.

The following assumptions about the nurse-patient interactions may be helpful.

First, assume the patient wants this to be a good interview if it is advantageous to her and her baby. One need not worry about pulling information from the patient. She will want to tell you anything that will help make her pregnancy better. She may not know what is best to tell the nurse or doctor.

Second, the interview will be more successful if the nurse first tells the patient why she is being interviewed. Parents of first babies especially desire and need information, since they know little of what to expect from this kind of encounter with a health worker.

Third, it is the responsibility of the nurse to put the patient at ease. The nurse must be warm, open, and accepting if the patient is to feel comfortable and reciprocate. The focus should be on looking forward to meeting a new person and anticipating the advantages for both participants. The nurse is going to meet a person undergoing one of nature's most fascinating processes—reproduction—and will have the opportunity to be a participant and observer. The patient requires a knowledgeable advocate in this experience. Both have the opportunity for personal growth and understanding.

Fourth, realize that most women have some ambivalent feelings about being pregnant. Few events in our lives have all positive ramifications and no negative ones. If you remark about how happy she must be, she may not feel that she can say anything about being unhappy. Unhappiness may be very real, even when it is a planned pregnancy. The new baby means having someone completely dependent who takes, takes, takes, and gives very little in return. Many people today, in a culture which values independence and freedom, find this a difficult adjustment.

Fifth, the responsibility for clarity rests with the nurse. To fulfill this obligation one must use all of the senses to detect signs of misunderstanding. This means watching eye and facial expressions as well as body movements. It means telling the patient the nurse may not always be clear and to please question the nurse if this occurs.

THE NURSE IN THE INTERVIEW

If all goes well, the nursing interview meets the needs of the nurse and the patient. It may sound strangely self-centered at first, but the nurse must be introspective and think about why the interview is taking place before it begins. The following paragraphs discuss areas of thought the nurse might like to pursue before interviewing:

The nurse must first meet the patient. If the nurse really does not enjoy meeting new people and discussing the concerns of the patients, this will be communicated in some way to the patient. Nurses go into nursing predominantly because they care for people. Allow yourself to relax and enjoy this meeting with this particular person. Do not think of other patients or how many have yet to be seen; concentrate on the person you are talking with. Listen to what the patient is telling and asking you.

The ability to communicate both verbally and nonverbally is necessary for the nurse to be successful. This knowledge will help to convey to the patient that you want to be with her, that you are relaxed, and that she is important and you have nothing that is more important than her at this time. Privacy maintained by the nurse is an assumed prerequisite.

Listen with your eyes, ears, feelings, even your intuition. If you have a hunch, check it out. If there is something that makes you feel a patient is not comfortable with you, try to find out why. You may even need to have someone else follow a particular patient if there is some barrier to communication. Consulting another colleague may provide valuable answers in some situations. If you see a patient with tightly clenched hands, you might assume she is tense or nervous. Do not leave it there—the patient may be telling you something. Tell her what you see, and ask if you are interpreting it correctly. It may free the patient to ask an embarrassing or worrisome question.

It is helpful if nurses understand themselves and the mechanisms of nurse-patient relationships. Bermosk speaks of those attitudes of warmth, acceptance, objectivity, and compassion as necessary for effective interviewing.[5] In the personal area of maternity nursing, these are especially important. How do we demonstrate these attitudes to patients? Perhaps by smiling, introducing yourself, making sure you hear and understand her name and explaining why the interview is taking place. The nurse and patient should mutually set the goals. Nurses should be tolerant, remembering not to be annoyed when required to explain something in more than one way to a patient. Remarking that you may have difficulty clarifying certain information may make the patient feel more relaxed and able to ask questions in return.

THE PATIENT IN THE INTERVIEW

Many factors about the patient influence the interview, the stage of pregnancy being one. Most of the concerns or questions she has during the first trimester have changed by the third trimester. Figure 16-3 indicates many of the areas commonly discussed when seeing patients in various trimesters. These time spans are not definite but demonstrate the usual times when they are of concern to many patients. The nurse in turn tries to give the information prior to the time the patient needs it. Many of the times are influenced by physiological changes in the body. For example, body image may be more significant in the third trimester, when the body form is dramatically changed. At times body image is so important and so threatened by pregnancy that this might be what concerns the woman the most on her first visit to a health care facility.

This situation occurred when a model sought prenatal care. She and her husband had planned to work for 2 more years before starting a family, and she was concerned about her career. They were dependent on both their incomes to maintain their present life-style. She had many questions on her first visit to the clinic. For example, would dieting hurt her baby? How soon after the baby was born would she be able to regain her figure, or would there be permanent changes? To help her find alternatives and allow her to make choices freely and participate in planning her care was very pertinent. This exemplifies some of the individuality necessary in planning patient care.

The patient's values about babies and families and about pregnancy itself all influence what information is needed and how it is best presented. A general guideline to follow is to allow the patient to question and lead the interview as much as possible. This will often tell you of the patient's value system and how you may best introduce information.

Where the family gets health information is another factor directly affecting the patient's perception of pregnancy. What kind of experiences do the patient's parents talk about when babies are discussed? Everyone develops ideas, perceptions, and values related to pregnancy, labor, and delivery. When families were larger and communities smaller, much of this was gained from family members, especially mothers, sisters, and grandmothers. Today there is still much influence from parents, but it is tempered by educational, cultural, and peer contact. No matter where values and perceptions originate, they will influence the pregnancy experience. With this in mind it is often wise to ask the family what their mothers said about having babies. You will

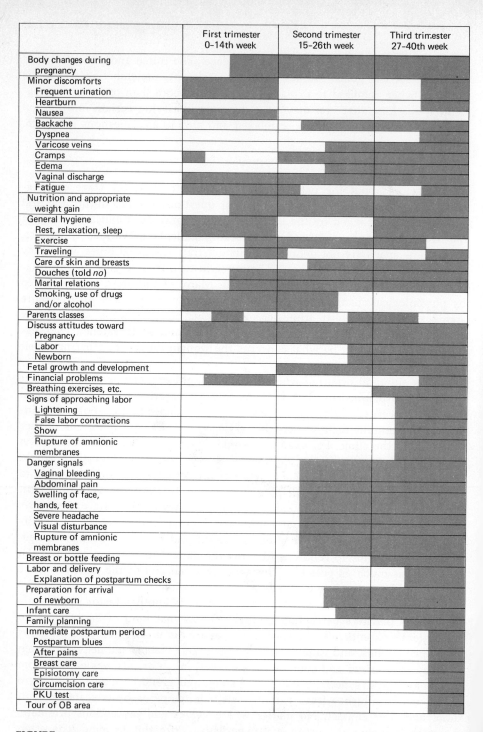

FIGURE 16-3

This bar graph demonstrates the approximate times during pregnancy a woman will experience concerns or need information in each category. From this data, a plan for teaching is made to present the information prior to her need, enabling the patient to better understand and be prepared for her experience.

get a variety of replies, from "pure hell" to a "joyous fulfilling experience." Allow the patients to elaborate on what their parents told them and, more important, ask what they thought of what their parent said. If the woman's mother had a bad labor and delivery, does she expect the same experience? How does she think it would be best to handle her fear? What is she afraid of? Being alone? Pain? Death? Something being wrong with the baby? It is wise not to dwell on apprehension but to leave the subject open for discussion. Be sure to allow enough time and opportunity for the patient to express herself.

Family resources and how she is accustomed to using them are an influential factor. If she and her mate regularly use written resources when they want to know something, she may wish to read some of the books written for prospective parents. As a consequence, she may have fewer questions than someone who is used to getting information by word of mouth. The latter may need special sessions with more time for questions and more generous use of pictures and demonstrations.

Our society often assumes everyone knows how to be a parent, but "mothering" and "fathering" behavior is learned. Many men and women unconsciously perform these roles the way their parents performed. Many women are astounded that when the baby arrives they do not have an overwhelming feeling of being a mother. When new mothers are with someone they trust, they often admit, "It doesn't seem real," or "I don't feel like a mother." Because it is assumed to be so natural, it is usually up to the professional to introduce learning behaviors in anticipation of the new role to help prepare the parents. Often they need to know that they will learn, that the baby will not break, and that it is normal not to "feel like a parent" right away.

THE HUSBAND IN THE INTERVIEW

The nurse's first contact is usually with the patient, but including the man in the relationship and plan of care may be very helpful. Ideally the plan of care is developed by the family, the nurse, physician, and possibly social workers and dietitians.

Nurses often state that when they ask the man if he wants to come into the interview he refuses, so they seldom include him. This may be because he does not know what is going to happen and nonverbally gets the message his presence is not necessary. Nurses might find men less reluctant to join the interview if they really make an effort to include them. This could be a significant step toward real family planned health care. A word of caution: There may be reasons the man does not want to be included, such as his cultural values. He may regard childbearing as feminine and feel threatened if he must be included. Perhaps he is not the father of this child. Maybe he really does not want to be there because of other interests. Choice should be maintained, but the opportunity to participate should be encouraged. He may want to be included later and should be offered the opportunity to join the conversation each time he accompanies the pregnant woman. One of the most pertinent reasons a man often does not accompany the woman to a clinic is the time of day. Most men work and do not want to give up a day's pay to accompany her. If we feel seeing both parents is important, maybe we should be making efforts to have evening maternity clinics.

If there appears to be some difficulty regarding the man's understanding and support of the pregnant woman during pregnancy, the nurse should suggest the patient bring him along on one of her visits to allow the three of them to talk. This may provide the opportunity to clarify the psychological and physiological changes pregnancy brings which are best dealt with by both parents when they are more knowledgeable and can be more patient with each other.

THE INITIAL INTERVIEW

The goals of the initial interview in order of priority are:

1 To establish a relationship
2 To obtain information
3 To give information

If a reciprocal relationship is not established, the interviewer will not have an accurate perception of the patient, and the patient will not be able to assimilate the information given at this time. With this in mind, the steps in the initial interview are:

1 Meet the patient and introduce yourself.
2 Explain the purpose of the interview.
3 Ask the patient to tell you how her pregnancy is progressing. Let her tell all she wants.
4 Listen to the patient. Be attentive; ask questions based on the information or cues she has given you.
5 Follow through on information she has given you. Clarify points of misunderstanding.
6 Find out how the woman feels now, physically and emotionally, in her pregnancy and how she has been coping until now.
7 Offer information pertinent to the trimester of pregnancy she is in. Ask how she is coping with the expected changes depending on the progress of her pregnancy (refer to Figure 16-3 for areas pertinent to that stage of the pregnancy).
8 Ask if you may explain the services of the clinic. If she answers to the negative, offer to explain during her next visit.
9 If she shows interest, explain the routine of seeing the doctor, the physical, the regular checks she will have each time she comes to the

clinic, the regular discussion of her progress, and the offering of information.

10 Close by asking for more questions and by making sure she does not leave without having her questions answered.

FOLLOW-UP INTERVIEWS

The pattern of nurse-patient interviews subsequent to the initial encounter and establishment of the relationship may be as follows:

1 Greeting.
2 Ask how she is getting along. If she gives the polite social answer of "being fine," ask about specific concerns. An example might be, "Are you still so tired?"
3 Let her explain what she is doing, what she is coping with, e.g., what she has done to cope with the early morning nausea she had last time she was in.
4 Ask about problem areas pertinent to that particular time in her pregnancy such as weight, diet, or discomfort.
5 After answering her questions, again offer information and resources she may not have asked about in areas related to that time in her pregnancy or the near future.
6 At each visit (at the end if it has not been brought up) offer information on her physiological changes and care and fetal growth and development.

As one can see, the key is to put the patient at ease, answer her questions, and then introduce new information so she will know what to expect as she goes through each period of her pregnancy.

Ethics

Ethics in health care sounds very old-fashioned and is often taken for granted. Certain ethics should pervade our practice every day. Confidentiality does not mean everything said by a patient is "top secret." It does mean this information should be used for the purpose for which it was given. We can tell patients that the reason we need to know things is so that we can help in their plan of care. Patients should be able to assume that health personnel will not gossip about them and that personal information will not be discussed where other people will overhear. Some of the expectations regarding information are set when the nurse explains that the purpose of talking with them is to establish a written plan of care.

If one refers to the earlier section in this chapter covering the categories of information included in the assessment of the patient, one will see many areas of very personal information. If this information is not respected and safe with the personnel gathering and using it, such persons should not be involved with patients. In some group situations in which parents share their experiences very personal information is revealed, but this is at the prerogative of the patient. The nurse should not take this freedom without the permission of the patient involved.

Establishing a relationship means setting the ground rules or expectations of the relationship so each will know how to behave and what to say. Health personnel who deal with very personal information are "breaking the rules" if good judgment is not used. There are certain ethical guidelines for the interpersonal relationship itself. Nurses learn about ethics in their philosophy classes, but the direct contacts in which these ethics are practiced with patients provide the opportunities to develop good relationships supported by genuine concern and respect for human dignity.

THE PLAN FOR OFFERING INFORMATION

In counseling and teaching during pregnancy some subjects fall automatically into trimesters. Other items of information for discussion may be important to the patient at different times, depending on the patient. General times when certain topics are usually important to the mother are listed in Figure 16-3. If a woman asks about something, it is discussed at the time she asks. An example might be sexual intercourse. Many young couples think they may hurt the baby and have questions regarding abstaining. If the nurse has put the family at ease, often this will be brought up by the patient. This is a very personal area and one which concerns all patients. The nurse should be well versed in information on this subject and should not be embarrassed by the question. If the nurse shows embarrassment, the patient will probably not want to be the cause of more embarrassment and will refrain from asking personal questions in the future. The interviewer should assess how comfortable the woman or couple is, and if they do not ask about intercourse, this information should be offered. (See Chapter 19.)

It is believed that the best learning occurs when the patient indicates a readiness for it, but there must be some consideration for the patient who does not know what to ask the nurse. The following areas of discussion can be introduced by the nurse even if the patient does not request the information.

Subjects introduced during the first trimester
Nutrition and basic diet information
Minor discomforts with comfort measures
    Frequent urination
    Nausea
    Vaginal discharge
    Fatigue

General hygiene
    Rest, relaxation, and sleep
    Employment
    Travel
    Douches
    Exercise
    Marital relations
    Smoking, drugs, or alcohol
Parents classes (attendance is usually recommended during the third tri-
    mester; many classes have strong emphasis regarding preparation
    for labor and delivery which may mean poor recall and application
    if taken too early)
Attitudes toward pregnancy
Fetal growth and development (often introduced during either the first or
    second trimester)

Subjects introduced before or during the second trimester
Minor discomforts with comfort measures
    Backache
    Varicose veins
    Cramps
    Edema
General hygiene
    Care of skin and breasts
Parents classes
Attitudes toward expected child
Fetal growth and development
Danger signals (caution of what to look for and do)
Preparation for arrival of newborn
Infant care

Subjects introduced before or during the third trimester
Minor discomforts
    Frequent urination (different cause this time)
    Heartburn
    Backache
    Dyspnea
    Fatigue
General hygiene
    Rest, relaxation, sleep (different reasons)
    Travel
Parents classes
Attitudes toward labor and delivery
Financial problems
Breathing exercises

Signs of approaching labor
Breast- or bottle-feeding
Labor and delivery itself, what to expect
Family planning (contraception after baby born)
Explanation of immediate postpartum period
Tour of the labor rooms, delivery rooms, postpartum unit, the nursery, and rooming-in facilities

Although the above plan attempts to assure readiness, information is often introduced long before it is needed because of the keen interest of patients. An increasing number of prenatal books are aimed at prospective parents, and many women come to the interview armed with questions quite early in their pregnancy.

Through the interviews an assessment of the patient is made, and the care plan is varied to meet the individual needs of patients. The aim of a plan for giving information is to be a supplementary tool in the nursing process. As the nurse assesses the patient on each visit, she will gather data, validate it with the patient, develop a plan of action, validate the plan with the patient, and proceed with the plan, giving the information that the patient needs at that time and then evaluating the success of each interaction. This process of explore, act, and explore again is a continuous cycle, existing over several months in the relationship between the nurse and the pregnant woman plus her family. Through this process the nurse helps the family find the information and services they need and want. This process when properly executed also results in growth and increased understanding of how to deal with life problems by both the nurse and the client. The emphasis is on maintenance of health, early detection of complications, and preventive measures. The nurse plays a key role as the advocate, counselor, and teacher of families in maternity settings.

THE MEDICAL ASSESSMENT

The first time a patient sees the physician a thorough "work-up" of the patient is usually, but not always, done. Some women spontaneously abort during the first trimester, and if this is a possibility, the physician might wish to delay the thorough history and physical exam. As the pregnancy progresses, the pelvic floor is also more relaxed, making it easier for a total examination, with a minimum of discomfort to the patient. The physician does want to establish that the woman is pregnant and get enough information to anticipate any problem. This means the total work-up is often done about the twelfth week after which a spontaneous abortion is not likely to occur.[6]

In the total medical assessment, a medical history is taken and a general physical examination is performed, including examination of eyes, ears, nose, and throat as well as breasts and pelvis. With a first pregnancy, the woman may not know what to expect and will feel more comfortable if the content of this initial visit is clarified. The physician wants an assessment of the expectant mother's general health. If she has an undetected problem, it is better to know and deal with it now rather than to have it appear later in her pregnancy when it might be difficult for both her and the unborn child.

Heart disease, kidney disease, and diabetes are problems which may exist undetected and would be dangerous during pregnancy. When these underlying diseases are known, steps can be taken to make the pregnancy as safe and nontraumatic as possible for the mother and the unborn child. A basic knowledge of her condition early in pregnancy also gives the physician a more accurate perspective from which to view any complications. The medical history section of the sample antepartal record (Figure 16-1) gives a list of the many disease phenomena and conditions the physician needs to know about.

Medical Antepartal Record

The medical antepartal record has five major parts which greatly influence the initial medical assessment:

1 The family's medical history
2 The patient's medical history
3 Her previous menstrual and obstetric history
4 The history of her present pregnancy
5 The physical examination

From these areas of appraisal, modifications in the prenatal plan of care will be developed, if necessary. Examples of how information in each of these five areas might alter the general plan are as follows:

1 If there is or has been diabetes in the family, it might be decided to test the patient thoroughly with a glucose tolerance test to determine if she is a borderline diabetic, in which case the pregnancy might precipitate the development of symptoms.
2 If the patient is Rh negative and her husband is positive, blood tests might be planned to watch for an erythroblastotic baby.
3 If she has had a previous pregnancy with complications, additional laboratory tests might be indicated, as well as the initiation of parent counseling.
4 If, in this pregnancy, the patient is having some bleeding and abdominal pain, bed rest may be ordered. Pregnancy tests may be reordered in case she has had a missed abortion and is no longer pregnant.

5 If they find the patient has syphilis, treatment is initiated, and the patient is seen more often than once a month in the first two trimesters (many of these specific problems will be covered in more detail in Part V, Complications of Childbearing and Childrearing).

In the past, a patient was interviewed by the physician for the appropriate historical data on the medical record. Other allied health personnel have also been used to interview patients and procure these data. Some health facilities are now trying patient-prepared historical data, using various questionnaires, card sorts, and even computers. All of these have been instituted to save time and yet maintain accurate records. We will probably see all of these systems, and more, used at various times in the future.

The historical data of the record provide information for areas of special attention during the physical examination. This information cues the physician to possible problems and signs and symptoms to watch for. When completed there should be a summation of possible complications in the record to provide everyone working with the patient with a total picture of the patient.

Pelvic Examination

At one time a patient always had a nurse or other female in the room when a pelvic exam was performed. This is often not the case now unless the physician anticipates some difficulty or assistance is needed in performing a procedure. In making an assessment of a patient and deciding whether the nurse's presence is necessary, several factors may be considered. These would include the patient's need for support and information, the age and marital status of the patient, whether it is the first pelvic exam, whether pain is anticipated or pathology is suspected, and the patient's apparent level of understanding and apprehension. Language barriers, learning difficulties, and mental retardation also pose dilemmas in helping the patient.

The nurse's role is to ask the patient to disrobe, drape her to prevent exposure, explain what to expect and why the pelvic exam is done, and help the patient understand how she may participate by relaxing. When the pelvic muscles are tight and tense, the physician cannot accurately assess the condition of the pelvic organs, and the patient will feel more discomfort. Nurses try various means to help the patient to relax. Different suggestions often help different patients. A nurse might ask a patient to place her hands on the middle of her chest and relax them. Tell her to breathe through her mouth and not hold her breath. Ask her to allow her knees to fall to the sides when her feet are in the stirrups. Concentrating on moving her toes, relaxing her ankles, and making her stomach soft also may make the exam easier for her. There are other suggestions, and you will find which ones seem to help you as you work with different patients and observe their reactions.

The nurse should always ask the patient to empty her bladder before the pelvic exam. Patients are asked to provide a urine specimen to be tested for albumin and sugar when they arrive at the clinic. Unless the woman has been waiting a long time, a full bladder usually should not be a problem.

Pelvic Measurements

The safety of a child passing through the birth canal is dependent on the size and shape of the pelvis. Abnormalities or irregularities may indicate the need for a cesarean section delivery. Pelvic measurements may be taken at any time. Usually they are done in the latter part of the pregnancy when the perineal tissues are soft and internal measurements cause less discomfort for the woman. Both internal and external measurements may be taken. A pelvimeter is used for the external measurements from which an estimate is made of the pelvic inlet and outlet. The diagonal conjugate, the distance from the symphysis pubis to the sacral prominence, is measured through an internal, manual pelvic examination. X-ray pelvimetry is usually done very late in pregnancy when an exact measurement is needed. X-ray procedures early in pregnancy may harm the fetus. If chest or other x rays are required for some medical problem, care should be taken to shield the fetus with a lead apron. (See Chapter 17).

General Prenatal Care

General prenatal care for most women follows a routine pattern after the initial history and physical and establishment of a plan of care. This pattern is demonstrated in Figure 16-1. This type of record is established to show any physiological changes that may occur during the progression of the pregnancy. Fluctuations of any degree often signal some type of complication. The signs and symptoms are interrelated and must be evaluated in the context of the total patient situation. The goal is to find problems early enough to prevent serious complications.

The patient usually sees a physician once a month until the eighth month, then every 2 weeks until the ninth month, and then once per week until she delivers. This, of course, is altered if there are complications or in those women who are considered high risks.

The cardinal checks done on each routine prenatal visit include the blood pressure, weight, edema, urine protein, and sugar. The hemoglobin is checked three to four times during the pregnancy.

Fetal circulation puts an added burden on the woman. Because of the extra tissue requiring perfusion, there is an increase in circulating fluid volume with some dilution of hemoglobin which is more slowly remedied by the increased production of cells. A high concentration of hemoglobin is needed to provide necessary oxygen for both mother and fetus. Most women are advised to take iron supplements throughout their pregnancy, since the increased iron required is difficult to get by diet alone.

Antibody titers are done on Rh negative women. The antibodies that build up in the mother's blood against the Rh positive baby usually do not rise appreciably until after the fourth month, although this varies from person to person. This is especially true if the woman has experienced more than one pregnancy. These titers are usually started about the fourth month, but the schedule varies with each physician's mode of practice.

Usually the only physical examination done on these routine visits is to palpate the abdomen, check the height of the uterus, and listen to the fetal heart rate. This brief physical plus the above checks will usually indicate any need for further exploration.

Weight gain, increased blood pressure, proteinuria, dizziness, persistent headaches, epigastric pain, and blurred vision may signal toxemia, one of the more complex complications of pregnancy. Bleeding, cramps, or abdominal pain early in the pregnancy might indicate a threatened abortion. If there are signs that the pregnancy is not proceeding normally, a pelvic examination may be performed. Indications might be bleeding, pain, or failure of the uterus to enlarge. Another reason for an early pelvic exam is a history of an incompetent cervix which might require a Shirodkar procedure.

Nursing Care in Medical Assessment

The nurse may work with the physician in different capacities during the medical assessment. The content of the patient's encounter with the physician may be explained, and the nurse prepares the patient for the physical exam, assists the physician with the procedures, and may act as chaperone and support to the patient.

The extent to which the nurse becomes involved in patient assessment varies greatly. In some clinics and doctor's offices, it is recommended that nurses make the assessment and refer those patients with complications to a physician. In others, little nursing participation is desired. Patients from these clinics and physician's offices often see a nurse for the first time when they enter the hospital! Patients who have had this type of experience and had a later experience with nurse involvement highly favor nursing participation. Women seem more informed and prepared to actively participate in the childbearing process when nurses have been appropriately involved. Nurses have moved into many health maintenance roles, and it would seem very natural for them to have an increasingly active participation in prenatal care.

REFERENCES

1 United Nations: Demographic Yearbook, 21st issue, Statistics Office of the United Nations, New York, 1970, p. 576.
2 Ibid., p. 578.

3 Lewis, Charles E., and Barbara A. Resnik: "Nurse Clinics and Progressive Ambulatory Patient Care," *New England Journal of Medicine*, 277:1241, December 7, 1967.
4 Anderson, Edith: "Today's Parents and Maternity Nursing," in Betty Bergerson et al. (eds.), *Current Concepts in Clinical Nursing*, Mosby, St. Louis, 1967, p. 362.
5 Bermosk, Loretta Sue: "Interviewing: A Key to Therapeutic Communication in Nursing Practice," *Nursing Clinics of North America*, 1(2):208, June 1966.
6 Hellman, Louis M. et al.: *Williams Obstetrics*, Appleton-Century-Crofts, New York, 1971, p. 494.

BIBLIOGRAPHY

Anderson, Edith: "Today's Parents and Maternity Nursing," in Betty Bergerson et al. (eds.), *Current Concepts in Clinical Nursing*, Mosby, St. Louis, 1967, pp. 355–363.

Apgar, Virginia: "Drugs in Pregnancy," *American Journal of Nursing*, 65(3): 104–105, March 1965.

Bates, Barbara: "Doctor and Nurse: Changing Roles and Relations," *The New England Journal of Medicine*, 283(3):129–134, July 16, 1970.

Beebe, Joyce E., et al.: "Bench Conferences in a Large Obstetric Clinic," *American Journal of Nursing*, 68(1):85–87, January 1968.

Berggren, Helen J., and Dawn A. Zagornik: "Teaching Nursing Process to Beginning Students," *Nursing Outlook*, 16(7):32–35, July 1968.

Bermosk, Loretta Sue: "Interviewing: A Key to Therapeutic Communication in Nursing Practice," *Nursing Clinics of North America*, 1(2):205–213, June 1966.

Bishop, Barbara E.: "First OB Nurse Visit—A Tool of Assessment," unpublished paper, 1971.

Cahil, Imogene D.: "Mutual Withdrawal: The Nurse and the Low Socioeconomic Mother," in Betty Bergerson et al. (eds.), *Current Concepts in Clinical Nursing*, Mosby, St. Louis, 1967, pp. 365–371.

Clark, Ann L.: "The Unwed Mother: Design for Nursing Intervention," in Betty Bergerson et al. (eds.), *Current Concepts in Clinical Nursing*, Mosby, St. Louis, 1967, pp. 400–406.

Fitzpatrick, Elise, et al.: *Maternity Nursing*, 12th ed., Lippincott, Philadelphia, 1971.

Fodor, John T., and Gust Dalis: *Health Instruction: Theory and Application*, Lea & Febiger, Philadelphia, 1968.

Hellman, Louis M. et al.: *Williams Obstetrics*, Appleton-Century-Crofts, New York, 1971.

Hennel, Magdalena: "Family-centered Maternity Nursing in Practice," *Nursing Clinics of North America*, 3(2):289–298, June 1968.

Horowitz, Mardit Nancy: "Psychologic Effects of Education for Childbirth," *Psychosomatics*, 8:196–202, July–August 1967.

Lesser, Marion S., and Vera R. Keane: *Nurse-Patient Relationships in a Hospital Maternity Service*, Mosby, St. Louis, 1956.

Lewis, Charles E., and Barbara A. Resnik: "Nurse Clinics and Progressive Ambulatory Patient Care," *New England Journal of Medicine*, 277:1236–1241, December 7, 1967.

McCoffery, Margo Smith: "An Approach to Parent Education," *Nursing Forum*, 6(1):77–93, 1967.

McCulley, Lee B.: "Health Counseling of Women," *Nursing Clinics of North America*, 3(2):263–273, June 1968.

Peplau, Hildegarde E.: "Professional Closeness . . . ," *Nursing Forum*, 8(4):342–360, 1969.

Preparation for Labor: Breathing and Relaxation Techniques, Minnesota Department of Health, Division of Special Services, Section of Maternal and Child Health, Minneapolis, Minn., March 1969.

Rubin, Reva: "Maternity Care in Our Society," *Nursing Outlook*, pp. 519–521, July 1963.

———: "Cognitive Style in Pregnancy," *American Journal of Nursing*, 70(3):502–508, March 1970.

Scott, Diane W.: "Crisis Intervention," in Betty Bergerson et al. (eds.), *Current Concepts in Clinical Nursing*, Mosby, St. Louis, 1967, pp. 392–399.

Smith, Dorothy M.: "A Clinical Nursing Tool," *American Journal of Nursing*, 68(11):2384 and 2388, November 1968.

Standeven, Muriel: "What the Poor Dislike about Community Health Nurses," *Nursing Outlook*, 17(9):72–75, September 1969.

United Nations: *Demographic Yearbook 1969*, 21st Issue, Statistics Office of the United Nations, New York, 1970, pp. 575 and 578.

Weidenbach, Ernestine: "Family Nurse Practitioner for Maternal Child Care," *Nursing Outlook*, 13(12):50–52, December 1965.

———: "The Nurse's Role in Family Planning," *Nursing Clinics of North America*, 3(2):355–365, June 1968.

17 | PHYSIOLOGICAL CHANGES DURING PREGNANCY

Ruth Ann Lambert

Pregnancy is a normal physiological process which necessitates adaptation of the various body systems of the pregnant woman to accommodate growth and development of the fetus. This adaptation is evidenced by many common and predictable changes; yet each pregnant woman experiences every pregnancy differently, and it affects how she thinks, acts, and feels.

The duration of pregnancy has been referred to variously as 10 lunar months, 40 weeks, 280 days, or 9 calendar months. Actually, the average length of pregnancy is approximately 267 days. This variation is explained by the clinical dating of pregnancy based on subjective evidence of the last menstrual period, while embryological dating is based on the time of ovulation. Ovulation occurs 2 weeks before the next menses.

A method commonly used to estimate the length of pregnancy is Naegele's rule: Count back 3 months from the first day of the last menstrual period (LMP) and add 7 days to arrive at the estimated date of confinement (EDC). Thus, an LMP of December 1 will give an EDC of September 8. This method has been demonstrated as accurate within 10 days in 80 percent of all deliveries.

FIRST TRIMESTER

Traditionally, pregnancy has been divided into three periods, or trimesters, which are each approximately 3 calendar months in length. Although pregnancy is a continuous and progressive process, each trimester serves as a landmark for particular stages of expected maternal changes and fetal development. During the first trimester the phenomenal events which follow fertilization and progress into the fetal period seem to overshadow the changes experienced by the newly pregnant woman. Nevertheless, these changes are important because they indicate the adjustments of the woman's body which are necessary to support a healthy and viable pregnancy.

Fetal Development

The first trimester spans the three stages of fetal development. The *period of the ovum* encompasses the first 2 weeks following fertilization. The *period of the embryo* extends from the period of the ovum through the eighth week. The *period of the fetus* begins after the eighth week and continues throughout the remainder of intrauterine life. The third month of pregnancy is the first fetal month.

FERTILIZATION

Pregnancy is initiated by fertilization, which occurs in the outer end of the fallopian tube. The mature ovum, produced at ovulation and deposited through the fimbriated opening of the tube, is surrounded by spermatozoa soon after coitus. It is believed that ovulation, coitus, and fertilization are almost synchronous, possibly occurring within 24 hours, because of the limited life-spans of the male and female gametes. The outer covering of the ovum, the corona radiata, is denuded by one or a combination of the following: action of the tubal mucosa, smooth muscle activity of the tube, and enzyme action of the spermatozoa. The remaining covering of the ovum, the zona pellucida, is penetrated by one sperm; the pronuclei of the ovum and sperm approach each other and join, and fertilization is accomplished. Fertilization reconstitutes the diploid number of chromosomes, determines the chromosomal sex of the zygote (the single cell structure which results from fertilization), and initiates cleavage.

CLEAVAGE

The series of rapid mitotic cell divisions which follows soon after fertilization is called *cleavage*. The many small cells which result from this process are called *blastomeres*. The zona pellucida retains the blastomeres, forming a small, solid, berry-like ball of cells—a *morula*. During the 2 to 3 days which follow fertilization the forming morula is propelled by ciliary action and peristaltic action of the tube through the lumen and into the uterine cavity.

BLASTOCYTE

While freely floating in the uterine cavity for a period of 3 to 4 days, the blastomeres cluster in one segment of the sphere. This cluster of cells is called the *inner cell mass*. Larger cells move to the periphery of the sphere, lining the zona pellucida, and enclose a fluid-filled space. The peripheral cells form the *trophoblast*. The fluid-filled cavity within the trophoblast is the *blastocyte, blastula,* or *blastodermic vesicle.*

IMPLANTATION

On or about day 7 following fertilization the zona pellucida disappears, allowing the trophoblast to come in contact with the endometrium. The usual area of implantation is high on the posterior wall of the uterus. The blastocyte seems to select a site between the openings of uterine glands over a capillary. *Implantation* occurs when the trophoblast adheres to the endometrial lining, penetrates the surface, digests, and erodes as it burrows deeply into the stroma. The blastocyte implants with the embryonic pole foremost. The *embryonic pole* is the location of the inner cell mass within the blastocyte.

Implantation occurs during the secretory phase of the menstrual cycle when the endometrium, under the influence of progesterone, becomes extremely vascular, succulent, and rich in glycogen. The endometrium becomes the *decidua* during pregnancy and is characterized by an exaggeration of the secretory phase. The stromal cells hypertrophy with further increase in the size and secretions of glands, coiled arteries become more tortuous, and arterioles lengthen and extend closer to the surface. As implantation proceeds, the decidua is differentiated in relation to the blastocyte. The decidua which lies beneath the implanting blastocyte is the *decidua basalis*; the *decidua capsularis* covers the implanting blastocyte; and the remaining lining of the uterine cavity is the *decidua vera*.

On or about day 8 following fertilization the trophoblast differentiates into two layers. The inner layer is the *cytotrophoblast*, or *Langhans' layer*, and consists of clearly delineated cells; the outer layer, the *syncytiotrophoblast*, is syncytium, that is, the cells have no clearly defined boundaries.

At about this time the trophoblast begins production of the pregnancy hormone, *chorionic gonadotrophin*. This glycoprotein substance acts on the corpus luteum to produce and maintain the corpus luteum of pregnancy which, in turn, maintains the production of estrogen and progesterone during the early weeks of pregnancy. The hormone progesterone becomes *pregnanediol* during pregnancy. Chorionic gonadotrophin is found in the serum and urine of pregnant women within 10 days after fertilization and is responsible for the positive findings in biological tests for pregnancy as early as 2 weeks after the first missed period. The rate of production of this hormone (CG) slowly increases during the first month and then rapidly increases to reach maximum production between the 60th and 70th days. It then gradually decreases to a level reached at the beginning of the second trimester and is maintained at this level throughout the rest of pregnancy.

It has been believed, since early studies, that the source of production of chorionic gonadotrophin was Langhans' layer, or the cytotrophoblast. However, recent studies have identified the syncytiotrophoblast as the source, indicating that this division of trophoblast is responsible for the production of all placental hormones—chorionic gonadotrophin, estrogen, and pregnanediol. These studies further suggest that the cytotrophoblast is the source of all trophoblastic cells—cytotrophoblast and syncytiotrophoblast.

As implantation continues, both layers of the trophoblast, which surround the blastocyte, thicken. The syncytium proliferates more rapidly over the embryonic disc, which is in contact with the decidua basalis. The digestive and erosive properties of the syncytium are evidenced as it continues to invade and replace decidual tissue. As the syncytium replaces decidua, small openings, or *lacunae*, occur in the syncytium and soon coalesce into a communicating network. About 12 days following fertilization the eroded capillary walls allow maternal blood to flow into the lacunae, which are lined with syncytium.

Meanwhile, columns of cytotrophoblast penetrate into the syncytium; these fingerlike projections of cytotrophoblast covered with syncytiotrophoblast are the *villi*. Shortly thereafter mesodermal cells from the inner surface of the cytotrophoblast migrate to and line the core of the villi. These cells are the primitive source of capillary formation in the villi. By the 15th day implantation is complete, and placental formation continues.

PLACENTATION

With the advent of the primitive sources of circulation the trophoblast becomes the *chorion* and the villi become *chorionic villi*. Early in the third week these villi, with capillary-forming mesodermal cores, are surrounded by lacunae-riddled syncytium. Maternal circulation reaches the lacunae through eroded capillaries. This represents the primitive status of placental circulation.

During the following weeks the fate of the villi differs in relation to the decidua with which they are in contact. The villi in contact with the dicidua basalis proliferate and assume a leafy appearance. This is known as the *chorion frondosum* and is the fetal component of the placenta. The remaining villi in contact with the decidua capsularis are gradually denuded, and this area is called *chorion laeve*, or *bald chorion*. During the ensuing weeks the connecting labyrinth of lacunae which surround the villi becomes the *intervillous spaces*. Later the chorion frondosum develops into 18 to 20 treelike structures, called cotyledons, which project from the chorionic plate and are surrounded by the intervillous spaces. Both cotyledons and the chorionic plate contain arterial and venous circulation which is fetal in origin.

EMBRYO

Concurrent with implantation and placentation the inner cell mass differentiates into a bilaminar *embryonic disc*. The inner germ layer is the *entoderm*, and the outer germ layer is the *ectoderm*. The embryonic disc is suspended between two cavities: the amnion, which is in contact with the ectoderm above; the secondary yolk sac, which is in contact with the entoderm below. Cells migrating from the inner surface of the cytotrophoblast fill the cavity of the blastocyte, forming a loose network called the *extraembryonic mesoderm*. Large cavities soon develop in this network, forming a new cavity called the *extraembryonic coelom*. The extraembryonic mesoderm persists as a lining of the trophoblast; it surrounds the embryonic disc with the amniotic cavity and the yolk sac and connects the caudal end of the embryonic disc with the trophoblast. This strand of mesoderm is known as the *body stalk*. The trophoblast and the mesodermal lining and the peripheral villi become the *chorion*—the outermost of the fetal membranes.

The end of the second week marks the beginning of the *period of the embryo*. At this time the primitive streak appears in the midline of the embryonic disc and indicates the cephalocaudal axis of the embryo. Early in the third week cells migrate from the primitive streak between the ectoderm and the entoderm to form the third germ layer, or the *mesoderm*. The embryonic disc is now trilaminar, and the ovum is now an embryo.

These germ layers give rise to all the various organs and systems of the body. The ectoderm contributes to the development of the entire nervous system, central and peripheral; the sensory organs; glands; and epidermis, including hair, nails, and enamel of the teeth. The mesoderm contributes to the formation of the dermis, the skeleton, the connective tissue, the vascular system, the urogenital system, and most skeletal and smooth muscles as well as the spleen and suprarenal glands. The entoderm develops into the epithelium of the digestive and respiratory tracts, eustachian tubes, and tympanic cavities; the bladder; and such organs as the liver, pancreas, thyroid, parathyroid, and thymus.

The amniotic cavity grows rapidly during the early embryonic period. It gradually encloses the embryo on all sides, in a purse-string-like manner, and ensheaths the body stalk, which will soon become the *umbilical cord*. This accomplishes the immersion of the embryo in the amniotic fluid within the *amnion*, the inner fetal membrane.

The events of the embryonic period are worth restating. The period extends from the end of the second week through the eighth week but begins with the differentiation of the trilaminar embryonic disc. It includes the dramatic events of embryonic development, which appears to entail a series of foldings, tube formations, outpouchings, inpouchings, openings, and closings, resulting in formation of the human body structures and systems with all their complexities. This occurs simultaneously with implantation, beginning placental function, and differentiation of fetal membranes. In spite of the extensive amount of development accomplished during the embryonic period, the growth rate is also remarkable.

Some growth occurs associated with implantation as a result of the activity of the syncytium. The just visible ovum increases in size to 1.5 mm, which includes the total chorionic sac, by the end of the second week. By the end of the fourth week the chorionic sac measures about 20 mm and the embryo measures about 5 mm. At the end of the embryonic period the embryo measures about 30 mm and weighs about 1 Gm.

FETUS

The end of the eighth week initiates the *period of the fetus*, which spans the three trimesters of pregnancy. The fetal period is marked by few, if any, new structure formations, and the subsequent development consists primarily in the growth and maturation of the existing structures.

During this first month of fetal development the head is still large, but the elongating neck raises the chin from the thoracic wall. Limbs are small with fingers and toes. Eyes are lidless when the period begins, but lids develop and fuse before the end of the month. Ears, nose, and mouth are recognizable. Internal structures, including the genitals, can be identified, but the external genitals continue to differentiate. Beginning ossification is present in some bones. At the end of the first trimester the fetus weighs about 20 Gm and is about 9 cm in length.

PLACENTA

Although placenta formation is a continuous process, the final developmental structures are not evident until the end of the first trimester. The cotyledons develop from the chorion frondosum, which evolved earlier as a restricted but complex version of the villi. *Restricted* refers to the limitation of area of the chorion in contact with the decidua basalis, and *complex* refers to the replacement of the simple fingerlike projections of the villi with the branchlike formation of the chorion frondosum. The *cotyledons* are treelike structures projecting from the chorionic plate and surrounded by intervillous spaces. Both the cotyledons and the chorionic plate contain definitive arterial and venous circulation which connects with the umbilical arteries and veins and terminates in a fine capillary network at the periphery of the cotyledons. Projections of decidua basalis extend from the basal plate toward the chorionic plate and incompletely separate the cotyledons, allowing for communication between the intervillous spaces. These *placental septa*, as they are called, contain the openings through which maternal circulation reaches the intervillous spaces. The placenta is small at the end of the first trimester, but it contains all the structures found when it reaches its maximum size during the fifth month.

The placenta is a complex organ, and researchers frequently identify new data related to it. The basic function of the placenta is to act as a transfer site where nutrients, oxygen, and other selected substances needed by the fetus are obtained by diffusion from the maternal circulation in the intervillous spaces to the circulation of the cotyledon. The fetal waste products are excreted in reverse order of this process.

FETAL MEMBRANES

By the end of the first trimester the amnion obliterates the extraembryonic coelom and fills the chorionic cavity. The chorion in turn almost fills the uterine cavity. The two fetal membranes remain in contact for the remainder of pregnancy.

Maternal Adaptation

The pregnant woman undergoes profound changes during pregnancy, but the onset is usually unheralded. The signs and symptoms of the first trimester indicate the occurrence of change, but the positive clinical evidence is not available until the middle of pregnancy.

PRESUMPTIVE SYMPTOMS

Subjective symptoms reported by the pregnant woman are presumptive.

Cessation of menses, or *amenorrhea*, is one of the more important symptoms of pregnancy. It is occasioned by the presence of the hormone chorionic gonadotrophin, secreted by the trophoblast. Chorionic gonadotrophin acts on the corpus luteum during the early weeks to maintain production of estrogen and progesterone, thus maintaining the endometrium and preventing menstruation. After one or two missed periods, especially in combination with other symptoms, many women are assured of their subjective diagnosis of pregnancy. It is considered as presumptive, clinically, because of the variety of factors which affect the menstrual cycle.

The nausea and vomiting of early pregnancy are sometimes referred to as *morning sickness*. It occurs in about 50 percent of all pregnancies. It is often limited to one period of the day, usually mornings; begins after the first month; and extends over 6 to 8 weeks. It is believed to be associated with the invasive activity of the pregnancy and change in carbohydrate metabolism. It is presumptive clinically, because nausea and vomiting are associated with many conditions. It becomes highly presumptive when it occurs in a woman who has been well and has missed a period.

Frequency of urination is due to irritability of the bladder. This may be caused by the increased anteflexion of the uterus with displacement of the cervix and stretching of the base of the bladder.

A feeling of fullness or tingling in the breast is due to hormonal influences.

PRESUMPTIVE SIGNS

The objective findings of an examiner are called signs. Signs are termed presumptive when they are considered the least reliable of the findings.

Changes in the breasts are enlargement and a tracing of bluish veins under the skin, which may be evident as early as the fourth week of pregnancy. Nipples also enlarge, become more erectile, and there is increased pigmentation of the areolae. Montgomery's follicles, the sebaceous glands throughout the areolae, gradually hypertrophy and become slightly elevated. Colostrum may be expressed during the third month. Breast changes are significant in a first pregnancy but have less value during subsequent pregnancies.

Chadwick's sign is the bluish-purple discoloration of the vulva, vagina, and cervix due to circulatory congestion in the pelvis which occurs in pregnancy. It occurs between 8 and 12 weeks.

PROBABLE SIGNS

Probable signs of pregnancy have greater reliability than the presumptive signs but are still not positive signs.

Hegar's sign is the softening and compressibility of the isthmus of the lower uterine segment. It is due to the hyperemia in the pelvis. It is elicited by bimanual examination—the isthmus is compressed between the fingers in the anterior fornix and the hand on the abdomen behind the uterus. It may be evident as early as 6 weeks and is the most reliable sign during the first trimester.

Goodell's sign is the softening of the cervix and is also due to increased congestion. It is observed in the sixth week in primigravida and even earlier in the multigravida.

Braxton Hicks contractions are painless, intermittent contractions which are believed to occur in 3- to 10-minute intervals as early as 8 weeks.

Biological tests for pregnancy are probable signs. The chorionic gonadotrophin in the urine of pregnant women causes the positive results. Findings are evident after the first month and have a 90 to 95 percent accuracy rate.

OTHER BODY CHANGES

The *uterus* changes in form, size, consistency, and position during the first trimester. The flat, pear-shaped uterus rounds out to a globular form. Enlargement is steady and rapid, the consistency is soft and spongy, and the walls become softer and thicker. An increase in anteflexion causes the body of the uterus to lay on the bladder. The *shape and size* is due to uterine accommodation to the growth of the contents of the uterine cavity. *Enlargement* is also due to hyperemia and increase in muscle fibers. Change in *consistency* is due to congestion. During the third month the uterus rises out of the pelvis to allow for growth of the fetus and expansion of the uterus and thus relieves the pressure on the bladder.

During the second month the *mucous plug*, a thick, tenacious mucus, gradually fills the *cervical canal. Vaginal secretions* are profuse, thick, white, and crumbly during the first trimester. The increased acidity of these secretions, due to lactic acid, probably serves as a protective barrier against organisms requiring an alkaline medium.

Basal body temperature remains constant for more than 2 weeks following fertilization and then gradually decreases. It is believed to be due to progesterone maintenance and may contribute to lethargy and tiredness during early weeks.

Pelvic joints, sacroiliac, and symphysis pubis become more relaxed, perhaps because of the effects of the ovarian hormone *relaxin. Blood volume* increases during the third month, and fat content of plasma becomes elevated. Metabolic changes occur as evidenced by a gradual falling of the basal metabolic rate. Blood sugar tends to be low, there is a loss of nitrogen content, and carbohydrate metabolism is disturbed. A weight gain of 2 pounds is expected. Mouth secretions have a high degree of acidity and may lead to increased salivation. The cause is unknown.

SECOND TRIMESTER

The second trimester of pregnancy is characterized by rapid fetal growth, and relative good health, and a feeling of well-being in the pregnant woman.

Fetal Development

At the beginning of the second trimester the fetus has distinct facial features; the eyelids remain fused, and the head is large but more proportionate to the body. The fingers and toes have beginning nail growth. During the next month *lanugo*, a fine, downy hair, covers the body, sex is distinguishable, *meconium* is present in the intestines, and muscles begin to contract. The skin is red and transparent, and all vessels are visible. The heart beat is strong. Ossification of bones develops further.

During the fifth month deposits of *vernix caseosa*, a white, cheeselike substance, is found on parts of the fetal skin. Meconium increases in amount and bulk. Iron deposits from the mother are stored. Enamel and dentine for the teeth is deposited. Eyelashes and eyebrows are present, hair on the head is scanty, and lanugo is more abundant. Movements are stronger and more frequent. The skin is still red but less transparent. The head is still large, but body proportions are closer to normal.

By the end of the second trimester the skin is red, thin, and wrinkled; eyelids are separate, and vernix caseosa is more abundant. Very human in appearance, the fetus weighs about 1½ pounds, and his total length is about 12 inches. Major body systems are still immature and require further maturation, but an occasional fetal survival has been reported.

The placenta reaches full maturity and maximum growth by the fifth month of pregnancy. The placenta continues to produce the hormones which support pregnancy until term. The hormones are chorionic gonadotrophin, estrogen, and pregnanediol.

Maternal Adaptation

The physical changes and signs present during the second trimester include the positive signs which facilitate the clinical diagnosis of pregnancy.

POSITIVE SIGNS

The irrefutable positive sign of pregnancy is the presence of *fetal heart tones*. These are heard during the fifth month of pregnancy and range between 120 and 180 beats a minute. Another positive sign which can be seen, felt, and heard by the examiner is *active movements of the fetus*. It is possible to palpate these movements as early as 12 weeks. During the fourth month the *fetal parts* can be differentiated by palpation, another positive sign. X-ray visualization of the fetus is possible during the fifth month.

OTHER PHYSICAL CHANGES

During the second trimester the *uterus* again changes in size and shape. The globular shape of the first trimester changes to ovoid as the uterus increases in size and rises up into the abdominal cavity, reaching the umbilicus during the fifth month and continuing to rise during the sixth. The lower uterine segment is drawn up into the body, and anteflexion disappears. Growth rate is greatest in the fundus. Growth of the uterus is due to the growth rate of the intrauterine contents as well as the thinning of the uterine walls after the fifth month. At the end of the trimester the uterus is felt as a soft, fluid-filled sac.

Between the 16th and 32d week *ballottement* is present. Tapping the fetus with a finger inserted in the vagina causes the fetus to rise in the amniotic fluid and then rebound to the original position.

Blood volume increase during this trimester is greater during the fifth month. This increase in circulation increases the cardiac output. The increase in plasma is greater than the increase in cells, resulting in the so-called pseudoanemia of pregnancy. At about this time the free hydrochloric acid and gastric acidity decrease, and this decreases the pregnant woman's potential to absorb iron.

Basal metabolism rises especially during the fifth month because of the increased growth of the fetus. Nitrogen retention increases to meet the needs of the enlarging uterus, developing breasts, and fetal growth.

Skin changes which occur usually at midtrimester include vascular spiders, erythema of the palms of hands, and deposits of pigment on forehead, nose, and cheeks, called *chloasma*, or the *mask of pregnancy*. These disappear after the termination of pregnancy. The linea nigra and striae gravidarum persist as faded lines after pregnancy is terminated.

Quickening usually occurs between the 18th and 20th weeks. The fluttering movements of the fetus are perceived by the pregnant woman. Braxton Hicks contractions, the intermittent uterine contractions, persist throughout the second trimester.

THIRD TRIMESTER

The third trimeser is characterized by further fetal growth and preparation for termination of fetal status. The pregnant woman anticipates the termination of pregnancy.

Fetal Development

As the third trimester begins, the fetus is red and wrinkled with little fat deposits in his lean body. He weighs about 2 pounds and is 12 inches long. During the ensuing months of development, fat is increasingly deposited to fill out and round out the fetal body, lanugo gradually disappears, hair on the head increases, nails grow to the tips of the fingers, and vernix caseosa is abundant. At the end of the trimester the fetus weighs about 7 pounds, his length is about 20 inches, the redness of his skin has faded, wrinkles have smoothed out, fat deposits are present with good body proportions, and the fetus is ready for delivery.

At birth the *fetal circulation* undergoes some specific changes as the lungs replace the placenta as the organs for gaseous exchange.

The nutrient-carrying oxygenated blood reaches the fetus from the placenta through the *umbilical vein* which enters the body of the fetus through the abdominal wall. It then divides into two branches: one small branch goes to the portal vein through the liver to the vena cava via the hepatic vein; the larger branch, the ductus venosus, goes to the vena cava directly. The vena cava carries mixed blood above the hepatic vein, arterial blood from the placenta, and venous return from the lower extremities. The blood from the inferior vena cava enters the right atrium of the heart, passes through the *foramen ovale*, to the left atrium, to the left ventricle, to the aorta. Blood from the superior vena cava enters the right atrium and goes to the right ventricle and the pulmonary artery. The lungs need only a small amount of blood for nutrition during fetal life; therefore, the largest amount of blood is shunted from the pulmonary artery, through the *ductus arteriosus*, to the aorta. Blood from the aorta goes to the body organs and the *hypogastric arteries*, which connect with the *umbilical arteries* through which the blood reaches the placenta.

With the advent of birth, the expansion of the thoracic cage triggers the change which results in a dramatic increase in pulmonary circulatory function and gradually obliterates the obsolete fetal structures. The increased pressure in the left side of the heart effects closure of the foramen ovale; the ductus arteriosus obliterates and becomes the ligamentum arteriosum. The cutting of the cord eliminates the need for the umbilical vein and arteries; the distal ends of the hypogastric arteries undergo atrophy, and the ductus venosus becomes the ligamentum venosum.

Maternal Adaptation

UTERUS

During the last trimester growth of the uterus keeps pace with fetal growth. Elasticity of the uterus increases, further strengthening the uterus and allowing greater stretching. The walls thin out and incorporate the lower uterine segment. The blood volume of the uterine vascular system encompasses one-sixth of the total circulation at term.

The uterus reaches the ensiform appendix in the ninth month; this contributes to the difficulty in breathing experienced during the last trimester. Frequently in the primigravida the uterus lowers itself and becomes fixed in the brim of the pelvis. This descent is called *lightening*. It occurs about 2 weeks before term in the primigravida, probably because of muscle tone. It is believed that the intrauterine pressure directs the presenting part into the stretched and thinned-out lower uterine segment, and the relaxation of the pelvic joints, sacroiliac, and symphysis pubis enables the uterus to sink into the pelvic brim. Good muscle tone aids in engagement—fixing of the presenting part in the pelvic brim. Sagging muscles are associated with an unengaged presenting part.

OTHER CHANGES

Breathing becomes difficult during the third trimester because of the upward pressure from the uterus on the diaphragm. The longitudinal diameter of the chest is somewhat shortened, but a compensatory widening of the horizontal dimension occurs, increasing the vital capacity. Breathing difficulties are relieved by lightening, but pressure on the bladder results. The vagina becomes more relaxed, the mucosa thickens, connective tissue is looser, and muscle cells hypertrophy—all in preparation for labor.

Pregnant women find this trimester the most difficult to cope with. Weight gain is a major concern. The average distribution of the weight gain at the end of pregnancy is shown in the following table.

Structure	Number of pounds
Fetus	7
Placenta	1
Fluid	2
Breast	3
Uterus	2
Protein storage	4
Blood volume	4
Total	23

Physiological changes in pregnancy are continually being studied and investigated to provide more knowledge about this complex developmental process. It is imperative that nurses actively participate in this quest for new knowledge as well as utilize new learnings in practice.

BIBLIOGRAPHY

Abramson, H. (ed.): *Symposium on the Functional Physiopathology of the Fetus and Neonate*, Mosby, St. Louis, 1971.

Bookmiller, M. M., and G. L. Bowen: *Textbook of Obstetrics and Obstetric Nursing*, 4th ed., Saunders, Philadelphia, 1963.

Davis, M. E., and R. Rubin: *DeLee's Obstetrics for Nurses*, 17th ed., Saunders, Philadelphia, 1962.

Eastman, N. J., and L. M. Hellman: *Williams Obstetrics*, 13th ed., Appleton-Century-Crofts, New York, 1966.

Fitzpatrick, E., S. R. Reeder, and L. Mastroianni, Jr.: *Maternity Nursing*, 12th ed., Lippincott, Philadelphia, 1971.

Greenhill, J. P.: *Obstetrics*, 13th ed., Saunders, Philadelphia, 1966.

Ingelman-Sundberg, A., C. Wirsen, and L. Nilsson: *A Child Is Born*, Delacorte, New York, 1966.

Marcus, S. L., and C. C. Marcus (eds.): *Advances in Obstetrics and Gynecology*, vol. I, Williams & Wilkins, Baltimore, 1967.

Patten, B. M.: *Human Embryology*, McGraw-Hill, New York, 1968.

Wiedenbach, E.: *Family-centered Maternity Nursing*, 2d ed., Putnam, New York, 1967.

Williams, P. L., and C. P. Wendall-Smith: *Basic Human Embryology*, Lippincott, Philadelphia, 1966.

18 | NUTRITION DURING PREGNANCY AND LACTATION

Joan E. Carter

Over most of recorded history, special attention has been given to the diets of pregnant women. Some kinds of food have been restricted or prohibited. Other kinds of food have been regarded as necessary to ward off catastrophe for the mothers or their infants. Restrictions seem to have had strong appeal in ancient times, and they have parallels in modern times, in both primitive and highly developed societies. Even today, some of the views concerning maternal nutrition have little more scientific basis than did the views of the ancients.[1] *

There are many factors affecting the outcome of pregnancy. Interrelated with nutrition are such things as age of the mother, birth interval, birth order, socioeconomic status, educational level, and psychological and physiological factors as well as the previous nutritional status of the woman throughout her lifetime.

This chapter was written by Joan E. Carter in her private capacity. No official support or endorsement by the Department of Health, Education, and Welfare, Health Services and Mental Health Administration, is intended or should be inferred.
* *Maternal Nutrition and the Course of Pregnancy* by the Committee on Maternal Nutrition, Food and Nutrition Board, National Academy of Sciences, has been used as the main reference source for much of the discussion in this chapter.

There is considerable evidence which demonstrates that women who are inadequately nourished during pregnancy tend to have more complications than women who were adequately nourished. Similarly, there is convincing evidence that babies born of well-nourished women are healthier than babies born of poorly nourished women.

IMPORTANCE OF NUTRITION DURING PREGNANCY

Strong evidence of the relationship of maternal nutrition to the outcome of pregnancy is reported in the following studies.

Frequently cited studies during World War II point to a definite relationship between the adequacy of the woman's diet and the outcome of pregnancy. In a report by Antonov[2] on children born during the siege of Leningrad in 1942 during which time both the quantity and quality of food were poor, he reports an incidence of 41.2 percent premature births during the period of food shortage compared with 6.5 percent when food was not so scarce. Newborn mortality for prematures was 30.8 percent, whereas for full-term babies it was 9 percent. Stillbirths more than doubled during this period. Antonov concluded that severe quantitative and qualitative nutritional deprivation of the woman decidedly affects the development of the fetus and the vitality of the newborn. During the wartime food shortage in Holland, Smith reports widespread amenorrhea among the women and a markedly reduced birth rate.[3, 4] Infants conceived before the months when food was short but born during the hunger period were significantly below expected heights and weights; Smith suggests that this can be correlated with maternal nutrition during the last trimester of pregnancy. He reported a slight increase in prematurity.

Burke and her coworkers[5, 6] found in a study at Boston Lying-In Hospital that every stillborn, every infant who died within a few days of birth (except one), all prematures, all functionally immature infants, and the majority of infants with congenital malformations were born to women with very inadequate diets. In this study the diets of the women and the condition of the infants were evaluated. The woman's diet was rated as "excellent," "good," "fair," or "poor." The infants at birth and during the first 2 weeks of life were rated by pediatricians who had no knowledge of the mothers' dietary ratings. The ratings of the infants were then correlated with the ratings of the mothers' prenatal diets. They found that when the maternal diet had been excellent or good that 95 percent of the infants were in excellent or good condition, and only 5 percent were in fair or poor condition. On the other hand, when the maternal diet had been poor only 8 percent of the infants were in excellent or good condition, but 65 percent were in poor condition, and 27 percent were in fair condition.

In a later study by Jeans et al. of 404 pregnant women in a Midwestern state, it was reported that all the stillbirths, all the neonatal deaths, and all the infants with congenital anomalies were born to women whose diets were poor or very poor.[7] Also, the incidence of prematurity rose sharply with the decrease in nutritional status of the woman, and the premature infants born to poorly nourished women were smaller and weaker than premature infants born to better nourished women.

Just as adequate nutrition is an important factor in maintaining good health throughout life, so it is during pregnancy. Adequate nutrition is needed to provide for the expectant mother's maintenance during pregnancy and to provide for the growth and development of the fetus. For the woman to be well nourished throughout her life and for her to maintain a good diet during pregnancy would help ensure safe, healthy pregnancies and healthy babies.

SPECIAL CONCERNS IN PREGNANCY

Toxemia

The etiology of toxemia is still not clearly understood. Many factors have been associated with the development of toxemia, including diabetes, chronic hypertension, the physiological immaturity of young primigravidas, multiple pregnancies, and nutrition. The exact relationship of nutrition to toxemia has not yet been fully clarified. The nutritional factors most generally associated with toxemia are calories and sodium.

Even though it has been commonly accepted that overweight women and those who gain excessive weight during pregnancy are more apt to develop toxemia, there is little evidence to substantiate this position.

> The idea that limitation of weight gain by caloric restriction protects against toxemia goes back to the observed reduction in the incidence of eclampsia in Germany and Austria-Hungary during World War I. Because of war-imposed scarcity of meat and fats, pregnant women gained less, and it was concluded without further study that a restricted diet was protective. Caloric restriction to limit gain in weight during pregnancy became widely advocated as a means to prevent toxemia and many other complications of pregnancy. The idea found its way into textbooks of obstetrics and was widely adopted by the medical profession. Seldom has a medical idea with such a basis (hearsay evidence) been applied so widely and subjected to so little scientific study.[8]

Tompkins reports nearly twice the incidence of toxemia in women who are markedly underweight than in those who are overweight.[9] He reports that failure to gain an average amount of weight during the second trimester is associated with a relatively high probability of developing toxemia. Tompkins also reports that an excessive weight gain of 9 to 10 lb at the end of pregnancy for extremely underweight women is compatible with minimum risk of developing toxic symptoms. [10]

The Committee on Maternal Nutrition recommends an average weight gain of 24 lb during pregnancy which is commensurate with a better than average course and outcome of pregnancy. [11] "Preventing this gain is particularly deleterious for underweight women. . . ." They stress the importance of the rate of weight gain and recommend a gain of 1.5 to 3.0 lb during the first trimester and a gain of 0.8 lb per week during the remainder of pregnancy. The committee agreed "that there is no advantage to be gained by prescribing weight reduction regimens for obese patients during pregnancy either for improving the course of the pregnancy or for contributing to the women's general health." [12] It was the consensus of the committee that any attempts at weight reduction should be delayed until after pregnancy.

Another common practice which should be questioned is the routine limitation of salt during pregnancy. Certain animal experiments have demonstrated an increased need for sodium during pregnancy. This may also be true for humans. Additional research is needed in this area. The Committee on Maternal Nutrition agreed that the practice of routinely restricting sodium during pregnancy and using diuretics at the same time is potentially dangerous.

Pregnancy in Adolescents

Special consideration needs to be given to the adolescent and her nutritional needs. Adolescents have a disproportionately large number of low-birth-weight infants. Neonatal, postneonatal, and infant mortality rates are much higher for infants born to adolescents. The pregnant adolescent is at an increased risk since she has to meet the needs for her own growth, which is not yet complete, plus the additional needs of the developing baby.

Complicating the problem is that teen-age girls, from reported studies, are consuming diets low in iron, calcium, vitamin A, and vitamin C. Many teen-agers may enter pregnancy in a questionable nutritional state. A good diet is especially important for the pregnant teen-ager in order to ensure adequate nutrients needed for her growth and maturation as well as those required by the pregnancy. Attention must be given to calorie, protein, and calcium intake, for each is critical to growth.

NUTRITION NEEDS DURING PREGNANCY AND LACTATION

Since pregnancy is normal, a pregnant woman's nutritional status and her diet should be thought of as contributions to a normal process leading to the birth of a healthy, full-term baby; they should not be thought of as a means of forestalling or treating possible complications. [13]

TABLE 18-1
RECOMMENDED DAILY DIETARY ALLOWANCES

Adult (age 22–35)	Calories	Protein, Gm	Calcium, Gm	Iron, mg	Vitamins			
					A, IU	B_1, mg	B_2, mg	C, mg
Nonpregnant	2000	55	0.8	18	5,000	1.0	1.5	55
Pregnant	2200	65	1.2	18	6,000	1.1	1.8	60
Lactating	3000	75	1.3	18	8,000	1.5	2.0	60

SOURCE: *Recommended Dietary Allowances*, 7th rev. ed., Food and Nutrition Board, National Research Council, 1968.

During pregnancy and lactation there is an increased need for nearly all nutrients. The recommended amounts of nutrients discussed in this section are based on the Recommended Daily Dietary Allowances, revised in 1968, as established by the Food and Nutrition Board, National Research Council.[14]

The recommended daily dietary allowances for a woman from twenty-two to thirty-five years of age when nonpregnant, pregnant, and when lactating are shown in Table 18-1 and are graphically illustrated in Figure 18-1. Following is a brief discussion of selected nutrients.

Calories

Calories provide energy and are needed for basal metabolism, synthesis of body tissue (growth, maintenance, pregnancy, and lactation), physical activity, bodily process, and to maintain thermal balance. The allowances for calories are established with the objective of providing sufficient energy to maintain body weight or support growth at levels consistent with health and well-being.

During pregnancy there is an increased need for calories to provide energy necessary for the building of new tissue in the placenta and fetus and for the increased work load imposed on the body by pregnancy. An additional 200 calories per day are recommended during pregnancy, and this is consistent with a weight gain of approximately 24 pounds. As has been mentioned previously, weight reduction should not be undertaken during pregnancy.

During lactation, additional calories are needed to supply the needed energy for milk production. Approximately 120 calories are needed for the production of 100 ml of milk. Since the amount of milk produced varies with individual women, the caloric intake would vary also. Assuming an average yield of 850 ml of breast milk per day, an additional allowance of 1000 calories per day is recommended by the National Research Council.

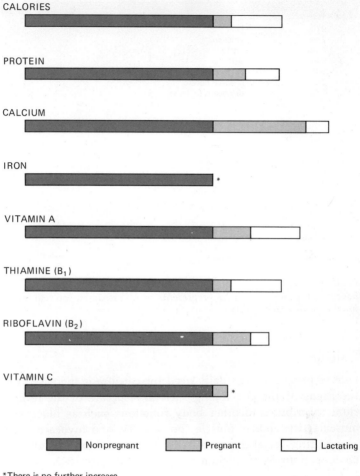

CALORIES

PROTEIN

CALCIUM

IRON *

VITAMIN A

THIAMINE (B₁)

RIBOFLAVIN (B₂)

VITAMIN C *

☐ Nonpregnant   ☐ Pregnant   ☐ Lactating

*There is no further increase

FIGURE 18-1
Percentage increases of nutrients during pregnancy and lactation for adult women between the ages of twenty-two and thirty-five.

Protein

Protein is needed to provide for growth of the fetus and for the development and maintenance of the various systems of the body. An adequate protein supply is needed for repair and maintenance of the expectant mother's own body tissue. The National Research Council recommends an additional 10 Gm of protein per day during pregnancy.

An additional 20 Gm of protein per day is recommended during lactation to meet the needs for milk production. Sources of protein are shown in Figure 18-2.

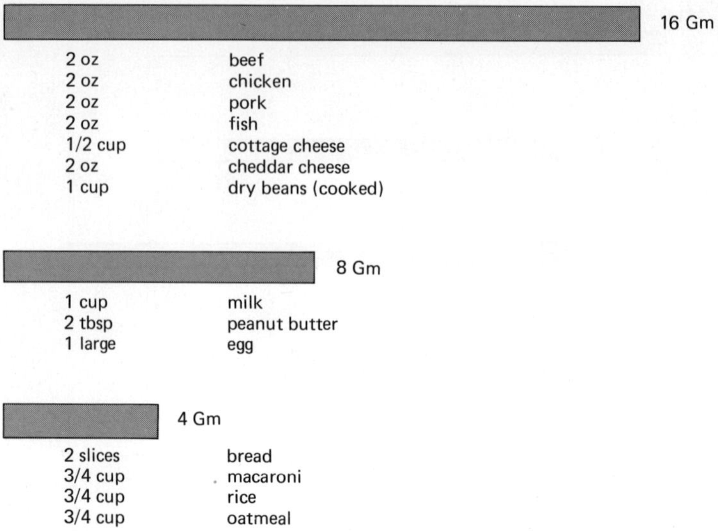

16 Gm

2 oz	beef
2 oz	chicken
2 oz	pork
2 oz	fish
1/2 cup	cottage cheese
2 oz	cheddar cheese
1 cup	dry beans (cooked)

8 Gm

1 cup	milk
2 tbsp	peanut butter
1 large	egg

4 Gm

2 slices	bread
3/4 cup	macaroni
3/4 cup	rice
3/4 cup	oatmeal

FIGURE 18-2
Sources of protein. Each bar represents an approximate protein value for the foods listed below it.

Calcium

During pregnancy the daily need for calcium is increased by 0.4 Gm to meet the needs of the developing skeletal structure of the fetus. In addition, calcium contributes to other body functions such as blood coagulation, neuromuscular irritability, muscle contractility, and myocardial function.

During lactation an additional 0.5 Gm of calcium per day is recommended. Sources of calcium are shown in Figure 18-3.

Iron

Iron is a constituent of hemoglobin and of a variety of enzymes. During pregnancy a daily intake of 18 mg of iron is recommended by the National Research Council. An adequate supply of iron during pregnancy is needed to maintain the expectant mother's hemoglobin level, to supply a reserve of iron for her use immediately after delivery, to furnish the infant's developmental requirements, and to provide him with a reserve of iron to be drawn on after birth.

The recommendation for women in the childbearing age is also 18 mg of iron per day. This amount of iron intake, the National Research Council reasons, should provide sufficient stores so that supplementation during pregnancy is not necessary. The Committee on Maternal Nutrition, on the other hand, recommends iron supplementation during the second and third tri-

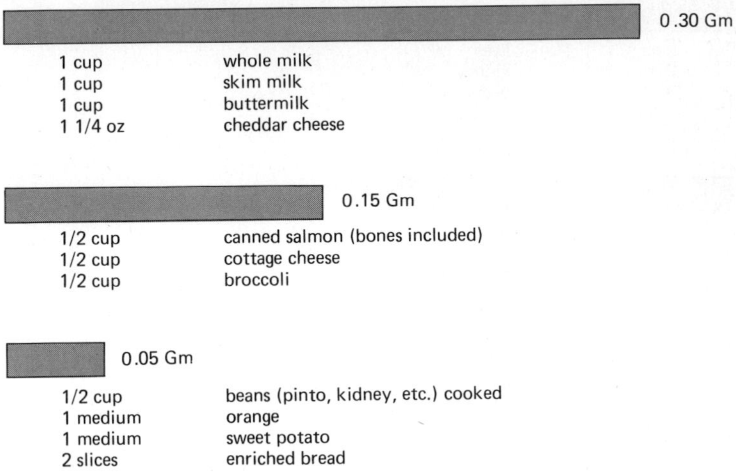

		0.30 Gm

1 cup	whole milk
1 cup	skim milk
1 cup	buttermilk
1 1/4 oz	cheddar cheese

		0.15 Gm

1/2 cup	canned salmon (bones included)
1/2 cup	cottage cheese
1/2 cup	broccoli

		0.05 Gm

1/2 cup	beans (pinto, kidney, etc.) cooked
1 medium	orange
1 medium	sweet potato
2 slices	enriched bread

FIGURE 18-3
Sources of calcium. Each bar represents an approximate calcium value for the foods listed below it.

mesters to help increase maternal hemoglobin concentrations and to protect maternal iron stores. During lactation the recommended iron intake is also 18 mg per day.

It is extremely difficult to meet the recommended allowance for iron; therefore, continued emphasis should be placed on encouraging the use of foods high in iron. Sources of iron are shown in Figure 18-4 (p. 342).

Vitamin C (Ascorbic Acid)

Vitamin C has multiple functions in the human body. It aids in maintaining the integrity of capillary networks and is essential for the health of gums and teeth. It is also essential for the production of an intercellular cement-like substance which is necessary for the support of cartilage, bone, muscles, and other tissues. The National Research Council recommends an increase of 5 mg per day during pregnancy and lactation. Sources of vitamin C are shown in Figure 18-5 (p. 343).

Vitamin A

Vitamin A is an essential factor in cell growth and development, in tooth formation, in normal bone growth, and for the integrity of the epithelial cells, including the uterus. The National Research Council recommends an additional 1,000 IU of vitamin A during pregnancy to provide for the nutritional well-being of the rapidly growing fetus.

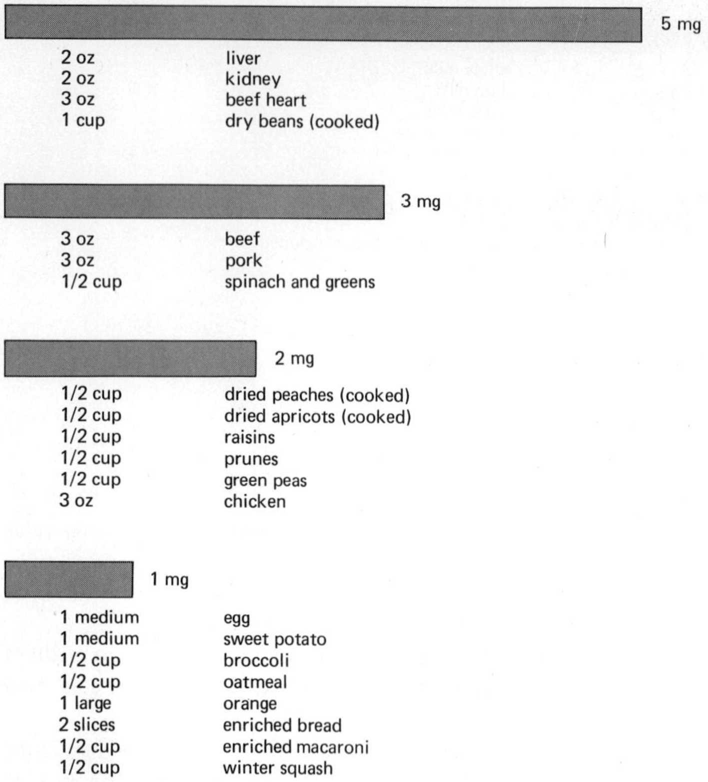

5 mg

2 oz	liver
2 oz	kidney
3 oz	beef heart
1 cup	dry beans (cooked)

3 mg

3 oz	beef
3 oz	pork
1/2 cup	spinach and greens

2 mg

1/2 cup	dried peaches (cooked)
1/2 cup	dried apricots (cooked)
1/2 cup	raisins
1/2 cup	prunes
1/2 cup	green peas
3 oz	chicken

1 mg

1 medium	egg
1 medium	sweet potato
1/2 cup	broccoli
1/2 cup	oatmeal
1 large	orange
2 slices	enriched bread
1/2 cup	enriched macaroni
1/2 cup	winter squash

FIGURE 18-4

Sources of iron. Each bar represents an approximate iron value for the foods listed below it.

During lactation an additional 3,000 IU are recommended to help ensure the nursing baby an ample supply of vitamin A. Sources of vitamin A are shown in Figure 18-6 (p. 344).

Vitamin B₁ (Thiamine)

Thiamine plays an essential role in the metabolism of carbohydrate. The need for thiamine increases as the caloric intake increases. The National Research Council suggests an increase of 0.1 mg consistent with the recommended increase in calories. Sources of vitamin B₁ are shown in Figure 18-7 (p. 345).

Vitamin B₂ (Riboflavin)

Adequate tissue function is dependent on sufficient amounts of riboflavin. The vitamin functions as a coenzyme concerned with tissue oxidation and respira-

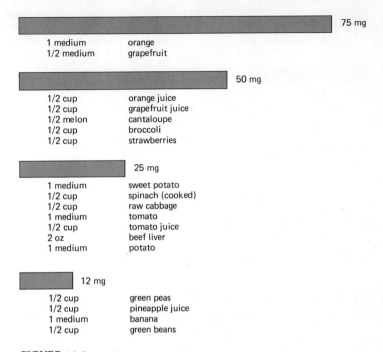

1 medium	orange
1/2 medium	grapefruit

1/2 cup	orange juice
1/2 cup	grapefruit juice
1/2 melon	cantaloupe
1/2 cup	broccoli
1/2 cup	strawberries

1 medium	sweet potato
1/2 cup	spinach (cooked)
1/2 cup	raw cabbage
1 medium	tomato
1/2 cup	tomato juice
2 oz	beef liver
1 medium	potato

1/2 cup	green peas
1/2 cup	pineapple juice
1 medium	banana
1/2 cup	green beans

FIGURE 18-5

Sources of vitamin C. Each bar represents an approximate vitamin C value for the foods listed below it.

tion and is involved both in protein and energy metabolism. An increase of 0.3 mg per day during pregnancy is recommended by the National Research Council. This is based on the estimated increase in metabolic body size resulting from the growth of the fetus and accessory tissues.

During lactation an additional daily intake of 0.5 mg is recommended. This is based on the amount of riboflavin excreted in the milk. Sources of vitamin B$_2$ are shown in Figure 18-8 (p. 346).

Vitamin D

Vitamin D promotes retention and utilization of calcium and phosphorus and is necessary in the formation of bones and teeth of the fetus. Vitamin D can be acquired either by ingestion or by exposure to sunlight, which activates a substance present in the skin.

On the basis of present evidence, the National Research Council recommends 400 IU of vitamin D during pregnancy and during lactation for both adults and teen-agers. Food sources of vitamin D include milk fortified with vitamin D, fish, egg yolk, and liver.

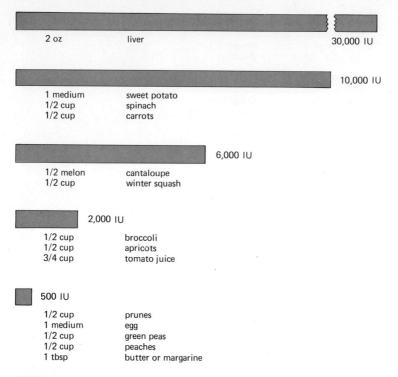

2 oz	liver

30,000 IU

1 medium	sweet potato
1/2 cup	spinach
1/2 cup	carrots

10,000 IU

1/2 melon	cantaloupe
1/2 cup	winter squash

6,000 IU

2,000 IU

1/2 cup	broccoli
1/2 cup	apricots
3/4 cup	tomato juice

500 IU

1/2 cup	prunes
1 medium	egg
1/2 cup	green peas
1/2 cup	peaches
1 tbsp	butter or margarine

FIGURE 18-6
Sources of vitamin A. Each bar represents an approximate vitamin A value for the foods listed below it.

Iodine

Iodine is an essential nutrient and should be included in the diet. The use of iodized salt should be encouraged. This is even more important for women living in areas where the soil and water are deficient in iodine.

FOODS TO MEET NUTRITIONAL NEEDS DURING PREGNANCY AND LACTATION

There are several combinations of foods which will provide the needed nutrients during pregnancy and lactation. One guide to the selection of foods to meet these nutrient requirements is the basic four food groups. Modifications on the selection of foods and combinations of foods may have to be made in order to make suggestions acceptable to individuals. For this reason, it is important that the person doing the nutritional counseling be familiar with the nutrient contributions of each food group so that appropriate substitu-

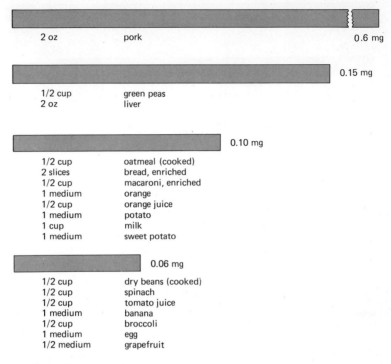

2 oz	pork	0.6 mg

0.15 mg

1/2 cup	green peas
2 oz	liver

0.10 mg

1/2 cup	oatmeal (cooked)
2 slices	bread, enriched
1/2 cup	macaroni, enriched
1 medium	orange
1/2 cup	orange juice
1 medium	potato
1 cup	milk
1 medium	sweet potato

0.06 mg

1/2 cup	dry beans (cooked)
1/2 cup	spinach
1/2 cup	tomato juice
1 medium	banana
1/2 cup	broccoli
1 medium	egg
1/2 medium	grapefruit

FIGURE 18-7
Sources of vitamin B_1. Each bar represents an approximate vitamin B_1 value for the foods listed below it.

tions can be made. Table 18-2 (p. 347) outlines the basic four food groups, recommended number of servings during pregnancy and lactation, foods included in each group, and what constitutes one serving in each group.

NUTRITION COUNSELING

Recognition of nutrition as a component of nursing care has been accepted since the days of Florence Nightingale. In her many writings it was evident that she recognized that food played an important part in a person's health and well-being. She encouraged nurses to accept their responsibility in this area of nursing.[15]

The nurse has many opportunities to provide nutritional guidance to expectant and lactating mothers. The nurse sees the woman at regular intervals—in the office, in the clinic, and in the home—and is in a good position to know and understand individual family situations, thereby making nutrition teaching more meaningful.

Young pregnant women are one of the groups which are most often will-

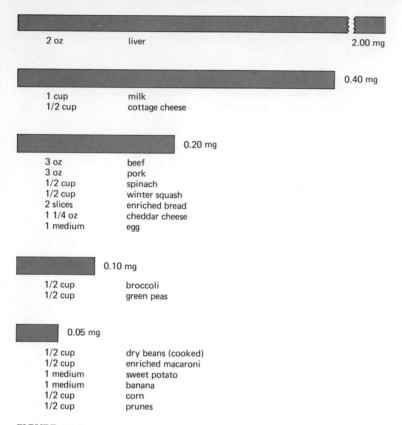

2 oz	liver	2.00 mg
1 cup	milk	0.40 mg
1/2 cup	cottage cheese	
3 oz	beef	0.20 mg
3 oz	pork	
1/2 cup	spinach	
1/2 cup	winter squash	
2 slices	enriched bread	
1 1/4 oz	cheddar cheese	
1 medium	egg	
1/2 cup	broccoli	0.10 mg
1/2 cup	green peas	
1/2 cup	dry beans (cooked)	0.05 mg
1/2 cup	enriched macaroni	
1 medium	sweet potato	
1 medium	banana	
1/2 cup	corn	
1/2 cup	prunes	

FIGURE 18-8
Sources of vitamin B_2. Each bar represents an approximate vitamin B_2 value for the foods listed below it.

ing to make changes in their dietary habits. Their interest in having a healthy baby is usually high. Nutrition advice presented at this time is most likely to be well received.

Nutrition advice must be geared to the expectant mother's previous food habits and to her purse, or it will not be used. The meanings and significance of food to individuals should be considered when counseling regarding a change of dietary habits. To most people, food is not merely a matter of nutrition and caloric value. There are many things that enter into the choices that a person makes when it comes to his dietary practices. A whole series of reactions, complexes, and emotions are maintained about food. A person may or may not be aware of these factors.

Cultural, religious, and economic factors affect a person's choice of food, as well as customs, habits, likes and dislikes, and availability of food. These

TABLE 18-2
BASIC FOUR FOOD GROUPS

Milk group

Contribution:	This group is a leading source of calcium and an important contributor of high-quality protein and riboflavin. Also provided are other vitamins and minerals.
Recommended servings:	Pregnancy, 3 servings Lactation, 3½–4 servings
Foods included:	Milk—whole, nonfat, buttermilk, evaporated, dry Cheese—cheddar type, Swiss, cottage Ice cream
Count as one serving:	1 cup (8 oz) whole, nonfat, or buttermilk ½ cup undiluted evaporated milk 3–4 tablespoons dry milk 1¼ cups cottage cheese 1½ ounces cheddar type or Swiss cheese 1½ cups ice cream

Meat group

Contribution:	This group is important for the protein it provides. In addition, many of the foods supply considerable iron, thiamine, riboflavin, and niacin.
Recommended servings:	Pregnancy, 3 servings Lactation, 3 servings
Foods included:	Beef, veal, lamb, pork, poultry, fish, variety meats such as liver, heart, kidney Eggs Dry beans, dry peas, lentils, nuts, peanut butter
Count as one serving:	2 ounces of lean cooked meat, poultry, or fish, all without bone 2 eggs 1 cup cooked dry beans, dry peas, or lentils 4 tablespoons peanut butter

Vegetable and fruit group

Contribution:	Vegetables and fruits are valuable because of the vitamins and minerals they contain, especially for vitamins C and A.
Recommended servings:	Pregnancy, 4–5 servings Lactation, 5 servings (Included in these servings should be a source of vitamin A and vitamin C)
Foods included:	*Vitamin C* Good sources—Grapefruit, grapefruit juice, orange, orange juice, cantaloupe, mango, papaya, strawberries, broccoli, green peppers, sweet red peppers, green chili peppers Fair sources—Tomatoes, tomato juice, honeydew melon, watermelon, asparagus tips, raw cabbage, collards, kale, mustard greens, potatoes and sweet potatoes, spinach, turnip greens

TABLE 18-2 *(Continued)*

Vitamin A

Dark green and deep yellow vegetables and a few fruits —apricots, broccoli, cantaloupe, carrots, chard, collards, cress, kale, pumpkin, spinach, sweet potatoes, turnip greens and other dark green leaves, winter squash

Other fruits and vegetables, including potatoes

Count as one serving: ½ cup of vegetable or fruit, or a portion as ordinarily served, such as 1 medium apple, banana, or orange, or half a grapefruit

¾ cup fruit or vegetable juice

Bread and cereal group

Contribution: This group furnishes worthwhile amounts of thiamine, iron, niacin, and smaller amounts of other vitamins and minerals.

Recommended servings: Pregnancy, 4–5 servings

Lactation, 4–5 servings

Foods included: All breads and cereals and baked goods that are whole grain, enriched, or restored; cooked cereals, ready-to-eat cereals, cornmeal, crackers, flour, grits, macaroni, spaghetti, noodles, rice, rolled oats, tortillas, quick breads, and other baked goods if made with whole grain or enriched flour

Count as one serving: 1 slice bread

1 ounce ready-to-eat cereal

½–¾ cup cooked cereal, cornmeal, grits, macaroni, noodles, rice, or spaghetti

factors which affect food patterns cannot be overlooked when counseling if the advice offered is to be accepted and utilized. Nutrition counseling should be made as individualized as possible.

In discussing nutrition education for the expectant mother consideration should be given to the prospective father. Frequently he has a strong influence on what the family eats. He may need to be convinced of the importance of an adequate diet for his wife. Effective nutrition education during this time could very well change food habits for the better and start the family on the road to better nutrition.

People in low-income groups often do not eat adequate diets. Some will need assistance in obtaining additional food. The nurse needs to be aware of the resources available in the community. The nurse can help these families avail themselves of programs such as food stamps, commodities, or other supplemental food programs. In addition, the nurse can provide assistance in planning an adequate diet from lower cost foods which will provide the needed nutrients. Some things which can help extend the food dollar are planning menus in advance and shopping according to the plan, taking advantage of specials, and purchasing large sizes and in quantity if storage permits. Emphasizing the taste appeal and nutritional value rather than the cheapness of foods is often more successful.

In order to be effective in nutrition counseling the nurse needs to have a good understanding of the four food groups discussed previously and what contributions are expected from the various groups. This is important so that the nurse can help the expectant mother make appropriate substitutions. For example, calcium tablets are not a nutritionally acceptable substitute for milk, since they do not supply the protein and vitamins, particularly riboflavin, found in milk. When a pregnant woman does not drink milk for one reason or another and calcium tablets are being taken, nutrition counseling should be directed toward helping her find adequate sources of the other nutrients she is not obtaining from the tablets.

How can dietary practices of expectant and lactating mothers be improved? Modifying an individual's dietary practice is difficult but not impossible for the enthusiastic nurse who truly believes that adequate nutrition is essential to the prolonged health and well-being of the mother-to-be and her baby. The expectant mother is not likely to follow diet suggestions unless she considers them important. Diet recommendations should be accompanied by an explanation of why they are made and then discussed in terms of how the recommendations can be fitted into her usual food pattern. Then the diet suggestions have a better chance of being accepted and followed.

Some suggested steps in nutrition counseling which have been found to be useful are listed below.

1 Obtain as much information as time permits on present food practices, including methods of preparing food, likes, and dislikes.
2 Evaluate the nutritional adequacy of the diet.
3 Support the good features of the diet.
4 Recommend and explain a few needed changes in problem areas. Suggest foods that will be as acceptable as possible to the family. Explain how these recommendations might be carried out, for example, in new recipes.
5 Involve the patient in the decision to change.
6 Follow through on suggested changes with additional recommendations if necessary.

Resource people can be of help to the nurse and should be utilized in efforts to provide nutrition guidance. The nutritionist or dietitian has knowledge of nutritional needs of pregnant and lactating women, nutritive value of foods, cultural food practices, and food budgeting. They are excellent resources which the nurse should seek out.

SUMMARY

There is considerable evidence that nutrition is an important factor during pregnancy and has an influence on the health of the woman and her baby. It is clear that a well-balanced diet containing sufficient amounts of all the nutrients is essential. The following points should be considered:

An average weight gain of 24 lb during pregnancy is recommended. The suggested rate of weight gain is 1.5 to 3.0 lb during the first trimester, and 0.8 lb per week during the remainder of pregnancy.

Special attention should be given to the nutritional needs of pregnant adolescents.

The underweight woman who becomes pregnant needs special attention.

Weight reduction regimens should not be undertaken until after pregnancy.

Routine restriction of salt during pregnancy is questioned.

The nurse has an important contribution to make in nutrition counseling of pregnant and lactating women.

REFERENCES

1 Committee on Maternal Nutrition, Food and Nutrition Board, National Research Council: *Maternal Nutrition and the Course of Pregnancy*, National Academy of Sciences, Washington, D.C., 1970, p. 1.

2 Antonov, A. N.: "Children Born during the Siege of Leningrad in 1942," *Journal of Pediatrics*, 30:250–259, 1947.

3 Smith, C. A.: "Effects of Maternal Undernutrition upon the Newborn Infant in Holland (1944–1945)," *Journal of Pediatrics*, 30:229–243, 1947.

4 Smith, C. A.: "The Effect of Wartime Starvation in Holland upon Pregnancy and Its Product," *American Journal of Obstetrics and Gynecology*, 53:599–608, 1947.

5 Burke, B. S., V. A. Beal, A. B. Kirkwood, and H. C. Stuart: "Nutrition Studies during Pregnancy," *American Journal of Obstetrics and Gynecology*, 46:38–52, 1943.

6 Burke, B. S., S. S. Stevenson, J. Worcester, and H. C. Stuart: "Nutrition Studies during Pregnancy. V. Relation of Maternal Nutrition to Condition of Infant at Birth: Study of Siblings," *The Journal of Nutrition*, 38:453–467, 1949.

7 Jeans, P. C., M. B. Smith, and G. Stearns: "Incidence of Prematurity in Relation to Maternal Nutrition," *Journal of the American Dietetic Association*, 31:576–581, 1955.

8 Committee on Maternal Nutrition: op. cit., p. 176.

9 Tompkins, W. T., and D. G. Wiehl: "Nutritional Deficiencies as a Causal

Factor in Toxemia and Premature Labor," *American Journal of Obstetrics and Gynecology*, 62:898–919, 1951.

10 Tompkins, W. T., D. G. Wiehl, and R. M. Mitchell: "The Underweight Patient as an Increased Obstetric Hazard," *American Journal of Obstetrics and Gynecology*, 69:114–123, 1955.

11 Committee on Maternal Nutrition: op. cit., p. 183.

12 Ibid.

13 Ibid., p. 3.

14 Food and Nutrition Board, National Research Council, *Recommended Dietary Allowances*, 7th ed., revised 1968, National Academy of Sciences, Washington, D. C., 1968.

15 Cooper, L. F.: "Florence Nightingale's Contribution to Dietetics," *Journal of the American Dietetic Association*, 30:121–127, 1954.

19 | SAFETY AND ACTIVITIES DURING PREGNANCY

Mary B. Johnson

Most of the advice given to patients about activities and safety during pregnancy deals with the physical aspects, but the emotionality inherent in each aspect cannot be denied. Pregnancy is both a physiological state and an emotional experience. Maintenance of the best possible physical condition is one of the prime goals of prenatal care. However, the health team's efforts cannot be directed to the physiological needs alone. Emotional care and understanding by professional health personnel are necessary in order to treat the patient within the totality of her pregnancy. Good prenatal care considers the woman as an individual within her specific medical and social situation.

The nurse usually works within one of three settings—a private doctor's office, a clinic, or in the community. Wherever the work setting is, nurses must identify the population of patients with which they are working before they can begin to advise women about their activities and safety during pregnancy. Age, marital status, habits, motivation, levels of knowledge, socioeconomic level, and many more factors will influence the nurse's approach to patients.

The initial contact between the nurse and patient is important because it may set the tone of their relationship for the duration of that woman's pregnancy. The nurse should be a sympathetic listener, a friend, and a resource person. Not only a thorough knowledge of the physiological and psychological aspects of pregnancy are needed, but also a recognition on the part of nurses as to their own feelings in relation to pregnancy, motherhood, sex, and feminity. Insight, not intimidation, is the key to establishing a role as a caring, resourceful person.

The nurse's role is to augment the obstetrician, not to displace his philosophy and advice. There is considerable difference of opinion concerning the details of management of pregnancy. The directions given here are basically generalities. Within a health care setting, the physician and nurse consider the patient as an individual with a unique pregnancy.

EMPLOYMENT

Today women of childbearing age are a major factor in the labor force, and it is difficult to say "yes" or "no" when a patient asks if she should continue working. Realistic adjustments in her mode of life must be made if employment is physically or mentally jeopardizing her health or pregnancy. Some of the most important factors involved are economic, psychological, and physical. The order of importance of these factors will vary with each patient and even with each subsequent pregnancy.

Many women are not content to stay home, and others are simply unable to quit because of their financial situations. Whether she is unmarried or has a husband who is in school or is unemployed, her job and salary become very important. Also, many women today intend to pursue their careers after pregnancy and see having the baby as a temporary stopping point in that career. Today many companies have lifted severe restrictions on pregnant workers, but the patient should check to see if she needs a work approval letter from her physician or if it will be necessary to resign after a certain period. Working up to and including the seventh month of pregnancy is a very common practice. Many hospitals do not have time limits, and nurses often work up to their date of delivery. One obstetric nurse worked in the delivery area while having contractions, gave report, went home and picked up her suitcase, and returned to check herself into the labor area.

Women work not only for the money but also as a "mental health break," as one patient with small children described it. Conversely, women who stay at home feel this is their last chance to be themselves and capture time alone with their husbands. Both points are valid, and the individual feelings of each woman are to be carefully considered. A woman who works must realize that the physical and mental strains of pregnancy should not be imposed upon her coworkers. Also, more careful grooming and a larger wardrobe are often expected of women who work outside the home.

Whether a woman works at home or outside, she must be aware of her physical activities and how they affect her and her fetus. Ideally she should

1 Avoid physical strain and not work to the point of fatigue.
2 Know the correct ways to lift and carry objects.
3 Avoid occupations involving toxic substances.
4 Take adequate rest periods either at home or at work.
5 Consider restrictions made by her physician to decrease her amount of physical work or strain. These recommendations might be made with the knowledge of a previous history of obstetric complications.

In general, long hours of physical work should be avoided. This includes standing or sitting for hours at a time, rotating night shifts, heavy lifting, and jobs requiring a delicate sense of body balance. Pregnant women do not have a ready reserve of energy upon which to fall back. Instead they become fatigued easily and are unable to regain their usual energy level as quickly.

Correct methods of lifting or carrying will decrease possible physical strain. By squatting or kneeling, bringing objects as close to the body as possible, and lifting from the legs, strong thigh muscles are used and back strain can be avoided. Instead of lifting children, have them climb onto a footstool and then onto the lap. Activity at home may be just as strenuous as at any outside position or job. A fall is basically the same whether it is from a stepladder while painting the nursery or from a chair at the office.

Occupations which involve toxic substances are to be avoided. Industrial workers especially should be urged to contact their company physician or nurse about possible hazards in connection with their work. The following is a partial list of toxic substances considered to be dangerous during pregnancy. It was compiled by the Maternal Child Health Service of the United States and stated in their *Standards for Maternity Care and Employment of Mothers in Industry.*

Aniline
Benzene and toluene
Carbon disulfide
Carbon monoxide
Chlorinated hydrocarbons
Lead and its compounds
Mercury and its compounds
Nitrobenzene and other nitro- compounds of benzene and its homologues
Phosphorus
Radioactive substances and x rays
Turpentine

Rest during work, either at home or in the office, is important for every pregnant woman, even if it is only a chance to elevate her feet for 10 minutes and regain some of her lost energy.

For women who have a previous history of not carrying a baby to term or who show a tendency to abort, the physician may advise rest as a necessity, and she may be encouraged to work only part time or to quit work altogether.

EXERCISE

As with employment, exercise should never be carried to the point of fatigue. Women who are pregnant do not have their normal resilience and do not recover as easily from physical exercise. Women who previously felt rested an hour after a game of tennis may need half a day to recover during pregnancy. Walking outdoors at a good brisk pace seems to be the most universally recommended exercise. Exercise of any kind is beneficial and ideally should be combined with fresh air and sunlight. Patients should be asked about their usual amount of activity, and it must be decided which activities should be increased or decreased. This also will change between the early and later periods of pregnancy.

The strenuous sports such as tennis, golf, skiing, horseback riding, backpacking, or canoeing should not be condemned immediately but should be individually considered for each patient. Pregnancy is not a reason to drastically change a way of life, but women should be warned that their sense of balance and timing may be altered by their increasing size. Many physicians do advise against taking part in active sports in which there is a greater likelihood of a direct blow to the abdomen. Exceptions are, of course, made. One woman went skiing during her seventh and eighth months with the blessing of her obstetrician, himself an avid and expert skier. Another woman, with no obstetric complications, continued to raise and train horses until late into her pregnancy.

Body-slimming exercises need not be stopped because of pregnancy and a disappearing waistline. Modified knee bends, sit-ups, or stretches as well as shoulder-relaxing exercises are usually allowed but must again be considered in relation to the individual patient and her pregnancy. Women who have never been active or exercise-minded should be cautioned against starting strenuous exercise regimens or taking up new sports at this time, not only because of a certain inherent clumsiness, but also to avoid pushing themselves to the point of fatigue.

SLEEP, REST, AND RELAXATION

During pregnancy it is not just extra sleep at night that is needed, as so many women believe, but an entirely new pattern of rest and relaxation. Besides an adequate amount of sleep each night, she should try to nap or rest for a half hour every morning and afternoon. Obviously not everyone can follow this schedule, especially the woman who works during her entire pregnancy or who is the mother of other small children.

"Rest and relaxation" is an individual concept, and what it means to each woman must be carefully defined before any attempts are made to modify her schedule of activities. Age, nervous disposition, marital status, culture, and normal activities must all be considered with each patient.

Flexibility is perhaps the key word in counseling pregnant women about resting; it can be explained that relaxation not only means sleep but the ability to sit down alone, elevate her feet or relax tense muscles, and simply do nothing for a while. This method of relaxation can help overcome some of the discomforts of pregnancy. Elevating the legs on a chair or even up against a wall or headboard may be recommended to help overcome edema or varicosities. Sims's position may be advised for vulvar or rectal varicosities.

Emotional rest is just as important as physical rest. The woman's physical activity is changed, but she also senses and reacts emotionally to many more things. Sounds seem louder, smells seem stronger and are sometimes nauseating, taste sensations change, and small annoyances may produce unwarranted irritation or anger.

Physically, sleep may be a problem, especially in the last trimester. Digestive discomforts and frequency of urination contribute to sleeplessness, as do nightmares and fears. The protruding abdomen itself is usually a major cause of discomfort. There is virtually no harmful position in which to sleep, but the most comfortable is usually on the side with a pillow under the top knee which has been brought forward. The pillow can also be used to support the abdomen if this is comfortable.

TRAVEL

Common sense is probably the best thing for patients to take along on trips or vacations. Some of the most commonly asked questions are, "How long can I stay?" "What precautions should I take along the way?" "Does it matter how I get there?"

The old myth about pregnant women not traveling far from home was disproved soon after World War II when it was shown that no significant increase in abortions occurred in wives of military personnel who followed their husbands all over the world.[1]

With a patient who has no apparent or anticipated obstetric complications, the time spent away from home is not as important as the fact that there will be a physician nearby in case of complications. For prolonged stays, arrangements should be made for another physician to see her on a regular basis until she returns home. If possible, no long trips should be planned during the last trimester in order to avoid delivering in a strange hospital where her obstetric history is unknown.

Each patient's individual pregnancy must be considered when advising her about traveling. Often patients delay "asking" permission from their obstetrician until just before they leave. Urge patients to have their vacation plans approved earlier. Advise them also to take along only those medications prescribed specifically for them by their obstetrician. If travel ordinarily makes the pregnant woman nauseated, her physician should be informed of this fact.

Since indigestion and heartburn do not enhance a vacation, special care should be taken with what and how much are eaten and drunk. The amount, of course, also depends on how weight-conscious both the patient and her physician are.

Means of Transportation

For women who are prone to "travel sickness," the train or airplane is probably the best choice. Railroads have no restrictions on carrying pregnant passengers and provide comfortable travel in either the day coach or the sleeper. Air travel, especially during the first trimester, has caused controversy on the basis of questionable fetal hypoxia during this formative period. Well-pressurized commercial airlines, as opposed to small private planes, are to be recommended. Some airlines have restrictions on carrying pregnant women; restrictions for domestic and foreign flights may also differ. Some airlines require letters with differing amounts of information from the physician before they will allow the woman to fly with them.

Air travel may be faster, but bus and car travel offers the advantage of frequent rest and bathroom stops. Advise patients not to try to finish their trip all in one day. Rest stops every 100 to 200 miles will help to eliminate stiffness, cramping, and poor circulation. A rest stop should include stopping the car, getting out and walking around, going to the bathroom, and elevating the feet periodically.

Driving

As long as the pregnant woman can comfortably sit behind the wheel there is no reason for her to stop driving. During the last trimester for obvious reasons she should be advised not to drive alone at night or in uninhabited areas. You might suggest that pregnancy is a very poor time to learn to drive, not only because of the inherent clumsiness of some pregnant women but also because beginning drivers are more prone to accidents.

Seat belts are another controversial matter among obstetricians. Although the rare case of uterine rupture has been reported due to a seat belt, seat belts definitely decrease the possibility of maternal mortality in severe car accidents.[2] Seat belts should be recommended and should be worn low, comfortably under the abdomen and in conjunction with a shoulder strap if possible. Both belts must be properly adjusted—not too tight and not pressing high against the neck or abdomen.

Vaccinations

The question of vaccinations is important in view of the widespread travels undertaken by many pregnant women these days. The diseases a woman may be exposed to must be considered when making travel plans and when considering the possibilities of pregnancy.

Vaccinations are a precaution but are questionable at the same time. Many live viruses are able to cross the placental barrier and infect the fetus. Therefore, all routine immunizations with live vaccines are to be avoided during pregnancy. The following list of vaccinations is based upon reports of the Advisory Committee on Immunization of Infectious Diseases of the American Academy of Pediatrics as reviewed by *The Medical Letter on Drugs and Therapeutics.*[3]

Smallpox: Vaccinia virus given during pregnancy can occasionally infect the fetus. Fetal vaccinia has almost always been associated with primary vaccination. Thus, primary vaccination should only be used in essential cases because of exposure in an endemic area.

Mumps and measles: These live viruses should never be given to pregnant patients.

Rubella: This virus vaccine has been shown on occasion to infect both the placenta and the fetus, the significance of which is uncertain. Pregnancy is a contraindication for administration of the live rubella vaccine.

Yellow fever: This is a live virus that should be given to pregnant patients only if there is a very great risk of exposure.

Poliomyelitis: Since polio has almost been irradicated in this country, immunization during pregnancy is rarely indicated.

Cholera: This killed bacterial vaccine should be given only if there is a danger of infection. There has been no convincing documentation of an abortogenic effect.

Other vaccines and tests: No recommendations were made by the Advisory Committee about vaccination against influenza, epidemic typhus, and typhoid. Tetanus and diphtheria toxiods are considered safe. The tuberculin and histoplasmin tests are also permissible.

The fact that the occasional fetal abnormality due to vaccinations cannot be ruled out leaves one definite course open to physicians and nurses; urge patients to have necessary immunizations before pregnancy and then allow the correct amount of time following immunization before conceiving. This precaution as well as avoiding exposure to the diseases will help reduce problems with infections and possible risks to the child's health and development. General good health is also a major factor in reducing threats to fetal development in that it reduces chances for infection or disease. Pregnant patients should be urged to report every illness to their physician no matter how minor it may seem to them.

DENTAL CARE

It is a common misconception that the baby absorbs calcium from the mother's teeth or jawbone. It should be explained to the patient that a proper diet will supply the baby with all the calcium and other necessities for healthy teeth and bones.

The baby's teeth are already developing during the second month of pregnancy and by about the sixth month the permanent tooth buds have started to form. Heredity is the major determinant of tooth size and shape, but the diet, health, and activities of the pregnant patient can affect their quality. Good dental health at all times goes without saying, but especially during pregnancy. Gums may have a tendency to bleed more readily and may appear somewhat red or swollen at times. Nausea, acid regurgitation (heartburn), omission of brushing the teeth (maybe because of gagging), excessive salivation (ptyalism), and changing day-to-day eating habits are all conducive to dental problems during pregnancy. Usually conditions that have gone unattended give the impression that pregnancy in itself aggravates dental problems.

The dentist should be informed early in pregnancy of either the possibility or the actuality of pregnancy. Dental visits, and especially any extensive work, should be discussed with the dentist and obstetrician so that they can decide together the best time for dental work and the safety and choice of drugs and anesthetics. Very seldom is dental work contraindicated, but extensive elective work may have to be postponed. The most favorable time for dental work is from the fourth to the seventh month.[4] The baby is well along in development and, just as important, the patient is usually feeling much better, less nauseated, and yet is not so pregnant that she cannot sit for a period of time.

Dental x rays, a diagnostic procedure, should be postponed until the latter half of pregnancy.[5] When used properly in connection with a lead apron over the abdomen, the dental x-ray machine should have no adverse affects with its small 1½-inch beam aimed only at the face.

X RAYS FOR DIAGNOSTIC PURPOSES

Occasionally obstetric patients rebel at the idea of x rays taken during their pregnancies. These women have heard many of the misconceptions regarding all forms of irradiation, including such examinations as the routine antenatal chest x ray.

In a recent guide to good practice of x-ray examinations prepared by the American College of Radiology, it was stated that the optimal period of examinations of the abdomen and pelvis of women of childbearing age is the first 14 days after the onset of the menstrual cycle. At this time patients are definitely not pregnant. Routine antenatal chest x rays may be taken at any time with a lead apron over the abdomen, but the procedure is usually delayed until after the sixth month.

Obviously when the woman is definitely pregnant the physician must make a choice as to the urgency of the procedure. For example, if the patient has active gastrointestinal bleeding, there would be very little question as to the need for a barium enema and upper gastrointestinal series, even in the first trimester when the fetus is the most susceptible. The radiologist should be informed of the pregnancy so as to shield the abdomen with lead apron if possible and also to minimize the level of radiation. If the pregnancy is undetermined and the x-ray procedure has been performed, usually there is little to worry about, since the radiation dose for most procedures is relatively small. However, in the case of extremely large dosage from a particular procedure or combination of procedures, experts should be consulted about the amount of radiation to the fetus and possible hazard to fetal development.

SMOKING AND DRINKING

Alcohol is usually not prohibited during pregnancy, although cocktails and beer are very high in calories. Taste is a sensation that changes with pregnancy, and many women find themselves unable to drink alcohol in any form. The quantity of alcohol in one or two drinks is eliminated rapidly from the bloodstream, and therefore only small quantities reach the fetus. The secondary effects of alcoholism, however, may lead to fetal underdevelopment because of maternal malnutrition.

Smoking, unlike drinking, may affect the child more directly.[6] Nicotine is absorbed in the bloodstream and passed to the fetus by means of the placenta. The amount absorbed, of course, depends on the amount inhaled. Some experts feel that this causes no more than a harmless increase in fetal heart rate, and yet others feel that it may somehow lead to fetal underdevelopment. Size of infants at birth is probably affected by the number of cigarettes smoked per day. Very heavy smokers—those who smoke more than one pack a day—seem to have smaller infants than nonsmoking mothers. There is still a great deal of controversy in recent literature regarding the possibility of stillborns, fetal abnormalities, prematurity, or maternal complications caused by smoking. For general health reasons, perhaps pregnancy is a good time to urge patients to try to stop smoking; many are nauseated in the first trimester and cannot tolerate the smell or taste of cigarettes anyway.

MATERNITY CLOTHING

Maternity fashions have changed greatly over the past few years. Clothing today is practical, attractive, and nonrestricting. To avoid constriction around the waist, dresses or tops should be hung from the shoulders and should not have tight elastic around the waistline. The importance of properly fitting girdles, brassieres, and shoes should be discussed with patients.

Usually a girdle is a deterrent to complete comfort, since many pregnant women feel as though they are encased in an elastic strait jacket. The properly fitted maternity girdle may be a necessity, however, for the woman who has always worn a girdle or who needs extra support for stretched muscles due to multiparity. The patient should lie on her back to put on the girdle and hook or adjust it starting from the bottom. It should not be so tight that when she sits up it is very constricting or uncomfortable. After the fourth or fifth month, backache may be relieved for some women by proper abdominal support, but it must be pointed out to patients that girdles do not prevent striae or stretched muscles.

Pregnant women should buy properly fitting and supportive brassieres in one cup size larger than usual. This is especially true for those women who have large pendulous breasts. These patients may even find that it is necessary to wear a breast support to bed at night.

Tight bands or garters tend to accentuate any varicosities or edema of the lower extremities. Garter belts or the more commonly worn panty hose are much safer and easier to wear.

The postural changes of pregnancy may be aggravated by either very high-heeled or very flat shoes. Both accentuate poor posture and may contribute to backache and fatigue. Low-heeled, comfortable shoes are advised, but high heels can be worn on occasion if the woman is aware that she may be inclined to tip forward due to the increasing size of her abdomen.

GENERAL HYGIENE

At one time tub baths and intercourse were prohibited during pregnancy because it was thought that water or semen readily entered the vagina and could cause infections harmful to the fetus. This concept has been largely negated today.

Bathing

There are now no restrictions on bathing during pregnancy unless the membranes have been ruptured, and then tub baths are strictly prohibited. Caution patients that they are not as agile during the later months and are more prone to fall. Rubber mats on the floor of the bath or shower and even hand rails are to be recommended. The temperature of the bath or shower is not a matter for concern, as long as it is comfortable to the expectant mother.

Douching

Douching is very rarely needed and should be done during pregnancy only when recommended by the obstetrician. Vaginal discharge or irritations should be mentioned to the physician. He may recommend more frequent change of underwear, suppositories, or a douche. Nylon underwear and panty hose, which so many women wear today, have the irritating effect of retaining heat in the perineal area and preventing the evaporation of normal perspiration, thus providing an incubator effect for organisms in the discharge. Sometimes just changing to cotton underwear, bathing daily, and keeping the vaginal or perineal area as dry as possible helps to clear the irritation. Douche bags, when prescribed and with the correct solutions, should be held low to decrease the force of gravity and should be inserted no more than 2 to 3 inches into the vagina. The patient may be seated on the toilet instead of in the bathtub, a very awkward position under any conditions. Hand bulb syringes should never be allowed as they could theoretically introduce air into the vagina, resulting in emboli. Other methods of introducing air into the vagina have resulted in documented cases of fatal air emboli in pregnant women.[7]

INTERCOURSE

Many couples and physicians in the past have believed that intercourse during pregnancy would harm the baby or the mother. Misconceptions such as this and ignorance about sex in general, and sex during pregnancy in particular, are still found today in this sexually open and permissive culture. At one time intercourse was prohibited for all 9 months of pregnancy or on the date of the expected period, but these beliefs have been shown to be without any factual foundations. Today the main restrictions that most physicians adhere to are no intercourse if the membranes are ruptured or if the patient is bleeding or threatening to abort. Patients with a history of repeated abortions may be advised to restrict intercourse during certain times of the pregnancy.

The openness of the physician and the nurse counseling the patient about sexual matters is clearly of the utmost importance. Patients may be reluctant to ask these rather personal questions unless the doctor- or nurse-patient relationship is good. If the nurse is a woman, she may be consulted for information because she may have had similar experiences. Because she will be utilized as a resource person, the nurse must take steps to prepare herself thoroughly for this role. Besides knowing the physiological and psychological aspects of sexuality, the nurse, if a woman, must also examine herself in regard to her own feelings in relation to pregnancy, sex, and her own femininity before she can successfully function as a resource person to others. If a man, the nurse must be able to empathize and establish a rapport with the pregnant woman he is counseling. Just as important is a good understanding of the physician's own philosophy about intercourse and his population of patients. Some doctors are restrictive during the last month and this of course is entirely based on the individuality of the patient and her pregnancy. Some patients also have a greater inherent risk of venereal disease and infection, and this group may be limited in the last month in contrast to those less vulnerable and better informed.

The nurse should be also aware of patients who are unable to communicate their questions, whether from embarrassment, ignorance, or cultural factors. Misinformation may promote silence or misunderstanding within the counseling situation. At some point it may become simply a volunteering of information in an interested, matter-of-fact, open-ended manner. Listening and reflecting within the conversation becomes essential. Encourage couples to communicate with each other about their feelings regarding their changing sexual relations. Then, hopefully, they will feel free to ask professional health personnel those questions they themselves cannot answer; this will help to clarify misconceptions and misunderstandings regarding intercourse.

Misunderstandings which have led to restriction of sexual activity during pregnancy include the following: pregnant women are uncomfortable and do not enjoy intercourse at this time; the membranes may rupture because of penile thrusts; an orgasm, which causes uterine contractions, might bring on early labor.

Some women have a decreased desire for intercourse during pregnancy. It may be uncomfortable, or it may be seen as unnecessary, since she is already pregnant. An unexplained aversion to her husband may occur and must be explained as a temporary idiosyncrasy accompanying the new condition of pregnancy. Many women for whom contraception was a hindrance find sex more enjoyable now, and their desires and responses may be heightened. This is especially true after the third month.

The membranes are so well protected by the cervix and mucus that they would be very difficult to rupture. Fear of infection caused by rupture of the membranes during intercourse is an old misconception. This concept dates back to the preantibiotic period in medicine and is largely negated today. Depending on the dilation of the cervix and the immediacy of delivery, the couple may be advised to restrict intercourse altogether or to restrict the depth of penetration.

Orgasm has not been definitively shown to bring on premature labor. Uterine contractions occur regardless of what causes the orgasm—masturbation or natural or artificial intercourse. Cases have been reported of labor onset immediately after orgasmic experience, however.

With conservative, traditional medical counseling, intercourse might formerly have been completely restricted for 4 to 6 weeks before birth and for

6 weeks postpartum; the couple would eventually resume sexual relations after a period of 3 months. Understandably, many couples did not adhere to this advice. Guilt feelings about this might lead to a subsequent lack of communications or problems with the marriage during pregnancy. Men often do not understand the prolonged period of restrictions and are not willing to endure this period of abstention; subsequently, some men look elsewhere for their sexual gratification.[8]

The couple's perception of their sexual relations plays a major part in the determination of their familial roles and subsequent sexual enjoyment. Men, as well as women, may experience lessening sexual drives during the third trimester. Pregnancy and childbirth also create emotional problems for the expectant father; some even experience symptoms of pregnancy along with their wife. Some men see pregnancy as a verification of their virility, and yet others see it as a test of their masculinity.

Women may equate the act of intercourse with an act of love, and during pregnancy intercourse may become a symbol of protection or of reaffirmation of her femininity or basic sexuality. This, of course, varies with every marriage and is dependent on such factors as age, marital status, culture, and basic feelings about this particular pregnancy. A woman may begin to look at her husband not only as a lover and provider, but also as the father of her child. Thus, new familial roles begin to be defined. The fact that the woman carries and nurses the child casts her into an essentially nurturing role and the man into a protective or supportive role. These roles, however, are changing and overlap to some extent within current cultural concepts.

Frequency of intercourse and positions are the decision of the couple, within the restrictions set by the physician. Frequency will change with the alteration in desire, and positions will have to be modified during the later part of pregnancy. In the last trimester, many women find it more comfortable astride the man or in a side-by-side position. Gentleness, use of lubricants if necessary, and avoidance of uncomfortable positions are to be endorsed. Mutual petting can be substituted during periods of forced abstinence. Couples should be cautioned, however, about unusual sexual activities that might be dangerous during the last weeks of pregnancy. There have been a few accidental deaths reported as a result of air emboli caused from precoital oral-genital contact.[8] Substitute sexual acts, if actual intercourse is prohibited, should be clearly specified.

SUMMARY

1 Work during pregnancy is medically acceptable within restrictions set by the obstetrician and the employer.
2 Exercise is permissible, but not to excess.
3 Sleep, rest, and relaxation are all very different concepts and may sometimes be seen as a medical necessity.

4 Travel, as well as all drugs and vaccinations, must be approved by the obstetrician.
5 Dental work is permitted with the joint cooperation of the dentist and the obstetrician.
6 X rays of pregnant women should be done only when necessary and then only with adequate shielding.
7 Cigarette smoking by the pregnant woman may be detrimental to the fetus.
8 Moderate drinking is acceptable if tolerated by the patient.
9 Tub baths are forbidden when membranes are ruptured, but there are no other restrictions on bathing.
10 Maternity clothes should be practical, attractive, and nonrestricting.
11 Douches are rarely needed and are permissible only upon advice of the physician.
12 Intercourse is a subject that should be individually considered for each patient within her medical and familial situation.

Not only is a thorough knowledge of the physiological and psychological aspects of pregnancy needed to counsel pregnant women about safety and activities during pregnancy, but also nurses must recognize their own feelings in regard to pregnancy, motherhood, sex, and femininity. Their role within the clinical setting is to augment the physician in his treatment and advice to individual patients.

REFERENCES

1 Guilbeau, J. A., and J. L. Turner: "Effect of Travel upon the Interruption of Pregnancy," *American Journal of Obstetrics and Gynecology*, 66:1224, 1953.
2 Crosby, W. M., and J. P. Costiloe: "Safety of Lap-belt Restraint for Pregnant Victims of Automobile Collisions," *New England Journal of Medicine*, 284:632–636, March 1971.
3 Drugs and Therapeutic Information, Inc.: "Safety of Immunizing Agents in Pregnancy," *Medical Letter on Drugs and Therapeutics*, vol. 12, no. 5 (issue 291), March 6, 1970.
4 Alk, Madelin (ed.): *Expectant Mother*, prepared in cooperation with the American College of Obstetricians and Gynecologists, Trident Press, New York, 1967.
5 United States Department of Health, Education and Welfare: *X-ray Examinations. . . . A Guide to Good Practice*, prepared in connection with the American College of Radiology, Maryland, 1971.
6 O'Lane, J. M.: "Some Fetal Effects of Maternal Cigarette Smoking," *Obstetrics and Gynecology*, 22:181–184, August 1963.

7 Aronson, M. E., and P. K. Newson: "Fatal Air Embolisms in Pregnancy Resulting from an Unusual Sex Act," *Obstetrics and Gynecology*, 31:127, July 1967.
8 Masters, W. H., and V. E. Johnson: *Human Sexual Response*, Little, Brown, Boston, 1966, chap. 10.

BIBLIOGRAPHY

Fitzpatrick, E., et al.: *Maternity Nursing*, 12th ed., Lippincott, Philadelphia, 1971.

Guttmacher, A. F.: *Pregnancy and Birth*, Viking Press, New York, 1962.

Hall, Robert E.: *Nine Months Reading: A Medical Guide for Pregnant Women*, rev. ed., Doubleday, New York, 1963.

Hellman, L. M., J. A. Pritchard, and R. M. Wynn: *Williams Obstetrics*, 14th ed., Appleton Century Crofts, New York, 1971.

Israel, S. L., and Isadore Rubin: *Sexual Relations during Pregnancy and Post-delivery Period*, Sex Information and Education Council of the United States, study guide no. 6, 1967.

Liley, H. M. I., with Beth Day: *Modern Motherhood: Pregnancy, Childbirth and the Newborn Baby*, Random House, New York, 1961.

Maternity Center Association: *Preparation for Childbearing*, 3d ed., Maternity Center Association, New York, 1971.

Montgomery, W. P., et al.: "The Tuberculin Test in Pregnancy," *American Journal of Obstetrics and Gynecology*, 100:829–831, March 15, 1968.

Peterson, W. F., et al.: "Smoking and Prematurity," *Obstetrics and Gynecology*, 26:775–779, December 1965.

Pugh, W. E., and F. L. Fernandez: "Coitus in Late Pregnancy," *Obstetrics and Gynecology*, 2:636, 1953.

Rubovits, F. E.: "Traumatic Rupture of the Pregnant Uterus from 'Seat Belt' Injury," *American Journal of Obstetrics and Gynecology*, 90:828–829, 1964.

Seacat, M., and L. Schlachter: "Expanded Nursing Role in Prenatal and Infant Care," *American Journal of Nursing*, 68:822–824, April 1968.

Zabriskie, J. R.: "Effect of Cigarette Smoking during Pregnancy," *Obstetrics and Gynecology*, 21:405, 1963.

20 | PREPARATION FOR CHILDBIRTH

Patricia A. Banasiak and Marya M. Corcoran

EVOLUTION OF CHILDBIRTH PROGRAMS

Historical Perspective

Everyone who comes to the experience of childbirth is prepared. The crux of the matter is whether the preparation is positive and realistic or negative and inaccurate. Preparation occurs throughout all life experiences and is influenced by family, church, school, and peer relationships. Without the word "childbirth" ever being used, a definite impression can be given to the young child whose mother says, "What I went through to have you, and look at what you're doing to me!" The nature of the preparation, then, becomes a primary concern for nursing, since it affects the entire maternity cycle. In order to assist patients in this endeavor, it is important to assess where we have been, determine where we are now, and map the course for future developments in the practice of childbirth education.

Prior to the 1900s, childbirth usually occurred at home. One need only recall an old movie or novel in which childbirth took place. The scene depicted was that of the laboring woman at home with the old family physician or midwife in attendance. If other children were present it was the husband's responsibility to keep them occupied. The father's paramount task, however, was to boil water in preparation for the birth. It should be noted that the quantity of water boiled far exceeded that which probably could be used. In any event, the entire family tended to be involved, in some way, with the arrival of the new baby.

Preparation for the new arrival, though probably not formally discussed in the family, took place nonetheless. The agrarian society, prior to this century, provided much of the sex education in its most natural settings. Since it was common to raise animals, even in the city, children learned about reproduction and birth as a normal, natural part of life. The knowledge acquired about animals was transferred to humans. Pain was experienced, but it was not the singular focal point during pregnancy, labor, and delivery.

The turn of the century brought many changes in childbirth practices. Concern over maternal and infant mortality rates grew, and hospitalization for childbirth became the trend. The advantages which were offered in the hospital were countered with several disadvantages. On one hand, a woman could expect to have her baby in an aseptic environment. In the efficient, sterile hospital, however, the father was recognized solely for his ability to provide transportation and to finance the event. He managed to bring his wife to the hospital at the onset of labor and returned 10 to 14 days later to pay the bill and take his family home. The woman shared her labor room with several other laboring women under the strict supervision of hospital personnel. From the moment of birth, the baby was whisked to the nursery to be cared for by efficient experts. The mother was completely removed from any involvement with her new baby, and only the more progressive hospitals allowed even a visiting period for the mother and her infant. The baby was cared for on a rigid schedule; and upon discharge from the hospital, the mother had little or no idea of who her baby was and what was involved in his care.

Hospitalization also offered the mother more analgesia and anesthesia than were practical at home. She was assured a comfortable, if not unconscious, labor. Regardless of her needs or wishes, she was medicated. In an attempt to make the experience a comfortable one for the patient, and a manageable one for the nurses, medications were given singly or in combination. The desired effects became complete unawareness of the discomfort and total amnesia about the event. With the woman completely medicated and safely attended by the nurses, the doctor could conduct his practice, to be summoned only at the time of delivery. And woe be to the nurse who did not get the doctor there in time!

The homecoming was another noteworthy event. The mother, father, and new baby were united after approximately 2 weeks of hospitalization. The mother and father had to reestablish their relationship, and the baby was a stranger to both of them.

Since the parturient woman was kept on complete bed rest for the duration of her hospitalization, she was naturally weak upon her return home.

Any children who were at home, as well as other young women in the family, learned through conversation and through their own observations that childbirth was incapacitating, if not painful.

Formalized preparation for childbirth was virtually nonexistent. Since the entire experience was managed for the woman, there was no need for her to have knowledge of anything aside from how to recognize the onset of labor. That preparation was frequently limited to the simple, but unsettling, statement, "You'll know."

A shortening of the hospital stay and an increase in the mother's involvement, at least in the feeding of the infant, occurred in the 1940s. It might be noted, however, that this trend evolved more from the hospital's need than from concern for family relationships. The increased birth rate and the decreased number of hospital personnel due to World War II made previous practices impractical.

During the 1950s the father was once again recognized as a member of the family. The demands of fathers returning from the war, as well as changes in medical and nursing education, fostered his inclusion during the hospital stay. The father became a more familiar sight at the bedside of the laboring woman. Unprepared as he might be, the frightened father stood there bravely.

Today's practices are influenced by historical developments. Although 90 percent of all births presently take place in the hospital, several factors may create a return to planned childbirth at home. Among these factors are the skyrocketing cost of hospitalization, the desire of couples to avoid the mechanized, unnatural hospital setting, and the evolution of different family structures with a greater emphasis upon shared experiences. In addition, the couple who plans for childbirth at home retains some measure of control over this significant event.

SELECTED CHILDBIRTH PRACTICES

It is impossible to deal with the subject of preparation for labor and delivery without some mention of pain, since this is the general expectation of the childbirth experience. Reduction or elimination of the discomfort has been a vital component of obstetrical management and, thus, the focus of programs of preparation. A thorough understanding of the variability of pain response is necessary for cogent guidance and support of those involved in childbearing. The subject of pain can consume an entire book and more, but the important point to emphasize is the complexity and the individuality of response to pain. Numerous studies over the years have only served to underline the complexity of pain. It is clear that there is a physical stimulus and a psychic modification and that multiple factors influence both aspects in any given person. Since there are no universal characteristics which define pain, there can be no set prescription for a means of pain relief. In its complex nature, one finds the reason for the wide variety of means employed to alleviate the pain of childbirth.

Pharmacological Intervention

As hospitalization for childbirth became the rule rather than the exception, women began to rely heavily on analgesia. The concern of practitioners to combat the discomforts of childbirth went hand in hand with the rapid development of pharmacological agents. Hospitalization, with its concomitant equipment and trained personnel, provided the environment conducive to a pharmacological approach. Large doses of depressant and amnesic drugs were administered to the patient, and unconscious labor became the trend. The most popular physican was one who would guarantee that his patients would not experience any pain in labor.

In addition to medication for labor, a general inhalation anesthetic was frequently administered for delivery. It was discovered, however, that the chemical agents utilized passed into fetal circulation with deleterious effects to the infant. Both the type of agent and the large amounts used contributed to the high perinatal morbidity and mortality rates. As concern for maternal and infant well-being grew, techniques were developed aimed at the reduction of pharmacological intervention which might be harmful. As so often is the case, the pendulum swung, the trend took a complete reversal, and one fear replaced another. Rather than a fear that drugs might be withheld, women now feared that drugs would be administered which would endanger their babies. For some women, all energies were directed toward achieving that state of physical and/or psychological preparation which would eliminate any need for medicinal relief.

The Read Method

Dr. Grantly Dick-Read was responsible for the original natural childbirth movement in England. The basis of this program was that childbirth was a normal physiological occurrence and as such should not be painful. Dr. Dick-Read believed that the experienced pain of labor and delivery was mental in origin. He attributed the cause of pain to culturally induced fear and anxiety. His writings, and the writings of both those who supported him and those who denigrated him, demonstrate that he had a persuasive personality. Dr. Dick-Read, who was described as an evangelistic crusader for his program, utilized every conceivable means of publicizing his beliefs. He widely incorporated emotional and sentimental phraseology which added to the impact of his pronouncements. The basic premise of the Read method, introduced to the United States by Dr. Thoms of Yale, centered around the triad of fear-tension-pain. The belief was that fear of labor and delivery was a learned response. This fear created tension and was responsible for the pain which occurred. Dr. Dick-Read's program, and the publicity which it received, co-incided with other circumstances. The concern of physicians for the welfare of women and their unborn babies and the genuine desire of women to be more involved in the birth process contributed to the spread of this program. Utilizing the premise of fear-tension-pain, the Read method attempted to break up this syndrome through education, psychological training, and physical conditioning.

The physical exercise component of the Read method was largely due to the work of Helen Heardman, a physiotherapist in England, who strongly supported Dr. Dick-Read's contentions. She believed, as he did, in the necessity of a healthy, positive mental attitude in the prospective mother. In addition, she advocated a vigorous program of physical education in preparation for parturition. Thus, through the combined efforts of Dr. Dick-Read and Mrs. Heardman, education, psychological training, and physical exercise to enhance relaxation comprised the original natural childbirth program.

Education was aimed at preparing prospective parents thoroughly in the anatomy, physiology, and process of pregnancy, labor, and delivery. Along with presentation and discussion of factual material, the Read approach included demonstration and practice of exercises to foster relaxation and to condition muscles involved in the birth process. Another component part of the Read method was the group process. Emphasis was placed upon deriving support from other group members as an inherent part of the program.

Read technique exercises were intended to prepare a woman physically for the muscular work of labor. They were designed to increase the elasticity of perineal muscles, to exercise the pelvis and back, and to foster the general improvement of circulation in the pelvic region. Among the exercises included to fulfill these objectives were tailor-sitting, squatting, kneeling, and pelvic rocking. Some authorities believed, however, that exercises which involved the pelvic girdle might damage the symphysis and lumbosacral joints.

Breathing exercises in the Read methodology included slow abdominal breathing, diaphragmatic breathing, and panting. Slow abdominal breathing was used primarily for the first stage of labor. This technique was aimed at raising the abdominal wall off the contracting uterus. Its purposes were to reduce the discomfort created by opposing forces and to promote general relaxation. Diaphragmatic breathing, to expand the ribs sideways, was said to enhance comfort in late active labor prior to pushing. Panting was included in the breathing techniques to avoid a forceful, rapid expulsion of the infant. Read proponents cautioned against excessive use of panting, since it might lead to hyperventilation and its resultant problems.

The nurse's role with Read preparation was one of teacher, demonstrator, and coach. With medical guidance and approval, the general format and guidelines for the program were established, and the nurse generally was responsible for implementing the program. Classes were geared to the presentation and discussion of factual components, and a period was allotted for demonstration and practice of the exercises. The nurse became vital as a coach—encouraging, explaining, and restating goals throughout the program. Attempts were made to carry through this same role once labor began, either by the same nurse or by other nurses equally grounded in the theoretical and technical aspects. Obvious areas of difficulty arose. An uninformed practitioner, or one who did not share an attitude of value in the approach, might fail to continue the support and guidance in the manner familiar to the patient. An overly enthusiastic nurse might become so involved in the goal of successful achievement that she might fail to correctly assess the patient's status. The nurse might also fail to utilize any measures other than that of cheering the patient on. Another problem lay in the consistency of the support. It was generally agreed that consistent sustainment in labor enhanced the patient's ability to progress more positively. With hospital personnel traditionally working a scheduled shift and the unpredictability of either the onset or the termination of labor, many contacts with multiple approaches might occur throughout the course of one labor.

However, aspects of the Read approach could be readily instituted with patients in labor who had never been instructed in the techniques and who did not need to have the techniques labeled as such. Relaxation positions and slow abdominal breathing assisted patients in reducing tension. This created a quieting approach which generally enhanced patient comfort.

Dr. Dick-Read's philosophy and approach were both stoutly defended and soundly denounced. In general, the strongest resistance arose from the all-or-none attitude engendered by the proponents of natural childbirth. For women who viewed training for childbirth as the panacea, disappointments stemmed from several sources. Women might need medication for parts of their labor, but since they were not prepared for this, they considered either the program or themselves worthless because neither had achieved their aims. Many a skeptical doctor allowed his patient to prepare for natural childbirth, only to follow his own practiced regimen of medication once the patient was hospitalized. Practitioners who were the strongest proponents of the Read method often withheld medication when it was not only necessary but crucial for the patient.

Although Dr. Dick-Read never proposed that analgesics or anesthetics be withheld, an attitude prevailed that to utilize such assistance was the ultimate failure of a woman in her most supreme achievement. Dr. Dick-Read repeatedly stated that medicinal support could be utilized, but the focus of his approach and the words which he used gave quite another message. Repeatedly in his own writings appear such phrases as "ability to endure" and "artificial aids." This terminology conveyed very clearly that such assistance should not be needed, and thus many would not dare to request medication.

Another facet of the all-or-none approach was the belief that any patient was suited to this technique, regardless of her physical or psychological constitution. Some women selected this means because it was the thing to do rather than because they believed it to be either necessary or rewarding. Little emphasis was given to the disadvantages or the need for alternatives, and as a result, many physical and psychological traumas were attributed to natural childbirth.

A report by Dr. Paul A. Bowers revealed that the women who availed themselves of the Read technique could generally be categorized into four groups. A large group appeared to be medically allied in some way. A second group perceived natural childbirth as a superior intellectual activity. The other two groups included women whose friends wholeheartedly recommended the approach and those with borderline or actual mental illness who viewed natural childbirth as a form of therapy.[1]

In the first group (those with some health orientation), many understood the program thoroughly, accepted it for themselves, and demonstrated a high rate of success. There were also, however, those with this orientation who suffered through it silently with what appeared to be success but only because they believed this behavior was expected of them. Another aspect is illustrated in the following example:

At a time when the Read method was highly favored in a given hospital, a clinical psychologist encouraged his wife to utilize this method. They arrived at the hospital to share the labor experience. What truly was shared, however, was in doubt. He was extremely enthusiastic about the classes, the exercises, and the labor. She said little, but when she experienced a mild contraction, she appeared tense and clenched her fists. For a while she attempted to smile and to show enthusiasm. Before labor progressed very far, however, she dissolved into tears with complete loss of control. She begged not to have "to go through with it." Her husband apologized to the hospital staff for his wife's failure. He was utterly dejected when his wife was heavily medicated and he was asked to leave the labor room. His wife was greatly relieved to receive medication for labor and general anesthetics for delivery. Later, she was extremely upset, because she knew she had disappointed her husband.

In the group of those who chose natural childbirth, there were those who actively engaged in preparation and who achieved their goals successfully. There were also those who believed that it was easy to perform in the prescribed manner with little or no preparation. Unfortunately, this group did not always meet their goal, which resulted in feelings of failure and/or guilt.

In the group which selected this method by endorsement, success was more likely if they grew to accept the method for themselves. Many who began the program because of another's endorsement failed to complete the program of preparation.

In the group of women with borderline or actual mental illness were those with perhaps the greatest liability in accepting this approach. Their reasons for selection were complex or negative, and for many, irreparable scars occurred. One example was the type of woman who utilized this approach to punish herself or to punish her husband. His *expected* presence precluded any relief from witnessing his mate's "suffering."

In general, it might be said that the highest predictor of successful achievement lay in the woman's motivation for selection of this technique. The woman who chose the Read method and who believed in its appropriateness for *herself* was far more likely to achieve its goals.

Regardless of which aspects of the Read method remain valid, acceptable, or usable, Dr. Dick-Read must be recognized as a pioneer in the movement for preparation for childbirth. Conscious, cooperative labor and family involvement have many of their roots in the Read method, and Dick-Read established the mental component of childbirth. This awakened many practitioners to the need for incorporation of psychological aspects into a responsible, safe, therapeutic practice of obstetrics.

The Psychoprophylactic Method*

The terms psychoprophylaxis and Lamaze are often used interchangeably to describe a method of childbirth preparation based on Pavlov's principle of conditioned reflex training. Psychoprophylaxis, which means mind prevention, is the more precise term; Lamaze, however, being an easier word to pronounce, is used more frequently.

Psychoprophylaxis was developed by Russian scientists who were interested in achieving childbirth without pain. These scientists postulated that through stimulus-response conditioning during pregnancy women could learn specific behaviors (controlled breathing and active relaxation) which they would automatically use during labor and delivery to eliminate the pain associated with childbirth. The method was practiced with great success in Russia and through the efforts of Dr. Fernand Lamaze became equally popular in France. Dr. Lamaze, a Paris obstetrician, became acquainted with the method while attending an obstetric conference in Russia. He and his associates modified the original method by adding a rapid, shallow type of breathing. This particular type of breathing has received strong criticism because it often results in hyperventilation which can cause problems for both mother and baby.

The method spread quickly throughout many European countries and stimulated much scientific research. In the United States, psychoprophylaxis gathered a following through the appeal of Marjorie Karmel's book, *Thank You, Dr. Lamaze*, which was published in the early 1950s. The method also encountered strong opposition in the United States from medically trained people largely on the grounds that it advocated painless childbirth. The concept of painless childbirth was not consistent with empirical observation.

* This section was prepared by Rose S. LeRoux.

Studies by anthropologists have shown that in all cultures in all parts of the world, women may experience pain during childbirth. The study of pain is complex; little is precisely understood about pain perception and pain thresholds among individuals. Due to the complexity of pain phenomena and to the abundance of pharmacological agents available for the relief of childbirth pain in the United States, it was thought unnecessary to condition women to have babies. The strong resistance to the Lamaze method itself and the people who tried to proselytize it in the United States may have been partially a product of American cultural orientation. Some members of the health professions viewed suspiciously women who chose to employ one of the "natural childbirth" methods because often they refused analgesics or anesthetics. They were suspected of being martyrs who were so committed to the method that they would suffer needlessly and unknowingly jeopardize safe obstetric care. Their personality characteristics were frequently scrutinized. The concept of suffering or sacrificing for an important goal may have been foreign to the thinking of an American "drug-oriented" society in which pain or emotional discomfort was readily relieved by medication. Little attention was given to other possible ways of relieving discomfort and enhancing awareness experiences. The Lamaze patient was well educated as to what to expect during labor and delivery and insisted on the type of care she wanted. This also may have had an unsettling effect on medical personnel.

In spite of resistance, the movement continued to grow. In 1960, interested physicians, nurses, physical therapists, and parents formed a nonprofit organization to further the goals of the psychoprophylactic method of preparation for childbirth during the antepartal and labor and delivery periods. The organization was called the American Society for Psychoprophylaxis in Obstetrics (ASPO) and presently has member chapters throughout the United States. The growth of the method is partly due to the satisfaction of the women who have had babies by the Lamaze method and to their zeal to have other women learn about it; it is also due to the support and leadership provided by interested professionals.

Although psychoprophylaxis has been modified throughout the years, the basic concepts of the method remain the same: *education* and *training*. The educational component of the program includes learning about childbirth. This portion generally includes content on the anatomy and physiology of the reproductive system and extensive study of the labor and delivery process. Effort is made to replace misinformation and superstition with valid scientific information. The training part of the program consists principally of learning controlled breathing and neuromuscular exercises. The pregnant woman is taught that instead of responding to a contraction by becoming tense and rigid, she must deliberately decontract (relax) her muscles. At the same time she must institute a series of breathing patterns according to the phase of labor she is in; she utilizes a different type of breathing during the effacement, dilatation, transition, and expulsion phases. Because the training sessions must take place during pregnancy, the patient practices responding to an imagined stimulus (uterine contraction). The patient simulates a uterine contraction by contracting an arm or leg muscle while simultaneously relaxing other muscles. The conditioner informs her as to what phase of labor she is in and she practices the controlled breathing she has been taught. The patient learns exactly what to expect at every step during labor and delivery and precisely what her role is. There is some question about how much actual conditioning takes place in the absence of direct stimuli (uterine contractions). Contracting the muscle of an arm or leg can hardly give the uninitiated primigravida an idea of the true intensity of a uterine contraction. The total length of labor is stressed and the patient becomes more realistic as to the amount of time involved in the process of having a baby.

The patient's husband is included in the classes. If there is no husband or if he is not presently available, a family member, a friend, or a nurse may be taught how to coach the patient through labor and delivery. The monitor is taught to remind the patient to breathe properly and to decontract her muscles. The monitor provides comfort measures such as wiping the patient's face with a cold cloth, offering ice chips, changing the patient's position, and massaging the patient's back with a light fingertip massage called effleurage. The patient receives positive reinforcement during labor that she is doing well. A physician usually presents a class on the possible complications that may occur during labor and delivery and how they are managed. The physician also discusses what types of analgesics and anesthetics he may use.

In the United States, the concept of "painless childbirth" has gradually given way to the concept of "education for childbirth." Empirical evidence has demonstrated that some women have easy labors and some women do not. Patients learn that having a baby is not like entering a contest in which one succeeds or fails. They are taught that analgesics and anesthetics are administered when necessary according to their individual needs and the discretion of their obstetrician. Although some studies indicate that women trained by the Lamaze method require less medication during childbirth, there is much controversy concerning the physiological mechanism by which the method reduces the perception of pain. Apparently the element of distraction plays an important part. It has long been observed that people intensely absorbed in activity are less sensitive to painful stimuli. It has been postulated that when many stimuli are sent to the cerebral cortex, the cortex will respond only to the strongest stimuli. Therefore, if during a uterine contraction a series of activities are carried out which require the complete attention of the patient, the perception of the contraction as a "pain" will be diminished. Adherents of the Lamaze method seem to refer more to the satisfaction they have experienced during childbirth than to the presence or absence of pain.

The method has become very popular with the well-educated population. Educated people are oriented toward taking classes, and it may seem natural o them to "learn" how to have a baby. They have had some control over events in their lives, and this method teaches them how to "stay in control." The fact that the husband is included in the preparation and has a definite role appeals to those couples who wish to share in a meaningful way their preparation for parenthood. Very little is known regarding the use of the method with people in lower socioeconomic groups.

It is the patient's prerogative to select the method of childbirth preparation which most appeals to her. The Lamaze method will appeal to some people, while hypnosis or some other procedure will appeal to others. The nurse can enable the patient to select a way of childbirth most appropriate for her by informing the patient of methods available and by careful counseling.

Hypnosis

Hypnosis is one of the oldest techniques known to the medical world. Its origins were in the spiritual realm where it was the province of the temple priests and mystics to employ hypnotic techniques. Within the health care system, it has been considered both beneficial and inappropriate, sometimes simultaneously.

Authoritative sources clearly demonstrate that hypnosis is a powerful and effective anesthetic agent. There have been repeated demonstrations of its use in obstetrics.

Certain obvious advantages exist with hypnosis. For any patient with a pathological condition which contraindicates the use of pharmacological agents, hypnosis can be utilized to provide a comfortable, controlled labor and delivery. It can also be a useful tool for the upset or disturbed patient. When hypnosis is not completely effective, only minimal analgesia or anesthesia is generally required.

Hypnosis requires skilled application and judicious use. In some settings where hypnosis is utilized, no interaction or noise of any kind is permitted. Many authorities agree, however, that the approach to the hypnotized patient in labor is one of quiet, unstartling commands and reassurance. This approach will enhance, not disrupt, the hypnotic state.

All patients are not suited to the technique of hypnosis, and there are obvious dangers if it is used indiscriminantly. One such danger, mentioned repeatedly, is that by removing the ability to perceive pain one removes a first-line defense mechanism of the body. The description of pain perceived by the patient can be a valuable diagnostic aid. Pain is often the signal of impending danger, such as in the instance of uterine rupture. Another frequently voiced objection to the use of hypnosis is the time requirement. Hypnosis requires training for the practitioner and is time-consuming for both the practitioner and the patient in the conditioning phase. Another challenge to its obstetric use is that although the patient is not under pharmacological influence, she may remain unaware of and be a nonparticipant in her labor and delivery. Proponents of the use of hypnosis point to the possibility of producing a state of waking hypnosis in which the patient is able to converse, interact, follow instructions, and participate with awareness in her own labor and delivery.

Hypnosis and the Read technique are intertwined in almost all of the literature. Dr. Dick-Read repeatedly denied that his method was hypnosis because a friend of his who was a hypnotist said it was not. Most authorities, however, maintain that the Read method is a form of hypnosis in that it utilizes the same basic approach and techniques. Dr. Dick-Read himself referred to some of his patients as being in a "trance from the beginning of their labor until the end." Other observers maintain that any of the psychophysical methods for relief of childbirth pain are in fact hypnosis. They cite the quiet, repetitive pronouncements to patients that their labor is not painful and that they are doing well as examples. According to them, this approach has a hypnotic effect upon the patient. Buxton carefully distinguishes between hypnosis, which artificially produces sleep, and "hypnotic effect" whereby a person may be profoundly affected although he is not asleep.[2] Some have always considered hypnosis quackery and therefore unsound for use in medicine. It is, however, regaining its popularity and is worthy of consideration.

PREPARATION FOR CHILDBIRTH TODAY

Factors Influencing Preparation

In recent years, there has been a steady increase in the number of formal programs to prepare parents for the childbirth experience. It is noteworthy that the growth of programs has been largely due to their acceptance by the public. Although many professionals currently attest to the necessity and value of such preparation programs, resistance to this movement remains observable. Many who deal with prospective parents demonstrate their disapproval of the involved, knowledgeable parent who intends to participate in the childbearing experience. There are many reasons for such attitudes among doctors and nurses alike. Often, professional practitioners believe that by virtue of their education and experience, they are more qualified to select what is best for the patient, including how she should bear her babies. It would appear that patient involvement represents a threat to some egos, and many who resist the movement feel that they are being asked to surrender their professional control. For some practitioners, it is more convenient for parents not to be concerned with details of process and care. The "I'll handle everything for you" approach often demonstrates that it is easier for the practitioner not to be bothered by questions and explanations. A third attitude is reflected by professionals whose experiences and education engender other beliefs. Their statements, such as "Why should a woman suffer to bear her child?" and "Why should any man want to witness his partner's pain and suffering?" are the antithesis of the philosophy held by parents who desire understanding of and participation in their childbirth experience.

Advances in professional education have fostered inclusion of parents in more of the activities surrounding childbirth. Prospective parents frequently attend the physician's office together, and even in the clinic setting it is more usual to see parents together for regular antenatal visits. Parents are being referred to existent childbirth education classes offered in the community, and it is increasingly common for hospitals to offer programs of antenatal education. Many private doctors have begun to provide programs of preparation for childbirth, usually under the guidance of the office nurse or nurse associate.

The influence of the mass media has been great and has stimulated the public's demand for increased preparation. Lay publications, movies, and television have presented their own, often one-sided and biased, views. An avalanche of popularly consumed articles offer simplified and glorified approaches to childbirth. Through communication media, false interpretations and misconceptions may arise. The overzealous endorsement of some professional practitioners also contributes to misnomers and misconceptions. These misunderstandings in many instances only serve to do more harm than good to the general premise of prepared childbirth.

Peer influence cannot be minimized. It is often observed that a close friend's or a neighbor's experience is given more credence than the explanations offered by professionals. Even a very positive recital of the wonders of the childbirth experience can be very detrimental. When the listener only hears the end result, with no assessment of the reality of such an approach for her, her experience frequently bears no resemblance to what she had expected.

Two of the familiar approaches, namely Read and Lamaze, acquired the titles of natural childbirth and painless childbirth, respectively. Inherent in the terminology "natural childbirth" is the idea that any medicinal or mechanical assistance defeats the naturalness of the event. If the goal of unassisted labor and delivery is not met, extreme frustration is likely. Resistance to appropriate medical intervention jeopardizes maternal and fetal welfare. "Childbirth without pain," on the other hand, conveys the impression that a certain practiced regimen abolishes the discomforts associated with childbirth. This descriptive, simplified terminology, applied to each program, often defeats preparedness for the realities of labor and delivery.

Whether programs had their origin in professional practice or in popular demand, all programs directed toward preparation for childbirth share similar goals or ideals. Essentially, these programs are aimed at reducing the amount of drugs needed and increasing the satisfaction of participants.

Current Practices

Purists in a given approach still exist within professional ranks. Many preparation programs are practiced as they were originally developed. Today's approach, however, is moving away from rigid adherence to a given technique. Programs sponsored by educational institutions, public health agencies, and hospitals are more likely to be representative of a combination of techniques tailored for the needs of those enrolled.

The objective of increasing satisfaction is now being met by judicious combinations of techniques and pharmacological agents, rather than by the ability to tolerate labor and delivery by technique alone. Adherence to the belief that ultimate femininity lies in an unmedicated labor and delivery has given way to goal achievement through more realistic and appropriate means. The administration of analgesics and anesthetics need not negate the achievement of conscious, cooperative childbirth. Regardless of the technique utilized, all authorities agree on the value of education to reduce anxiety and to enhance involvement in the childbirth experience.

Education to eradicate needless or unfounded fears is certainly valid. Programs of preparation attempt to provide knowledge and understanding in a realistic, factual way. In addition to facts, most preparation programs include exercises to achieve physical or psychological conditioning. No single rationale or purpose exists for the exercise component in childbirth education. All psychophysical programs include these techniques, and claims have been made that exercises shorten labor, reduce pain, and avoid complications. Although no such obstetric effectiveness has been proven, authorities do agree that exercise contributes to general physical and mental health. Some women state, however, that the sole value of the exercises for them was one of distraction.

Relaxation techniques are frequently utilized as supportive measures with the patient in labor. Posture and positioning are vital to both comfort and relaxation, since they reduce the stress and strain on muscles. The ability to control breathing can enhance relaxation or may simply provide distraction.

Anticipation of pain heightens anxiety. Anxiety intensifies pain perception. The terminology which is utilized when a person is under stress can contribute to heightening or lessening this stress. An expectation can be created through word selection. Thus, avoidance of repeated reference to pain and the utilization of less charged words is likely to evoke a positive, relaxed response. Terminology selection is also vital in the collection of accurate data. Asking the patient to describe what she feels is more likely to elicit her perception of sensations than asking her, "How often are your pains?" or "Are you in pain?" The number of women who deny that contractions are painful is noteworthy, but they do admit that the accompanying sensations such as backache, tingling, pressure in the groin and vagina, and radiating sensations along the thigh do give rise to their discomfort in labor.

Each individual and each couple come to the experience of childbirth with unique and complex backgrounds. All have differing expectations, fears, and states of preparedness. Regardless of the approach or means of preparation, the primary goal remains one of a safe outcome for the parents and the baby. The ultimate goal is to accomplish satisfaction with dignity. Achievement of this goal is enhanced by a knowledgeable nurse who is sensitive to the needs of others. Sensitivity necessitates self-awareness and an honest recognition of the impact of attitudes and values upon others.

The following examples illustrate divergent patient and personnel expectations:

A young husband was with his wife during her labor with their second child. No visible expressions of discomfort were observed in the wife, and by all measurements she was well established in active labor with frequent moderate to firm contractions. The husband did not fit the expected pattern of a supporting, backrubbing, coaching helpmate, but rather appeared to agitate consistently and "pick an argument" with his wife. A continuous bantering, bickering interaction was noted. A nurse who was well schooled in the Read technique was concerned about what she perceived to be lack of husbandly support. She encouraged the husband to leave his wife and go to supper. The nurse failed to note that there had been no hostility or anger observed in the couple's interaction. The wife was quite active in joining, and at times initiating, the interchange. Within minutes of the husband's departure, the wife became restless, grimaced and stated, "Oh, the contractions are much stronger now." The labor pattern was unchanged, but her perception was different. Apparently, a familiar pattern of behavior had been utilized successfully for those involved. It was disallowed because of the nurse's perceptions and expectations.

A nurse related the story of how change in approach affected her own labor awareness and behavior. Admitted in labor to a busy unit at a time when most of the patients were heavily medicated, she met a great deal of resistance and intolerance to her "natural childbirth" ideas. She was highly motivated to participate in the birth of her baby and well educated in the theory and techniques. She described her first hours of labor as hours spent busily defending her right to her own means. There were hours of continuous battle with an unkind, rough resident who considered her to be quite "nuts." She has little recall of this part of her labor. She stated that she was too busy fighting and being angry to be physically uncomfortable. At the time a different resident came on duty, she was amazed and thrilled to find a compassionate, supportive person. He demonstrated the approach which she believed to be important for success. Almost immediately, she became extremely uncomfortable and perceived her labor as quite painful. In this instance, apparently the distraction of the battle and the sudden change in approach had unpredicted effects.

An appropriate and meaningful childbirth experience is one which considers the needs, desires, and capabilities of a given family unit. The family-centered approach has been developed in an attempt to meet these needs. "Family-centered" is often interpreted to mean a shared labor and delivery experience, rooming-in, and breast-feeding as a natural follow-up. While it is true that these experiences are very often related and extremely rewarding for some parents, it is appalling to see that this is the only interpretation of a family-centered experience. Focus on familial needs recognizes that each family unit may "share" in different ways. When agreed upon mutually, selected experiences can be more rewarding than the total package. Insistence upon a prescribed set of activities denies the family's right to determine what is meaningful to them. Too often, under the guise of family-centered, a hospital really provides a staff-centered program. It is based upon their beliefs and facilities with little or no deviation from a stated program permitted.

Much emphasis is given to preparing a family unit for the birth experience of their first child. It may have many ramifications which influence future experiences. However, more intensive preparation is often necessary for the multiparous family, since the strongest influence on attitudes and beliefs is the previous childbirth experience. If this experience was difficult or frightening, positive attitudes will be more difficult to achieve than with a family in which no such sensitization has occurred.

Assessment of the individual or group to be prepared is vital in planning and implementing any program or technique. Perusal of a program, however, frequently demonstrates that it is based upon practitioner beliefs with little or no regard for the needs of the participant. It is true, of course, that the learner does not always know what he needs to know. It is also true, however, that he cannot and will not learn until his initial needs are met. "The primary purpose of education is not reassurance, but honest recognition of anxiety and examination of the realities on which it is based."[3]

An increasingly larger segment of the childbearing public demands education. The age of ignorance and alienation is being replaced by the era of personalization and involvement. Mass means of care for patients in labor are giving way to more personalized and individualized approaches. Large labor rooms are being modified to hold one or two laboring women. Provision for fathers as an integral part of the team of attendants is a more accepted practice. The hospital is coming to realize its responsibility to provide safe, humane, personalized care.

What the hospital has yet to do is to assume responsibility for more far-reaching, inclusive parent education. This is demonstrated in the adherence to preparation for childbearing to the exclusion of childrearing. Preparation for parenthood is not totally the hospital's province; however, there are those aspects which are appropriately the hospital's responsibility.

Programs aimed at preparation have grown over the years. Programs of education which encompass all aspects of family life are beginning to evolve.

Implications for Other Preparation Programs

The sensible approach to preparation for childbirth is that which concerns itself with the attitudes, values, and beliefs of the participants. It attempts to allay unrealistic fears, to provide means of coping with unavoidable fears and stress, and to promote selection of techniques which best meet the needs of each individual and family group.

Obviously, preparation is most effective if it occurs throughout one's life. Our ultimate aim is to increase its consistency and accuracy which would foster its occurrence as a normal part of life. This type of preparation would bring any participant to the actual reality of pregnancy with basic, factual knowledge and healthier, more positive attitudes. Even with improved preparation, fear and misconceptions may continue to create problems. With this background, however, the realities and the specifics relative to the problem could be handled more easily and quickly. If all who are now involved in childbirth were adequately prepared, there would be fewer fantasies and misconceptions in the succeeding generation. The point here is not to devalue programs of preparation, but rather to emphasize the need for utilizing knowledge and techniques toward the most satisfying experience possible within the therapeutic milieu of each patient.

We are, however, a long way from that point. Many people have not benefited from explanations and education which could have enhanced their childbirth experience, regardless of the approach. When we begin to appraise the needs of patients and their families more honestly, we will begin to identify what constitutes minimally adequate, if not totally satisfying preparation. In order to satisfy the needs of patients primarily and professional practitioners secondarily, we must begin to look at who is involved in programs of preparation.

Programs for prepared childbirth have historically been structured for the typical married couple. Repeated references to "husband" and "wife" cement this impression. Although partners were involved in creating the child, for a variety of reasons there may be no future involvement of the male. Yet absence of the male because of death, separation, or disinterest frequently provides the reason for a woman's exclusion from some programs. The usual rationalization is that it would be uncomfortable for *her*. Must the presence of a husband be the ticket of entry into these programs? Whose comfort are we *really* considering? Since single parenthood may give rise to problems, is this not all the more reason for professional assistance? Emphasis needs to be placed on the fact that absence of marriage or of a partner need not exclude the patient from such programs.

We have begun to include husbands in the activities related to childbirth. We are much slower to include *fathers,* as opposed to husbands, and are particularly resistant to the inclusion of significant others who fit neither the husband nor the father category. It may be a male friend, father, mother, aunt, or other close friend whose role interaction with the pregnant woman is most significant. If this relationship is one which provides support in times of stress and crisis, does it not follow that presence or involvement at the time of labor and delivery might be not only permissible but beneficial? If so, then to increase the value of this interaction, the significant other(s) may need to be part of the preparation. All contacts of a patient need not move into the hospital setting with the parturient woman, but again, assessment of a given situation provides the basis for evaluating what is shared by whom.

If preparation is to be meaningful for parents, it appears logical that professional practitioners and parents need to work together in formulating and implementing a practical, rewarding experience. Establishing an appropriate approach includes the citation of possible alternatives which may be accepted by either patient or practitioner requirements. Thus, the elements of defeat inherent in the failure to meet a prescribed regimen are less likely to occur. In this way, ultimate professional responsibility for the safety and welfare of those concerned is in no way jeopardized. Most patients are relieved to have realistic, safe decisions made for them. Difficulties arise when no rationale is given for decisions and all rights in the decision-making process are denied the patient.

Prior to the fact of a given experience, it seems irrational and dangerous to espouse an approach that will require *no* adaptation. Each individual who arrives at the time of childbirth is unique. So, too, is each program or technique of prepared childbirth a unique entity with its own strengths and weaknesses. Thus, it is impossible to dictate one means of preparing for childbirth.

The very nature of pregnancy can be a predictor of readiness to learn. Thus, the timing and sequence of content will influence the effectiveness of learning. Thorough understanding of the physical and psychological aspects can increase awareness of when critical issues are likely to emerge. According to Reva Rubin,

> There is indeed a cognitive style in pregnancy, one of inconclusive questioning and uncertainty. Two sets of questions and an underlying sense of uncertainty alternate during the course of the pregnancy to effect, in harmony with the biological changes, progressive developmental stages of pregnancy.
> One set of questions is concerned with time within the life space, the

other with a personal sense of identity. Both sets of questions are salient to a sense of feminine identity.[4]

Early in pregnancy, the physiological changes which create gastrointestinal problems and fatigue, accompanied by the disquieting thought of pregnancy as a fact, hardly provide the impetus to become prepared for labor and delivery. At this time, efforts are most appropriately geared toward assisting resolution of the *reality* of the pregnancy.

In the second trimester, when physical symptoms are usually not problematic, there is a general sense of well-being. This period affords an opportunity to begin to deal with the realities of pregnancy. Now the focus is upon impending role change for the parents, and plans for the event of childbirth begin. If diapering or bathing an infant is a learning activity, it serves as a vehicle for trying on this impending role. This is a valuable tool in assisting role transition, but it should not be confused with the belief that learning to handle, bathe, and diaper an infant has been achieved. This learning can only occur when their infant is a reality. Thus, it belongs properly with activities aimed at establishing parent-infant relationships in the postpartum period.

The third trimester of pregnancy generally brings a return of discomforts, a sense of physical and emotional burden, and a more introspective manner. Educational and supportive techniques now can be directed toward expression of the impatience and fears. These can assist the identification of appropriate coping means. The aim here, late in pregnancy, is to assist the family in garnering reserves which will enable them to tolerate the threats of labor and delivery.

Preparation for childbirth can foster internalization of the impending occurrence with acceptance of its realities. Through a learning experience which increases problem-solving skill, participants can come to trust in their own ability and cope with both the predictable and unpredictable aspects of childbirth. Trust in oneself fosters trust in others involved and in the interventions which may become necessary in a particular situation.

The selection of appropriate resources by each person is to be applauded in the quest for prepared childbirth. Patients and practitioners respect each other's rights and responsibilities through prior awareness and knowledge of what those rights and responsibilities entail. An adequately prepared patient arrives at the time of labor and delivery with a sense of dignity and control which is usually maintained regardless of unforseeable events.

FUTURE PROGRAMS IN CHILDBIRTH PREPARATION

One of the best opportunities for preventive medicine is in the field of obstetrics. Antenatal care has long demonstrated its effectiveness in reducing perinatal mortality. Thus, it is conceivable that through a program of *preven-*

tion rather than intervention, the crisis of childbirth might be reduced or perhaps eliminated.

Within the childbirth experience lies an excellent opportunity to demonstrate continuity of care and comprehensive services. There can be no doubt that assisting families, of whatever constitution, ultimately affects society at large. It is long overdue that we of the profession assume more leadership in the preventive aspects which we know are possible.

Too often we discharge our responsibilities to parents with a miniature course in labor and delivery and the traditional baby bath. Our larger responsibility is the assistance of each parent in the assumption of his parental role.

Various programs which have been developed have attracted given segments of society but have failed to contact all strata. Those who avail themselves of these programs are generally the more advantaged or more informed. To reach those who are uninformed, untouched, and alienated becomes our goal.

In order to accomplish this goal, health care professionals must abandon their restrictive approach to care. Community resources can help us learn what approaches and methods will be accepted. We can look for guidance to colleagues who continue to experience success in the community. Honest evaluation of success and failure can assist in the identification of health care services to be provided.

The nurse who engages in parent education needs to be well prepared in all aspects of childbearing and childrearing. A background in the physical, behavioral, and social sciences which encompass growth and development is vital. It is mandatory that this nurse have knowledge and experience in various teaching methods as well as an understanding of the cultural variations in a particular community. These are the qualifications necessary to help parents clarify issues through a problem-solving approach, rather than making decisions for them.

It is predicted that the next decade will see the continued development of out-of-hospital services with more concentration on health and less preoccupation with illness. This trend demands the development of new roles for nurses and greater efficiency in their utilization.

> There is a new role for tomorrow's nurse. She could in the next decade or two be responsible for the health of families in the community and for their nursing care in the hospital if a member of the family required this specialized nursing service. . . . This new nurse would move freely from the home to the hospital and back. She would become the family's nurse and her main concern would be *health*.[5]

Traditional means of operating must be abandoned—the old must give way to the new, more rational, more efficient. The nurse is envisioned as an independent practitioner who would be accountable to the physician for a specific medical regimen but who could also prescribe for the nursing needs of the patient and her family. As an independent practitioner the nurse will utilize the nursing knowledge, experience, and expertise of all colleagues and will provide consultation when it is sought. These nurses will give direct patient care if this is the need, and will act as liaisons between the hospital and the community. Above all, they will be responsible to and for their patients and accountable to the profession.

REFERENCES

1 Bowers, Paul A.: "Natural Childbirth," *Medical Clinics of North America*, 39:1789–1799, November 1955.
2 Buxton, C. Lee: *A Study of Psychophysical Methods for Relief of Childbirth Pain*, Saunders, Philadelphia, 1962, p. 53.
3 Bruce, Sylvia J.: "Do Prenatal Educational Programs Really Prepare for Parenthood?" *Hospital Topics*, p. 106, November 1965.
4 Rubin, Reva: "Cognitive Style in Pregnancy," *American Journal of Nursing*, 70(3):502, March 1970.
5 Mussallem, Helen K.: "The Changing Role of the Nurse," *American Journal of Nursing*, 69(3):515, March 1969.

BIBLIOGRAPHY

Auerbach, A. B.: *Parents Learn through Discussion: Principles and Practices of Parent Group Education*, Wiley, New York, 1968.
Bowers, Paul A.: "Natural Childbirth," *Medical Clinics of North America*, 39:1789–1799, November 1955.
Bruce, Sylvia J.: "Do Prenatal Educational Programs Really Prepare for Parenthood?" *Hospital Topics*, pp. 104–106, November 1965.
Buxton, C. Lee: *A Study of Psychophysical Methods for Relief of Childbirth Pain*, Saunders, Philadelphia, 1962.
Chabon, Irwin: *Awake and Aware*, Delacorte Press, New York, 1966.
Chertok, L.: "Psychosomatic Methods of Preparation for Childbirth," *American Journal of Obstetrics and Gynecology*, 98:698–707, July 1967.
Dick-Read, G.: *Childbirth without Fear*, 2d rev. ed., Harper, New York, 1959.
Fielding, W., and L. Benjamin: *The Childbirth Challenge: Common Sense versus "Natural" Methods*, Viking, New York, 1962.
Fitzpatrick, E., S. Reeder, and L. Mastroianni: *Maternity Nursing*, 12th ed., Lippincott, Philadephia, 1971.
Hoff, Florence E.: "How Any Nurse Can Help," *American Journal of Nursing*, vol. 69, no. 7, July 1969.

Hommel, Flora: "Natural Childbirth—Nurses in Private Practice as Monitrices," *American Journal of Nursing*, vol. 69, no. 7, July 1969.

Karmel, M.: *Thank You, Doctor Lamaze*, Lippincott, Philadelphia, 1959.

Maternity Center Association: *Seminar on Childbearing and Family Life: Prelude to Action*, The Maternity Center Association, New York, 1969.

Mead, Margaret: *Cultural Patterns and Technical Change*, The New American Library of World Literature, New York, 1955.

Mussallem, Helen K.: "The Changing Role of the Nurse," *American Journal of Nursing*, 69:514–517, March 1969.

Rubin, Reva: "Cognitive Style in Pregnancy," *American Journal of Nursing*, 70:502–508, March 1970.

Sclare, A. B.: "Psychoprophylaxis in Obstetrics," *Nursing Times*, 61:1373–1374, October 1965.

Tanzer, Deborah: "Natural Childbirth: Pain or Peak Experience," *Psychology Today*, October 1968.

Vellay, P., and A. Vellay: *Témoinages sur l'Accouchement sans Couleur*, Editions du Senil, Paris, 1956.

Yahia, C., and P. Ulin: "Preliminary Experience with a Psychophysical Program of Preparation for Childbirth," *American Journal of Obstetrics and Gynecology*, vol. 93, no. 7, 1965.

21 | EMOTIONAL CONSIDERATIONS FOR THE PREGNANT FAMILY

Vivian Littlefield

In recent years it has been recognized that it is essential to treat the entire family when one member is ill and to consider the family as a whole when attempting to promote emotional health,[1] and the emphasis in maternity nursing also is on family-centered care. It seems appropriate to consider the entire family as "pregnant" when one is concerned with emotional needs. Each family member in his own way is *expectant* of a change in the family makeup as well as a change in his role within the family. The response of each family member will in turn influence the response of all other members. The preparation period during pregnancy is important for each family member in different ways and will have an important influence on the emotional environment of the "new" family after the birth of the baby. The type of support and guidance a family receives during the preparation period of pregnancy will most likely influence the family's ability to cope with the stress of pregnancy and to be prepared emotionally to provide a healthy environment for its newest member. (See Figure 21-1.)

Although the health professions have not always been overly concerned with emotional needs during pregnancy, since safety has of necessity taken precedence, some professions are beginning to recognize the importance of doing more than providing physically healthy mothers and babies. The rec-

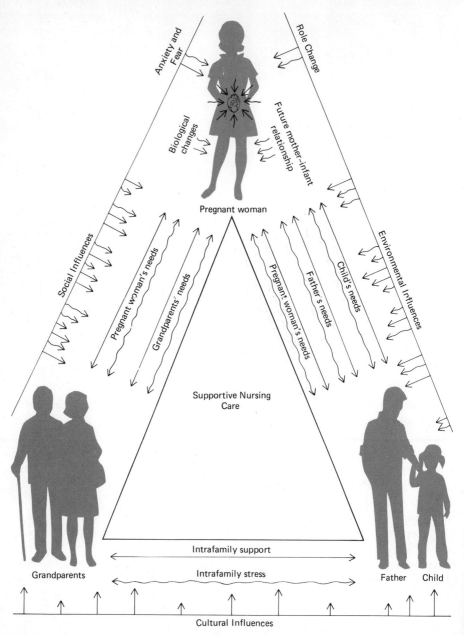

Anxiety and Fear

Role Change

Biological changes

Future mother–infant relationship

Pregnant woman

Social Influences

Pregnant woman's needs

Grandparents' needs

Child's needs

Father's needs

Pregnant woman's needs

Environmental Influences

Supportive Nursing Care

Grandparents

Father   Child

Intrafamily support

Intrafamily stress

Cultural Influences

FIGURE 21-1

This diagram indicates the influence of each family member's needs on the needs of other members during pregnancy. The supportive role of the nurse in assisting each family member (primary and extended) in coping with stressful situations is indicated by the triangle in the center.

ognition that child battering, mental illness, and many psychosomatic illnesses result from unhealthy mother-infant-family relationships has made it important to promote mental health and to detect emotional illness during pregnancy and in new family relationships. There is some evidence, too, that many of the complications of pregnancy such as habitual abortion, hyperemesis gravidarum, pseudocyesis, toxemia, prematurity, and prolonged labor are emotional in origin, or are at *least* enhanced by stressful emotional situations in the pregnant woman's biopsychosocial environment.[2, 3, 4] There is also evidence that suggests that the emotional stress of the pregnant woman may have some influence on the fetus in utero and on his behavior at birth and may cause congenital abnormalities.[3] If this is true, it becomes essential to promote psychological health in the pregnant woman and her family unit.

In addition to the emotional stress that pregnancy can bring to the family, there are various sociological, economic, cultural, and environmental situations that can influence the amount of stress present during pregnancy; these situations also influence the family's ability to handle the stress that the biological and psychological changes bring about in the family members individually and as a whole. Such additional stresses include poverty, marital difficulties, inadequate living conditions, and difficult work situations. In evaluating the emotional needs of a family, all of these factors must be considered so that the family can be helped to cope more effectively with the various stresses present. This can be done by helping the family eliminate or decrease various stressful situations, or by enhancing the family's ability to cope with stressful situations. Nursing especially has the opportunity and should be prepared with appropriate intervention "tools" to assist the family in this respect.

It seems that the professional nurse is in an extremely important position to provide emotional support to the pregnant family, by virtue of educational background and job situation, which often puts the nurse in contact with the pregnant woman in the clinic, hospital, and/or doctor's office as well as in the pregnant woman's home. But perhaps more important is the fact that of all the professional workers who assist the pregnant family, the nurse has a psychological and sociological closeness that other health professionals often lack. Caplan believes that this "closeness" is a unique function of nursing. He sees this as an extremely valuable tool in relating to the pregnant woman and her family. He suggests that the "wise sister role" of nurses allows patients to be more free in their relationships with nurses and to more readily trust them with their problems and concerns.[5]

In order to provide "emotional support" for the pregnant family the nurse needs knowledge of the biological and physical changes that pregnancy initiates in the expectant woman. In addition to this knowledge, the nurse must understand the needs of other family members facing these changes in the pregnant woman and what is involved in assuming a new role in the family. The nurse cannot overlook cultural influences on reproductive beliefs and patterns as well as how *all* of these factors interact to influence the emotional tone and feeling of the family.

This chapter will attempt to provide a basis of knowledge about the emotional changes of pregnancy and how they influence the pregnant woman. First the emotional needs of the pregnant woman will be considered in some detail; then the needs of significant others will be explored. How these needs are interdependent on each individual member and how the family handles the stress to cause conflict or comfort will be discussed. Throughout this discussion some suggestions will be made concerning appropriate intervention by the nurse in order to assist the family to cope in an appropriate way. Some attention will then be given to the emotional situations that are pathological. A chart has been prepared that will assist the nurse in detecting possible emotional situations that may be unhealthy for the pregnant woman, the infant, or the family.

THE PREGNANT WOMAN—CHANGED AND CHANGING

Biological and Physical Changes That Influence Emotional Needs

Pregnancy is a biological state which causes changes in the woman's chemical and physical environment. These changes in hormones and physical appearance have a great influence on the woman's emotional needs and state. Among the physiological changes initiated by conception are changes in protein metabolism, carbohydrate metabolism, level of electrolytes, blood volume, and amount of body water as well as numerous endocrine changes in the thyroid gland, pituitary gland, and ovaries. There is an increased production of estrogen and progesterone.[6] According to Benedek, Caplan, and Richardson, all of these changes are important in producing the "pregnant personality," or what is termed "the mood of pregnancy." Some of the most common changes that are present during pregnancy are the woman's general introversion, passivity, and primary narcissism (the increase in the energy which a woman turns in on herself during pregnancy). It is felt that these traits of pregnancy are due to the increased production of progesterone.[7] The reader is referred to a text on physiology and Chapter 17 of this text for a more complete picture of the physiological changes taking place.

Again, it is important to be aware of the interaction of the physiological changes and how they are received by the pregnant woman through her individual psychological makeup and her cultural and sociological background. Depending on her psychological and sociological background, these physiological changes may or may not cause additional stress. Whether or not she chose to be pregnant also influences her emotional acceptance or rejection of her condition and all the changes that are taking place within her body. Her methods of resolving previous psychological developmental stages also influence the way she views pregnancy and her changed emotional state.

In addition to introversion, passivity, and primary narcissism, other changes due to the biological state of pregnancy are changes in sexual desire, mood swings, emotional lability, irritability, increased sensitivity, and changes between the equilibrium of the ego and the id. There are also emotional changes as a result of change in body image. All changes of course may not be present in every woman or, if present, may not be a problem of severe degree, depending on the individual family situation.

INTROVERSION AND PASSIVITY

One of the most common changes in the emotional response of many pregnant women is their introversion and passivity. The need to rest, to do quiet things, and a lessened interest in previous activities may be frustrating to the woman or to her family. One patient described this feeling as being "detached" from others and from the situation. If the pregnant woman knows this introversion is a possibility, she is less likely to be frustrated by it. However, if she is not aware of this "turning-in," she could become concerned about her lack of interest in things she was previously enthusiastic about. Passivity and introversion are less acceptable to some women, and often husbands, mothers, and relatives are somewhat confused and concerned by the change.

Some women become more outgoing, or extroverted, during pregnancy. They are also more active. These women state they feel better than at other times. This appears to occur less frequently than introversion, but since it is a possibility, one should think of the consequences or confusion of both patient and family as well as friends or an employer when the pregnant woman's personality is "different" from what it was previously.

PRIMARY NARCISSISM

Primary narcissism is also a trait of pregnancy that is perhaps frustrating to family and friends. This trait, however, can be viewed as an important protective mechanism. It causes the woman to consider her own needs during pregnancy and to begin to love the fetus as an extension of her own body. The woman who is busy caring for others and doing for others at her own expense is assisted to care for herself in a more appropriate manner in order to maintain pregnancy at a more optimal state. The self-centeredness that is often evident is at times upsetting to the pregnant woman or to various family members, relative to their degree of dependence on her before pregnancy. At any rate, this is an extremely important change for the nurse to consider, since it might be frustrating to the family, the pregnant woman, or to other health workers who ask the mother to follow certain regulations regarding rest, activity, or nutrition for the baby. The pregnant woman is concerned about *her* needs and the restrictions that pregnancy may place on *her*. It is highly possible that the nurse who understands this need might be more effective in getting the pregnant mother to follow necessary medical, nutritional, and physical requirements since it is the nurse who understands how the pregnant woman may view these restrictions. The nurse can help put restrictions in the context of being beneficial for the pregnant woman herself, rather than *always* placing emphasis on doing everything "for the baby." If the nurse feels guilty about giving extra attention to the pregnant woman, who seems to be healthy and well and appears somewhat self-centered, it should be considered that this giving to the pregnant woman is helping her prepare psychologically for giving to her child.

CHANGES IN SEXUAL DESIRE

If one spends time talking with the pregnant woman about her concerns, it becomes clear that there are changes in sexual desire. Some women indicate their best sexual experiences are during pregnancy; others indicate little interest in sex during pregnancy. Obviously, this change in sexual desire is likely to cause emotional stress on the part of the pregnant woman as well as her husband. Anticipatory guidance concerning these changes in sexual desire is certainly needed early in pregnancy with assurance to both parents that this is quite common. It is easy to see that a combination of introversion, passivity, and narcissism coupled with decreased sexual desire might increase the family stress. It is possible that one can visualize the various problems encountered by each family member when varying degrees of these changes occur. Visualize how this mood of pregnancy might be accepted differently by families with different sociocultural backgrounds. Cultures which accept a more sedentary role for women and which value passive personalities may accept the mood of pregnancy better than the young, mobile middle-class American family which encourages the wife to have a career of her own and values a more outgoing, aggressive female personality. Consider cultural or religious patterns that may have a bearing on the mood of pregnancy.

Mood swings, emotional lability, irritability, and increased sensitivity have been said to be a part of the mood of pregnancy. The degree to which the patient is irritable and overly sensitive is individual and is influenced by the woman's basic personality, her level of emotional and physical maturity, and her desire to be pregnant. The fact that such changes are possible is probably difficult for the family to handle. In Dr. Bradley's book, *Husband-coached Childbirth*, he writes to husbands, "Let us . . . explore in detail the problem of living with pregnant women. Let's face it, they're nuttier than a fruitcake! . . . A pregnant woman is a changed and ever-changing woman. She gradually not only looks different but she feels different and acts different."[8] This colorful way of getting the idea across to the husband perhaps indicates the difficulty one has adjusting to the mood swings and the fact that a woman during pregnancy is "different" and at times unpredictable.

INDIVIDUAL DIFFERENCES IN RESPONSE TO PREGNANCY

Some emphasis should be given to the variables that influence the degree to which a given woman responds to the biological changes. Anyone can observe a number of pregnant women and detect much variance in the amount of introversion, irritability, and sensitivity as well as the other traits of pregnancy. One important variable is the woman's previous emotional makeup.

One author indicates that women who were, prior to conception, demanding, complaining, unstable, and unable to adapt to changes or stress were found to be moody, uncooperative, self-indulgent, self-pitying, and full of somatic distress during pregnancy. Likewise, those rated stable during pregnancy were generally rated stable during everyday life.[9] There were exceptions to the rule, however, and so we must realize that a relatively stable and mature woman may experience a fair amount of emotional stress during pregnancy. Another variable that influences individual response to pregnancy is whether or not the woman wanted to become pregnant.

AMBIVALENCE TOWARD PREGNANCY

Dr. Gerald Caplan has done much research on the emotions of pregnancy and has found that 80 percent of the women who become pregnant admit they are disappointed and anxious when they find that they are pregnant.[10] Dunbar indicates that even those women who wanted to become pregnant have doubts when they actually accomplish their goal.[11] This ambivalence results from many complex factors and may be expressed in some of the mood swings, nausea and vomiting, increased anxiety or various somatic symptoms such as constipation, diarrhea, disturbed sleep, or overeating.

Although there is disagreement in the literature concerning the origin of the somatic symptoms during pregnancy, psychosomatic theory indicates that emotional stress can be portrayed in physical symptoms. Emotional influence seems highly possible in the most common physical symptoms of early pregnancy—nausea and vomiting. Although most authors agree that there is a physiological basis for this symptom, an example will illustrate this point. Some American Indian cultures do not have a term for morning sickness, and few of the women in this culture had this manifestation in early pregnancy. However, when members of this culture moved to California, they developed the symptoms of nausea and vomiting during early pregnancy.[12] When nausea and vomiting is excessive, as in hyperemesis gravidarum, this is interpreted by many authorities as a symptom of severe emotional distress. Deutsch's description of the vomiting of pregnancy is perhaps the most psychologically oriented. She says that vomiting tries to rid the mother-to-be of the child, but a triumphant feeling (that the fetus is still intact) after emesis represents the conflicting wish to keep the child.[13] Other authors indicate that the psychological origin of vomiting in pregnancy is due to undesired sexual relations or to an undesirable relationship between the pregnant woman and her mother.[14, 15] Regardless of the origin of the physical symptoms of nausea and vomiting, almost all authors agree that emotional stress can increase the symptoms or prohibit effective treatment of such symptoms. This emotional influence is an important fact for nurses to remember when nausea and vomiting are problems for patients.

It seems appropriate at this point to discuss a theory based on the wholeness of man or the idea that man is more than the sum of his parts. This implies that one cannot fully comprehend man (or a pregnant woman in this instance) until one considers how all his "parts"—psychological, social, and physical—interact with each other to make him more than either of these alone. It becomes evident that as we study emotional aspects of pregnancy, these cannot be considered in a void without considering how the woman's physical makeup responds, what environment she lives in, and what her sociocultural and religious background is. All of these influence the way she perceives the emotional stress and the action she will take to handle it. Women in some cultures respond to pregnancy as an illness, while others change their pattern of living very little as dictated by the cultural expectations. In a regular maternity clinic the nurse will observe patients who have varying ideas of pregnancy.

ORAL TONE OF PREGNANCY

Another important trait of the pregnant personality is the oral tone or, as Chertok indicates, the emphasis on "hypersomnia, interest in food, greed, dependence, and susceptibility in relation to the environment."[16] This need obviously will cause conflict when restrictions are placed on food intake. Caplan indicates that patients often disagree with the dietitian over diet because of this emphasis on oral needs as well as the fact that these needs, coupled with the revival of conflicts between mother and child, are not conducive to having the pregnant mother follow the dietitian's advice. Better results were obtained when the diet for the pregnant woman was given to her by the obstetrician as a medical prescription.[17] This information should indeed have implications for nursing, especially if the nurse finds difficulty in persuading a patient to follow dietary advice.

Disequilibrium between Ego and Id

Now, let us return to Dr. Bradley's remark to husbands that the pregnant woman is "nuttier than a fruitcake." This remark refers to the changes between the equilibrium of the ego and the id. Caplan, Montagu, and Guttmacher indicate that psychological development is relived during pregnancy, and the pregnant woman works through developmental tasks she was unable to solve in appropriate ways in the past. Caplan describes this as allowing a "great deal of id material to come to the surface."[17] During this time fantasies, needs, and repressed wishes become conscious. In any other situation, this would only happen when a person was psychotic. However, the difference between the pregnant woman and the psychotic is that the pregnant woman is aware of reality. This reworking of old conflicts is thought to help the woman become a more mature individual. What a good preparation for motherhood if this is in fact the case! However, problems may arise if the pregnant woman shares these ideas with family members or health workers who fail to realize this aspect of pregnancy. Caplan also believes that many of the pregnant woman's fears are linked to old conflicts becoming conscious. Some of the fears he mentions that are a result of this reworking of old conflicts are dying during childbirth, giving birth to a monster, or fear that the baby may die.[18] Depending on the support given during pregnancy, the environmental stress present, and the maturity of the pregnant woman, this reworking of earlier developmental stages may or may not be a positive situation. Nevertheless, it brings with it anxiety and emotional needs that are not clearly evident on a conscious level. Therefore, even though the pregnant woman and her family seem to be in a fairly stable life situation during pregnancy, there may be unconscious conflicts that cause anxiety. This could perhaps cause the nurse to miss many of the patient's cues for need of support and help if the nurse did not consider that there may be anxiety present in the pregnant woman without obvious cause.

The nurse's responsibility in handling this ego-id disequilibrium is to be aware that all types of comments may be made by the pregnant woman that might not be said or tolerated at other times. In this respect one could help the mother discuss how she will handle psychosexual development in her own children. Also, by not being shocked by the ideas the mother brings up, such as "hating" her mother or various sexual difficulties, the nurse can allow the mother to "work through" these problems without unnecessary anxiety. Caplan indicates he thinks this is the reason that many obstetricians and nurses avoid talking with and working with pregnant mothers on a closer level.[19] He believes that nurses and obstetricians are upset by the kind of things that pregnant women talk about openly. If the nurse indicates anxiety about the topics the pregnant woman wants to discuss, it might be difficult for the patient and the nurse. The nurse who teaches pregnant women in groups should have some knowledge and appreciation of these psychological factors of pregnancy. The pregnant woman, as a result of the changes taking place, can handle the ideas that are now hers. The nurse, social worker, or student may be somewhat unprepared and unable to handle these ideas comfortably.

Physical Change and Body Image Conflicts

Physical changes occurring during pregnancy also affect the pregnant woman's concept of self and influence her response to pregnancy. The reader is referred to some resources on body image and its influence on the individual. Many authors indicate that there is always some change in body image during pregnancy. The degree of difficulty perceived by the pregnant woman will depend on many things: the degree of threat that change in body image presents to her; the views of her family, friends, neighbors, and others of her sociocultural background; and her acceptance of pregnancy. The change in physical state may or may not cause her emotional stress. If the pregnant woman's husband is continually reminding her of her size or awkwardness, this is likely to have an influence on her. If, on the other hand, the husband views her pregnant state as a manifestation of his manliness and reminds her of her beauty, the threat of body image change may be less stressful. A survey of current dress and the resultant advertising for such dress for pregnant women will give the reader an idea of the general acceptance of pregnancy. Is there excessive desire to hide the presence of pregnancy or to emphasize it?

Role Change and Its Influence

In addition to the mood changes, the changes in personality, the weakening of defenses, and the change in body image, there is the overriding factor of a change in role that pregnancy is preparing the mother to assume. Regardless of the pregnant woman's desire to change her role from wife to mother, from first-time mother to second-, third- or fourth-time mother, she must at the close of pregnancy assume a new role. This of course may bring countless psychological problems and conflicts.

INFLUENCE OF PSYCHOLOGICAL DEVELOPMENT

The pregnant woman's previous development psychologically will influence her readiness to assume the role of mother. The pregnant woman is now entering the developmental stage of generativity versus stagnation, according to Erikson.[20] At this point in her psychological development, the woman and her husband need to be psychologically prepared to guide and care for their children. The pregnant woman's ability to give to others and to sacrifice her own needs will perhaps influence the psychological stress mothering has for her. Her society's and subculture's acceptance of motherhood and the role of women will have had its influence on her and on how stressful pregnancy is for her. The family situation and the degree of support and acceptance she receives will certainly either minimize or enhance her needs in regard to "taking-on" the mothering role.

TAKING-ON THE MATERNAL ROLE

Reva Rubin has described role change during pregnancy and how the woman experiences this change psychologically. She has taken Mead's "taking-in the role of other" and Sarbin's "adopting-the-ways-of-others" and has studied how the specific role of mother is assumed. [21, 22]

The various methods used by the woman during pregnancy in order to take-on the mother role are identified by Mead and Sarbin as (1) play, (2) fantasy, (3) empathy, and (4) copying. [22] Rubin indicates that this process is "a quiet, continuous process, but not a passive one." She also relates that the underlying motivation for taking-in is the "intent to become." [23]

Observing actions of a group of pregnant women in a doctor's office, in a prenatal clinic, or at a neighborhood gathering for coffee, for that matter, will reveal a number of these taking-in activities. The pregnant woman may be wearing maternity clothes before they are necessary to accommodate her new shape. She establishes friendships with pregnant women in various stages of pregnancy and mimics their behavior. She offers to baby-sit for friends, relatives, or acquaintances so that she can "try-on" the role of mother. She may decide to adopt a pet to practice her mothering activities. One pregnant woman attempted to adopt a pet during late pregnancy and was told by a pet adoption agency to come back *after* her baby was born! They had had too many pregnant women who wanted a pet to "practice mothering," and who, after the baby arrived, returned the pet!

Another way the pregnant woman prepares for mothering is to fantasize how it will be. This talking about and exploring how they will behave when the baby does certain things gives the nurse an excellent opportunity for anticipatory guidance concerning infant care, what babies need psychologically in the form of mothering, and what kinds of problems arise for the new mother. As the mother suggests positive acts of mothering that assist the infant to gain a sense of trust, the nurse can reinforce their behaviors. As the pregnant woman mentions behaviors that do not necessarily create a healthful environment for the baby, the nurse can suggest other behaviors that would be better. By helping the pregnant woman explore what she will do in problem areas of infant care, such as crying, illness, or feeding problems, the nurse can help the mother prepare a variety of solutions for mothering. This process is beneficial to the pregnant woman and provides her with opportunities to maximize her coping ability to assume a new role.

In order to more fully understand this taking-on process, let us look at it more closely. (A complete discussion of Rubin's five operations can be found in Chapter 25.) In the earliest stages of pregnancy *mimicry* was the method women used to assume the mother role as observed by Rubin. Also, each time she approached a new stage of becoming a mother—childbirth or child-rearing—she returned to this process of mimicry. After these women had experiences trying-on this role, they took on the mothering role by a process identified as *introjection-projection-rejection*. In this process, there was a selective process which adapted those behaviors that were best suited for her own situation and personality.[24] For example, the pregnant woman may say, "My sister left her baby in the crib with his bottle propped up, but I couldn't do that. He might choke, and I will want to hold my baby." This statement would offer opportunity for the nurse to reinforce the pregnant woman's choice of action.

Another important aspect of taking-on the mothering role as seen by Reva Rubin is the "letting-go" of the former role that is "incompatible with the aspiration of the maternal role."[25] Again, the choice of the patient to be in this situation (pregnant) will make a great deal of difference in the difficulty with which she lets go of former roles. Previously, it was mentioned that the pregnant woman's desire to be pregnant influences her response to the changes taking place. This is also true of the difficulty or ease with which she lets go of former roles. Regardless of her desire to be pregnant, however, the pregnant woman will most likely have ambivalent feelings about giving up old roles. Miss Rubin indicated that most women have difficulty in this respect. The pregnant woman actually grieves over her loss of role. This grieving is a "review in memory of the attachments and associated events of a former self. This memory of details of former self helps to loosen the ties with that self."[26]

Perhaps an example will be helpful. A pregnant woman recently indicated how she and her husband packed away the various articles of his school days and her work days in a trunk in preparation for becoming parents. Parenthood in this situation necessitated his becoming the financial support of the family. This was described as a ritual during which there were tears as they remembered experiences in this past life together. After this experience, this couple seemed to move very rapidly and more easily into doing the things necessary to prepare for parenthood. It should be noted that this pregnancy was planned for many years to be at this point in time. This process of letting-go is not pathological but therapeutic and necessary for the mother, and perhaps the father, if the parent role is to be assumed. This grieving is often seen on the postpartum unit, and the new mother is not able to move into mothering activities until this psychological step is well advanced.

One might speculate as to the most appropriate time to work through this letting-go process. Should the pregnant woman begin this during pregnancy? Should she be encouraged by the nurse to begin this process? It is highly possible that many women should be encouraged to begin thinking about their new role so that it is not so difficult to move into it after the birth of the baby. Other women indicate little readiness for this process during pregnancy. It is also possible that naturally, or as a course of pregnancy, the mother will begin this process, and some assistance and encouragement will be all that is needed. The number of women on the postpartum unit who have not begun this grieving process seems to indicate that some research is needed into the most conducive way to support and encourage this process so that the patient has the least amount of stress and does work through this in an acceptable way that does not impede her assuming the mothering role.

This process of letting-go was demonstrated very vividly by a young, attractive, immaculately groomed mother who had given birth to a little girl 2 days previously. She was in a rooming-in unit, and various efforts had been made to assist this mother in learning how to care for her infant. However, her fingernails were of such length that she could not handle the baby, pin the diaper, or bathe the baby because the staff feared she would hurt her baby. There were quite a few nurses who were critical of this new mother. "Why doesn't she cut those fingernails?" The nursing student who had been working with the young mother had an understanding of the letting-go process and of the patient's difficulty in giving up her former role and accepting her new role, and she listened with understanding and assisted with baby care the mother could not do. On the last hospital day, the new mother asked for scissors and cried while she was cutting her beautifully manicured nails. The student accepted this and provided opportunities for the new mother to care for the baby that morning. She performed the tasks well and when the student later made a home visit, the student reported that she was "mothering well."

It should be noted that this letting-go process is not limited to the pre-pregnant state—that is, grieving over loss of one's status as a bride, professional woman, or single girl—but that the mother who has previous children is affected by the loss of a relationship with her youngest child as the baby. Rubin's study revealed that women pregnant for a second time do grief work over the prepregnancy state *as well as* over the relationship with their first baby. Third- and fourth-time mothers grieve over loss of financial income and independence that a job might have offered them.[26] One mother who was having difficulty giving up the relationship she had with her first child said, "Will I have enough love for this new baby? Will my son suffer because my attention is elsewhere?" Obviously, the timing of the second, third, and fourth pregnancy will affect the degree to which this is a problem. Also, relating to one husband and one child is different than relating to one husband and two or more children. The mother wonders if she will be able to meet all the needs of the family.

Reva Rubin indicates that the ability to perform the tasks of mothering is facilitated if the grieving process as well as the taking-in process is complete. In light of this idea, it would seem important to help the mother work through this process quickly so that she can care for her new baby as soon as possible because our system of maternal care requires the mother to function as a mother very soon after the baby's birth. Since grandparents are often far away, there is less help for the new mother and she has less time to take-in and let-go before taking-on the mothering role. We need to look at how our mobile families, stripped of grandparents, and the short hospital stay cause stress as well as how the stress can be lessened.

However, the question of the most appropriate time for moving through the taking-on process needs to be researched. What actions or support by nurses would facilitate this process? Rubin's observations indicate that this grief work occurred sporadically, that it was only tentative during pregnancy, and that it was only complete or most often brought to some sort of resolution after 3 to 4 weeks with a baby. Is this necessary? Could appropriate support and encouragement in this process of the mothering role be facilitated? Would it then be easier for the mother to care for her baby during the first few weeks?

MATERNAL ROLE ACHIEVEMENT

Specific behavior by the pregnant woman indicates she has assumed the identity of mother. Knowing these behaviors should be most important to the nurse in order to ascertain if the woman is prepared psychologically for her new role. Role achievement can be said to be accomplished when:

1 The pregnant woman refers to mothering activities as *I* without reference to models.
2 The tense used in describing her actions as a mother is *present* rather than *future*.

If childbirth is imminent and there are *no* signs that role identity is progressing in the pregnant woman, this should alert the nurse to watch for problems as the new mother assumes this role after the birth of her baby.

The role of the nurse in helping the mother to take on the mothering role during the antepartal period is summarized in the following list:

1 Provide opportunities for the pregnant woman to express her concerns about mothering and to discuss what she will do as a mother.
2 Provide opportunities for the process of mimicry, role play, fantasy, and introjection-projection-rejection by offering group classes, and encouraging interchange among patients in clinics, doctor's offices, or in neighborhood groups.
3 Provide appropriate reading material concerning mothering activities and use anticipatory guidance concerning appropriate activities necessary in the care of newborns.
4 Encourage the pregnant woman to express the difficulty she will have in giving up former roles.

5 Encourage the family to be supportive and to understand that the grieving process involved in giving up former roles is normal and important to the pregnant woman psychologically.
6 Be open and non-judgmental when the woman expresses ambivalent feelings or if she has difficulty assuming the mothering role.
7 Assess the mother's progress in taking-on the mothering role and relay this evaluation to the postpartum nursing staff so that they can be supportive and provide opportunity for this process to take place after the baby arrives.

Establishment of Mother-Infant Relationships

SELF-LOVE AND ITS INFLUENCE

Pregnancy is a time for the pregnant woman to begin to establish a relationship with her child. Previously it was mentioned that the pregnant woman was narcissistic. This turning-in of energy on herself is a process that allows her to love the fetus as an extension of her own body. Each woman develops a feeling for the fetus in an individual manner. Caplan indicates that the more narcissistic a woman is, the easier she develops love for the fetus.[27] If the pregnant woman develops such a feeling for the fetus, she comes to feel the fetus has a personality and a relationship with her. She may name the fetus, ascribe various traits to it, and talk about the fetus as if he had feelings, needs, and wishes. Usually the fetus is not seen as a person until after quickening.

RELATIONSHIP WITH THE FETUS

Observation of pregnant women reveals that they have varying degrees of feeling for their fetuses. Some women have no feeling or a negative feeling for their fetuses. Caplan indicates this is a negative sign, for it usually carries over to the newborn. After the baby is born, women who have developed a feeling for the fetus in utero seem to move into positive mother-infant relationships more readily. One exception to this sometimes occurs when the baby does not match the expectations the mother had of her future baby. In other words, if the baby is of the opposite sex than that which she wanted, is of a different personality, is quiet and passive rather than active and aggressive, or has a defect that is disturbing to the mother, she may not develop a feeling for the baby as quickly as she might have if the baby "fit" her imagination.

Since there is usually a *time lag* between the birth of the baby and true maternal feeling for that baby, the pregnant woman needs to be aware of this during pregnancy so that she does not feel there is something wrong with her when she does not love her baby immediately. This maternal love can develop a few hours to several weeks after the baby's birth and usually comes on suddenly. A number of factors influence the onset of maternal love. Some of these factors are:

1 The relationship the mother had with the infant as a fetus.
2 The type of labor and delivery experience, including fatigue, response to large amounts of medication, or postpartal complications.
3 The fit of the child to her needs and desires.
4 The pregnant woman's personality.
5 Cultural expectations of the family unit.
6 Hospital routines that keep mother and baby apart.

Since women have fantasies about this baby during pregnancy, Caplan contends that nurses can pick up clues and predict problems in the future mother-infant relationship by listening to their fantasies. Table 21-1 indicates the various clues and the possible predictions that the nurse might make.

A CIRCULAR REVERBERATING PROCESS

Other areas that help the nurse assess the future mother-infant relationship are the amount of impersonal references she makes to the fetus. If the pregnant woman does not think of the fetus as human, speaks of the fetus as "it," and has not given any thought to a name for the infant even in late pregnancy, this may be a clue to problems in the early postpartum period. It should be stressed, however, that any prediction of a relationship prenatally will need to be verified; the opposite conclusion may be drawn once the baby arrives because the relationship then becomes a circular, reverberating process between two individuals. Whether a positive or negative relationship develops depends on each individual—mother and baby—meeting or not meeting the needs of the other.

For example, the mother's attitude toward the fetus may be judged as negative because of her talk about the fetus, lack of naming him, or not making any preparations for the baby as well as complaints about "it" kicking her and disturbing her sleep. When the baby arrives, the baby is a boy. Her culture indicates the importance of having a boy. Her husband is pleased with this and becomes very supportive, and the baby responds extremely well to feeding and the mother's caretaking activities. This negative feeling portrayed during pregnancy will probably develop into a positive one. Therefore, any indication on the part of the nurse that there may be a negative mother-infant relationship should be resolved once the baby has arrived. It is also possible that the future relationship between mother and baby is predicted as being positive, but because the baby does not fit the mother's expectations, as well as various other situations, the relationship does not

TABLE 21-1
FANTASIES OF PREGNANT WOMEN ABOUT THE FETUS

Fantasy	Predictive value
Regarding age of the baby, the pregnant woman sees the baby as an infant 4 to 5 months old.	If she *always* talks of the infant as older than a newborn baby, there may be problems during early infancy.
The pregnant woman's daydreams about the fetus revolve around what the child will be when he is grown.	The pregnant woman may not see the child as an individual but may attempt to meet her own ambitions through the child.
The pregnant woman talks of the baby as *always* a boy or *always* a girl.	Problems may arise if the child is of the opposite sex. Better if the mother is ambivalent about the sex in her fantasies.
The pregnant woman knows *exactly* what the baby is like.	She may not be able to see the baby as he is, with his own needs and personality.
After the baby is born, the new mother pictures a "marvelous baby" beyond all estimates of people around her.	The new mother may be unable to see his real needs.

SOURCE: Developed from Gerald Caplan, *Concepts of Mental Health Consultations, Their Application in Public Health Social Work*, Children's Bureau, Washington, D.C., 1959.

develop. The nurse must be alert for negative relationships during pregnancy and after the baby is born.

The student of nursing may ask, "Why is it important to predict problems?" The importance of knowing if all will be well with a particular mother, infant, and family is emphasized because of the problems that may result if this mother-infant relationship is negative. The mother is all-important to the infant. She is essential not only to his physical health but also to his emotional health and development. Exploration of Bowlby's studies of the failure of infants to grow and mature normally without mothering even when all aspects of their physical needs were met emphasizes the need to detect faulty mother-infant relationships early so that steps can be taken to correct the situation *before* there is severe damage to the infant.[28] Even if the situation is not as drastic as in what is called *the battered child syndrome*, it may deprive the infant of adequate love to meet his needs so he can establish his sense of basic trust; this in turn causes a less than healthy emotional personality.

Disordered Mother-Infant Relationships

Let us now look at some of the results of disordered mother-infant relationships and discuss some of the clues to these relationships that will assist the nurse in detecting the possibility of such relationships in pregnancy.

Leo Kanner indicates that "in our civilization there are three types of maternal rejection of the baby: open hostility and neglect, perfectionism, and overprotection."[29]

OPEN HOSTILITY AND NEGLECT

The first category, open hostility and neglect, includes such problems as the battered child syndrome, the child's failure to thrive, abandonment, and all degrees of parental neglect. One author has called this lack of love for the infant, "psychological miscarriage."[30]

It is often hard for the beginning student in nursing as well as experienced nurses to recognize the scope of the problem in psychological miscarriage. It is possible to discount behaviors of pregnant women or new mothers that indicate an incapacity to love and care for their babies. It is indeed difficult to suspect a prospective mother of the possibility of battering or abusing her child. Perhaps a few statistics from Miss Morris's article, "Psychological Miscarriage," will be helpful to point out the fact that the problem actually occurs more frequently than previously suspected.[30] Miss Morris reports that there are from 50,000 to 70,000 children who are neglected, battered, and exploited every year. Another 150,000 children are in foster homes for these same reasons, and from 8 to 10 percent of all school children in one 20-county study were in need of psychiatric examination and some type of treatment for their problems. Kempe also refers to similar statistics which indicate that a proportion of the battered children die or suffer permanent brain damage.[31, 32]

Individual cases are equally upsetting as they actually point to the violence, deprivation, and dehumanization involved. Only one experience with a child who has been neglected or battered by parents is necessary for the student of nursing to become aware of the severe emotional problem involved. Also, since this problem is often one that is passed on from generation to generation, it becomes a cycle of dehumanization and pain that must be broken.

From a study of the battered child syndrome, it is possible to identify various clues during pregnancy that would be indicative of the possibility of such a problem. More research is needed as to more specific or predictive behaviors, however. Kempe suggests the possibility of using psychological tests and suggests that the pregnant woman should be asked, "What are some sources of worry and tension concerning your baby?" This question asked in an open, accepting, and interested manner may be fruitful in getting the pregnant woman as well as the father of the baby to share their feelings with the nurse about becoming parents.

Morris indicates several criteria that can be used to assess the adequacy of a mother's behavior during the early weeks of an infant's life. Although we are discussing pregnancy and its emotional conflicts, it is important to consider what a healthy relationship is. Then, as the nurse listens to the pregnant woman talk of herself as a mother or how she might behave under certain situations, clues could be picked up that would call for further observation once the baby has arrived. "Mother-infant unity can be said to be satisfactory when a mother can: find pleasure in her infant and in tasks for and with him; understand his emotional states and comfort him; read his cues for new experience; sense his fatigue points."[30]

The pregnant woman's description of the baby's needs may be a clue to her acceptance of a newborn's needs. The pregnant woman's expression of dislikes for the tasks of mothering also may be a clue to disunity. Her desire to know what might comfort her baby and her expression of her desire to do so would be positive clues.

Another clue to the possibility of abuse or battering is in the type of parental discipline as well as the parent-child relationship the pregnant couple experienced in their childhood. Any indications of severe emotional deprivation or severe punishment may be a clue to watch for such behavior in the pregnant couple. Kempe indicates that psychologists and social anthropologists recognize that "patterns of childrearing, both good and bad, are passed from one generation to the next in relatively unchanged form."[33] Constant worry about defects or injury to the child or fear that their infants may have diseases are also clues to faulty mother-infant relationships. If the mother expresses extreme dislike for the infant and his bodily functions of eating and defecating, this too may be a clue as to a disordered relationship. Expression of fear of her infant's natural dependent needs as well as expression of fear that their infant will die are also possible indications of a faulty future relationship between mother and baby.

PERFECTIONISM

The second disordered mother-infant relationship mentioned by Kanner is perfectionism. In such a relationship the mother is ambivalent about accepting her child, and as a result, the mother attempts to justify her negative feelings on the basis of the child's shortcomings and tries to make the child perfect, therefore acceptable. She overdoes everything—bathing, feeding, following instructions to the letter in various books—and she takes advice literally. She adheres to feeding schedules and early bowel training. Obviously, this will lead to frustration on the part of the child. Perhaps as the woman fantasizes about her performance as a mother, if she insists on specific, detailed advice, the nurse might detect clues as to the possibility of this problem. The nurse could help the pregnant woman to work out her ambivalence toward the child if this is not too disordered. Also, the nurse could explore the needs of infants and the fact that infants do not need to "fit textbook pictures."

OVERPROTECTION

Overprotection is another form of rejection, and clues to this possibility should be identified when possible. In this situation the mother overdoes because she feels guilty about resenting the pregnancy and blaming the child for her own disrupted goals. As the nurse interacts with pregnant women, an indication of strong resentment toward pregnancy and an indication that the mother feels she has to sacrifice everything for the baby is a clue to the possibility of overprotection. Extreme concern over every action of the baby is also a clue to the possibility of overprotection. The problem becomes more acute when the child grows up and is not allowed to break away from his mother and become independent.

Factors Influencing the Mother-Infant Relationship

There are a number of factors, other than the relationship with the fetus and rejection of pregnancy, that seem to influence the mother-infant relationship. It seems important to identify some of the factors that research and clinical observation have indicated may influence this relationship. If these factors are known, it is possible that the nurse may be able to assist in fostering positive relationships or to detect the possibility of negative relationships.

Some of these additional factors found in the literature are:

1 The psychological environment in which the pregnant woman grew up and the amount of love and attention she received
2 The support she receives from significant others during pregnancy and later in the role of mother[34]
3 The actual birth experience and how she is treated personally[35]
4 The degree of satisfaction she receives from the birth process itself[36]
5 The degree to which she has "taken-on" the maternal role and "given up" former roles that are in conflict with her mothering activities[37]
6 The type of baby she receives and the "fit" of this baby to her own needs and expectations (right sex, condition, emotional makeup)[38]

Morris identifies the difficulty a modern woman has in assuming the mothering role and establishing an effective relationship with her child when childbirth has become a "technical affair" that strips her of her individuality and her humanity. The hospital staff's attitude toward her seems to influence her feelings about her self-respect and her baby's worth.[39] She feels that lack of dignity and individualism is one reason women fail to attend prenatal clinics and come to the hospital late in labor.

In addition, hospital routines at times tend to interfere with normal taking-on behavior of mothering. Not only may the mother be delayed in this process when she is not allowed to see her baby, but the chance of picking up negative clues to a mother-infant conflict or of fostering positive relationships are not possible when the mother is not seen with her baby.

Indeed, more research is needed as to the clues that can be detected in pregnancy or before so that these parents can be helped. Nursing needs to become involved in research and clinical studies which predict faulty relationships on the known facts. Follow-up studies on these patients must then be done to ascertain if in fact such abuse or neglect does occur. It would be beneficial if such clues were picked up and further observations were made during the postpartum period as well as during the early period of child-rearing. If many of the clues mentioned were apparent, further observations could be made. Certainly the unborn baby and the parents would benefit from breaking the chain that perpetuates this condition if a situation of child battering or neglect was present. Not only must the nurse consider detecting faulty mother-infant relationships, but the nurse must also consider taking steps that foster positive mother-infant relationships by helping the mother and her family prepare emotionally for the new baby. This would involve encouraging the mother to talk about her relationship with her baby, facilitate the pregnant woman's mimicry, role play, fantasy, and establishment of identity. The nurse also should help the pregnant woman understand the infant's need for love, attention, and dependent care. All steps that help decrease stress associated with pregnancy and childbirth as well as increase respect for the individual's uniqueness will be positive steps in fostering positive mother-infant relationships. If the pregnant woman has accepted her new role, receives support from significant others who understand her changed needs, receives respect and support from prenatal care, and has a positive birth experience, it will be easier for her to give love and attention to her infant. A young student once equated the kind of care and family support a pregnant woman needs to foster positive mother-infant relationships to filling a cup—if the cup (i.e., pregnant woman) was filled to capacity, then it would overflow. This overflow was for the baby. (See Figure 21-2.)

Anxiety and the Nurse's Role

From the preceeding discussion, it is hoped that the reader will have become increasingly aware of the amount of anxiety that can be present even in the most "normal" pregnant woman. Pregnancy can be seen as a period of crisis, a period of increased vulnerability, or as one author described it, "a normal biological state, yet it tests the physiological and psychological reserves of [the] woman."[40] Various areas have been pointed out that cause emotional stress in the pregnant woman. Most of these areas of stress deal with the changed state due to pregnancy and do not identify other life stresses that may enhance any of these anxieties. These other stresses could be financial difficulties, marital difficulties, unwed status, family mobility, or indeed any difficulties that would cause stress at any other time. Pregnancy already taxes many of the patient's reserves; therefore, new stresses may cause more problems than they would at other times when the family is not pregnant.

It will be remembered that anxiety and emotional stress may come from previous developmental conflicts renewed, ambivalent feelings about the pregnancy itself, family and cultural background contributions, change in

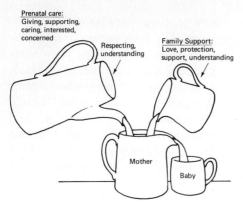

Prenatal care:
Giving, supporting, caring, interested, concerned

Respecting, understanding

Family Support:
Love, protection, support, understanding

Mother

Baby

FIGURE 21-2
Symbolic representation of the support and care that a pregnant woman receives "spilling over" into her ability to care for her infant.

role, biological changes that affect mood and body image, and change in sexual needs. In addition, there are fears associated with the labor and delivery process that include fear of pain, disability, and death.[41] The idea that a patient must go to a hospital to have a baby may indicate that birth is a difficult and painful procedure. Also, many patients hear of friends' and neighbors' labor and delivery experiences that are not always positive experiences. The practice of putting patients to sleep just before delivery also may have some influence on patients as they believe they missed "so many of the terrible things of childbirth." Cultural background also has much to say about the difficulty of labor and delivery. Of course, many tales of bad experiences are often reinforced because occasionally mothers *are* "cut, torn, and injured, [and] babies are born with congenital defects."[42]

ANXIETY ASSOCIATED WITH LABOR AND DELIVERY

Grantly Dick-Read's idea of the fear-tension-pain syndrome in labor perhaps indicates some of the problems that have arisen because of lack of knowledge and fear of the labor and delivery process. Dick-Read felt that if the fear was reduced, then the tension and resultant pain would be decreased. Since he has had success in providing a less painful labor and a better outlook for many patients, one could assume that helping the woman deal affectively with this aspect of reproduction would indeed benefit her greatly. Other psychoprophylactic methods of childbirth preparation have also had beneficial results in improving the patient's experience during labor and delivery. A number of studies have been done that indicate that prepared women, or women who have known what to expect during labor and delivery, have had a better experience during delivery and have felt more satisfaction in their achievement. Other studies have shown that if certain comfort methods were applied, then the pregnant woman was better able to handle the stress of labor.[44] Buxton's study of the various methods of preparation for labor and types of self-help methods during labor points out that information and certain techniques do improve the situation for the pregnant woman.[45] Other studies indicate that if the woman is helped to handle the stress of labor and delivery, she can more quickly and readily relate to her infant and assume the mothering role with less difficulty.

It is pointed out in the literature that the patient who is informed about what is to occur during labor and delivery is less likely to have increased stress. Knowledge of this as well as the fact that the patient may actually dread labor and not know what is to happen would be ample to encourage the nurse to provide some type of anticipatory guidance for the patient facing labor and delivery. It is doubtful if obstetricians will be able to supply enough information, since they are becoming more and more pressed for time with each patient. Nursing must take the lead in providing this information to patients. Often middle- or upper-income patients seek out this information by attending various classes, but the lower-income patient often does not; or when she does, it is not available to her. Also, experience with patients from lower-income levels in a clinic setting indicates that even when such classes *are* available they may not take advantage of the situation. A genuine effort needs to be made to discover what lower-income patients really want in the way of information and emotional support. This is often true for other patients as well. Charlotte Painter, a writer by profession, wrote an interesting book describing her feelings and experiences during pregnancy. Concerning her prenatal classes, Mrs. Painter writes of the nurse, who had just avoided the issue of pain in labor: "All her nice charts and graphs would have been more suited to a high school hygiene course." She says the "mothers were prepared . . . for something more fantastic than the bland fare that was offered."[46] This indicates that the nurse is not looking at what the patient needs but has already decided what she needs. It is extremely important for the nurse to understand the emotional situation as the pregnant woman sees it and to be willing to provide her with the kind of help and information she really needs rather than what is traditional in such classes. Readiness to learn is influenced by the emotional conflicts present that block learning. Timing is very important and should be based on the emotional state and needs of the participants of these classes. Mann had indicated that a number of parents who attended prenatal classes felt these classes did not prepare them for the task of parenthood.[47] Nonstructured group discussion classes are likely to be the best method for providing emotional support, since the nurse could meet each patient's need as it arises. The reader is encouraged to read about this nonstructured, patient-centered instruction.[48] Certainly the nurse must understand the emotional needs and changes occurring in the pregnant woman fully if nonstructured group discussion is to be provided.

OTHER CAUSES OF ANXIETY

Kroger has identified other areas that cause stress to the pregnant woman that have not been mentioned here. These are the pregnant woman's feeling of inadequacy and the possibility of her rejection of femininity, and the attempt of patients to live beyond their emotional capacity. He discusses many of the other things that we have mentioned here and indicates three areas that should be helpful to the patient:

1 Educate the pregnant woman about her condition.
2 Help the pregnant woman understand and accept her ambivalence toward her pregnancy.
3 Help the pregnant woman accept herself as she is.[49]

The text by Kroger entitled *Psychosomatic Obstetrics, Gynecology and Endocrinology* will be most valuable for the reader who is interested in the psychosomatic aspects of reproduction and gynecological problems.

In summary, then, the nurse's role with the pregnant woman is to identify anxiety, recognize its base, help her cope with it effectively, assist or support the pregnant woman and her family in reducing or eliminating this stress when possible, and to use anticipatory guidance to prepare the pregnant woman and her family for the changes, stresses, and problems that pregnancy may bring.

Cultural Influence on Pregnancy

In order for the nurse to be helpful to the family in reducing emotional stress, the nurse must understand how the cultural background of the family influences the response to childbearing. Some perusal of cross-cultural studies of how reproduction is handled in a variety of ways will call attention to the difference in beliefs and attitudes and the effect on the behavior of the family as well as its individual members. Because the culture also influences the nurse and the medical profession's beliefs and behaviors concerning reproduction, there is always the possibility of conflict between the patient and the caretaking professional that often causes emotional stress for the family. Observations have led us to recognize that cultural understanding can often make the difference between helping and turning away certain families. Therefore, it seems important to include a discussion of how culture does influence childbearing, and particularly pregnancy.

Niles Newton recognizes the importance that culture plays in determining behavior during the reproductive years. He says, "All known human societies pattern the behavior of human beings involved in the process of reproduction. Beliefs concerning appropriate behavior in pregnancy, during labor, and in the puerperium appear to be characteristic of all cultures."[50]

The culture influences such things as nutrition, spacing of children, what clothes should be worn, and what kind of help the pregnant woman should have during pregnancy, labor, and delivery. All of this patterning influences attitudes, thought processes, what kind of medical help is solicited, and what restrictions are adhered to during pregnancy.

In the chapter "Cultural Patterns of Prenatal Behavior" in the book *Childbearing—Its Sociocultural and Psychological Aspects*, Niles Newton and Margaret Mead indicate different cultural attitudes toward pregnancy in various areas (Table 21-2).

All of these aspects of the influence of culture may be seen in this country. They vary with the subculture, the area, and certainly with the individual family. If cultural beliefs differ between the medical and nursing staff and the patient, conflicts are bound to occur. If, for example, a woman sees pregnancy as a shameful situation, the emotional overtones will be different from those of a woman who sees the pregnant situation as proof of her husband's virility. If the nurse's view of pregnancy is different from that of the pregnant woman and the nurse fails to see the patient's point of view, the nurse may misread clues to problems or assume there are problems when, in fact, there are none.

Two other important aspects of the influence of culture on emotional needs are the family's view of reproduction in terms of privacy, and cultural beliefs concerning the couple's responsibility for the outcome of pregnancy. For example, some cultures stress that reproduction is a very private affair and seek to provide the pregnant woman with extreme privacy even from her husband, especially during birth. In other cultures, childbearing is a very open occasion and may be shared with many people. Certainly varying degrees of this privacy vs. total openness are apparent in our culture. It may be very stressful to some women to have so many medical personnel available and watching, while to other patients this procedure is perfectly acceptable. Also, it is important to be aware of how various individuals view roles of wife and husband during pregnancy and delivery. If the couple prefer privacy for the wife and the baby's father is uncomfortable being part of the delivery or any other aspect of pregnancy, it is important that they are not forced into "family-centered care" with the baby's father present during birth.

On the other hand, if the family sees pregnancy and birth as a family affair, it is unfortunate when we exclude fathers from classes, talks, and participation in the birth process. The consideration of the individual's beliefs about privacy is important because it can cause unnecessary stress to the couple. When the man's and woman's views of pregnancy differ, it is important to listen and help the couple to come to some form of compromise that is comfortable and not stressful for either.

Our culture believes that "the outcome of pregnancy and childbirth is of considerable public concern. It emphasizes the special value of each human infant and mother and their right to live and be cared for regardless of per-

TABLE 21-2
CULTURAL ATTITUDES TOWARD PREGNANCY

Cultural attitudes	*Possible areas of conflict*
Responsibility for fetal growth.	This attitude results in restrictions in dietary habits, sexual practices during childbearing, and guilt if all is not well when the baby is born.
Feelings of solicitude toward the pregnant woman.	This may influence the amount of attention and help the woman receives with her daily tasks. Conflicts may arise when cultural beliefs are vastly different from medical philosophy. Newton indicates that American culture seems to view pregnancy in light of pathology, since American obstetricians are so "obsessed with pathology" and can't see a woman who needs their services as not sick.[51]
Pregnancy as proof of sexual adequacy.	People of some cultures feel it is important to marry only *after* pregnancy occurs. Conflict may occur between cultures who hold this belief and middle-class health workers.
Pregnancy as a time of vulnerability and debilitation.	The pregnant woman is isolated and kept away from others. A certain degree of this is evident in some cultures in which the pregnant woman is kept from various activities and functions such as maintaining certain jobs and performing certain tasks.
Pregnancy as a time of shame and reticence.	Various cultures and *subcultures* do not tell that the woman is pregnant until she is "showing." Also, this view of pregnancy may have some influence on seeking medical help late in pregnancy or taking necessary precautions concerning certain aspects of care. This also may influence the person's attitude toward pregnancy. If this condition is something that is not talked about, then perhaps it is considered shameful. Such attitudes may cause some anxiety in the pregnant woman.[52]

SOURCE: Adapted from N. Newton and M. Mead, "Cultural Patterns of Prenatal Behavior," in S. A. Richardson and A. F. Guttmacher, *Childbearing—Its Sociocultural and Psychological Aspects*, Williams & Wilkins, Baltimore, 1967, pp. 164–171.

sonal qualities and defects."[53] Such an idea brings with it various emotional problems because when the outcome of pregnancy is abnormal, the couple often feels guilty. Some stress may occur when the pregnant woman and her family recognize the responsibility they have for caring for the child, regardless of such an outcome. Such a cultural belief may also result in increased stress if abortion is recommended or when genetic counseling has indicated that the couple should not have children because of some genetic problem. Those who do not hold this belief may not have as great a problem accepting abortion or intervention to terminate pregnancy.

In addition, culture influences the length of the transition period after birth. The transition period is the time of close relationship between mother and child before she takes on other tasks of primary importance. This total commitment to the newborn may last 4 to 5 years or a few minutes. It determines when the woman will get pregnant again and what type of activities she will assume while caring for her young child. Varying views in this respect may influence the family's choice of spacing children and may be in conflict with what is physically healthy for the woman. Emotional stress will result when views differ between partners as well as between the couple and the medical recommendations.

Our society, which insists that women have their babies in a hospital, conveys the idea that pregnancy is an illness. Also, the medical treatment of many of the discomforts of pregnancy also indicates to pregnant women that pregnancy is an illness. Various groups tend to promote "natural childbirth," physiological childbirth, and encourage the woman not to take any kind of medication during pregnancy. This conflict between practices may cause unnecessary stress as the pregnant woman and her family listen to various ideas about prenatal care. On the one hand, she is encouraged to seek all types of medical aid for her discomforts; on the other, she is told that having a baby is natural and not complicated. She may be made to feel guilty no matter which method she chooses, especially if the outcome of pregnancy is not normal. The various beliefs held by different generations also often causes conflict in practices if the extended family is assigned or assumes a caring role for the pregnant woman during pregnancy. This is often seen when the young pregnant woman refuses to follow medical advice that is based on scientific knowledge in preference for grandmother's advice.

The influences of culture, subculture, and geographic area are very complex, and the student of nursing should always be aware that each individual views reproduction in a different light. This view may in fact be the key to unlocking problems or to helping the family solve problems that are emotionally disturbing because of cultural beliefs about pregnancy which are different from the view of the health workers or institution. The nurse must help the patient come to some acceptable compromise when conflicts arise which jeopardize emotional health or physical safety. However, care should be taken to be absolutely certain that any advice or restrictions placed on the pregnant women and their families are absolutely important to health rather than the nurse's personal and cultural beliefs about childbearing.

A nurse encouraged a couple with four children to marry. This couple was already effectively caring for these children and was satisfied with their common law marriage. They could see no advantage to spending the money for a license or taking the time or effort to marry and were comfortable in the present situation. Stress seemed apparent when the nurse insisted they were wrong by not marrying. It would most likely be quite upsetting to know how much unnecessary stress has been caused by forcing cultural values on those who are not part of that culture. It is hoped that as nurses more fully comprehend the influence of one's beliefs and background on one's behavior that they will question traditional requirements for pregnant families and consider only health needs when making suggestions to the family about their care.

SIGNIFICANT OTHERS—THEIR NEEDS AND CONFLICTS

The Father

The role of the father during the reproductive period is culturally determined. Newton indicates that our culture emphasizes mandatory support mostly and excludes the father from the childbearing process.[53] A survey of the visiting practices in most maternity hospital units as well as opportunities for the fathers to attend "mother's" classes indicates that having a baby is a woman's business. However, many of the psychoprophylactic methods of preparation for childbearing now include fathers, and many of the maternity units have instituted family-centered maternity care. Fathers are becoming more involved and are learning to be helpful during labor. Some obstetricians have sessions for both the man and woman so that their questions can be answered.

Figure 21-3 shows an entire family coming to the antepartal clinic. What an opportunity to help the entire family with their individual needs and concerns! A number of institutions allow fathers in the delivery room so that they can share the birth of their baby. This often causes great conflict among staff members who are not attuned to the importance of including the father. Fear of contamination and of the father's interfering with routines are areas of concern. At any rate, in many areas the role of the father during childbearing is becoming more active and more involved. Some forward-looking professional workers have been extremely concerned about the father's needs during this time and have provided sessions for him to understand the change that is taking place in the woman as well as the changes in his role that will be required in his relationship with his child. We will now consider some of the emotional problems facing a father-to-be and make some suggestions as to the nurse's role in helping him cope in a positive way with what might be a stressful situation.

EMOTIONAL PROBLEMS FACING A FATHER-TO-BE

Changes in Wife

First of all, the husband must adjust to the changes taking place in his pregnant wife. She may seem different and may require more attention and be

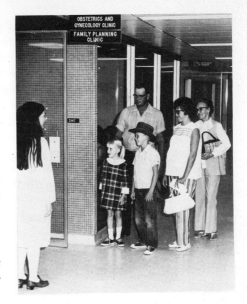

FIGURE 21-3
The entire "pregnant family" is visiting the clinic. This is a good opportunity for the nurse to identify needs of the significant others, as well as the pregnant woman, and enhance the family's coping ability and support of each other in preparation for a new family member. (*Courtesy of the University of Colorado Medical Center, Denver, Colorado*)

more sensitive than she was in the past. This indeed must be a difficult situation, especially if he was not aware that she may be changing. In addition to her personality changes, her changes in need for increased rest, and her turning inward, he might be frustrated by the change in her sexual drive, depending on his own needs and the type of change that occurs in his wife. Regardless of the degree of the problems involved in this adjustment to a "new" wife, he may need anticipatory guidance as well as a little empathy for his frustrations. He also will need some help in recognizing how important it is for him to give his wife additional attention and love during this time. It might be important to explain to him that he is helping his wife "store up for the baby." Even if the changes in the wife are minor or if they are pleasing to the husband, there are enough changes in role and for preparation for the baby to call for some adjustment on the part of the husband.

Rivalry Situation

Caplan indicates there may be a "rivalry situation" between husband and wife during pregnancy and the early period after the birth of the baby.[54] The wife may be receiving more attention from relatives or friends and, of course, from the obstetrician and the nurses. He may or may not have been prepared for the pregnancy at this time and the added responsibilities that he must assume may be stressful, depending on his job and career situation. He also may be upset by the idea of being "replaced" by the baby once it has arrived. If his wife is turning inward and has less interest in sex, this may reinforce his fears. The man's level of maturity, his desire to become a parent, and his job security all play a part in how he responds to his wife's pregnancy. His own background and the type of role model his father was or his friends are will most likely influence the type of role he assumes during pregnancy and during the birth process. His ideas about the husband-father role may be very different from his wife's ideas concerning his role, and this may cause conflict.

For example, perhaps the wife is attending parents classes that require a very active role of the husband. She is insistent that he become part of the group and participate in the birth process and be very active in baby care. If the husband in this situation is not at all comfortable with this role, as the men in his family have never participated in such activities and he does not feel this is a man's role at all, this may cause conflict and difficulty. The nurse could help the husband and wife understand each other's different needs and encourage them to work out a solution that would be acceptable to both.

Reactions to Wife's Fantasies

Caplan also mentions that the husband often is upset by the wife's fantasies and may feel there is something wrong with her. He, too, may be aware of many old wives' tales and may have a great deal of fear about the outcome of this pregnancy. He may be afraid of the damage that the birth may do to his wife as well as whether she will be as desirous sexually as she was before birth. He may have misconceptions regarding breast-feeding in this respect and may decide for his wife how she should feed her baby. Exploration of the husband's ideas regarding childbearing is important; if they are causing stress for him or for his wife, the nurse or doctor can clarify misconceptions and help the couple to understand each other's needs. Often providing the husband with this information and helping him understand his wife and know how to meet her needs will greatly decrease the amount of stress in the family situation during pregnancy.

Adjustment to a New Role

Because the role of father in our culture is not always well defined, it may be necessary to help the father assume the fathering role. Not much is written on what the fathering role should be and how the father assumes this role. Assumption is made that his role is to support his wife in the early stages of pregnancy and then later he is to relate to the child in some appropriate way. Nurses need to study the needs of the father and find appropriate ways that are helpful and supportive to the expectant father. It should be remembered in helping the expectant father to assume his role that it must be done in light of his cultural and socioeconomic background. The nurse must not insist that an expectant father perform a role that is acceptable to the nurse or the medical staff but must help husband and wife understand that they have to work out something that is comfortable for each of them. The more appropriate role for the nurse is to help the pregnant woman understand her husband's needs. Many women instinctively recognize the rivalry situation that is possible between the husband and the new baby and have ideas on how to handle this. Obviously, new babies do take a great deal of time, and usually the obstetrician restricts sexual activities for at least 6 weeks after birth. Therefore, the husband must forego some of his needs in order to establish his new family. If he has become sole provider of the family, this may place additional strain on him. The nurse who reminds the wife of these difficulties may help her avoid some of the stress that might otherwise prevent the husband from being understanding and supportive.

Grandparents

One must consider the needs and influence that the extended family members have on the pregnant woman. In some subcultures the grandparents and other relatives play a significant role during the childbearing period. If the nurse fails to recognize this, it may cause stress to her personally as well as to the family unit.

Perhaps an example will suffice to stress the importance of recognizing the needs of the grandparents. A young student was caring for a Spanish-American family. The pregnant woman was in her teens, and she and her husband lived with his parents. The student nurse visited this patient in the home after caring for the new mother in the prenatal clinic and on the postpartum unit. The young student had participated in teaching the young mother many aspects of childbearing and caring for a newborn baby prior to the patient being dismissed postpartally. Upon visiting in the home, the young nurse found that the new mother was not following her instructions but was instead caring for the baby as the grandmother directed. At times her infant care was in conflict with the nurse's instructions regarding bathing, proper clothing, and feeding schedules. She explored the situation further and learned that the young mother had been under a great deal of stress because of the conflict in ideas about the care of the new baby. She wanted to follow the young nurse's instructions, but when she did she upset the grandmother and her husband. The young nurse explored the importance of the needs of the grandmother and how change in baby care threatened the grandmother's feeling of competence. Working with the grandmother and letting her make decisions about changes helped this situation. In a way, the change in practices said to this grandmother, "You were not a good mother because you did this or that wrong." Since the young mother in this situation needed to depend on her mother-in-law because of the family structure and the role each played, she was constantly in conflict. Had the young nurse recognized the cultural and family individuality, she could have talked with the grandmother during pregnancy and before the new mother went home and included the grandmother in making plans for the newborn's care. This was possible because the grandmother was a frequent visitor to the antepartal clinic as well as the postpartum unit.

In our mobile society, many young parents are separated from grandparents and lack the help and support these family members provide. At such times the nurse may be needed to help the pregnant woman do more planning than would be done otherwise. Reva Rubin's study, mentioned previously, indicated that the mother of the pregnant woman was seen more as help and support than a role model by the pregnant woman. Absence of this support in our society for many women may be frustrating. Grandparents can often be helped to be very supportive of prospective parents and should be included in the family's plan of care when they are available.

Inclusion of the grandparents in prenatal instruction and in the current practices of the day may be important, since these practices are likely to be very different from those at the time they were raising children. Grandmothers who attend nonstructured classes for pregnant women can share ideas and experiences of infant care. Inclusion of grandparents in these classes or discussions gives the nurse opportunities to clarify misconceptions that these expectant grandparents may have that could contribute to the pregnant woman's anxiety. Some new ideas as to how these expectant grandparents may be educated and helped to be more supportive to the pregnant couple should be explored.

Emotional Considerations for the Unborn Baby

Any discussion regarding the emotional considerations for the family during pregnancy would be incomplete without some discussion of the influence of the emotional response of the pregnant woman on her unborn baby. Previously, such ideas might have been considered folklore or myth and not scientific. However, studies with animals and retrospective studies with humans have pointed to the possibility of the influences of emotions on the unborn baby. Some authors feel that clinical evidence indicates that emotional stress in the mother *does* have some influence on the unborn baby. Ferreina in his book *Prenatal Environment* says that "so much positive evidence has now been accumulated that the question is no longer about whether the pregnant woman's emotions have an impact upon the fetus but about the pathways, the nature, and the consequences of such an impact.[57] Ferreina reports in his book a number of studies that point to the fact that increased emotional stress can result in such congenital abnormalities as cleft palate, prenatal complications such as toxemia, habitual abortion, and hyperirritability of the infant at birth. These studies as well as some of the conclusions of M. F. Ashley Montagu in his book *Prenatal Influences* point out the need for further study of the effects of the emotional stress on the fetus. However, it is certainly not conclusive that such stress in the pregnant woman will cause problems that result in reproductive malfunction (toxemia, prematurity, difficult labor), congenital malformations, or disordered personality in the newborn infant. Certainly enough evidence has been gathered for one to consider this a possibility and to recognize that the emotional environment may be extremely important not only in terms of family stability but in terms of the infant's start in life.

DIRECT INFLUENCE ON FETAL DEVELOPMENT

It should be noted that many of the studies that point to the influence of maternal emotions on fetal development and conditions at birth are retrospective in nature, indicating that memory of the mother may be influenced by the outcome of her pregnancy. Such studies should be considered in this light and additional studies be undertaken. Montagu attempted a study with better controls; it was a current study with stress being determined before the baby was delivered. Since his methods were more scientific, his results should be considered more seriously. He found increased fetal activity when there was increased maternal stress and when this increased stress remained high over a period of weeks. Of the 61.5 percent babies who were hyperactive after birth, 38.5 percent had mothers with emotional disturbance during pregnancy.[56] What of the other babies who were hyperactive? What of severely disturbed mental patients who deliver perfectly normal babies? These and other questions arise when considering this subject. Ferreina found that pregnant women who had a greater fear of having a baby and who had extreme attitudes, as rated on a scale, had a baby who behaved in a deviant way. This was a double blind study with 163 mothers and infants and was statistically significant.[57]

INDIRECT INFLUENCE ON FETAL DEVELOPMENT

One can quote numerous studies which say that there is indeed the possibility of some emotional influence on the unborn baby. Some authors indicate that maternal activity and the response to stress in the form of overeating, smoking, and not following medical advice also are ways in which emotional stress can influence the newborn infant. These activities may be more accepted as ways in which maternal stress influences the baby. Therefore, this indicates the need for the nurse to help the pregnant woman cope with stressful situations more appropriately so that dietary restrictions and limitations of activity, when necessary, are not as difficult for her. Also, the nurse should help the pregnant woman in coping with minor discomforts of pregnancy such as nausea, diarrhea, leg aches, and constipation by advocating proper diet, exercises, and activity so that she does not seek medication to ease her anxiety and/or discomfort. The probability of causing defects in the unborn by taking drugs early in pregnancy is now an accepted fact. Since little is known about specific results of many drugs and individual response on the part of the mother and fetus, it is important to help the pregnant woman *avoid the use of medication* when at all possible.

When one considers the possible pathways of conveying maternal stress to the fetus, logically one recognizes the possibilities of the resulting influence on fetal development. This influence will, however, depend on the developmental stage of the fetus as well as the individual fetus's susceptibility to various stresses.

Montagu suggests that chromosomal anomalies fail to be expressed in fetal development if pregnancy proceeds in a favorable environment.[58] A favorable prenatal environment then is important in fetal development. Montagu also suggests that emotional disturbances in the male or female are capable of disordering spermatogenesis and ovulation. If this is true, then there is a possibility that the processes of cell division may also sometimes be thus affected. Montagu argues that if pseudocyesis is possible, why not abortion? The fact that psychotherapy alone is sometimes successful in habitual abortion also indicates the influence of the emotions on reproduction.

MECHANISM OF TRANSFER OF CORTICOSTEROIDS

Perhaps an explanation of the effects of stress and how these might be relayed to the fetus through the placental barrier, as described by Ferreina, will be helpful in indicating the possibility of emotional influence on the fetus. During stress there are high levels of corticosteroids as well as disturbances in plasma proteins in prolonged emotional problems. Also, there is often hyperventilation associated with anxiety. This, of course, changes the levels of oxygen and carbon dioxide present in maternal blood. It is possible that high levels of corticosteroids and changes in plasma proteins as well as lack of oxygen at various stages of pregnancy may in fact be beyond a level of tolerance for the fetus at his particular stage of development. One must explore the idea of individual differences for stress tolerance in the pregnant woman as well as in the individual fetus. Ability to tolerate such changes depends on individual susceptibility and the period of gestation during which the stress occurs.

The importance of the nurse's role in assisting the family to cope with stress during pregnancy is hopefully emphasized by this discussion of the effects of stress on the unborn baby. Being aware of the possibilities of how stress might influence the fetus directly through high levels of corticosteroids, maternal activity, and indirectly through behaviors and activities in the pregnant woman, such as overeating or not following medical advice, should make the nurse more determined to assist the family in appropriate ways that will reduce stressful situations. The reader is referred to the following texts for information concerning emotional influence on the fetus: Montagu,[4] Richardson and Guttmacher,[2] and Ferreina.[3]

Emotional Needs and Conflicts of Children

Other important family members to remember when considering the pregnant family are the children who are already a part of the family. Their needs for emotional support and education during pregnancy are great. Pregnancy can be a difficult time, or it can be a time for learning and growing, depending on how it is handled by the parents. The important variable to consider in determining the effect that a new brother or sister will have on these children is the age of the children when the additional family member arrives. The type of explanation given to the expectant child, the timing of the explanation, and the type and amount of preparation emotionally will again depend on the age of the child. The very young child will not be as aware of the change in his mother's body as the older child but may be somewhat upset by the emotional changes of his mother and in turn may respond by behavior that is regressive or frustrating to the pregnant mother. The young child also will be upset by the change in the household, such as preparation for the new baby, and will need to be prepared for this well in advance, especially if he is to change rooms or beds when the baby arrives. When the child *does* recognize the change in his mother's body and in the activity of her lap (fetal kicking), he should be given an explanation of what is going on and how the baby is growing in the mother's womb. Depending on his age and his questions, he should be given an explanation of what is happening as clearly and openly as possible. The advent of a new baby provides an extremely good opportunity to help the child with his sex education. The nurse may need to help the mother and father recognize the child's (or children's) needs and help them handle situations that may cause problems. Also, the recognition that a child may have ambivalent feelings toward the new baby is important because he may respond with aggression toward the baby or regressive behavior, and this in turn may be frustrating to the parents. The possibility of sibling rivalry should be mentioned during the course of pregnancy, since the parents should be prepared for it and armed with ideas as to how to cope with it. Also, some planning and proper timing are necessary so that the parents can prepare the child before the new baby arrives. Previously, it was mentioned that the woman who is pregnant for the second or third time must work through her grief at giving up the "baby" relationship with the last child. This is most likely difficult for the mother and obviously for the child, depending on his age. Some need to assist the parents to make plans and begin working through this stage would be helpful on the part of the nurse.

The Family—Each Individual's Influence on the Whole

Again reference is made to the idea of the wholeness of man, and this idea is applied to the wholeness of the family. The family is influenced by each individual's needs and conflicts. If one member is under stress, this is likely to influence the other members' amount of stress. As has been seen, pregnancy places different kinds of emotional stress on different members. The complexity of how this might influence other family members and in turn influence the individual should be considered when a plan of care is proposed by the nurse. Figure 21-1 demonstrates this idea of the effects of each member on other members. Each family member's individual strengths must be considered as well as how each member may be supportive to the other. It should not be the nurse who gives all the support, but it should be the nurse who guides and encourages the family to use their own coping mechanisms to support and help each other. After all, having a baby *is* a family affair! The nurse should assume a primary supportive role when no family member is capable of fulfilling such a role. Much of the nursing care during the reproductive period involves support of family strengths. Also, it would be impossible to provide adequate care without considering the entire family's needs and how they intertwine to influence other family member's needs. New ideas and new research are needed in how the nurse, through sociological and psychological closeness, can best intervene and assist families during the childbearing process.

Nursing Intervention in Meeting Emotional Needs

In this chapter various suggestions have been made as to appropriate nursing interventions to assist the family during the stages of pregnancy with various emotional problems. Previously in this text you have been given in-depth information concerning pregnancy, family needs and roles, the influence of the cultural background, and the physical stress that pregnancy poses for the pregnant woman and her family. In addition, the reader is referred to the chapter on nursing assessment for a more complete view of what is meant by nursing intervention. A summary follows, indicating what is involved in providing emotional support to the pregnant family. The nurse should:

1 Assess the emotional needs of the pregnant woman and her family. Some consideration should be given to assessing the pregnant woman's:
   a Response to the physical and chemical changes of pregnancy
   b Readiness for the mothering role
   c Need for supportive relationships with husband, parents, and in-laws
   d Cultural background's influence on her response to childbearing
   e Level of anxiety concerning childbearing, the birth process, and childrearing

f Future mother-infant-family relationships

g Amount of family support and help

h Environmental situation and its resultant stress on the pregnant family

i Behavior that is indicative of pathological emotional situation (see Table 21-3)

2 Make plans for nursing intervention that include enhancement of the family's coping mechanisms and assist the family in preparing emotionally for the new family situation. The ultimate goal should be a positive emotional climate for the new baby. The nursing tasks involved will include:

a Anticipatory guidance as to the course of pregnancy, the occurrences during birth, and the tasks of mothering and fathering

b Listening to fears and anxieties and taking some steps to eliminate stress that causes emotional overtones

c Supportive measures that assist the family in dealing with stress of an emotional nature or assistance in finding ways to eliminate stress that causes emotional overtones

3 Periodically evaluate how the family is coping with its pregnant state and reassess needs as they change as well as make plans for different intervention when planned nursing intervention is not decreasing stress.

Throughout the assessment process the nurse must be aware of predicting the high-risk family emotionally as well as physically. Some indications of pathological situations have been discussed, but because of the complexity of the emotional situations that could become pathological, Table 21-3 has been prepared to facilitate identification of pathological emotional stress.

Nursing intervention for a family who is pregnant can truly be a creative process, for there are many factors, variables, and individual needs to consider when planning and implementing that care. Hopefully, such intervention will assist the family in maintaining a more favorable emotional environment during the childbearing years so that the task of generativity is fully met. It is when such intervention is helpful that good obstetric nursing care becomes preventive pediatric care.

A word of concern and caution should perhaps be presented in a discussion of such lofty goals of preventive care. The fact is not that we shouldn't aspire to such heights, but that at the present time, research has not indicated those aspects of care that *actually* promote mental health or those factors that cause mental ill health. Much needs to be done in this respect, and nursing should be involved in discovering what can be done to promote emotional health. Caplan, in an introduction to *Prevention of Mental Disorders in Children*, perhaps says it most effectively:

TABLE 21-3
CHARACTERISTICS OF HIGH-RISK FAMILIES

Behaviors indicating possible severe emotional stress	Possible problem	Nursing role
Pregnant woman		
Nausea and vomiting continue beyond the first trimester.	Possible rejection of pregnancy. Depending on severity, can become hyperemesis gravidarum.	Observation and assessment of severity of symptoms. Awareness of any indications of rejection of pregnancy or other emotional stress. Inform physician. Assist patient with decreasing vomiting and stress. When advanced, help maintain food and fluid needs.
Reporting of a number of abortions prior to current pregnancy.	Habitual abortion which may have some basis in severe rejection of pregnancy.	Explore patient's feelings toward this pregnancy and previous pregnancies when appropriate. Convey this information to the physician. Assume supportive role indicated by psychiatric assessment.
Physical signs of toxemia, increased blood pressure, increased weight, edema, dizziness, albuminuria, etc.	Combination of physical and mental stress resulting in toxemia (etiology unclear). Can be enhanced by emotional stress.	Explore family situation to detect possible areas of emotional stress such as marital problems, financial stress, overwork, poverty, etc. Assist family in lessening stress and provide emotional "rest" as well as physical rest.
Extreme anxiety over pregnant state, childbirth, etc.	Misconception, unconscious conflicts, and lack of information.	Offer explanation of pregnancy and childbirth processes and assistance in helping patient and family cope with anxiety. Provide opportunity to attend classes, obtain literature, and explore feelings openly.
Verbal indication of inability to relate to new baby or expression of severe emotional deprivation and harsh discipline as a child.	Possibility of child battering or neglect or at least less than optimum relationship with new child.	Observations of the family situation and relating information to physician and child battering team if available. Make arrangements to explore further on postpartum unit and in early home situation.
Expression of difficulty in accepting maternal role and/or no evidence of taking-in or taking-on of this role.	Difficulty in mothering.	Explore patient's view of pregnancy. Help patient find opportunity to work through her negative feelings. Relate problems to obstetri-

Observation	Intervention
Evidence of attempted abortion.	cian and a psychiatrist if indicated. Follow-up observations on the postpartum unit to determine status.
Rejection of pregnancy and mothering.	Maintain a non-judgmental attitude, listen to patient, assist in eliminating guilt. Refer patient to obstetrician and psychiatrist for evaluation and possible therapy or therapeutic abortion.
Sleeplessness, excess irritability, anxiety, excessive depression or excitement, suspiciousness, preoccupation with trivia and tense agitation.	Relate symptoms to obstetrician and encourage pregnant woman to seek psychiatric help.
Psychoses of pregnancy. Usually occurs postpartally and is estimated to occur 1 in 400 to 1,000 pregnancies.	

Fetus

Observation	Intervention
Signs of fetal distress such as extreme hyperactivity, failure to grow, increase in heartbeat.	Relay observations to obstetrician. Explore with pregnant woman possible areas of stress. Help reduce stress.
Possible response to severe emotional stress in mother or family situation.	

Husband

Observation	Intervention
Extreme nonacceptance of wife's changes during pregnancy. Lack of support to wife and wife's increased stress because of this attitude.	Explore problems and misconceptions and provide anticipatory guidance and support so husband can support wife. Encourage seeking help from obstetrician, psychiatrist, or family counselor as indicated.
Misunderstanding, lack of maturity or inability to be a father figure.	
Indications of nonacceptance of role of father or background indicating possible child battering.	Explore problems, support and help in minor situations; if possibility of severe situation, refer to child battering team or psychiatrist.
Nonacceptance of father role and possibly faulty relationship to child, resulting in battering or neglect.	

Children (expectant)

Observation	Intervention
Regressive behavior, change in behavior, emotional anxiety (assessed in regard to age and normal areas of stress).	Anticipatory guidance *before* occurrence. Plan with parents considering age and individuality of child so as to decrease the amount of stress the child experiences.
Fear of replacement or change in environment as a result of change in room or bed and/or parent's stress.	

We cannot afford to sit back and wait for our lack of knowledge of the etiology of mental disorders in children to be remedied by many long years of patient research. Intensive research must be carried on, but it also seems important to survey relevant systems of etiologic theory and clinical experience and to attempt to arrive at a judgment regarding etiologic factors operating at a community level and also to plan for amelioration of the factors decided upon.[59]

Hopefully, nursing intervention will proceed along this course as it relates to emotional support for pregnant families. Attempts to detect emotional stress, help the family cope in the most appropriate way (according to knowledge), and evaluate the intervention and revise it are necessary. The challenge can be great to the student of nursing to find new ways to assist families to have a positive experience with childbearing in preparation for childrearing.

REFERENCES

1 Nathan, Ackerman, Frances L. Beatman, and Sanford N. Sherman: *Expanding Theory and Practice in Family Therapy*, Family Service Association of America, New York, 1967.
2 Richardson, Stephen A., and Alan F. Guttmacher: *Childbearing—Its Sociocultural and Psychological Aspects*, Williams & Wilkins, Baltimore, 1967.
3 Ferreina, Antonio J.: *Prenatal Environment*, Charles C Thomas, Springfield, Ill., 1969, p. 125.
4 Montagu, M. F. Ashley: *Prenatal Influences*, Charles C Thomas, Springfield, Ill., 1962, p. 169.
5 Caplan, Gerald: *Concepts of Mental Health Consultations, Their Application in Public Health Social Work*, Children's Bureau, Washington, D.C., 1959, pp. 264–265.
6 Ferreina: op. cit., pp. 23–31.
7 Caplan: op. cit., p. 46.
8 Bradley, Robert A.: *Husband-coached Childbirth*, Harper & Row, New York, 1965, p. 108.
9 Mason, Edward A.: "Emotional Reactions in Pregnancy—Are They Predictable?" *The Bulletin of Maternal Welfare*, pp. 18–22, March–April 1958.
10 Caplan, Gerald: "Normal Emotions in Pregnancy," *Briefs*, 21(3):35–39, March 1957.
11 Dunbar, Flondus: *Emotional and Bodily Changes*, 4th ed., Columbia University Press, New York, 1954.
12 Ferreina: op. cit., p. 127.

13 Deutsch, Helene: *The Psychology of Women*, Grune & Stratton, New York, 1944.
14 Newton, Niles: *Maternal Emotions*, Hoeber-Harper, New York, 1955.
15 Deutsch: op. cit., p. 405.
16 Chertok, Leon: *Motherhood and Personality*, Lippincott, Philadelphia, 1969, p. 32.
17 Caplan: *Concepts of Mental Health Consultations.*
18 Ibid., p. 53.
19 Ibid., p. 54.
20 Erikson, Erik: *Childhood and Society*, Norton, New York, 1963.
21 Rubin, Reva: "Attainment of the Maternal Role. 1. Processes," *Nursing Research*, 16(3):237–245, Summer 1967.
22 Rubin, Reva: "Attainment of the Maternal Role. 2. Models and Referrants," *Nursing Research*, 16(4):342–346, Fall 1967.
23 Rubin: "Processes," p. 240.
24 Ibid., p. 242.
25 Ibid., p. 243.
26 Ibid., pp. 243–244.
27 Caplan: *Concepts of Mental Health Consultations.*
28 Bowlby, John: *Maternal Care and Mental Health*, World Health Organization, Geneva, Switzerland, 1952.
29 Fitzpatrick, Elise, Sharon Reeder, and Luigi Mastroianni, Jr.: *Maternity Nursing*, 12th ed., Lippincott, Philadelphia, 1971, p. 199.
30 Morris, Marion C.: "Psychological Miscarriage: An End to Mother Love," *Trans-Action*, 3(2):8, January–February 1966.
31 Kempe, C. Henry, et al.: "The Battered-child Syndrome," *Journal of the American Medical Association*, 181:17–24, July 7, 1962.
32 Helfer, Ray E., and C. Henry Kempe: *The Battered Child*, University of Chicago Press, Chicago, Ill., 1968.
33 Kempe: op. cit., p. 18.
34 Caplan: *Concepts of Mental Health Consultations.*
35 Morris: loc. cit.
36 Littlefield, Vivian: *Maternal Satisfaction with the Birth Experience and Maternal-Child Adjustment*, an unpublished study presented to the graduate faculty of the University of Colorado School of Nursing, 1964.
37 Rubin, Reva: "Basic Maternal Behavior," *Nursing Outlook*, 9(11):683–686, November 1961.
38 Caplan: *Concepts of Mental Health Consultations.*
39 Morris: op. cit., p. 9.
40 Lewis, Couper: "Emotional Stress in Pregnant Women," *Nursing Times*, 57:79, January 20, 1961.
41 Kroger, William S.: *Psychosomatic Obstetrics, Gynecology and Endocrinology*, Charles C Thomas, Springfield, Ill., 1962, pp. 34–35.
42 Morris: loc. cit.

43 Dick-Read, Grantly: *Childbirth without Fear*, Harper, New York, 1953.
44 Littlefield, Vivian: *An Experimental Investigation into the Effects of Supportive Nursing Care on Primiparous Patients during Labor*, an unpublished study presented to the graduate faculty of the University of Colorado, 1964.
45 Buxton, C. Lee: *A Study of Psychophysical Methods for Relief of Childbirth Pain*, Saunders, Philadelphia, 1962, p. 102.
46 Painter, Charlotte: *Who Made the Womb*, The New American Library, New York, 1966, p. 88.
47 Mann, David, Luther E. Woodward, and Nathan Joseph: *Educating Expectant Parents*, Wolff, New York, 1961.
48 Auerbach, Aline B.: *Parents Learn through Discussion: Principles and Practices of Parent Group Education*, Wiley, New York, 1968.
49 Kroger: op. cit., p. 35.
50 Richardson and Guttmacher: op. cit., p. 147.
51 Ibid., p. 171.
52 Ibid., pp. 164–169.
53 Ibid., p. 163.
54 Caplan: *Concepts of Mental Health Consultations*.
55 Ferreina: op. cit., p. 25.
56 Montagu: op. cit., p. 176.
57 Ferreina: op. cit., p. 133.
58 Montagu: op. cit., p. 187.
59 Caplan, Gerald: *Prevention of Mental Disorders in Children*, Basic Books, New York, 1961, p. 7.

BIBLIOGRAPHY

Atkinson, Bernie Cain: "Educating Prospective Parents," *Nursing World*, 134:29–31, May 1960.
Baird, Sir Dugald: "The Social Aspect of Obstetric Practice," *Obstetric and Gynecological Survey*, 20:410–430, June 1965.
Caplan, Gerald: "Psychological Aspects of Maternity Care," *American Journal of Public Health*, vol. 47, pp. 25–31, January 1957.
Carty, Elaine A.: "My You're Getting Big," *Canadian Nurse*, 66:40, August 1970.
Clark, A. L.: "The Adaption Problems and Patterns of an Expanding Family: The Prenatal Period," *Nursing Forum*, 5:93–108, 1966.
Corbin, Hazel: "Meeting the Needs of Mothers and Babies," *American Journal of Nursing*, pp. 54–56, January 1957.
Donovan, Patricia, and Selma Landisberg: "Some Psychologic Observations of 'Educated Childbirth,'" *New York State Journal of Medicine*, 53:2504, 2510, November 1953.

Edelston, H.: "The Psychological Approach in Childbirth," *Nursing Mirror*, 116:53–55, April 1963.

Ely, Carol, Rosemary J. Diufio, and Elizabeth C. Koster: "Are Maternity Clinic Dropouts Necessary?" *Nursing Outlook*, pp. 41–43, July 1967.

Fitzpatrick, Elise, Sharon Reeder, and Luigi Mastroianni, Jr.: *Maternity Nursing*, 12th ed., Lippincott, Philadelphia, 1971.

Greengard, Joseph: "The Battered Child Syndrome," *American Journal of Nursing*, pp. 98–100, June 1964.

Gunn, A. D.: "The Normal Pregnancy," *Nursing Times*, 66:69, January 1970.

Harris, R. E.: "Mother and Child," *Nursing Times*, 58:1465, November 1962.

Haward, L. R.: "Some Psychological Aspects of Pregnancy," series in *Midwives Chronicle*, 82:12, January 1969; and March 1969; April 1969; May 1969; June 1969; July 1969; August 1969; September 1969; October 1969; November 1969.

Heicks, G. M.: "What Makes a Good Parent?" *Children*, 7:207–212, November–December 1960.

Helfer, Ray E., and C. Henry Kempe: *The Battered Child*, The University of Chicago Press, Chicago, Ill., 1968.

Horney, Karen: *Feminine Psychology*, Norton, New York, 1967.

"How Mother Affects Unborn Baby," *Woman's Day*, 33:12, July 1970.

Jacabziner, Harold: "Rescuing the Battered Child," *American Journal of Nursing*, pp. 92–97, June 1964.

Jefferies, Derek: "The Sequelae of Childbirth," *Nursing Mirror*, pp. 283–284, June 1963.

Josselyn, Irene M.: "Cultural Forces, Motherliness and Fatherliness," *American Journal of Orthopsychiatry*, 26:264–271, 1956.

Keane, Vera R.: "Maternity Care—From the Parent's Viewpoint," *Briefs*, 22(4):56–59, April 1958.

Kempe, C. Henry, Frederic Silverman, Brendt F. Steele, William Draegemueller, and Henry K. Silver: "The Battered-child Syndrome," *Journal of the American Medical Association*, 181:17–24, July 1962.

Klein, Henriette R., Howard W. Patter, and Ruthe B. Dyk: *Anxiety in Pregnancy and Childbirth*, Hoeber-Harper, New York, 1950.

Larsen, Virginia L.: "Stresses of the Childbearing Year," *American Journal of Public Health*, 56:32–36, January 1965.

Le Fever, John: "View from the Side of the Table," *American Journal of Nursing*, 63:67–69, June 1963.

Lesser, Marion S., and Vera R. Keane: *Nurse-Patient Relationship in a Hospital Maternity Service*, Mosby, St. Louis, 1956.

Martin, Purvis L., and Steward H. Smith: "Public Relations in Our Maternity Wards," *American Journal of Obstetrics and Gynecology*, 81:1079–1085, June 1961.

Maternity Center Association: *Meeting the Childbearing Needs of Families in a Changing World*, Maternity Center Association, New York, 1962.

McFarland, Margaret, and John Reinhart: "The Development of Motherliness," *Children*, 6:48–52, March–April 1959.

McKinlay, J. B.: "The Sick Role, Illness and Pregnancy," in P. J. M. McEwan, *Problems in Medical Care*, Tavistock Press, London, 1971.

Meek, L.: "Maternal Emotions and Their Implications in Nursing," *Registered Nurse*, 32:38, April 1969.

Newton, Niles: *Maternal Emotions*, Harper, New York, 1955.

Parsons, T.: "Sick Role, Illness and Pregnancy," in Elise Fitzpatrick, Sharon Reeder, and Luigi Mastroianni, Jr., *Maternity Nursing*, 12th ed., Lippincott, Philadelphia, 1971, p. 189.

Peplau, Hildegard: "Anxiety in the Mother-infant Relationship," *Nursing World*, p. 134, May 1960.

Pratt, Dallas, and Jack Neher: "Mental Health Is a Family Affair," *Public Affairs Pamphlets*, #155, Public Affairs Committee, New York, 1956.

Reeder, Leo: "Social and Cultural Meaning of Pregnancy," in Elise Fitzpatrick, Sharon Reeder, and Luigi Mastroianni, Jr., *Maternity Nursing*, 12th ed., Lippincott, Philadelphia, 1971, p. 174.

Rick, Oliver J.: "Hospital Routines as Rites of Passage in Developing Maternal Identity," *Nursing Clinics of North America*, 4(1):101–109, March 1970.

Rubin, Reva: "Cognitive Style in Pregnancy," *American Journal of Nursing*, 70:502, March 1970.

———: "Maternity Care in Our Society," *Nursing Outlook*, 11:512–521, July 1963.

Selye, Hans: *The Stress of Life*, McGraw-Hill, New York, 1956.

Senders, Virginia L.: "After Office Hours—An Academic Psychologist Looks at Nursing Care," *Obstetrics and Gynecology*, 14(6):817–824, December 1959.

Shaness, Natalie: "Psychological Problems Associated with Motherhood," *American Handbook of Psychiatry*, vol. III, Basic Books, New York, 1966.

Steele, R., and J. T. Longworth: "The Relationship of Antenatal and Postnatal Factors to Sudden Unexpected Death in Infancy," *Canadian Medical Association Journal*, 94:1165–1171, 1966.

Wallen, Paul: "Reactions of Mothers to Pregnancy and Adjustment of Offspring in Infancy," *American Journal of Orthopsychiatry*, 20:616–622, July 1950.

Warrick, Louise H.: "Femininity, Sexuality and Mothering," *Nursing Forum*, 8(2):212–224, 1969.

Weidenback, Ernestine: *Family-centered Maternity Nursing*, Putnam, New York, 1967, chap. 5, "Anticipatory Counseling and the Nurse," pp. 85–91.

Yankauer, Alfred, Walter E. Boek, Emma L. Shaffer, and Dorothy Clark: "What Mothers Say about Childbearing and Parents Classes," *Nursing Outlook*, 8:563–565, October 1960.

UNIT B
MANAGEMENT AND SUPPORTIVE CARE DURING LABOR AND DELIVERY

22 | THE FIRST STAGE OF LABOR

Elizabeth W. Sturrock and Sally Ann Yeomans

The first stage of labor will be discussed in this chapter. Complications and the basic anatomy, physiology, and mechanisms of labor will not be covered in this section; however, a thorough understanding of this material will facilitate the nurse's ability to make educated decisions. For this reason an extended bibliography at the end of this chapter includes references specific to human female reproductive anatomy, human pregnancy and labor, nursing care during pregnancy, and drugs and their effects on the expectant mother, the fetus, and the newborn.

DYNAMICS OF LABOR
Definition of Labor

Labor may be defined as rhythmic contraction and relaxation of the uterine muscles with progressive effacement (thinning) and dilatation (opening) of the cervix, leading to expulsion of the products of conception.

Labor can and does occur at any time during pregnancy but takes place most frequently at *term*, or about 40 weeks after the last normal menstrual period.

The Three P's

The labor process involves a relationship between the "three P's": the *powers*, or uterine contractions; the *pelvis*, including the size and shape; and the *passenger*, which includes the size, position, and presentation of the fetus as well as the bag of waters, or amniotic sac. Normal labor assumes that the powers are sufficient, the pelvis is adequate, and the passenger is of average size and is in a normal position. Complications of labor occur when there are problems with one or more of the P's.

Stages of Labor

Labor is divided into four stages:

First stage: From the onset of labor through complete dilatation of the cervix.

Second stage: From complete dilatation of the cervix through delivery of the infant.

Third stage: From the delivery of the infant through the delivery of the "afterbirth," or placenta.

Fourth stage: From the delivery of the placenta through the first hour postpartum. This is an arbitrary time during which the vital signs should stabilize and any tendency for immediate hemorrhage should be controlled. It is a critical period for every mother.

The first stage of labor has been further divided into *phases* to facilitate understanding of progress or lack of progress during this stage. These phases will be described later in this chapter.

Initiation of Labor

An unknown entity triggers labor. Possibilities include (1) interaction between the pituitary hormones, oxytocin, FSH, LH, and LTH; (2) the action of estrogen and progesterone from the corpus luteum of the ovary; (3) the placental hormone human chorionic gonadotrophin (HCG); (4) the size, weight, and maturity of the infant(s); (5) volume of the uterus; and (6) competency of the cervix.

Contractions

Uterine muscle does not lie dormant but contracts rhythmically in both the nonpregnant and pregnant states. As pregnancy progresses, the patient and examiner may feel the uterus contract and relax. Toward the end of pregnancy these contractions may be felt by the pregnant woman, particularly when she retires for the day, as an occasional episode or continuing for 1 to 3 hours. In fact, these Braxton Hicks contractions may frequently be rhythmical and of such duration as to cause the woman to think she is in labor. They stop, only to resume again later. The frequency, duration, and quality (or strength) of contractions must be *evaluated by the examiner's hand*, not by what is heard from the patient.

True versus False Labor

True labor contractions do get longer, stronger, usually more frequent, and depict some sort of a "regular" pattern. Each woman in labor has unique, individual contraction patterns. For example, these patterns may occur every 3 to 6 minutes and last for 40 to 60 seconds, or every 5 to 8 minutes and last for 30 to 90 seconds, or every 4 minutes and last for 50 seconds. The patterns may change as labor progresses.

False labor contractions frequently do not last over 35 to 40 seconds and do not become longer and stronger. Although they may occur frequently, they do not usually feel strong to the examiner's hand. They may stop abruptly or may gradually fade away. Cervical dilatation does not occur, but cervical ripening may. (See the section on Ripening below.)

Effacement

Cervical effacement is defined as the thinning of the cervix. Colloquially, the bottleneck gets shorter. Thus, the cervix is described as long (2 inches, or uneffaced), or a given *percentage* of effacement is stated: 50 percent effaced, 80 percent effaced, or completely effaced, which is often paper thin. The degree of effacement depends upon the examiner's evaluation and judgment. This estimation frequently varies considerably among examiners. As the uterine muscle contracts, the cervical tissue is pulled up into the lower segment. In the primigravida, this usually occurs prior to the onset of true labor, while in the multigravida, this often occurs concomitantly with cervical dilatation, as is shown in Figure 22-1.

Dilatation

Cervical dilatation is defined as the opening of the cervical os, the diameter of which is measured in centimeters; 10 cm is designated as complete dilatation. The head of a small infant may come through a smaller cervical opening, while the larger head may require a diameter larger than 10 cm.

Although the cervix of the primigravida does efface prior to labor, there is usually no *cervical dilatation* until labor is established. The multiparous cervix may dilate during the last few weeks of pregnancy so that she comes

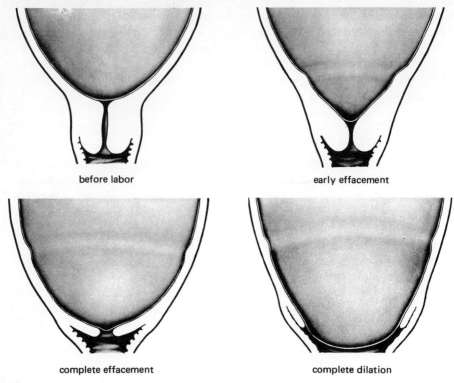

before labor

early effacement

complete effacement

complete dilation

FIGURE 22-1
Effacement in the primigravida usually occurs before dilatation begins.
(Used with permission from Ross Clinical Education Aid # 13, Ross Laboratories, Publisher.)

to labor with an *uneffaced or only partially effaced cervix 1 to 2 cm dilated*. (See Figure 22-2.)

Ripening

The term "ripe" cervix is often used. It is believed by some that the Braxton Hicks contractions help prepare the cervix, or ripen it, for the job ahead. The cervix moves from its posterior position during pregnancy to an anterior position, and the normally firm tissue softens considerably. The cervix may be described as "very pliable," "butter soft," or even "patulous," which indicates that the cervix is ripe.

The pregnant woman who comes to labor with an unripe cervix which is posterior, firm, and uneffaced with a closed cervical os is headed for a longer and possibly more difficult labor. A certain number of contractions and time are required to first ripen this cervix and then to efface and dilate it. These early contractions are experienced by some women as very sharp and hard.

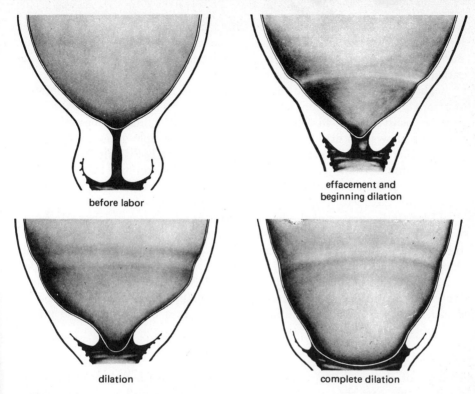

before labor

effacement and
beginning dilation

dilation

complete dilation

FIGURE 22-2
Effacement in the multigravida usually occurs concurrently with dilatation.
(Used with permission from Ross Clinical Education Aid # 13, Ross Laboratories, Publisher.)

The patient becomes discouraged when no progress in dilatation has occurred. If she understands the problem, she can better deal with the situation.

The Bag of Waters

Spontaneous rupture of the bag of waters, or the membranes (amniotic sac), may occur at any time: prior to the onset of labor, during first stage of labor, or during the second stage of labor just before delivery of the head. If not previously ruptured, it frequently ruptures as complete dilatation occurs, heralding the second stage of labor. In a multigravida, this may signify a quickly approaching delivery.

Upon rupture of the bag of waters, the fetal heart rate (FHR) should be checked *immediately* to determine any compression of the umbilical cord; a much slower, perhaps irregular, or very rapid rate may signify problems. Amniotic fluid is usually clear or milky white with flocculent particles of vernix. Meconium staining (yellow, old; green, fresh) signifies that the infant has suffered or is suffering some circulatory impingement. An exception is the infant who is in the breech position; these infants normally pass meconium during labor. Port-wine colored fluid signifies bleeding from a marginal separation of the placenta or from the cord.

There are two definitive tests to determine rupture of the membranes. A strongly alkaline reaction, or deep blue color, on nitrazine test paper indicates a positive result. In the fern test, the suspected fluid is smeared upon a slide and allowed to dry. A fernlike pattern is detectable on examination under the microscope. Interference with the results of both tests may occur if there is contamination with soap, blood, or vaginal secretions. Because cleansing agents are alkaline, a perineal shave should not be done until the nurse checks with the doctor regarding his desire to do such an examination.

Frequently rupture of the bag of waters heralds onset of labor. However, when labor does not ensue for 12 to 24 hours the chance of an ascending intrauterine infection is greatly increased. Likewise, when the presenting part does not fit well into the pelvis, prolapse of the cord may be a hazard. Bed rest is ordered, and vital signs (TPR, BP, FHR) of the mother and the fetus are checked. Prophylactic antibiotics are sometimes used. Labor may be induced to reduce chance of intrauterine infection of both mother and infant.

Descent

Descent of the presenting part refers to the downward and outward movement of this part through the pelvis. The normal, well-flexed head (vertex) twists and turns, flexes and extends to maneuver through the pelvis just as one might twist and turn a hand and flex or extend the fingers to get the hand into a jar. There are three planes, or obstacles involved in the descent stage: the pelvic inlet, the pelvic midplane, and the pelvic outlet. When the examiner can feel the presenting part at the level of the ischial spines, a midplane landmark, he knows the largest part of the head has come through the inlet. The head is thus engaged. The presenting part is also now at zero (0) station. When the vertex has descended to the perineum, the largest part of the head has usually passed the ischial spines, another obstacle. The head is now at a plus two (+2) station. Delivery of the head brings it past the third obstacle: the outlet, which is under the pubic arch, between the ischial tuberosities, and over the coccyx. A presenting part floating is referred to as a −5 station; *dipping* into pelvis is usually called a minus three (−3) station. Thus, any *minus* station refers to an unengaged presenting part. These *stations*, −5 to +5, are specified arbitrary points past which the presenting part passes in its trip through the pelvis. The numbers assigned to the stations are the number of centimeters the presenting part is above or below the level of the ischial spines. The greater the minus (−) value, the higher the presenting part is; the greater the plus (+) value, the lower and closer to delivery. (See Figure 22-3.)

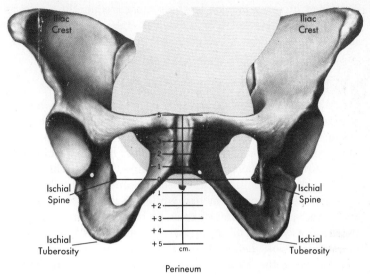

Ischial
Spine

Ischial
Spine

Ischial
Tuberosity

Ischial
Tuberosity

Perineum

FIGURE 22-3
Stations of presenting part (degree of engagement). The location of
the presenting part in relation to the level of the ischial spines is
designated as *station* and indicates the degree of advancement of the
presenting part through the pelvis. Stations are expressed in centimeters above (*minus*) and below (*plus*) the level of the ischial spines
(*zero*). The head is considered to be *engaged* when it reaches the level
of the ischial spines.
(*Used with permission from Ross Clinical Education Aid # 13, Ross
Laboratories, Publisher.*)

Lightening

In the primigravida, the head is often engaged at the onset of labor. In fact,
this may occur from a few days to several weeks prior to delivery, either
suddenly or over a period of several days. The patient may breathe more
easily but may have considerably more difficulty walking and may notice
urinary frequency due to pressure on the bladder. This process is called
lightening. An unengaged head may be cause for concern. Can this head enter
this pelvis? Is the fetal head too big or pelvic inlet too small? In the multigravida, a floating head (−5 station) is not unusual, although lightening does
occur for some a few days or perhaps a few hours prior to the onset of labor.

Show

Show is heavier vaginal mucus discharge, often blood-tinged, noticed as the
cervix begins to efface or dilate. The *mucus plug* occluding the pregnant cervix is most often discharged prior to admission. Some women have no show.

A sudden increase in bloody show most frequently occurs as the cervix goes to complete dilatation. An old wives' tale seems to merit mention: Bloody show heralds the onset of labor either within 24 hours or in about 2 weeks.

Duration of Labor

Every nurse will, sooner or later, be frustrated as to how to deal with such questions as: "How much longer will it be?" "Something surely must be wrong—I've never gone this long before!" "I can't take any more—help me!" "Why is it taking so long? My sister had hers in 5 hours." Experienced labor room nurses will have made some astute observations, albeit not 100 percent accurate. Why, for instance, do some women with short, mild, even irregular contractions precipitate in bed while the nurses sit wondering if they are in labor, and yet other women seem to have long, strong, frequent, regular contractions with little or no apparent progress? We refer you to Dr. Emanuel Friedman's book, *Labor: Clinical Evaluation and Management.* The relationship between the amount of cervical dilatation and the amount of time in which the dilatation occurs is significant. Friedman has shown that the progress of normal labor is slow at the onset, begins to pick up, reaches a maximum rate, and then slows somewhat just prior to complete cervical dilatation.

The tool for measuring this relationship is a graph on which *cervical dilatation* is plotted in relation to a *regular time sequence,* usually at hourly intervals. The normal curve is S, or sigmoid, in shape. (See Figures 22-4 and 22-5.)

Phases of Labor

The two major phases of the first stage of labor are

1 Latent: Longer with less progress; the "getting ready to move" phase. Starts with the onset of a regular contraction pattern.
2 Active: Normally shorter and a progress phase; divided into three sub-phases:
    a Acceleration phase: The "get going" phase.
    b Phase of maximum slope: The "go-go" phase of rapid progress.
    c Deceleration phase: The slowing down phase of very hard work, terminating in complete dilatation of the cervix.

The relationship between time and dilatation accomplished in the various phases should be noted. Table 22-1 denotes the *upper limits* of time allowed in the normal progress of labor. This is a good guideline for all persons involved in the care and management of laboring women.

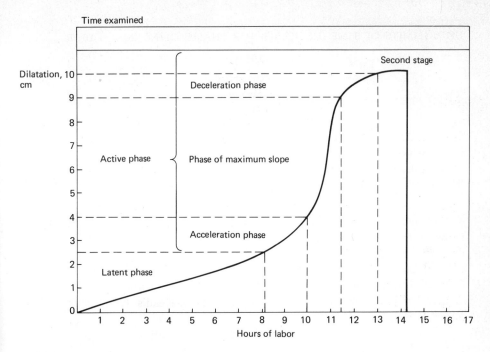

FIGURE 22-4

A sample of a normal S curve in a primigravida labor. The latent phase was 8¼ hours during which the cervix dilated 2½ cm. The total active phase lasted 5 hours.

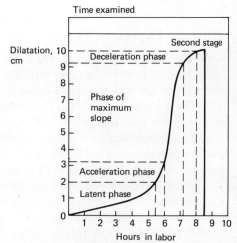

FIGURE 22-5

A sample of a normal S curve for a multigravida labor. The latent phase lasted 5½ hours, resulting in 2 cm dilatation. The total active phase was 2½ hours.

TABLE 22-1
UPPER LIMITS OF TIME (IN HOURS) FOR PHASES OF NORMAL LABOR

	Latent phase	Active phase			Total active phase	Total first stage	Second stage
		Acceleration phase	Maximum slope phase	Deceleration phase			
Primigravida	20	4	5	3	12	32	2
Multigravida	13	5	4	1	10	23	1

SOURCE: Values suggested by E. A. Friedman: *Labor: Clinical Evaluation and Management,* Appleton-Century-Crofts, New York, 1967.

Other terminology frequently encountered defines the phases of first stage labor as *early* (0 to 4 cm), *active* (4 to 8 cm), and *transition* (8 to 10 cm). For more detailed discussion of the graphic analysis of labor and the physiological phenomena associated with each phase, see Friedman's *Labor: Clinical Evaluation and Management;* Bonica's *Principles and Practice of Obstetric Analgesia and Anesthesia;* and Dick-Read's *Childbirth without Fear.*

Descent of the presenting part normally is a continuous process in labor. Friedman has shown that this descent increases during the active phase and reaches maximum descent in the deceleration phase of the first stage and in the second stage of labor.

It is no wonder that the patient seems most uncomfortable during the period just prior to complete dilatation: The cervix is being retracted over the presenting part, which is moving rapidly down. The contractions are often frequent, long, and strong at this time to accomplish these tasks. Physiologically, this is very hard work.

How the Expectant Mother Experiences Body Changes

Concomitant changes occur during labor. No woman ever experiences the labor process exactly the same way. Semantically, the use of "may" and "often" throughout the text alludes to these possible differences.

The primigravida will feel the lightening, or dropping, as the fetal head moves down into the pelvis suddenly or gradually. Descent has started. The engaging presenting part causes increased pressure on the femoral veins. This predisposes to increased dependent lower extremity edema and varicose veins because of the impaired venous return.

Sometime during the last month or two of pregnancy, the normal rhythmic contractions, now called Braxton Hicks contractions, are felt by some women as an intermittent backache, cramping sensation in the groin, pulling sensations in the upper thighs, or stretching just above the symphysis pubis. These irregular on-again-off-again contractions occur most frequently when the woman attempts to rest. Ripening as well as effacement of the cervix in the primigravida, or slight dilatation in the multigravida, is taking place. The woman's need for rest increases. A nap or two during the day is needed. Since her physical load is great, her sleep may be interrupted. The infant needs a chance to move about, which is more easily done when she is at rest.

As time of labor approaches, the normal vaginal mucus discharge frequently becomes profuse. This is often watery but should not be confused with a ruptured bag of waters.

With cervical dilatation, the protective mucus plug will become dislodged and a blood-tinged mucus show appears. The patient should arrive in the admitting room sometime soon.

Physiologically, the contractions of false and true labor are identical. False labor can only be diagnosed after the fact. False labor contractions can be frequent, every 2 to 3 minutes, but they seldom last more than 35 seconds. They may stop abruptly or gradually. Associated with these may be fetal activity. Every time the fetus moves or kicks, the uterine muscle contracts. Such uterine muscle irritability is common prior to the onset of labor. No matter how often or well the false labor dynamics are explained to women, they still express distress at having come to the hospital. "You are disappointed," we say, and the patient shares all sorts of remarks. The long awaited day has not come. To the frightened primigravida, false labor can be emotionally devastating. Fear of the unknown keeps her panic level high. Likewise, the multigravida who has had previous rapid labors does not wish to precipitate en route.

The Prepared Patient

Many women avail themselves of prenatal classes and may be well coached in breathing and relaxing techniques. The methods used will vary. Or the expectant mother may just naturally adapt some very effective method(s) of her own. Such techniques will be used prior to labor, practiced especially during periods of Braxton Hicks contractions. Not infrequently, these women are admitted to labor later than those who are unprepared. It stands to reason that these women may also have some ideas about how they hope their labor and delivery will be managed by the nurse and the doctor. Ask them. They will tell you, between contractions. Prior knowledge of the specifics of different methods taught in various geographic regions can be most helpful to nurses in working with labor patients.

INDUCTION OF LABOR

Medical induction is the initiation of labor by the attendant and includes any or all of several methods: (1) rupture of the membranes, (2) intravenous oxytocic drip, (3) "stripping of the membranes," (4) use of hormonal drugs (prostaglandins), and (5) intraamniotic instillations. The method most frequently utilized at term with a live baby, is oxytocin via intravenous drip, with or without concomitant artificial amniotomy. Careful evaluation of the pregnant woman's state of readiness is required. Considerations include gestational age and condition of the fetus, ripeness of the cervix, and the patient's physical and emotional condition. Table 22-2 lists the indications for medical induction of labor.

The Process

The process of medical induction varies in details from area to area and from physician to physician. Generally, the evaluated patient is "prepped" and an intravenous infusion is begun. An oxytocic is diluted in a second infusion which is "piggy-backed" to the original. The rate of infusion is titrated against the uterine response to the oxytocic agent. In this way, the oxytocin can be well regulated and rapidly controlled. The safest method of induction is use of an infusion machine, such as the Harvard Pump or Ivac Peristaltic Pump,* which delivers exact amounts of oxytocin intravenously via the

---

* The Harvard Pump is manufactured by Harvard Instrument Company, Dover, Massachusetts. The Ivac Peristaltic Pump is manufactured by Ivac Corporation, La Jolla, California.

TABLE 22-2
INDICATIONS FOR MEDICAL INDUCTION OF LABOR

Indication	Rationale
Maternal diabetes	The incidence of intrauterine fetal death increases as pregnancy progresses past the 36th week.
Toxemia of pregnancy (severe or uncontrolled)	The development of eclampsia or convulsive disorders puts both mother and infant at severe risk and must be prevented. Delivery of the infant is the overall cure for toxemia.
Rh incompatibility	This is a fast disappearing phenomenon. Erythroblastosis fetalis becomes more severe as pregnancy progresses and may be fatal to the baby.
Rupture of the membranes for 12 to 24 hours without spontaneous onset of labor	Ascending infection may cause intrauterine and fetal infection since the membrane barrier is gone.
History of precipitous labors	The usual assumption in this case is "once a fast labor, always a *faster* labor." The safest place to care for complications surrounding precipitous labor and delivery is the hospital.
Documented postmaturity of the fetus	Estriol levels are dropping, the placenta is insufficient for the demands placed upon it. The infant is at risk.
Pressing socioeconomic factors	This is difficult to define but usually jointly agreed upon by the mother and her physician.

piggy-back line into the direct line. This eliminates constant monitoring of the rate of infusion, but the setting of the pump must be checked frequently. (See Figures 22-6 and 22-7.) Patients at some institutions have been observed to adjust the oxytocin infusion rate higher in the mistaken belief that they would be safely reducing the time they must spend in labor. It is always important to explain the procedures to patients along with the warning that the physician is setting the rate at a level which is as effective as possible within safe limits. Also, the nurse should inform the patient that the rate will be increased by the physician as rapidly as is consistent with safe care.

Artificial rupture of the bag of waters, amniotomy, may be performed prior to or at the same time the infusion is begun, or it may be deferred until 4 or 5 cm dilatation is reached. Amniotomy alone may stimulate initiation of labor, but it must be remembered that amniotomy is a "point of no return." Once the membranes are ruptured, delivery should be carried out within 24 hours to lower the likelihood of intrauterine infection. Upon rupture of the bag of waters, whenever this occurs, artificially or spontaneously, the nurse's *first* action should be to *auscultate* the fetal heart rate and evaluate it. If the umbilical cord prolapses, the rate will slow drastically. Any substantial in-

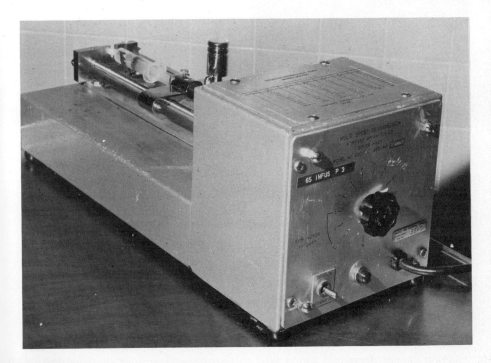

FIGURE 22-6
The Harvard Pump regulates the flow of medications via a piggy-back line into the direct intravenous infusion line.

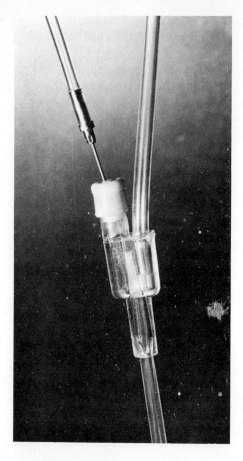

FIGURE 22-7
A second intravenous line can be added to an already running infusion line by insertion of the needle from IV number 2 into the rubber cap or tube available on the tubing of IV number 1.

crease or decrease, more than 20 beats per minute, or any irregularity of the fetal heart rate should be reported immediately to the physician.

Nursing Care and Responsibilities

Nursing responsibilities during medical induction include all those functions performed during spontaneously initiated labor, plus keeping close watch on the vital signs every 15 to 30 minutes, perhaps more frequent rectal or vaginal examinations to assess progress or lack of progress, careful recording of the foregoing, and maintenance of the direct intravenous line. Contractions occurring more often than every 2 minutes or lasting longer than 1 minute may be indicative of impending tonic uterine contraction. Tonic uterine contraction causes decreased blood flow to the placenta and, at the least, causes hypoxia and distress to the fetus. If not corrected, it can lead to uterine rupture, which frequently leads to fetal and/or maternal death. Tonic uterine contraction with a partially dilated cervix may lead to cervical laceration and precipitous delivery. In the event the physician is absent from the patient's room, the nurse should turn off the oxytocin infusion and notify the physician of this action and rationale. Electronic monitoring of contractions and fetal heart rate, if available, is indicated in *all* induction procedures. (See section in this chapter on Electronic Monitoring.)

The 1969 edition of *Standards for Obstetric-Gynecologic Hospital Services*, established by the American College of Obstetricians and Gynecologists, had the following to say about the use of oxytocics in the labor room:

> These drugs should be administered to undelivered patients only upon written order of the physician. Obstetric nursing personnel may assist in the observation of undelivered patients who are receiving oxytocic drugs but should not be expected to assume complete responsibility. A qualified obstetrician should be constantly available in the labor area. Should he leave, the oxytocic must be stopped until he returns.

Any nurse or student nurse functioning in an intrapartum area should be aware of this statement and adhere to it in all instances in which oxytocics are administered to undelivered patients.

Augmentation

The obstetrician may decide to augment or stimulate an already established "poor quality" labor, that is, ineffectual labor wherein there is no diagnosed problem with the pelvis or passenger. The same procedural routines apply as for induction of labor.

The nurse must watch for bleeding carefully and judiciously for at least 12 hours after delivery. Following induction or stimulation, the uterus has a strong tendency to relax, causing immediate or delayed hemorrhage.

PAIN RELIEF

Psychological Preparation

Psychological and physical preparation for labor appears to significantly reduce the amount of medications pregnant women require. The unprepared patient may often respond to knowledge, teaching of relaxation and breathing techniques, and reassurance. The nurse must be aware of the type (or lack) of preparation each patient has and supplement this verbally, nonverbally, and by nursing actions directed to both the patient and her family. Avoidance of traumatic and emotionally charged terms and substitution of low-key phrasing can be of assistance in decreasing or preventing anxiety in the patient.

Some traumatic terms	Less traumatic substitutes
"Pains"	Contractions, tightening of the uterine muscles
Pain, hurt	Discomfort, stretching or pulling sensations, pressure, uncomfortable
Blood, bleeding, bloody show	Red-tinged mucus, pink-streaked show, red, pink or brownish discharge

These substitutions do not mislead the patient, but by reducing the emotional overlay associated with more traumatic terms, nurses can avoid inducing anxiety in otherwise nonanxious patients. Nurses can also avoid reinforcing anxiety and negative emotional responses in anxious patients.

Pharmacological Preparation

Use of drugs of any kind during labor is a serious undertaking. The nurse must be aware not only of the direct effects of the specific medications on the pregnant woman, but also of both the direct and indirect effects upon the fetus. It should go without saying that the nurse must be thoroughly familiar with these aspects of drug administration and of the specific drugs to be offered during labor. On many occasions, the timely use of sedatives, tranquilizers, narcotics, or local analgesia will speed labor as well as make the parturient more relaxed, comfortable, and cooperative. See Table 22-3 for a summary of some of the most important effects of some of the drugs in use. This table is not all-inclusive, nor does it relieve the nurse or student nurse of the responsibility of *looking up each drug administered*.

The use of amnesics, such as scopolamine, is outmoded in modern obstetrics; it is only of historical interest.

ELECTRONIC MONITORING

Philosophy and Rationale

One of the newest concepts in obstetrics is the use of electronic devices for monitoring frequency, intensity, and duration of contractions and for continuous recording of fetal heart rate patterns. It should be obvious that continuous monitoring of the fetus is more accurate, in terms of detecting fetal distress, than is periodic evaluation with a fetoscope. Intermittent stethoscopic monitoring during labor and delivery, when the fetus is at the highest risk of the entire pregnancy, allows detection of only gross changes in the fetal heart rate and therefore provides little useful information. Only ominous changes are likely to be detected by fetoscopic or stethoscopic monitoring as usually practiced.

It has been determined that simultaneous graphic recording of the fetal heart rate and uterine activity can give an accurate picture of the status of

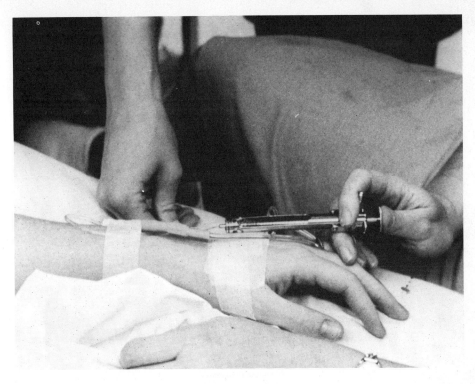

FIGURE 22-8
Medication may be ordered to be given intravenously via an existing intravenous line.
It should be delivered *slowly* at a rate of approximately 1 cc per 3 to 5 minutes.

the fetus. Drs. Roberto Caldeyro-Barcia, Edward H. Hon, and Konrad Hammacher, among others, have documented the relationship of certain patterns during labor and the resultant neonatal condition, as evaluated by Apgar Score. The reader is encouraged to refer to publications by these authors for discussion of fetal heart rate patterns, their interpretation, and appropriate nursing and medical intervention. However, in the absence of the physician and theoretical knowledge of these patterns, any time the fetal heart rate deviates more than 20 beats per minute from the base line or dips to below 100 beats per minute, appropriate nursing response includes (1) administration of oxygen to the parturient, (2) turning her to her side, and (3) notification of the physician. The reader is also referred to the operation and interpretation guidelines that each company publishes and distributes with their monitors.

Contractile status, although most accurately determined via intrauterine catheter monitoring, can be determined by external monitoring also. The fetal heart rate can also be determined by external monitoring, although the accuracy is impaired and electrical interference can be a problem.

TABLE 22-3
DRUGS ADMINISTERED DURING LABOR

Drugs	Effects and side effects (maternal)	Effects and side effects (fetal)	Placental transmission	Effects on labor
Narcotics: Morphine Demerol Nisentil Leritine Dolophine Levo-Dromoran Numorphan Dilaudid Heroin	Onset analgesia is 10-30 min after IM and 3-5 min after IV administration. Adequate analgesia for 2-4 hours. May cause respiratory depression, bradycardia, tachycardia, or orthostatic hypotension. Often cause nausea and vomiting. May lead to urinary retention.	Cause depression and narcosis in the fetus and newborn which may be severe with excessive use or with other depressant factors present.	Rapid for nearly all.	May slow labor if given too early. May enhance labor if given in optimum amount and in active labor.
Barbiturates: Seconal Nembutal Phanodorn Delvinal Phenobarbital Amytal	Sleep, sedation, mild tranquilizer, mild antiemetic. In large doses, produce depression of respiratory and circulatory functions.	No apparent depression of the newborn, but rate of recovery from birth asphyxia may be depressed for 2 to 4 days, as may infant's attention span. Potentiate action of narcotics thus may contribute to narcosis.	Rapidly. Blood levels quickly adjust to equilibrium with maternal blood levels.	Excessive doses may cause slowing of labor, especially in early or latent phases.
Ataractics (tranquilizers): Phenothiazines Thorazine Phenergan Sparine Trilafon Compazine	Sedation, ataraxia, mental and physical relaxation, decrease in nausea and vomiting during and following labor. Potentiation of narcotics, though some have antianalgesic effects. Respiratory depression; occasionally ataxia, athetoid-like movements, and bizarre neurologic reactions.	Some of these may depress the fetus due to the potentiation of narcotics.	Readily crosses placenta with blood levels equalizing rapidly with maternal levels.	Either no effect documented or slight to moderate decrease in duration of labor.
Propanediols: Miltown Equanil	Ataraxia, and mild amnesia when used with Demerol. Urticaria and pruritis (low incidence).	No effects or side effects measured.	Readily. Same as phenothiazines.	None measured.
Diphenylmethanes: Atarax Vistaril	Sedation, ataraxia, mental relaxation. Reduces amount of narcotic needed for pain relief; reduces incidence of vomiting. No significant side effects.	None noted.	Readily. Same as phenothiazines.	None noted.

TABLE 22-3
DRUGS ADMINISTERED DURING LABOR (Continued)

Drugs	Effects and side effects (maternal)	Effects and side effects (fetal)	Placental transmission	Effects on labor
Local blocking agents Lidocaine Mepivacaine Procaine Chloroprocaine Piperocaine Hexylcaine Tetracaine Dibucaine	*Paracervical:* Interrupts uterine pain pathways but does not relieve perineal pain. If injected intravenously, may cause severe systemic reactions: convulsions, vascular collapse, and sudden death. Hematoma may occur if vessels are accidentally damaged. *Pudendal:* Perineal anesthesia when properly executed.	*Paracervical:* Transient fetal bradycardia. Low Apgar scores associated with paracervical block. Sudden fetal death may occur if accidental injection into fetal scalp or cranial cavity. Sudden absorption of the drug into the maternal system may lead to fetal distress or death due to the rapid placental absorption.	Readily.	Slow and may stop labor if given in latent phase. Mild inhibition of contractions may occur, lasting for approximately 30 min. Rate of dilatation is not affected.
	Systemic reactions may occur; accidental sciatic injection will result in leg anesthesia; hematoma may occur, as may puncture of the rectum. Vascular collapse and death may follow accidental vascular injection.	*Pudendal:* Does not depress infant when properly administered. Severe fetal depression may result if intravascular injection is accomplished.	None if not injected into the maternal vascular system.	Interrupts pushing reflex when properly executed. Patient must be coached to bear down with her contractions. Overdose impairs contractions.

SOURCE: J. J. Bonica: *Principles and Practice of Obstetric Analgesia and Anesthesia*, vol. 1, Davis, Philadelphia, 1967. For a good description and drawings of the considerations of paracervical block and pudendal block, the reader is referred to this excellent standard text.

External Monitoring

External monitoring is accomplished by application of one or more sensing devices (transducers) to the expectant mother's abdomen by means of straps. Such application is frequently the responsibility of nurses employed in the intrapartum area. The sensing devices detect the onset of the contractions, their intensity and duration. Electric impulses from these transducers then translate the information onto a moving graph paper so that a continuous, wave-like pattern is seen on one side of the graph paper and represents the contractions. The fetal heart rate is also detected and translated into electronic impulses and then to the graph paper, and this pattern is plotted against the labor pattern. Certain decelerations and accelerations are significant when in response to uterine contraction.

One drawback to the external monitoring is that patients doing abdominal breathing to help them cope with their contractions find it extremely

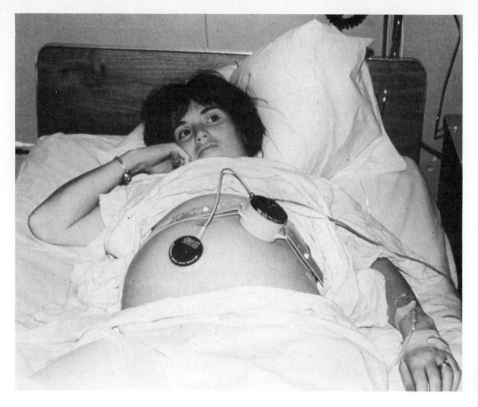

FIGURE 22-9
External monitoring is via transducers (sensing devices) applied to the abdomen with straps.

difficult to breathe deeply. If the straps are too loose, however, the transducer will not pick up the contraction or monitor the fetus. Correct placement of the transducer(s) for comfort and accuracy is a legitimate nursing function.

Internal Monitoring

Internal monitoring means that sensing devices are introduced directly into the uterus. The contraction transducer is a special fluid-filled catheter which transmits exact pressure in terms of centimeters of water to the monitor. The fetal monitoring device is a pronged scalp electrode which is embedded in the fetal scalp by the physician and transmits the electrocardiogram of the fetus to the graphic display. Internal monitoring is more comfortable for the patient insofar as breathing and position changes are concerned. However, she must use a bedpan to empty her bladder when the intrauterine catheter is used,

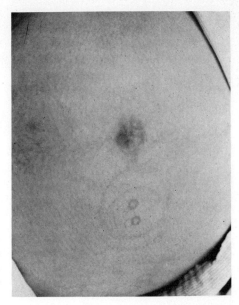

FIGURE 22-10
A common problem with external monitoring is marks left on the patient's abdomen. These marks finally faded 6 hours after the monitor was removed. There was no abdominal edema present. With abdominal edema, marks may last as long as 8 to 12 hours.

rather than get up to go to the bathroom. The transfer to the delivery room from the labor room must be planned prior to urgent need.

Nursing Care of the Monitored Parturient

Before caring for patients who are to have fetal monitoring during labor, it is of utmost importance for the nurse to be acquainted with the proper application and operation of the particular unit in use. An inservice education unit is available at most institutions which utilize monitoring devices. If such a program is not available, a conference with a representative of the company which manufactures the unit is helpful. The representative can supply reference materials and can demonstrate the mechanically correct way of applying and operating the unit. Further discussion with and demonstration by members of the medical and nursing team who are particularly successful in obtaining optimum results will also be helpful. Once the theory of operation is known, the next step is supervised use of the monitor.

Continuous electronic monitoring of the labor contractions and the fetus should free the nurse to give more and better *direct assistance to the expectant mother.* Explanation of the monitor, emphasizing the benefits to be gained by its use, is essential to the psychological well-being of the patient. Any family members who are present should be included in the discussion. All questions should be answered as completely as possible, and the answers should allow for the level of understanding of the questioner.

No matter whether she is being monitored internally or externally, the

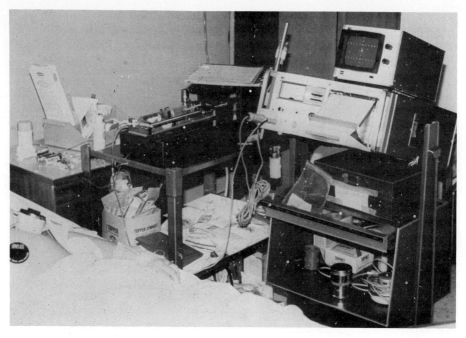

FIGURE 22-11
The patient is frequently confronted with a barrage of electrical equipment, usually mounted on stands containing the supporting supplies and equipment.

patient should not be left on her back for the remainder of her labor except by specific order of the physician. Patients try to cooperate. They are afraid to move with imposing straps and wires in place. Although readjustment of the transducers is a common necessity with external monitoring when the patient moves, internal monitoring should not be affected. Nurses should *cheerfully* readjust the abdominal transducers and note on the graph paper any changes in position.

There is a tendency among both medical and nursing personnel to "nurse the machine" to the exclusion of the patient and her family. Units with nursing station readout consoles strongly encourage "patient care from the desk." Unless there is definite evidence of fetal distress, observation of the graphic display at 15-minute intervals is sufficient. To avoid the temptation of "monitor nursing," the volume, if there is one, can be turned down and the face of the machine turned away from the nurse. During the time the nurse takes the pulse and blood pressure, a reading from the monitor can also be taken and fetal distress patterns identified, if present. More frequent spot checks may be obtained if there are any questions or concerns on the part of the nurse, parturient, or her family. Another method of handling the situation is for the nurse's back to be toward the machine while sitting with the parturient; the nurse can turn to observe the readout at predetermined intervals.

Operation of Electrical Equipment

With more and more electrically operated equipment being used in modern hospitals for monitoring and treating patients, a word concerning safe operation of electrical equipment is appropriate at this time.

Improper use of monitoring devices and other equipment may lead to electrocution of the patient, a family member, or other hospital personnel. The following guidelines must be adhered to in all instances when electrically operated equipment is to be used:

1 If more than one piece of equipment is used for one patient, they should all be plugged into the same power receptacle if possible.
2 The attendants should avoid touching more than one piece of equipment at a time and should avoid touching widely spaced portions of the same piece of equipment.
3 Personnel should avoid touching metal surfaces of such items as pipes, other pieces of equipment, or plumbing fixtures.
4 A three-prong outlet and plug should be used in all cases.
5 *Never* break off the grounding prong of a three-prong plug. If a suitable outlet is not available, call the engineering department and *do not use that piece of equipment* until an appropriate outlet or outlet adapter is available.
6 If there is any *tingling* sensation upon touching the patient or any equipment attached to her, all devices *not necessary to life support* of the patient must be unplugged *immediately* and the situation reported to the physician and the hospital engineer.

For more details and theory, the reader is referred to an excellent booklet, *Using Electrically-operated Equipment Safely with the Monitored Cardiac Patient*, published by Hewlett-Packard Company, Waltham, Massachusetts. Although directed to those dealing with coronary intensive care unit patients, the information will benefit any person working with electrical devices of any kind.

NURSING CARE DURING LABOR

Philosophy

A healthy baby should be delivered to a healthy mother in as safe and satisfying a way as possible.

Nursing care during labor presupposes the necessity that the nurse has a thorough understanding of (1) the anatomy and physiology of reproduction; (2) mechanisms of labor; (3) complication of labor; (4) some principles of human reactions to stress; (5) basic concepts of Lamaze, Dick-Read, and psychoprophylactic preparation for childbirth; and (6) basic concepts in the nursing process.

Nursing responsibilities include (1) evaluation and reporting of signs and symptoms denoting progress and any deviations from normal, (2) techniques in physical care, and (3) emotional and physical support. Nursing actions should be based upon sound judgment in relation to presenting situations.

Admission

The first contact made with a pregnant woman may be upon her admission in labor. Specific relevant information *quickly* obtained broadens the framework of understanding and allows the nurse to assess needs more easily and accurately, incorporate appropriate action, and validate the results. In short, to *quickly* recognize the pregnant woman as an individual who presents some degree of ability to cope within her present physical condition is one of the first objectives of intrapartum care.

What immediate information would be most helpful to nurses which would enhance evaluation of the patient's status? What procedures are required by the physician and by the hospital? What are some of the more commonly used orders and routines from which nurses work? Some women are admitted well along in labor; a priority checklist may be helpful. Tables 22-4 and 22-5 indicate admission and emergency priorities, respectively.

If labor is well advanced, the patient may be unable to void. If very active and moving, don't bother to weigh her. If an enema is mandatory, stay with her—preferably use the bedpan in bed. Notify the physician immediately of rupture of membranes or any urge to push or marked increase in show. These mothers frequently have elevated blood pressure.

Open-ended questions give the expectant mother an opportunity to express herself in any direction she wishes. Nurses may need to validate information by asking some specific questions. Knowledge gained in this manner should dovetail appropriately and pinpoint inconsistencies.

For example, the patient appears happy but tired. The nurse may remark, "You appear happy now, but also tired." The patient says she is so happy that she is finally in labor. She had so much energy today; she cleaned the whole house, rearranged all the furniture, and cooked a special meal for her family. Specifically, the nurse asks her when she last slept. She answers that she went to bed at 10:00 P.M. but never got to sleep since her usual bedtime contractions did not stop after an hour as usual. The nurse may wonder if she is really in labor. Overwork and even fatigue may be the cause of extended painful Braxton Hicks contractions which could terminate in false

TABLE 22-4
ADMISSION PRIORITIES

Activity	Priority*	Follow-through
A History from patient		
1 Pregnancy status	1	
a 4 digit		Full term, premature, abortions, number living children
b 2 digit		Gravida, para
c Estimated date of confinement		Estimated date that her doctor told her; what she thinks if there is a discrepancy
2 If single—keeping baby?	1	If not keeping: *a* Who is handling (label record inside and out)? *b* Does she wish to know sex and/or weight? *c* Does she wish to see baby? *d* Does she wish to care for in the hospital?
3 Plan to bottle- or breast-feed?	2	Some mothers wish to breast-feed on the delivery table or within the first postpartum hour.
4 Allergies, especially to drugs or food	1 & 2	*Label chart front and inside.*
5 Varicose veins Hemorrhoids	1	Chart—may not use stirrups if varicose veins are present.
Vulvar varicosities		May not shave if vulvar varicosities present.
6 Kidney or bladder infection during this pregnancy?	3	Still a problem? Watch for problems postpartum. May be the cause of premature labor or false labor.
B Labor status		
1 When last slept	3	If patient is fatigued at onset of labor, plans should be made by the doctor and nursing staff regarding resting the patient.
2 Contractions	1	
a Started when?		Time since no interruption in contractions.
b Now?		Check and time as you talk. Chart.
c Where does she feel discomfort? Front, back, both?	**3**	Be prepared to give anticipatory guidance.
d Keep written record.		Memory is short, patterns are not always regular.
3 Bag of waters	1	
a Intact	Before doing prep.	Chart.
b Ruptured		Chart.
(1) When, what time, which day?		Prior to admission or any time thereafter and most frequently when cervix becomes completely dilated if not before. Check fetal heart rate and notify doctor. Chart description of color, odor, and amount immediately.
(2) Gush or leak? Uncontrollable?		
(3) Color?		
(4) Odor?		

TABLE 22-4
ADMISSION PRIORITIES (Continued)

Activity	Priority*	Follow-through
4 Show	1	
a None or normal discharge		
b Blood-tinged mucus		Normal
c Frank blood or clots		Bed rest. No enema until the doctor is notified. Check amount, save evidence. No vaginal or rectal exams.
C Vital signs		No matter how fast she's moving, get the pulse, blood pressure, and fetal heart rate for a base line.
1 Weight	2	
2 Temperature, pulse, respirations	1 & 2	
3 Blood pressure	1	
4 Fetal heart rate	1	
D Woman's preparation for childbirth Ideas of what she expects, classes, tours, etc. Knowledge of and bias for or against medication.	3	Should know in order to follow through with her. Also, the well-prepared woman may be admitted well along in labor. What type anesthesia?
E Special procedures		
1 Admission urine— usually clean catch if possible	4 & 5	Hospital routine and status of labor will determine.
2 Perineal shave	4 & 5	Hospital routine and status of labor will determine this. Know hospital procedure and doctor's routines regarding none, partial, or complete.
3 Enema	5	Doctor may order. You may discover from patient that she has been having diarrhea. Check with the doctor prior to giving. If bag of waters is ruptured, check with the doctor. Analgesia, especially narcotics, may render the mother incapable of expelling the enema.
4 Shower	4 & 5	If available and time permits and patient desires.
5 Special blood work	4 & 5	Some hospitals and doctors want admission complete blood count or hematocrit values. Antibody titers are usually obtained on Rh negative women.
6 Intravenous fluids	4 & 5	Some doctors and hospitals automatically start intravenous infusions on all labor patients. Know hospital procedure and be prepared.
7 Amniotomy (artificial rupture of membranes)	4 & 5	Occasionally done on admission or any time thereafter—know procedure.

TABLE 22-4
ADMISSION PRIORITIES (Continued)

Activity	Priority*	Follow-through
8 Labor stimulation or induction	4 & 5	Patients may be admitted for this.
F Review prenatal chart or patient medication ID card if available for:	3	
1 Blood type and Rh	1	Especially at or prior to delivery. Cord
2 VDRL date and result		blood needed for the Rh negative mother's
3 Last hematocrit recorded		delivery.
4 Illnesses during pregnancy	3	Chart; health team conference.
5 Special comments or problems	3	Chart; communicate to staff.

* Priority:
1 As soon as possible   3 As appropriate   5 Routine procedure of hospital
2 Before taking action   4 On order of physician

labor. It is not unusual for a patient to have this excess energy just prior to labor. She is usually very happy early in labor and often says she has had contractions every time she tried to rest for 1 or 2 hours for the past week to month. These contractions often ripen the cervix, that is, cause softening of the tissue, bring the cervix anterior, and allow cervical effacement to occur. The cervix of the multigravida may also dilate 1 to 2 cm with Braxton Hicks contractions. The nurse may think: She may well be in early labor. I need to feel each contraction and help her conserve her energy since she comes to a hard job already tired. I'll ask her if the bag of waters has ruptured or whether she's had any show. Or, if indeed this is false labor, I will need to

TABLE 22-5
EMERGENCY PRIORITIES

Priority	Base line
1	Vital signs, especially pulse, blood pressure, and fetal heart rate. Axillary temperature if very uncontrolled.
2	Pregnancy status: 2 digit and estimated date of confinement.
3	Ask if married. If not, ask if she is planning to keep baby.
4	Plan to bottle- or breast-feed (do not give lactation suppressants if breast-feeding).
5	Does she have any allergies, especially to medications?
6	Time contractions started—character now, interval, and duration.
7	Bag of waters ruptured (look as you ask)?
8	Bloody show or frank bleeding—look, note brightness of blood.
9	Check for blood type, Rh, VDRL, and hematocrit.

determine what she understands about false labor, how she feels about it, and possibly help her to recognize her need for and ways of getting rest periods to prevent overfatigue.

The admission charts should be helpful. Note that the logical order of procedures does not always coincide with the priority order of procedures.

Timing of Contractions

Timing of contractions can only be done appropriately by palpating the contraction, although how the patient reacts and what is said are certainly important. Are her reactions consistent with what is felt? Contrary to what is seen and heard so often, *regular contractions* mean a regular contraction *pattern*. "Come to the hospital when your contractions are regular and 5 minutes apart," the doctor says. The mother is admitted to the emergency room, babe in arms, saying, "You said when they got regular, but they never got regular!" She is not lying. When the doctor asks if her contractions are regular she responds, "No, but the *pattern* is!" If contractions *are* regular, this implies a regular pattern also.

Contractions are best evaluated by the nurse on the fundus of the uterus by spreading slightly relaxed cupped fingers lightly and equally over the fundus. As the contraction begins, the uterus not only becomes tense, firm, or even hard from muscular contraction, but the midline uterus rises up and away from the patient's spine with a gradual rise and fall pattern. The deviated uterus may be held in the midline to observe this. Some nurses may have a tingling or crawling sensation in the hand as the uterus rises. There is a sensation of the uterus rising into the palm of the hand.

The *length* or *duration* of a contraction is the length of time the contraction is palpable. The *frequency* of contractions is the time interval from the beginning of one to the beginning of the next. The *intensity* of the contraction is measured by the degree of indentability of the uterine muscle during the contraction. This procedure is often uncomfortable for the patient and care must be taken. The nurse should try to indent the fingers into the uterus gently but firmly during the height of the contraction. The intensity evaluated by the nurse may not coincide with what the patient perceives. It may not coincide exactly with the evaluation of another nurse, either, for it is a subjective evaluation.

Do not massage or knead this uterus. The patient's skin or the uterus itself may be very tender. The nurse's hand should be kept in place during and between several contractions. How well relaxed is the uterus between contractions? How active is the infant? It should not be necessary to point out that the examiner's hand is directly against the skin of the patient's abdomen. There is nothing (sheet, gown, undergarment, etc.) between the nurse's hand and the patient's abdomen. Contact must be skin-to-skin, or the subtle changes during a contraction may not be perceived.

The nurse must record data about the patient's contractions. Memories are short, shorter without experience. All sorts of labor patterns and frequencies have been documented. It is true that normally contractions become closer, longer, and stronger as progress is made, but there always will be exceptions.

Contractions over 90 seconds long should be reported as should those occurring less than 2 minutes apart.

Bladder Care

The bladder should be kept emptied, for even a small amount of urine can be the cause of severe discomfort. A full bladder also inhibits descent of the presenting part. When able, the patient may prefer to use the bathroom or a bedpan on a chair in her room. This position change can be relaxing.

Vital Signs

The temperature should be taken every 4 hours. An axillary temperature will suffice if the patient is very active. Early signs of an infectious process or simple dehydration will be detected earlier than later. An efficient nurse automatically checks the patient's pulse frequently. A rate over 100 may be cause for concern. Any sudden rise, however, should be investigated further and reported. Most institutions have routines for checking blood pressure and fetal heart rate. A sound rule for checking these signs is better too often than not enough. The more active the labor, the greater the chance for fetal distress. The fetal heart rate most often cannot be heard during a contraction. It slows then, but should recover within 30 seconds following a contraction. Although most authors suggest finding the fetal back, then listening over the back or chest area, try listening through the umbilicus first, since there is less maternal tissue through which to hear. Either lateral lower flank area is also a good choice.

Check the patient's pulse as the fetal heart rate is auscultated to be sure that it is the fetal heart rate and not the patient's pulse that is heard. Make this a routine habit.

The blood pressure often rises during active labor. Take the blood pressure between contractions at least every hour, more often if there are problems or if it is steadily rising.

Vaginal and Rectal Examinations

Student and many staff nurses may never perform these examinations; those who must will learn by repeated practice.

Either examination will provide information on the condition of the cervix as well as position and station of the presenting part. Certainly the

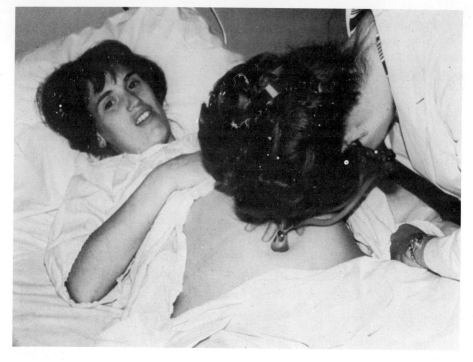

FIGURE 22-12
The fetal heart rate should be obtained a minimum of every 30 minutes during active phase.

vaginal examination allows far greater accuracy as well as access to the membranes in order to evaluate their status.

It is particularly important to keep any rectal secretion from entering the vagina since *Escherichia coli,* normal flora of the bowel, becomes hostile to mother and infant if introduced into the vagina or uterus.

Procedures for vaginal examinations are designed to prevent cross contamination by cleansing the introitus and perineum to permit entry of fingers of sterile gloved hand while avoiding the introduction of hostile bacteria. The soundest cleansing method is simply one wipe from the front to back with tissue or sponge; *discard and repeat* as necessary.

Examinations will be facilitated if the expectant mother is encouraged to relax and breathe deeply during the examination.

Supine Hypotensive Syndrome

In this disorder, the patient cannot lie flat on her back because she becomes light-headed, nauseated, perspires profusely, and may faint. These are signs of circulatory shock. This position allows the enlarged uterus to exert enough pressure on the abdominal aorta and the inferior vena cava to cause the problem. When the patient's blood pressure is sufficiently lowered, placental insufficiency, or lack of blood flow, occurs and can be hazardous to the infant. This patient must either be kept off her back or have her backrest sufficiently elevated to avoid the problem.

Communication Barriers

Cultural differences within the patient and professional populations may pose critical communication barriers for all concerned.

The clinic nurse hears a patient complain of "vomicking" all day. Is she saying "vomiting"? Clarify what happens when she vomits. This may be excess mucus, often in relation to heartburn.

When asked if she has had any bleeding early in pregnancy, a patient states she has had "clogs" for a couple of days, then "strings" for a week. What is she saying? Has she had clots? What size were the clots and what did they look like? "Strings" may mean mucus. Ascertain if they were blood-tinged, the color, and amount. Was it enough to warrant wearing a pad?

Still another mother complains of "itching in her privates." Itching of the vulva, perineum, and vagina usually is due to monilia or trichomonas vaginitis. Odor, amount of discharge, and color, as well as microscopic examination or culture of the suspected discharge, can help the nursing diagnosis.

An anxious pregnant woman keeps asking about "contraptions." Does she mean contractions? Ask what she is referring to. One mother was referring to wrist straps and stirrups in the delivery room.

A Spanish-American parturient repeatedly moans, "Dolor, dolor, dolor." Dolor in Spanish means pain.

"Mamma mia!" expresses what?

An older Navajo Indian woman who speaks broken English remains unresponsive verbally or emotionally. Why? This is a cultural response. Unknown individuals are sometimes not recognized for as long as 3 days. Help is not acceptable to many.

A woman having desultory latent phase contractions vehemently states she *is* in labor! Why the vehemence? Maybe she is in labor or maybe her astrologer told her this is the best day for her baby to be born; or maybe her husband thinks he's had enough of her complaining.

The words bowel movement may not be understood by some patients. What words do these patients use for bowel movement?

Value Systems

How do nurses respond emotionally and/or verbally to the following:

A thirty-six-year-old, separated, Appalachian female, now gravida X para IX, on welfare for 16 years, refuses tubal ligation because she desires more children.

> A Jehovah's Witness parturient is found to have a hematocrit of 20 percent and refuses administration of any blood products.
> A Navajo woman refuses to prepare for diagnosed twins.
> An unwed mother is giving the baby up for adoption but requests to feed and care for the infant while in the hospital.
> A married woman plans to give up a legitimate baby for adoption.
> A couple demands to see their anomalous stillborn.
> A mother of five blatantly states she does not want this infant.
> A patient admits to an attempted criminal abortion early in this pregnancy.

The preceding situations involve logical responses by these women or parents in relation to their culture, knowledge, or judgment. In the Navajo culture, twins are considered very bad luck. This mother responds by disowning both or caring for only one. The woman who does not want her sixth child may be totally unable to care for this added burden, while the mother of ten may find childbearing her primary gratification in life. Religious stigma can be powerful, as in the case of the Jehovah's Witness who expressed her refusal for a transfusion.

Just as the patient brings her own background of experiences, her self-image, and concepts to the labor experience, so the nurse brings an entire range and background of experiences, concepts, and self-image. Within these limits, each interacts with the other. Expectations of behavior on the part of the nurse or patient and the perceptions involved in the responses of the other will influence how the patient will respond to the stress of labor and how the nurse will in turn respond to the patient and her actions.

The family of the patient, when present, will influence the patient's experience and response in either a positive or negative manner. It is one of the responsibilities of the nurse to detect the strengths and weaknesses in familial relationships and utilize them to the best advantage for the patient.

Nurses are not asked to change their value systems, but to be aware of the infinite combinations in the value systems of others. It is much easier to understand these differences if the reasons for them can be understood. Thus, the nurse in an intrapartum area should be familiar with the value systems and beliefs of subgroups within the community.

The Difficult Patient

A mother of two, with no prenatal care, is admitted at 32 weeks' gestation with severe toxemia. She is told, "You deserve the mess you're in. If you'd come to clinic it wouldn't have happened." Frustration and conflict arise here, since toxemia is treatable, and the inherent problems can often be controlled, but not without care.

A terrified teen-ager in very early latent phase screams with every contraction and sobs without control between them, calling constantly for her mother. She is told by the frustrated nurse, "If you are old enough to get pregnant, you are old enough to go through labor without all this fuss." A value judgment. Guilt for some is handled through suffering. Where is her mother? Could she come? Could she help her daughter? Can the nurse help as a substitute?

A very anxious, tense patient screams out of control during transition and refuses all attempts of support. She is told, "You certainly are not co-operating very well." She breaks into tears, further frustrating the staff. Screaming may reduce the tension, fear, and loneliness experienced at this time. Stay with her, encourage her on the good job she is doing. Concentrate on the positive aspects of her behavior. They are there if the nurse looks for them.

The apparently uncooperative, screaming woman sets our nerves on edge and can render us incapable of dealing constructively with the situation. Puni-tive behavior, while recognized as an immature method of handling our own frustrations, may seem to be the action of choice at a given moment. This is not so. A much better solution is:

1 Try to remove yourself from the situation until you yourself are under control—take time to think.
2 Ask yourself: What is this patient trying to tell me? Screaming and crying are forms of communication frequently expressed as a result of intense frustration, disappointment, fear, or any combinations of these. Likewise, the normal patient has a need to vent and to be heard.
3 Ask yourself: What do I know about this patient? What have I ob-served about her which would lead me to think she might be frus-trated, disappointed, or afraid? List the possible reasons.
4 What processes of labor might cause these problems?
  Fear of not understanding what is happening.
  Fear of being alone.
  Frustration because she's not doing or is unable to do what she thinks she ought to do.
  Frustration because she feels she's not understood and is unable to express herself.
  Frustration because several different people have told her differing stories about what's happening.
  Disappointment because she has not delivered yet while others have come and gone.
5 Ask yourself: Does she really want to scream and cry? Usually not, if she can help it. She would rather remain in control of herself and cope in a more socially and emotionally acceptable manner.
6 Therefore, any effort we make to help this woman gain or regain con-trol is usually very much appreciated. Likewise, honest efforts to ac-

cept patient behavior signifies understanding and is equally appreciated.

7 Plan:

 a Verbalize acceptance of the patient as a person, and nonverbally express acceptance by hand contact to hand or shoulder with a smile: "It's O.K."

 b Confront her with a known fact or observed behavior such as: "You appear tense and uncomfortable" or "I wonder if you're really very afraid."

 c Plan to wait and listen. The spoken truth may open the door to truths your patient has been unable to express. Fears of a dead or malformed baby, being "cut open," and dying are not uncommon during the very active phase of labor. Fear of being left alone compounds the problem. Verbalization of these fears may be impossible.

 d Plan to help her with any nursing technique you consider might be helpful, such as breathing or a backrub.

 e Evaluate your results.

 f Plan to remain with her or tell her when you leave, when you expect to return, and how she can call for you.

The Nurse's Role

To the young or inexperienced nurse, the labor and delivery area may pose a very real threat. Often the anxiety level is so great that the nurse is unable to function effectively. The experienced nurse finds this exciting area a challenge. This nurse is secure with knowledge of the labor process and is often very capable in dealing with the needs of parturients and their families. This nurse can anticipate the outcome of a situation and will be prepared to handle it. Such security is gained through a combination of textbook knowledge and experience. Nursing judgments are made on a basis of scientific knowledge and principles and previous experience with heavy reliance on scientific principles.

Although all nurses should understand the basic principles of labor and delivery, not everyone will enjoy working in this area. The better prepared nurses are to cope with presenting situations, the more they can enjoy the responsibilities and inherent rewards. It is recommended that nurses read information on labor and delivery, nursing during labor, and drug administration during labor and delivery. The information on nursing care and support during labor in *Family-centered Maternity Nursing* by Ernestine Wiedenbach is especially recommended as a background to functioning in the labor and delivery area. Nurses should become very familiar with the labor and delivery unit in which they work, the mechanics of the unit, what procedures are done and how, where things are stored, and how laboratory work is accomplished. Know the total charting system well. In this way, frustration levels are reduced. Nurses are then more able to interact with the laboring woman. Listen to the patient and then listen some more. Do remember to encourage her during and following contractions.

MISCELLANEOUS NURSING TIPS

Nurses should not talk to or expect the patient to talk during a contraction. Turn off glaring overhead lights when not needed. Untuck the top covers to give the patient freedom to move her feet. Leave the emesis basin out so she can get it quickly if sudden, overwhelming nausea strikes in the nurse's absence. Pin or clip the call bell securely to the bottom sheet within easy reach. Keep the perineal area as clean and dry as possible to prevent contamination of the vagina by rectal bacteria. A clean, dry perineum also makes the patient more comfortable. It is better not to use a peri-pad unless it is merely laid under her, since the patient's activity may dislodge it and provide the contamination the health team is trying to avoid. Change underpads often enough to keep the patient dry. Ice chips, when permitted, are appreciated. Antichapping lipsticks, petroleum jelly, or other sturdy ointment will reduce dry lip discomforts.

It is not statistically true that the woman laboring with the breech presenting may expect a hard labor. However, she may experience a somewhat harder delivery of the after-coming head. A head under the ribs causes more discomfort which can be alleviated by raising the backrest. Meconium staining of the amniotic fluid is expected with breech presentations. Prolapse of the cord between irregular boundaries of the fetal legs is more common. The nurse must be alert to this. A presenting foot moves up and down and can give an incessant urge to push. But the woman must *not* push. Although the smaller extremities and buttocks may come through a partially dilated cervix, the head will not. She must understand the problem and cooperate fully if she is to deliver a live infant. Fortunately, this is a rare problem. The fetal heart rate usually will be heard high, at the umbilicus or perhaps above. Compression of the fetal head during a contraction does slow the rate which, again, usually returns to normal in 30 seconds.

Multiple pregnancies may go undiagnosed until after the fact. If in premature labor, the woman may be very much concerned about the chances of survival, cost of care, anomalies, etc. These labors may be somewhat longer but not necessarily harder. Incidentally, picking up two separate heartbeats is really difficult unless a Doppler device is used, and even then, this may not be 100 percent accurate.

This is a good time to explore a misconception women have regarding hard labor versus long labor. A long labor to women often means a hard labor. The length of labor does not define the frequency, duration, or intensity of contractions for a given labor. A labor may be longer because the contractions are farther apart and milder. Likewise, a short labor may be really hard when relentless hard contractions keep pounding away.

THE NURSE'S "BAG OF TRICKS"

The "bag of tricks" which are carried around by experienced nurses frequently are not learned in textbooks. Neither are most of these tricks documented by research, but they frequently work. Let us explore a few.

Cold Feet

Cold feet frequently go unnoticed, even by the patient. The nurse should feel the woman's feet. She may feel hot, yet her feet are cold. Warm them, wrap them in a warm bath blanket, and notice how the patient becomes more relaxed. Warming the feet may also help relieve or prevent leg cramps or the "shakes" frequently encountered during transition.

The Bedding

Plastic-covered pillows and mattresses are uncomfortable for patients. They are hot. Labor is hard work, and the patient is often overheated. Extra bedding between the patient and the plastic helps. A tepid sponge bath may help. This need not be a big procedure, but can be done lightly and quickly.

If the hospital supplies two or more pillows to each labor bed, this is fortunate. Extra pillows can be of immeasurable comfort to the laboring woman in helping her to find a comfortable position by supporting the back, abdomen, or leg(s). She may wish to lie on her stomach, and the pillows can then be used to take the weight off her uterus by being positioned under her hips and breasts.

Positioning

In many labor rooms, women lie flat on their backs to accommodate nursing and medical care. Most laboring women seem to be more comfortable in some other position. The parturient may wish (1) the backrest higher or lower or a pillow under the knees, (2) to be turned on one side or the other with or without the backrest up, (3) to sit on the side of the bed or in a chair, (4) to be up walking for a period, or (5) to be on "all fours," on her hands and knees, in bed to facilitate pelvic rocking. The last position might be accomplished on the floor if appropriate padding and protection is placed on the floor for the patient to kneel on.

If the woman wishes to be up walking, and the membranes are ruptured, she may do so only if the presenting part fits snugly in the pelvis and is well applied against the cervix. Otherwise, a prolapsed cord may result.

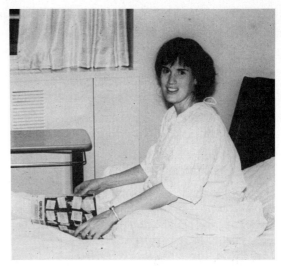

FIGURE 22-13
At any time during labor, the patient may relax in any way most comfortable to her.

FIGURE 22-14
Being out of bed and walking about may be helpful to the patient, both in terms of comfort and in terms of stimulating the onset of active phase. Even with ruptured membranes, the patient may be allowed up, providing the presenting part is engaged and well applied to the cervix.

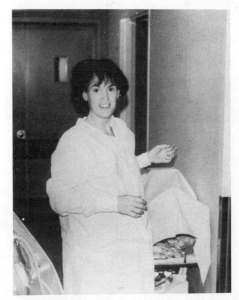

The patient may have had a rectal or vaginal examination, had the fetal heart rate checked or a fetal monitoring device attached, and then may have been left flat on her back, where she dutifully remains. Such a position may be actively hazardous if this patient suffers from the supine hypotension syndrome. In such a case she *must* sit up or turn on her side, or her blood pressure will drop ominously and she will become unconscious and go into shock. (For a more detailed discussion, see Hellman and Pritchard, *Williams Obstetrics*, pp. 259 and 452.)

Backaches and Backrubs

Backache during pregnancy is common; it can be devastating during labor. Most frequently this is a mechanical problem; a relationship between the mother's anatomical structures and the presenting part, often the head with the occiput in one of the posterior positions. During labor contractions, the stretch of the uterosacral ligaments increases the stress. Counterpressure (backrub) and counterstretch of opposing muscles and ligaments (pelvic rocking) can give fantastic relief. Likewise, heat or occasionally cool applications, or standing in a warm or hot shower will relieve the discomfort. While in the shower, the patient should have a metal chair against which to lean or on which to sit. The nurse should remain very close, as progress can occur rapidly. Side positions, an elevated backrest, sitting, or standing and leaning on a suitable solid object such as a bed or chair may help, especially during a contraction. Side lying positions may require upper knee elevation to take the pressure off the symphysis. A pillow or a folded sheet or bath blanket may be used for this purpose. Position changes are good both from a comfort standpoint as well as for consideration of circulatory dynamics.

There are as many ways to give a backrub as there are people to give them. By the process of trial-and-error, the most suitable method for a given mother will be found. Light, moderate, or firm pressure or rubbing over a smaller or larger area using the fingertips or palms may be discontinued at the end of a contraction or may be continued for a few seconds to a minute.

The patient should be instructed to inform the nurse what feels best, where, when, and for how long.

Breathing Techniques

Breathing techniques help the expectant mother keep her mind on something other than her contractions as well as providing anatomical and physiological aid to labor. Any method or combination of methods which provide these and help her to remain relaxed and in control of herself are appropriate. The nurse has the need to show and tell, but it is better to watch and listen first, not through just one contraction, but several, and then evaluate what is hap-

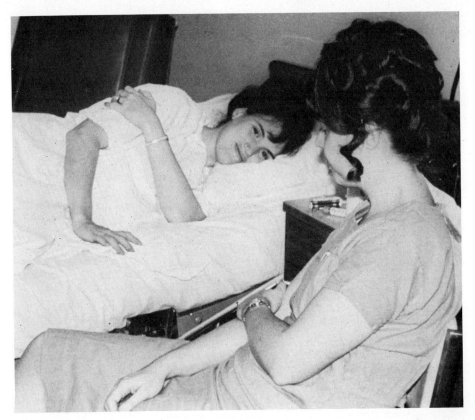

FIGURE 22-15
The nurse is simply sitting with the patient in latent phase. She is comfortable, sitting quietly, and does not feel she must carry on conversation. Her presence is reassurance enough at this time.

pening and make appropriate suggestions, one at a time. Build on the patient's strengths and change only what is not working. Nurses should stay at the bedsides of women in labor.

COMFORT AND POSITIONS OF THE PASSENGER

In many instances, the position of the presenting part, usually the occiput with vertex presenting, can be determined by observing the positions the patient chooses, the location of maximum discomfort, and the contraction pattern. Since internal rotation of the presenting part is one of the mechanisms of labor, some changes are expected in location of maximum discomfort, positions, and contraction patterns. Watch for them.

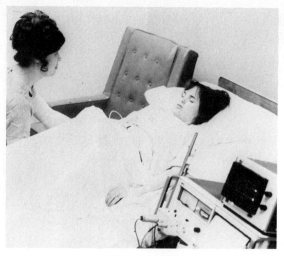

FIGURE 22-16
As active phase progresses, the nurse must frequently coach the patient with each contraction to
relax completely, to utilize the breathing techniques,
and to be encouraged regarding the progress she
is making.

Anterior Positions of the Passenger

The patient who chooses to lie on her back with the backrest elevated
slightly, who states her primary discomfort is over the symphysis down into
the groin area, and who has contractions which are equally long and strong
probably has the occiput in one of the anterior positions. Abdominal breath-

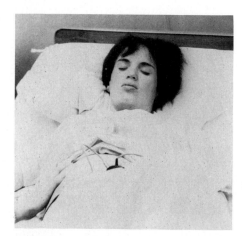

FIGURE 22-17
Between contractions in the transition
phase, complete relaxation is imperative.
Medication may be needed to assist this
relaxation. During contractions, the patient
is seldom completely relaxed unless under
the influence of local blocking.

ing often gives good relief during the contraction. Gently "lifting and holding" the uterus at the level of or just below the umbilicus can be helpful.

Posterior Positions of the Passenger

The woman who cannot lie on her back, complains of severe backache during contractions, and has a contraction pattern of one longer, stronger contraction and one or two shorter, milder contractions may have the vertex presenting in one of the posterior positions. Chest or costal breathing seems to be more beneficial here. It is statistically true that posterior labors are slightly longer, although not necessarily harder.

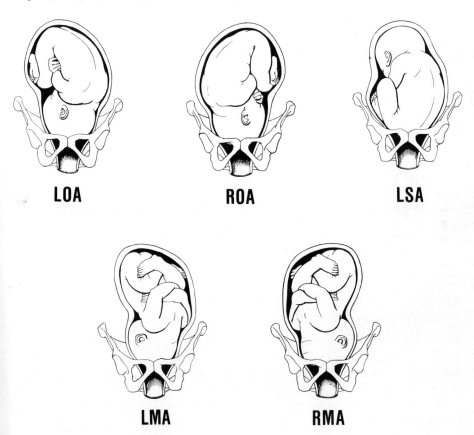

FIGURE 22-18
Fetus in anterior positions: LOA, ROA, LSA, LMA, RMA.
(Used with permission from Ross Clinical Education Aid # 18, Ross Laboratories, Publisher.)

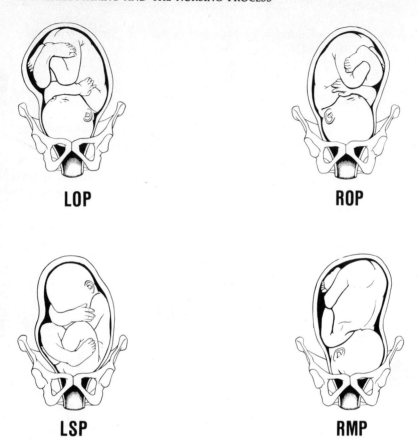

LOP **ROP**

LSP **RMP**

FIGURE 22-19
Fetus in some of the posterior positions: LOP, ROP, LSP, RMP.
(Used with permission from Ross Clinical Education Aid #18, Ross Laboratories, Publisher.)

Transverse Positions of the Passenger

When the vertex is in the occiput transverse position (not transverse lie), the mother is often more restless. She may roll back and forth with equal discomfort in back and in front. She cannot find a most comfortable position. She should be allowed to roll and move. This is her only comfort. The contraction pattern may be a combination of those discussed in the two previous paragraphs.

Assisting Progress

When the vertex is in either a posterior or transverse position, many obstetric nurses believe faster, better progress is made if the patient will lie on the

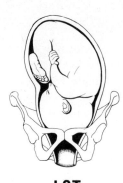 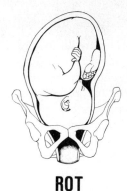

LOT   **ROT**

FIGURE 22-20
Fetus in some transverse positions: LOT, ROT.
*(Used with permission from Ross Clinical Education Aid # 18, Ross
Laboratories, Publisher.)*

side opposite the infant's back. Since the vertex usually rotates spontaneously
to an anterior position prior to birth, this side position may allow the normal
rotation to occur more quickly and easily. Another interesting observation
can be made: If the infant's back is on the maternal right side, the chances
of the vertex rotating to the posterior and then to the anterior are very good,
while with the back on the left side, the vertex often remains in the anterior
position.

Use of Medications

An increasing number of mothers- and fathers-to-be are attending preparation for childbirth classes. Medications are always discussed. In a few instances use of any medication during labor is strongly discouraged. Labor is
physically and emotionally very hard work. Any athlete can tell you that
excessive physical output may render him so physically exhausted as to make
complete and continued relaxation impossible. An example is the night tosser
who is too tired to sleep soundly. The body makes a desperate effort to relax
overtired muscles. Countercontraction and relaxation of muscles are accomplished as he thrashes about in bed. The laboring woman, particularly a
primigravida, may reach this point. Small amounts of appropriate medication
can assist the labor process, not hinder it. Whatever assists a smooth, normal
labor should also assure a more lively and vigorous infant. When known, the
patient's desires for or against administration of medication should be considered.

Fathers in Labor and Delivery

The trend toward father participation is steadily growing. Although some physicians and institutions hold steadfastly to the "no visitors" rule in labor rooms or no admission of husbands or male friends to the delivery room, others are adapting to changing times. Rooming-in is more available. More parents are saying, "We wish to participate together"—this is not an abnormal request. Considerable experience with fathers in attendance at delivery both in the home and in the hospital has been shared by the authors. An inebriated or psychotic man does not belong in the delivery room. Nor does the man belong in the delivery room who does not wish to be there. This leaves the majority, whose concern for their wives or women friends is real, and the support they provide is frequently superhuman. They share the greatest mystery of life, the birth of their infant.

Nourishment during Labor

It is inconceivable that such hard work should be expected to be accomplished without nourishment. Readily absorbable carbohydrates are the best choice, either orally, by intravenous fluids, or both. Fruit juice can cause gas pains. Hard candy or honey is usually well tolerated if permitted.

The "Shakes"

Uncontrollable shaking of the legs during the transition period and into the second stage can disrupt a woman's coping ability. The exact cause is unknown. (See Chapter 25 for a more detailed discussion of theories of the causes). Warm feet and legs seem to relieve the problem in many cases, as will stretching the legs out between contractions. Application of counterpressure to the feet of a straight leg upward or upon the flexed knees downward may help. *Be forewarned, it is hard work.* Shaking of the legs should not be confused with chilling in which some of the same signs are in evidence.

A Warning

Nurses who work in the labor and delivery area should be aware of the woman who says, "Don't touch me! Leave me alone. Get out!" Normally, this is an expression heard during the transition phase when the laboring woman desperately wants someone with her, not to bother her but to assure her that she is doing well. She may very well have a claustrophobic sensation that there is no escape, the walls are closing in, and that there is no place she can go. *Do not leave her alone.*

Pushing

A problem occasionally complicates progress of labor at 7 to 9+ cm dilatation which requires the extreme efforts of nurse and patient. No woman should be allowed to push until the cervix is *completely* dilated, not even at 9+ cm. Nurses and doctors often refer to the patient at this time as having an anterior lip remaining. This anterior lip may well be impinged under the symphysis, and it will become edematous if the patient pushes. It then requires more time to become retracted.

At this time the presenting part may have descended sufficiently to give enough pressure to cause a "need-to-push" sensation. Actually, a bulging amniotic sac can cause the same sensation. The patient must understand why she is not to push and be continuously encouraged to breathe, pant, or blow in any way she can during these contractions. The patient must not push. The more she is able to keep from pushing now, the more quickly the cervix will retract over the fetal head. Second stage will then begin and she can do what comes so naturally—push.

The Possible Precipitator

Everyone is concerned about the patient, usually a multigravida or grand multipara, who is expected to deliver her baby very rapidly.

This is a justifiable concern. The deceleration phase may be bypassed as the occiput descends and the cervix goes from 5 to 8 cm to 10 cm in one contraction. When this happens, the baby is frequently born with the next contraction. An astute observation of the abdomen here may provide a very valuable clue. Often the uterus appears to be riding to one or the other side of the abdomen. The baby will not be born with the uterus in this position. The uterus, prior to delivery, comes to the midline and stays there. Cervical dilatation may or may not provide a clue here. A baby is soon to arrive!

BIBLIOGRAPHY

N*l*S

Alexander, L.: "Rectals and Vaginals: The OB Nurse's Job?" *RN*, 29:39, February 1966.

Assumpta, Sister H. M.: "Abdominal Decompression during Labor," *Canadian Nurse*, 57:1132, December 1961.

Auerbach, Aline B.: "Meeting the Needs of New Mothers," *Children*, 2:223–228, November–December 1954.

Ball, H.: "Relieving Pain in Labour," *Nursing Times*, 61:638, May 7, 1965.

Barkla, P. C.: "New Concepts in the Management of Labour," *Midwives Chronicle*, 82:82, March 1969.

Beard, R. W., et al.: "Supine Hypotension Syndrome," *British Medical Journal*, 1:297, May 2, 1970.

Beazley, J.: "Labour Pain—How Much Are Midwives to Blame?" *Nursing Mirror*, 127:19, November 1, 1968.

Bejec, D. C.: "Natural Childbirth," *Philippine Journal of Nursing*, 36:111, March–April 1967.

Bender B.: "A Test of the Effect of Nursing Support on Mothers in Labor," *ANA Regional Clinical Conference*, p. 171, 1967.

———: "Taking the Drip out of Pitocin," *Nursing Mirror*, 121:188, October 22, 1965.

Benedek, Theresa: "Psychobiological Aspects of Mothering," *American Journal of Orthopsychiatry*, 26:272–278, April 1956.

Bergin, M. A.: "Monitoring the Fetal Heart," *Nursing Clinics of North America*, 1:559, December 1966.

Bethea, D. C.: "The Effect of the Shave on Infections in Maternity Patients," *Nursing Research*, 12:103, Spring 1963.

Bonica, J. J.: "Obstetric Analgesia and Anesthesia: Recent Trends and Advances," *New York Journal of Medicine*, 70:7079–7084, August 15, 1970.

———: *Principles and Practice of Obstetric Analgesia and Anesthesia*, Davis, Philadelphia, 1967.

———: *The Management of Pain*, Lea & Febiger, Philadephia, 1953.

Bradley, Robert: *Husband-coached Childbirth*, New York, Harper & Row, 1965.

Burnett, C. W. F.: "Foetal Distress during Labor," *Nursing Times*, 65:1579–1581, December 11, 1969.

———: "Obstetric Nursing Syllabus. The Female Reproductive Organs and the Breasts, Part 1," *Nursing Times*, 58:256, March 2, 1962.

———: "Obstetric Nursing Syllabus. Normal Pregnancy, Part 2," *Nursing Times*, 58:297, March 9, 1962.

———: "Obstetric Nursing Syllabus. Normal Labour, Part 3," *Nursing Times*, 58:331, March 16, 1962.

———: "Obstetric Nursing Syllabus. Normal Labour: Its Management, Part 4," *Nursing Times*, 58:363, March 23, 1962.

———: "Prolonged First Stage of Labour," *Nursing Times*, 65:1553, December 4, 1969.

Buxton, C. L.: "Breathing in Labour, the Influence of Psychoprophylaxis," *Nursing Mirror*, 120:viii, June 18, 1965.

Caldeyro-Barcia, R., et al.: "Diagnostic and Prognostic Significance of Intrapartum Fetal Tachycardia and Type II Dips," paper presented at the Symposium on Prenatal Life, sponsored by the Departments of Gynecology and Obstetrics, Harper Hospital and Wayne State University School of Medicine, November 1–2, 1967.

———, C. Mendez-Bauer, J. J. Poseiro, L. A. Escalona, S. V. Pose, J. Bieniarz, I. E. Arnt, L. Gulin, and O. Althabe: "Control of Human Fetal Heart

Rate during Labor" in D. E. Cassells (ed), *The Heart and Circulation in the Newborn and Infant*, Grune & Stratton, New York, 1966.

Cameron, S.: "The Nurse's Role in the First Stage of Labor," *Practical Nurse*, 14:30, January 1965.

————: "Support in First Stage of Labor," *Hospital Topics*, 43:99, September 1965.

————: "Supportive Care," *Canadian Nurse*, 61:26, January 1965.

Caplan, Gerald: *An Approach to Community Mental Health*, Grune & Stratton, New York, 1961.

————: *Concepts of Mental Health and Consultation*, Children's Bureau Publication no. 373, Washington, D. C., 1959.

————: "Psychological Aspects of Maternity Care," *American Journal of Public Health*, 47:25–31, January 1957.

————: "The Mental Hygiene Role of the Nurse in Maternal Child Care," *Nursing Outlook*, 2:14–19, January 1954.

Chalmers, J. A.: "New Concepts in the Management of Labour," *Nursing Mirror*, 127:20, November 22, 1968.

Clark, J.: "It's Different on the Receiving End," *Nursing Mirror*, 129:30, October 3, 1969.

Clark, R. B., et al.: "Neonatal Acid-Base Studies I. Effect of Normal Labor and Obstetric Manipulation," *Obstetrics and Gynecology*, 33:23–29, January 1969.

————: "Neonatal Acid-Base Studies II. Effect of a Heavy Medication–Narcotic Antagonists Regimen for Labor and Delivery," *Obstetrics and Gynecology*, 33:30–34, January 1969.

Clemence, Sister M.: "Existentialism: A Philosophy of Commitment," *American Journal of Nursing*, pp. 590–605, March 1966.

Cohen, S. N.: "Drugs That Depress the Newborn Infant," *Pediatric Clinics of North America*, 17:835–850, November 1970.

Corbin, Hazel: "Childbirth without Fear," *American Journal of Nursing*, pp. 392–393, June 1947.

Crawford, M. I.: "Physiological and Behavioral Cues to Disturbances in Childbirth," *Bulletin of the American College of Nurse Midwifery*, 14:13, February 1969.

Crowther, A. N.: "The Mystery of the Early-morning Stork. Circadian Rhythms in Childbirth," *Nursing Times*, 63:347, March 17, 1967.

Dalgarno, Imokel: "Psychoprophylaxis in Midwifery," *Nursing Mirror*, 118:571, September 25, 1964.

DeLee, S. T., and J. J. Duncan: "Training for Natural Childbirth," *American Journal of Nursing*, pp. 660–662, October 1949.

"Delivery Room Spectators and the Law," *Regan Report on Nursing and the Law*, 8:1, March 1968.

Denny, Frank: "The Dangerous Third Stage," *Nursing Mirror*, 118:9, April 3, 1964.

Dicker, K.: "Husbands in the Labour Room," *Nursing Journal of India*, 60:263, August 1969.

————: "Husbands in the Labour Ward," *Nursing Times*, 65:416, March 27, 1969.

Dick-Read, Grantly: *Childbirth without Fear*, Harper, New York, 1953.

————: *Introduction to Motherhood*, Harper, New York, 1950.

Dillabough, A. M., and E. L. Rosen: " 'Epidurals' Are Here to Stay," *Canadian Nurse*, 66:34, October 1970.

"Distended Urinary Bladder Impeding Passage of the Fetal Head," *Journal of Mt. Sinai Hospital*, 36:156–158, March–April 1969.

"Drugs in Normal Labour," *Drug Therapy Bulletin*, 5:75–76, September 15, 1967.

Dumoulin, J. G.: "Breech Delivery," *Nursing Times*, 67:825–827, July 8, 1971.

Dwyer, J. M., and W. A. Lynch: "Nursing Responsibility for Decreasing Maternal and Perinatal Mortality and Morbidity, Intrapartal Management, Part 2," *Hospital Progress*, 48:66, January 1967.

Estey, G. T.: "Natural Childbirth—Word from a Mother," *American Journal of Nursing*, 69:1453, July 1969.

Fairs, P. J.: "Relieving Pain and Discomfort in Labour, The Role of the Midwife," *Nursing Times*, 62:599, May 6, 1966.

Farill, M. S.: "Adolescent in Labor," *American Journal of Nursing*, 68:1952–1954, September 1968.

Fell, M. R.: "Induction of Labour," *Nursing Mirror*, 122:35, April 8, 1966.

————: "Prolonged Labour," *Nursing Mirror*, 126:29, March 22, 1968.

Fenton, A. N., and C. M. Steer: "Fetal Distress," *Hospital Medicine*, 1:34, October 1965.

Fitzpatrick, Elise, Sharon R. Reeder, and Luigi Mastroianni: *Maternity Nursing*, 12th ed., Lippincott, Philadelphia, 1971.

Forbes, R.: "Psychoprophylaxis," *District Nurse*, 10:74, July 1967.

Foulkes, J. F.: "Drugs Ancient and Modern in Obstetric Practice," *Midwives Chronicle*, 83:288, September 1970.

Friedman, E. A.: "An Objective Method of Evaluating Labor," *Hospital Practice*, 5:82, July 1970.

————: *Labor: Clinical Evaluation and Management*, Appleton-Century-Crofts, New York, 1967.

————: "The Functional Divisions of Labor," *American Journal of Obstetrics and Gynecology*, 104:274–280, January 15, 1971.

————: "Use of Labor Pattern as a Management Guide," *Hospital Topics*, 46:51–59, August 1968.

————, and M. R. Sachtleben: "Station of the Fetal Presenting Part: III, Interrelationship with Cervical Dilatation," *American Journal of Obstetrics and Gynecology*, 93:537, October 15, 1965.

————: "Station of the Fetal Presenting Part: II, Effect on the Course of

Labor," *American Journal of Obstetrics and Gynecology*, 93:530, October 15, 1965.

————: "Station of the Fetal Presenting Part: I, Pattern of Descent," *American Journal of Obstetrics and Gynecology*, 93:522, October 15, 1965.

————: "Station of the Fetal Presenting Part: V, Protracted Descent Patterns," *American Journal of Obstetrics and Gynecology*, 36:558, October 1970.

————: "Station of the Fetal Presenting Part: IV, Slope of Descent," *American Journal of Obstetrics and Gynecology*, 107:1031, August 15, 1970.

————, et al.: "Computer Analysis of Labor Progression," *Journal of Obstetrics and Gynaecology of the British Commonwealth*, 76:1075–1079, December 1969.

Garrey, M. M., A. D. T. Govar, C. H. Hodge, and R. Callender: *Obstetrics Illustrated*, Williams & Wilkins, Baltimore, 1969.

Gebhard, Paul H., et al.: *Pregnancy, Birth, and Abortion*, Hoeber, New York, 1958.

Gelb, Barbara: *The ABC's of Natural Childbirth*, Norton, New York, 1954.

Goetsch, C.: "Fathers in the Delivery Room—Helpful and Supportive," *Hospital Topics*, 44:104, January 1966.

Goodlin, R. C.: "Intrapartum Fetal Heart Rate Responses and Plethysmographic Pulse," *American Journal of Obstetrics and Gynecology*, 110:210–226, May 15, 1971.

Goodman, R. R.: "Psychological Support in Labor: A Supervisor's Views," *Hospital Topics*, 42:99, August 1964.

Goodrich, Frederick: *Natural Childbirth*, Prentice-Hall, Englewood Cliffs, New Jersey, 1957.

Graham, W. E.: "Routine Vaginal Examination of the Intrapartum Patient," *Journal of the Indiana Medical Association*, 61:610–611, May 1968.

Greenhill, J. P.: *Obstetrics*, 13th ed., Saunders, Philadelphia, 1965.

Hammacher, K.: "Diagnosis of Fetal Distress by Means of Cardiotocography (CTG)," Vth World Congress of Gynaecologists and Obstetricians, September 23–30, 1967, Sydney, Australia, Butterworth, 1967.

————: "The Clinical Significance of Cardiotocography," paper presented at the European Congress of Perinatal Medicine, March 28–30, 1968, Theine, Italy.

————: "The Diagnosis of Fetal Distress with an Electronic Fetal Heart Monitor," in *Intrauterine Dangers to the Foetus*, report of the Symposium, Prague, October 12–14, 1966, *Excerpta Medical Monographs*, Amsterdam.

————, et al.: "Foetal Heart Frequency and Perinatal Condition of the Foetus and Newborn," *Gynaecologia*, Karger, Basel, p. 349, 1968.

Harrison, G.: "Recent Advances in Obstetric Analgesia, Part 1," *Nursing Mirror*, 118:155, May 22, 1964.

Hellman, Louis, and Jack Pritchard (eds.): *Williams Obstetrics*, 14th ed., Appleton-Century-Crofts, New York, 1971.

Hendricks, C. H., et al.: "Normal Cervical Dilatation Pattern in Late Pregnancy and Labor," *American Journal of Obstetrics and Gynecology*, 106:1065–1082, April 1, 1970.

Hershey, M.: "Legal Side of Medical-Moral Issues," *American Journal of Nursing*, p. 103, June 1962.

Hoff, F. L.: "Natural Childbirth—How Any Nurse Can Help," *American Journal of Nursing*, 69:1451, July 1969.

Hommel, F.: "Natural Childbirth—Nurse in Private Practice as Monitrice," *American Journal of Nursing*, 69:1446, July 1969.

Hon, E. H.: "The Human Fetal Circulation in Normal Labor," in D. E. Cassells (ed.), *The Heart and Circulation in the Newborn and Infant*, Grune & Stratton, New York, 1966.

———: *An Introduction to Fetal Heart Rate Monitoring*, Harty, New Haven, 1969.

———, and R. H. Paul: *A Primer of Fetal Heart Rate Patterns*, Harty, New Haven, 1970.

Iorio, H.: "Effective Support during Labor and Delivery," *RN*, 25:70–74, February 1962.

Jackson, R. J. A.: "Prevention of Prolonged Labour," *Nursing Times*, 65:1331, October 16, 1969.

Jouppila, P.: "Faecal Impaction Preventing Engagement of the Fetal Head," *Annales Chirurgiae et Gynaecologie Fenniae*, 60:92–94, 1971.

Juzwiak, M., "A Common Sense Approach to Labor and Delivery," *RN*, 27:53, August 1964.

———: "An Intimate Look at Husband-coached Childbirth," *RN*, 29:45, December 1966.

Kantor, Hiekel: "To Shave or Not to Shave?" *Canadian Nurse*, 61:368, May 1965.

Karmel, Marjorie: *Thank You, Dr. Lamaze*, Lippincott, Philadelphia, 1959.

Kemp, S.: "The Dignity of Labour," *Nursing Times*, 66:1436, November 5, 1970.

Kreul, W.: "Mother and Child—Labor and Analgesia," *Wisconsin Medical Journal*, 68:170, February 1969.

Laine, J.: "Experience of the Use of Intranasal, Buccal and Intravenous Oxytocin as Methods of Inducing Labour," *Acta Obstetrica et Gynecologica Scandinavica*, 49:149–159, 1970.

Ledger, W. J.: "Graphic Analysis: An Aid in the Early Recognition of Abnormal Labors," *University of Michigan Medical Center Journal*, 33:266–269, November–December 1967.

Litz, A. W.: "Natural Childbirth," *Bulletin of the American College of Nurse Midwifery*, 13:28, February 1968.

Lorincz, A. B.: "Danger Signs in the First Stage of Labor," *Hospital Medicine*, 6:115, September 1970.

Lowenstein, A., et al.: "Digital Rotation of the Vertex," *Obstetrics and Gynecology*, 37:790–791, May 1971.

McCabe, Inga: "Natural Childbirth—A 'Most Thrilling Experience'" (pictorial), *RN*, 32:40, April 1969.

McKay, R.: "Obstetrics for Student Nurses. The Female Reproductive Organs and the Breasts. Part 1," *Nursing Mirror*, 115:i, December 14, 1962.

————: "Obstetrics for Student Nurses. Physiology and Management of Normal Pregnancy. Part 2," *Nursing Mirror*, 115:v, December 21, 1962.

————: "Obstetrics for Student Nurses. Physiology, Mechanism and Management of Normal Labour, Part 3a," *Nursing Mirror*, 115:v, December 28, 1962.

McLaren, J. B.: "Maternal Respiration in Labour," *Midwives Chronicle*, 83:112, April 1970.

Matousek, I.: "Fetal Nursing during Labor," *Nursing Clinics of North America*, 3:307, June 1968.

Matthews, A. E. B.: "Drugs in the First Stage of Labour," *Nursing Times*, 63:648, May 1967.

————: "Reflections on the Pain of Labour," *Nursing Mirror*, 118:550, September 18, 1964.

Mendez-Bauer, C., et al.: "Relationship between Blood pH and Heart Rate in the Human Fetus during Labor," *American Journal of Obstetrics and Gynecology*, vol. 97, February 15, 1967.

Milic, A. M. B., and K. Adamsons: "Fetal Blood Sampling," *American Journal of Nursing*, 68:2149, October 1968.

Miller, J. S.: "Return the Joy of Home Delivery with Fathers in the Delivery Room," *Hospital Topics*, 44:105, January 1966.

Montgomery, E.: "Coping with Pain—Felt or Fancied," *Midwives Chronicle*, 83:248, August 1970.

Moore, J., et al.: "Assessment of Obstetric Analgesic Therapy," *British Journal of Anaesthesia*, 43:772, July 1971.

Morton, J. H.: "Fathers in the Delivery Room—An Opposition Standpoint," *Hospital Topics*, 44:103, January 1966.

Murphy, A., "Natural Childbirth," *American Journal of Nursing*, 56:1298.

Novack, J. A.: "Psychological Support in Labor: A Nursing Educator's Views," *Hospital Topics*, 42:97, August 1964.

"Obstetrical Nursing," *International Nursing Review*, 4:12, January 1957.

O'Driscoll, K., et al.: "Prevention of Prolonged Labour," *British Medical Journal*, 2:477–480, May 24, 1969.

Oxorn, H., and W. Foote: *Human Labor and Birth*, Appleton-Century-Crofts, New York, 1964.

"Paracervical Block in Labour," *British Journal of Anaesthesia*, 42:657, August 1970.

Paynich, M. L.: "Cultural Barriers to Nurse Communication," *American Journal of Nursing*, 64:87–90, 1964.

Pence, P. D.: "A Long Labor," *American Journal of Nursing*, 61:101, August 1961.

Poppers, P. J.: "Overventilation during Labor," *Bulletin of the American College of Nurse Midwifery*, 13:4, May 1968.

Preuedourakis, C. N., et al.: "Bacterial Invasion of Amniotic Cavity during Pregnancy and Labor," *Obstetrics and Gynecology*, 37:459–461, March 1971.

Prigot, A., and C. T. L. Froix: "A Chemical Compound for Hair Removal: Use in Surgical and Obstetrical Patients," *Hospital Topics*, 41:103, February 1963.

Pugh, J. W.: "The Clean Non-Sterile Vaginal Examination in Labor," *North Carolina Medical Journal*, 30:48–53, February 1969.

"Reviewing: Diet, Detoxification, and Toxemia of Pregnancy," *Nutrition Reviews*, 21:269, 1963.

Richardson, Stephen A.: *Childbearing: Its Social and Psychological Aspects*, Williams & Wilkins, Baltimore, 1967.

Rodman, M. F.: "Drugs Used in Labor and Delivery," *RN*, 24:42, May 1961.

Rose, Patricia A.: "The High Risk Mother-Infant Dyad—A Challenge for Nursing?" *Nursing Forum*, 6(1):94–103, 1967.

Rubin, Reva: "Basic Maternal Behavior," *Nursing Outlook*, pp. 683–686, November 1961.

———: "The Family-Child Relationship and Nursing Care," *Nursing Outlook*, 12:36–39, September 1964.

Rutherford, R. N.: "Fathers in the Delivery Room—Long Experience Molds One Viewpoint," *Hospital Topics*, 44:97, January 1966.

Schaefer, G.: "Induction of Labor," *American Journal of Nursing*, 61:89, September 1961.

Schulman, H., et al.: "Variability of Uterine Contractions in Normal Human Parturition," *Obstetrics and Gynecology*, 36:215–221, August 1970.

"Sedation without Depression," *Pulse*, 15:13, no. 1, 1961.

Sheikh, G. N., et al.: "The Duration of Induced Labor," *Journal of Obstetrics and Gynaecology in the British Commonwealth*, 77:1070–1076, December 1970.

Shubeck, F., et al.: "Fetal Hazard after Rupture of the Membranes," *Obstetrics and Gynecology*, 28(1):22–32, July 1966.

Smyth, C. H.: "Foetal Heart Sounds: Their Significance for the Midwife," *Nursing Mirror*, 122:xi, June 3, 1966.

Steer, Charles M.: *Moloy's Evaluation of the Pelvis in Obstetrics*, 2d ed., Saunders, Philadelphia, 1959.

Stenchever, Morton: *Labor: A Workbook in Obstetrics and Gynecology*, Yearbook Medical Publishers, Chicago, 1968.

Surhis, Eleanor Brady: "The Importance of Listening," *Nursing Outlok*, 8(12):686–687, December 1960.

"The Effects of Labour on the Foetus and the Newborn," *Nursing Journal of India*, 57:15, January 1966.

Thoms, Herbert: *Childbirth with Understanding*, Charles C Thomas, Springfield, Ill., 1960.

Thornton, J. A.: "The Relief of Pain in Labour," *Nursing Times*, 61:1128, August 20, 1965.

Tipton, R. W., et al.: "An Index of Fetal Welfare in Labor," *Journal of Obstetrics and Gynaecology of the British Commonwealth*, 78:702–706, August 1971.

Tryon, P. A.: "Assessing the Progress of Labor through Observation of Patients' Behavior," *Nursing Clinics of North America*, 3:315, June 1968.

———: "Use of Comfort Measures as Support during Labor," *Nursing Research*, 15:109, Spring 1966.

Wajdowicz, E. K.: "Abdominal Decompression during Labor," *American Journal of Nursing*, 64:87, December 1964.

Watson, M.: "The Present Position of Pain Relief in Labor, Part 1," *Nursing Mirror*, 116:431, August 16, 1963.

———: "The Present Position of Pain Relief in Labor, Part 2," *Nursing Mirror*, 116:447, August 23, 1963.

Westgate-Smith, S.: "A Normal Confinement—Obstetric Patient Care Study," *Nursing Times*, 60:1136, September 4, 1964.

Wiedenbach, Ernestine: *Clinical Nursing: A Helping Art*, Springer, New York, 1964.

———: *Family-centered Maternity Nursing*, Putnam, New York, 1967.

———: "Family Nurse Practitioner for Maternal and Child Care," *Nursing Outlook*, 13(12):50, December 1965.

———: "Nurse-Midwifery: Purposes, Practice and Opportunity," *Nursing Outlook*, 8(5):256, May 1960.

Williams, B.: "Sleep Needs during the Maternity Cycle," *Nursing Outlook*, 15:53, February 1967.

Willis, T.: "Monitoring the Mother and Fetus during Labor," *Canadian Nurse*, p. 28, December 1970.

Wilson, Miriam: "Effects of Maternal Medications upon the Fetus and the Newborn Infant," *American Journal of Obstetrics and Gynecology*, pp. 818–825, March 15, 1962.

Wingate, M. B.: "Cautionary Obstetric Tales," *Manitoba Medical Review*, 48:188–189, May 1968.

Winkelbauer, R. G.: "Amniotomy: Its Role in Normal Labor," *Journal of the Maine Medical Association*, 62:8–9, January 1971.

Wood, C., et al.: "Fetal Heart Rate and Acid-Base Status in the Assessment of Fetal Hyposia," *American Journal of Obstetrics and Gynecology*, 98:62, 1967.

23 | THE SECOND STAGE OF LABOR

Betty L. Wilkerson

In assessing the woman in labor, the nurse should be keenly aware of the beginning of the second stage. This stage can be measured from the time the cervix is completely dilated until the baby is delivered. It is the period when the baby descends from the uterus through the birth canal and is expelled. The second stage of labor may last only 2 minutes or may take longer than 1 hour.[1]

The second stage includes many observable signs. The uterus changes in shape during the contractions. It becomes longer as a result of stretching of the lower uterine segment, and also because the fetus is lying in a more vertical position. At the same time the uterus is lengthening, it becomes diminished in the transverse and anteroposterior diameters.[2] The uterine contractions become longer, stronger, and more frequent. The woman in labor becomes increasingly anxious; she desires someone with her at all times. If there has not been a bloody show previously, it will now be in evidence as the cervix recedes. If bloody show has continued through labor, it now becomes increased in amount and in redness. This is caused by the rupture of capillaries in the cervix and also possibly from the membranes separating from the decidua in the lower uterine segment. The patient frequently becomes nauseated, with emesis occurring at the time of complete dilatation.[3] If the membranes have not ruptured previously, this may now occur. The patient indicates she has a desire to bear down. She may tell the nurse this, or she may begin to hold her breath and strain in an unconscious effort. She has the sensation of needing to urinate or defecate. A late sign is the characteristic "grunt" during straining or pushing which is readily ascertained and is usually followed closely by flattening of the perineum and rectal bulging.

The nurse or physician may examine the patient to confirm the early signs of the second stage. Depending on the physician and the hospital procedure, the patient may be examined either rectally or vaginally. She should then be transferred *unhurriedly* to the delivery room; "last minute" rushed trips should be avoided. The patient is already apprehensive, and this frantic activity adds greatly to her general uneasiness. The husband's anxiety will also increase at this time, particularly if he will not be coming to the delivery room. The parents-to-be need a brief moment to share words of encouragement, perhaps an embrace. The nurse should, if possible, offer the couple this privacy.

TRANSFER TO DELIVERY ROOM

The ideal time for transferring the patient to the delivery room is when the cervix is dilated 7 to 8 cm for a multipara, and when it is dilated completely for a primigravida. This, of course, varies with the individual patient and depends on how the labor has thus far progressed.

Should the patient have the urge to bear down during the time she is being transferred to the delivery room, the nurse quickly assesses the situation, and if delivery is imminent, the patient is coached to pant until the contraction is over. It is helpful if the nurse demonstrates how to pant by actually panting with the patient. This is done simultaneously with the transfer. When the patient has refrained from pushing and is safely placed on the delivery table, the nurse can truly appreciate how valuable panting has been.

During this period the nurse should create an atmosphere in which the patient develops confidence and trust in those caring for her, an atmosphere in which she feels accepted in her behavior and realizes she is a very special woman.

The nurse can demonstrate caring and enhance this feeling by simply explaining occurring events. The patient may need help in moving from the bed to the delivery table. The bed must be held securely against the delivery table as the patient transfers, otherwise it will roll away as the weight is shifted. She should be told why she needs to "scoot" to the section where the table separates. The stirrups must then be adjusted properly. The patient should draw her legs up, in a bent position at the knees. The nurse places the stirrups at the same height as the patient's knees. The length is also adjusted, according to the patient's leg. The stirrups must also be turned slightly outward, away from the site of delivery. The patient's legs are then "tried" in the stirrups after the adjustments are made to determine if they are properly fitted—and again they may be altered. If the stirrups are adjusted correctly, in height and length, the patient will be more comfortable, cramps in the legs may be prevented, and she will be in the proper position to push against her feet when bearing down during contractions (Figure 23-1). In the event that leg cramps do occur, the nurse straightens the patient's leg, slips one hand under the patient's knee, and then places the other hand against the patient's foot, causing the toes to be bent upward. The leg cramps generally disappear with this prompt action. The nurse should be sure that the stirrups are as comfortable as possible.

Hand bars should also be adjusted, but the wrist cuffs should not be fastened until the patient is cleansed for delivery. The wrist cuffs appear to be one of the most disliked parts of "having a baby." The patient states she "doesn't like being strapped down," or having to "wear handcuffs." There is probably a feeling of being deprived of independence and human dignity. At the time the cuffs are fastened, the patient should be told the reason for them, including the fact that this is to protect her and the baby from infection, since it is easy to forget and touch the sterile drapes.

SETTING PRIORITIES

The nurse in the delivery room has priorities to set. It is necessary to keep the patient as comfortable as possible, monitor fetal heart tones by watching the electronic monitor or by listening with a stethoscope, take the blood pressure, prepare the sterile supplies at the appropriate time, call the anesthetist, or have equipment available for the physician to insert a regional or local anesthetic. The nurse must prepare oxytocic drugs, perhaps watch an intravenous drip rate, prepare identification for the newborn, chart necessary information, assist the physician, monitor contractions by observing the electronic monitor and/or by palpation, and at the same time reassure and supply information to the patient.

The nurse reassures the patient best by talking slowly and exactly into the patient's ear, letting her know that she is progressing well and that her baby will soon be born. The nurse realizes the patient is very introverted at this time, and it is necessary to gain her attention to make her aware of what is going on about her.[4] This usually requires much repetition in helping her understand what is occurring during this stage of labor.

Meanwhile the nurse also assists the patient in bearing down with each contraction. She literally "bears down" with her, by telling her how to breath, how to push, and congratulating her in her endeavor. Although this normally occurs spontaneously when the cervix is completely dilated, the primigravida or the patient who is given a conduction anesthetic particularly may need assistance in this technique. One way to assist the mother is to explain that

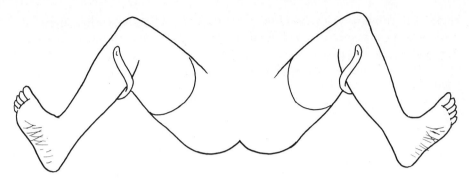

FIGURE 23-1
Stirrup position for delivery.

when the contraction begins, she should take a breath, exhale, then take another breath and hold it; at the same time she pulls back on the hand bars with her elbows flexed as though she were rowing a boat and attempts to bear down. Explain to the patient that she will have the same feeling as though she were passing a constipated stool. The nurse evaluates how the patient is progressing by observing if her neck is resting on her breast. Is she pulling back on the hand bars? Is she holding her breath properly and bearing down? Are her buttocks resting in a downward position? Is the perineum bulging? Is the rectal sphincter dilating? Is the baby's head yet in evidence? It is important that the nurse uses vocabulary the patient will understand during this coaching period.

The nurse must assess the frequency, duration, and intensity of the contractions; it is therefore necessary to palpate the patient's abdomen with the fingertips. By doing this, the nurse will be able to coach the patient to push more effectively during the acme of the contraction. For the best progression toward delivery, the patient should have several productive pushes to each contraction. Between contractions, the nurse assists the patient in relaxing. Comfort measures, such as keeping the perineum clean and dry, moistening the patient's lips, wiping her forehead with a damp cloth, and sometimes a brief backrub or sacral pressure should be used as appropriate.

When the contraction begins, the nurse again explains what to do, repeating the above instructions. It greatly encourages the patient to know she is doing what is expected, and that she is accomplishing the purpose. The patient should *always* be told when the baby's scalp becomes visible. Many delivery rooms have overhead mirrors which the patient may desire to use. She should be given the opportunity to make this decision.

During this stage of labor, the baby is flexing his head upon his chest for more room to move through the birth canal. He is also rotating internally. His head has entered the pelvis in a transverse position, and it must now rotate until the occiput is lying under the symphysis pubis. The next step entails the delivery of the head in an extended position, since the nape of th neck acts as a pivot. External rotation occurs following the delivery of th head, when the head rotates from the anteroposterior position back to the lef or right, depending on the original position. The shoulders are then delivere similarly to the head (Figure 23-2).

If the father is present, he may be helped to feel a real part of th delivery by showing him how to make the patient more comfortable. Ever effort should be made to include him in the proceedings. If he has attende childbirth classes, he may be waiting only for a word of encouragement t actively help his partner.

In the ideal situation, the same nurse has cared for this patient durin the course of her labor, and by the time of delivery she has become this pa tient's "nurse." This is a very close, personal relationship between the patien and the nurse, which also includes the father. They have come to *rely* on *thi* nurse; it is a time of real sharing, now that the culmination of their efforts i approaching.

NURSING CARE IN THE ADMINISTRATION OF ANESTHETICS

As the nurse assists the physician in administering anesthetics, explanatior of the birth process and preparation continues. Depending on the type o anesthetic the physician and the patient have decided upon, the nurse ap propriately assesses the situation and acts accordingly. If an ongoing epidura or caudal anesthetic has been used, the nurse anticipates a final perineal dose The necessary drugs and syringes are made available, and the nurse assist the patient in positioning. When the saddle block is the method of anesthesia the nurse asks if the physician wants the patient on her side or sitting up. Ir the sitting position, the patient rests her head on the nurse's shoulder, witł her feet resting on a stool or tailor fashion. The lumbar spine and the neck should be flexed in either position. If spinal anesthesia is planned, the nurse has the necessary equipment available and will position the patient on her side. When pudendal or local anesthesia is used, the patient is prepared for delivery and draped. If general anesthesia is chosen, the anesthetic and suc- tion machines must be at hand and the anesthetist must be in readiness.

When conduction types of anesthesia are used, the nurse is well aware of the possible complications which could occur. Close observations are made for signs of either systemic hypotension or respiratory paralysis. The blood pressure is taken every 5 to 10 minutes. If the patient becomes nauseated and the blood pressure suddenly drops and remains low, the physician would expect the nurse to increase the drop rate of an existing intravenous infusion to restore blood volume to the central circulation. This could also be done by elevating the legs, if feasible. The nurse might also be able to move the pa- tient to her left side to decrease vena caval compression, which would aid in

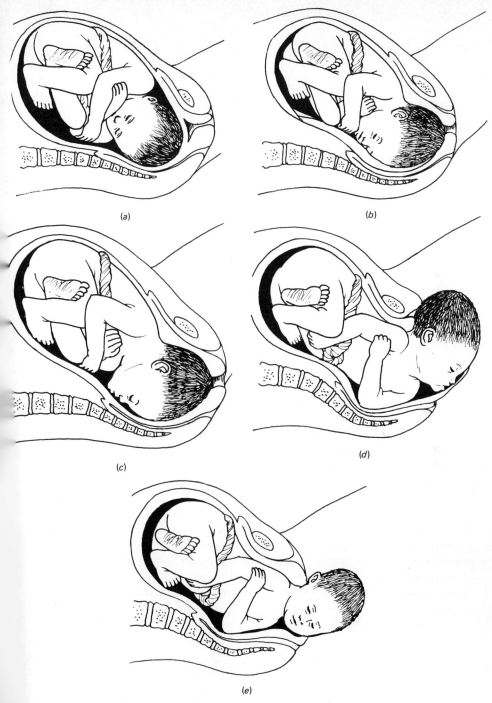

FIGURE 23-2
Mechanisms of labor. (*a*) Engagement, descent, flexion. (*b*) Internal rotation. (*c*) Extension beginning. (*d*) Extension complete. (*e*) External rotation (restitution).

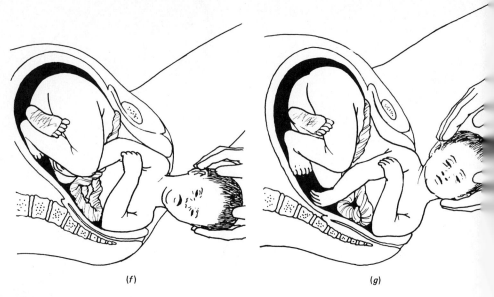

(f)   (g)

FIGURE 23-2 (Continued)
(f) External rotation. (g) Expulsion.
(From Ross Clinical Education Aid # 13, Ross Laboratories, Columbus Ohio.)

venous return from the lower extremities.[5] Occasionally, oxygen and a vasopressor drug may be used.

When general anesthesia is used, the nurse is cognizant that a pregnant woman's stomach can never be assumed empty and is watchful of signs of vomiting or aspiration. If vomiting occurs, the patient's head must be turned to the side to promote expectoration of vomitus and so that aspiration is prevented.

The nurse and/or the physician meanwhile continue to explain what is happening and to comfort the patient before and during these anesthesia procedures. A gentle pat or a squeeze of the hand indicates a real awareness of what the patient is experiencing. It is very frightening to the patient, and to the father if he remains with her, to see the equipment put in readiness for these procedures. The "unknown" causes apprehension and, again, simple explanation is vital. The patient must understand that the pain will soon be gone—though she is being made temporarily more uncomfortable perhaps during instillation of anesthetic.

PREPARATION FOR DELIVERY

When the time of delivery arrives, the nurse, who has previously adjusted the stirrups and hand bars for this patient, fastens the wrist cuffs and raises the patient's legs simultaneously for placement in the stirrups. Lifting the legs together is important to prevent straining of the pelvic ligaments. The nurse also uncovers the sterile tables, and completes the other tasks necessary immediately before delivery. If the father remains in the delivery room, a watchful eye is kept on his reactions. It is well to anticipate his needs, assist him to a stool, or perhaps assist him in leaving the room, if indicated.

The nurse prepares the patient for delivery by scrubbing the vulva and lower thighs. The general principle is to scrub from the labia outward, without retracing the movements. (Figure 23-3.) The nurse *never* removes the gloves and does not leave the end of the delivery table until replaced by the physician. She is responsible for observing the perineum and protecting the baby. In the meantime, the physician has scrubbed, gowned, and gloved for the delivery.

The patient needs the nurse's reassuring presence again at this time and will also need an interpretation of the actions expected of her. If the physician directs the patient, the nurse may nonverbally support the patient in her efforts by perhaps placing a hand on her shoulder or wiping her forehead. It is very difficult for the patient to respond when more than one directs her. She may have to be told when a uterine contraction is occurring, depending on the type of anesthetic being administered. She may need continuous help in bearing down, or a whispered, "It won't be long now." The nurse should anticipate when forceps are indicated and should have the physician's preferred type at hand.

As the infant's head separates the perineum, the physician prepares to slowly and guardedly deliver the head. He will most likely perform an episiotomy at this time to prevent the muscles and fascial structures from being stretched or torn. The episiotomy will also reduce possible injury to the bladder, urethra, and rectum. The patient should be forewarned when the episiotomy is done because it is possible she may feel pressure, or perhaps some pain.

The most frequent type of episiotomy performed today is the midline. It is a straight incision made in the middle of the perineum and is preferred because it anatomically heals more easily, causes less discomfort, is easier to repair, has a smaller blood loss, and dyspareunia rarely occurs.[6]

As the head widely distends the perineum, the Ritgen's maneuver is frequently used. The physician places a towel over the rectum and gently presses the baby's chin, while at the same time pressing downward on the occiput. The delivery of the head is thus controlled (Figure 23–4).

THE DELIVERY

The physician will strive to deliver the head between contractions to prevent lacerations. Upon delivery of the head, he quickly examines the infant's neck to ascertain if the umbilical cord is encircling it and, if so, slips it over the

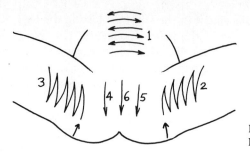

FIGURE 23-3
Perineal scrub before delivery.

head. If the cord is too short and tight, it must be clamped and cut im
mediately to prevent asphyxiation.

The anterior shoulder is delivered next, followed by the posterio:
shoulder. Suddenly, it seems the entire baby is born, and the physician is
removing excess mucus and fluid from the oropharynx. The infant generally
cries and the lungs promptly expand. At the time of the birth, the mother
should be told immediately the sex of the baby and should also be able to see
the infant as soon as possible. This is a time when the nurse can share with
the mother in her achievement and joy. It is a climactic moment for the
mother when the doctor holds the baby where she can see him. The nurse
must carefully note the exact time of birth for charting and for legal certification of the birth.

The length of time between delivery of the newborn and the clamping

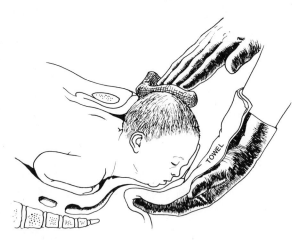

FIGURE 23-4
Ritgen's maneuver.
(From Elise Fitzpatrick, Sharon R. Reeder, and Luigi
Mastroianni, Jr., Maternity Nursing, 12th ed., Lippin-
cott, Philadelphia, 1971, p. 265.)

of the cord varies among physicians. Williams says the ideal time for the cord to be clamped is still unclear. He also states that an advantage from placental transfusion is the addition of approximately 50 mg of iron which would help to prevent later iron deficiency anemia.[7]

Babson and Benson believe that the umbilical cord should be clamped and cut 15 to 20 seconds following delivery and that the attendant should wait, holding the baby at the placental level, until the infant takes a breath or two. However, they do not believe the time period should be extended if a breath has not been taken.[8]

Preliminary findings by Moss, Duffie, and Fagan would recommend delaying clamping of the cord. Their evidence reveals that clamping of the cord before the beginning of respirations could be a factor in pathogenesis of respiratory distress syndrome.[9]

Taylor, Bright, and Birchard suggest late clamping of the cord may cause overinfusion with placental blood and feel the addition of blood from the placenta does not benefit the premature infant.[10]

The physician places two oschners or Kelly clamps on the baby's cord and cuts the cord between the clamps. After the cord is cut, either a clamp or a tie is securely placed approximately 1 inch from the baby's abdomen.

Many hospitals use the Apgar score for the evaluation of the newborn. This is done at 1 and again at 5 minutes following birth and includes evaluation of the infant's heart rate, respiratory effort, muscle tone, reflex irritability, and color.[11] The physician and/or the nurse determine the Apgar score and the infant's condition as well at the time of birth. It has been noticed that Apgar scores determined by the attending physician are often higher than the values supplied by a more objective attendant, such as a nurse or anesthetist. The evaluation must be noted on the chart (Figure 23-5). The infant is then placed on his side in a heated crib, since this position facilitates drainage of mucus secretions. The infant is dried in order to reduce loss of body heat through evaporation.

The room temperature in the delivery area is usually very low, since it is kept at the most comfortable level for physicians and attendants wearing scrub gowns. The newborn enters this extrauterine environment with a shock, since he is used to the comfort and warmth of the womb.

Various heating devices are available for preventing hypothermia in the newborn. The objectives are the same—in general, to maintain the infant's body temperature, which in turn affects the amount of oxygen consumed, aids in controlling apnea, and affects the acid-base balance. Another advantage of the modern heating devices is they are made in such a manner that the infant is still quite accessible for various necessary admitting procedures, such as resuscitation.

The nurse, while closely observing the infant, prepares to give the mother an oxytocic drug. This medication is usually given directly following the delivery of the placenta. Syntocinon, Methergine, Ergotrate, or Tocosa-

SIGN	0	1	2
Heart Rate	Absent	Slow Below 100	Over 100
Respiratory Effort	Absent	Slow Irregular	Good Crying
Muscle Tone	Flaccid	Some Flexion of Extremities	Active Motion
Reflex Irritability	No Response	Grimace	Cry
Color	Blue Pale	Body Pink Extremities Blue	Completely Pink

FIGURE 23-5
Apgar score chart.
(Photograph from "Apgar on Apgar" film sponsored by Gerber Products Co., 1967.)

mine are frequently used oxytocics. The mother should again be included and given an explanation of what the drug is and why it is being given. The nurse also palpates the fundus to determine if it is remaining firm.

At this time, the patient usually requires repair of the episiotomy, and the nurse places the necessary materials for the use by the physician, adjusts the overhead light, and proceeds to a more thorough assessment of the newborn.

A nursing assessment of the newborn generally includes the five Apgar ratings, plus observation to be sure the air passages are remaining clear and the following general considerations:

Are there three vessels in the umbilical cord (two arteries and one vein)?
Do the head and chest appear about the same size?
Does the baby appear physically mature?
Are there forceps marks?
Is there apparent bulging of the anterior fontanel?
What type of cry does the baby have?
Is there bleeding from the cord?

How does the skin appear—mature, immature, postmature?
Is there a caput succedaneum?
Are there gross abnormalities?
Does the anus appear normal?
Is there any jaundice?
Is the type of breathing remaining normal? Is there retraction?

The general admission procedure for the newborn also includes identification and prophylactic eye treatment. Identification usually consists of two bracelets for the baby, and one for the mother. These state the mother's name, physician's name, hospital number, sex of infant, date and time of birth. The baby's bracelets are placed on an arm and a leg (Figure 23-6). They are rechecked each time the baby is brought to the mother. Identification may also consist of taking the infant's footprints. Antibacterial agents are used to protect the infant from ophthalmia neonatorum with subsequent blindness. This is a requirement by all states, and penicillin, sulfacetamide, or 1 percent silver nitrate may be used. Silver nitrate and penicillin are the agents most commonly used.

Silver nitrate is supplied in sealed wax ampules, and an opening must be made in the ampule with a pin. The nurse opens the infant's eye and inserts 2 drops of the solution into the conjunctival sac. The nurse can turn the

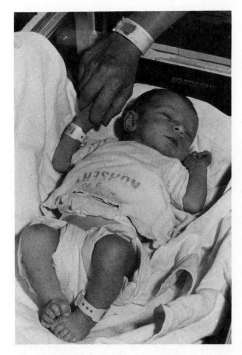

FIGURE 23-6
Identification bracelets.

infant's head away from the light which usually causes the baby to open his eyes spontaneously. The eyelids should be dried in order to facilitate opening of them manually. The procedure is repeated in the other eye, and after the medication has had contact for 2 minutes, the eyes are rinsed with normal saline or sterile water to remove the excess medication. Penicillin is supplied in ointment or ophthalmic drops. It is instilled in the manner of the silver nitrate, but no irrigation is necessary.

The infant is then ready to be admitted to the nursery. In transit, he should be shown once more to his mother and also shown to his father and/ or other family members. The nurse relates whatever vital statistics are available about the baby, and reassures the family that mother and baby are doing well, if appropriate.

Each woman in labor is very different. Each reacts differently to pain, each expresses fears differently, and each responds to the nurse differently. In the nursing process, these differences are determined, and each patient is evaluated as an individual. The nurse forms a plan of "how I can meet *her* needs." Sometimes, these initial plans are changed so the patient's needs can be more fully met. The nurse's actions always consider the patient and the baby's welfare. After the baby is born is an appropriate time to review the nursing care the patient received and evaluate what was good, what the nurse would change if the experience could be repeated, and what was gained by this family by the role the nurse played. Did the type of nursing help to make the delivery a truly meaningful experience for this family? By this type of evaluation, *maternity* nurses are born.

REFERENCES

1 Wiedenbach, Ernestine: *Family-centered Maternity Nursing*, Putnam, New York, 1958, p. 303.
2 Hellman, Louis M., and Jack A. Pritchard: *Williams Obstetrics*, 14th ed., Appleton-Century-Crofts, New York, 1971, p. 362.
3 Fitzpatrick, Elise, Sharon R. Reeder, and Luigi Mastroianni: *Maternity Nursing*, 12th ed., Lippincott, Philadelphia, 1971, p. 258.
4 Rubin, Reva: "Puerperal Change," *Nursing Outlook*, 9:754, 1961.
5 Fitzpatrick, Reeder, and Mastroianni: op cit., p. 232.
6 Hellman and Pritchard: op. cit., p. 425.
7 Ibid., p. 415.
8 Babson, S. G., and Ralph C. Benson: *Primer on Prematurity and High-risk Pregnancy*, Mosby, St. Louis, 1966, p. 81.
9 Moss, A. J., E. R. Duffie, and L. M. Fagan: "Respiratory Distress in the Newborn: Study on the Association of Cord Clamping and the Pathogenesis of Disease," *Journal of the American Medical Association*, 184:50, 1963.

10 Taylor, P. M., N. H. Bright, and E. L. Birchard: "Effect of Early Versus Delayed Clamping of the Umbilical Cord on the Clinical Condition of the Newborn Infant," *American Journal of Diseases of Children*, 98:650, 1959.

11 Apgar, Virginia: "The Role of the Anesthesiologist in Reducing Mortality," *New York Journal of Medicine*, 55:2365, 1955.

BIBLIOGRAPHY

Caplan, Gerald: *An Approach to Community Mental Health*, Grune & Stratton, New York, 1961.

Flowers, Charles E.: *Obstetric Analgesia and Anesthesia*, Hoeber-Harper, New York, 1967.

Greiss, Frank: "Obstetric Anesthesia," *American Journal of Nursing*, 71:67–69, January 1971.

Hilliard, Mary: "The Changing Role of the Maternity Nurse," *Nursing Clinics of North America*, 3(2):277–288, June 1968.

Lutz, Linda, and Paul Perlstein: "Temperature Control in Newborn Babies," *Nursing Clinics of North America*, 6(1):15–23, March 1971.

Matousek, Irene: "Fetal Nursing during Labor," *Nursing Clinics of North America*, 3(2):307–314, June 1968.

Tryon, Phyllis: "Assessing the Progress of Labor through Observation of Patients Behavior," *Nursing Clinics of North America*, 3(2):315–326, June 1968.

Williams, Barbara L., and Sharon T. Richards: "Fetal Monitoring during Labor," *American Journal of Nursing*, pp. 2384–2385, November 1970.

24 | THE THIRD STAGE OF LABOR

Vivian Littlefield

To be effective, complete, and patient-centered, nursing care should be goal-directed. This is particularly important in the third stage of labor, the placental stage, since the baby has just arrived and requires skilled nursing care that will establish him in his new environment physically, psychologically, and socially. The mother's care is extremely important, too, since this is the most dangerous stage for her because of the possibility of postpartum hemorrhage. In addition to these tasks, the nurse should encourage the mother to feel she has successfully accomplished a great task in giving birth to her new baby.

It is also during the third stage that most hospital routines require the completion of various charts and forms by the nurse. If the nurse does not have specific nursing goals in mind, nursing care may become disorganized and therefore incomplete. The rush and excitement often present in delivery rooms has lessened during the third stage, and if no complications arise, the nurse could relax and become busy with the numerous forms and reports required at this time unless there are specific goals in mind. Therefore, this chapter will identify specific goals, based on the needs of the mother, newborn, and family following childbirth, through the placental stage, and until the patient leaves the delivery room. Following the identification of these goals, the basic knowledge necessary to accomplish them will be presented as well as identification of various tasks that accomplish each nursing goal.

The overall goal in patient care during the third stage of labor should be *to provide as physically healthy a mother and infant as possible and encourage the establishment of the family unit.*

The third stage of labor, or the placental stage, begins with the birth of the baby and is completed with the expulsion of the placenta. During this stage the placenta separates and is expelled. This involves the forces of uterine contraction and intraabdominal pressure. The first hour immediately following the expulsion of the placenta has been termed the *fourth stage of labor.* This critical time *after* the expulsion of the placenta is the time postpartum hemorrhage, due to uterine atony, is most likely to occur.

In order to provide adequate care, or to set proper nursing goals, the nurse must know what is happening to the new mother and the newborn during this stage of labor. Since the needs of the newborn and his immediate care were covered in the previous chapter and will be further delineated in Chapters 28 and 29, goals for the newborn's care will only be summarized in this chapter. The nurse should remember that as care is given to the mother in the third stage, care for the newborn is going on concurrently. Often the nurse must set priorities of care between the mother and the newborn because of the problems that each might develop which require reordering of care. The nurse may need to call for assistance from other nurses or specialists, such as a pediatrician or obstetrician, when the situation indicates.

There are also several goals of nursing care that were begun prior to the third stage of labor and that the nurse must keep in mind as she carries out goals that are more specific to the third stage. Since the tasks involved in meeting these goals have been covered in previous chapters concerning labor and delivery, they will only be identified here for completeness. The goals that were begun previously and should continually be met are:

1 Prevention of infection in the mother and infant by strict aseptic technique.
2 Provision of safety for the mother and infant by maintenance of equipment, control of personnel in and out of the delivery room, proper administration of medications, proper positioning of the new mother, and proper care in handling the newborn.
3 Assistance to the obstetrician so that there is adequate equipment or information essential to providing adequate obstetric care.
4 Assurance of the maintenance of dignity and self-respect for the new mother, her husband (or significant other), and baby.

ESTABLISHING TWO SEPARATE INDIVIDUALS— MOTHER AND BABY

Nursing Knowledge Needed

The knowledge needed by the nurse to meet the goal of establishing two individuals, mother and baby, concerns the physiology involved in the placental separation and delivery. The nurse must know methods used to assist in the separation and expulsion of the placenta when this does occur naturally, and the problems that can result from inadequate placental separation and expulsion. By knowing the signs of inadequate placental separation, the nurse can detect any problems present and assist the obstetrician in solving them. The nurse also must know which drugs can be used to prevent hemorrhage, as well as the side effects of these drugs. The nurse needs to know why it is important for the entire placenta to be delivered and what the procedure is when it is not entirely delivered. By knowing these purposes and procedures, an explanation can be offered to the patient in the event the placenta is delivered incompletely. The nurse also needs knowledge of the technique by which the cord is cut and the physiology involved in this process.

After the baby is born, the uterus contracts at regular intervals. There

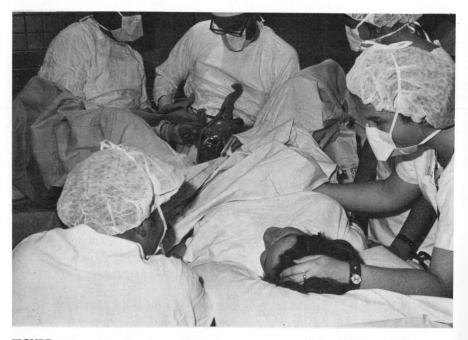

FIGURE 24-1

The climax for a family that has actively participated in the birth process. The nurse can do much to facilitate this participation. (*Courtesy of The University of Colorado Medical Center, Denver, Colorado*)

is less content without the baby, and consequently, the area of placental attachment is greatly reduced. This disproportion between the uterus and the placenta brings about a folding of the maternal surface of the placenta and causes separation to take place. Bleeding occurs in the placental folds and expedites placental separation. The placenta then moves into the lower uterine segment or upper vagina as an unattached body. The nurse should be familiar with these signs because it is often the nurse's responsibility to note the time of delivery of the placenta. The signs which suggest the placenta has separated are:

1 The uterus rises upward in the abdomen because the placenta has moved down into the lower uterine segment. Figure 24-2 indicates the shape of the uterus when this occurs.
2 If the umbilical cord protrudes 3 or more inches from the vagina, this also indicates that the placenta has descended.
3 The uterus assumes a globular shape and becomes firmer (Figure 24-2).
4 A sudden gush of blood often occurs and is the result of the separation of the placenta.
5 The cord fails to recede when the uterus is elevated.[1]

These signs of placental detachment appear from 1 to 5 minutes after the delivery of the infant. As long as the uterus remains firm and there is no excessive bleeding, the obstetrician waits until the placenta is separated. No massage is practiced before placental detachment since massage is usually futile and possibly dangerous.[2] The major goal of the obstetrician in managing the separation and expulsion of the placenta is to prevent unnecessary

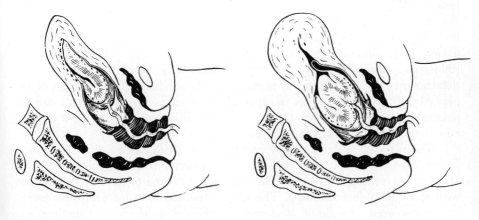

FIGURE 24-2
Shape of the uterus before and after separation of the placenta.
(From E. Stewart Taylor, Beck's Obstetrical Practice, 9th ed., The Williams & Wilkins Company, Baltimore, 1971, p. 199. By permission of the publisher.)

blood loss. This is accomplished by making sure that the uterus is firmly contracted and that the placenta is expelled as soon as possible.

Awareness that there are many raw places for the uterus to bleed helps the nurse understand the importance of the uterus contracting and becoming globular immediately after the placenta has separated. If the uterus relaxes after the placenta separates, then the chance of hemorrhage is great.

Once the placenta has separated, it must be expelled. This usually can be accomplished by the patient's bearing down in the same way as when she assisted with the birth of the baby. The mother at this point may be dozing, distracted from the birth process, or engaged in watching her newborn. The nurse should assist her in bearing down so that the placenta is expelled with the least amount of trauma. It has been stated that when the mother is involved and uses her own efforts, it prevents some of the fetal blood from the placenta from entering the maternal blood. This crossing of fetal blood into the maternal blood often occurs with manual assistance and causes sensitization of the maternal blood when the mother is Rh negative.

When the patient is anesthetized she cannot assist with expelling the placenta. Therefore, she must be assisted by the physician or, in some situations, by the nurse under the physician's guidance. This procedure is as follows: (1) palpate the fundus to be *certain* that the uterus is firm; (2) exert downward pressure with one hand on the fundus of the uterus; and (3) employ the placenta as a piston, and push the placenta out of the vagina.[3] This placental expression should be done with gentleness and without squeezing. If it is attempted when the uterus is boggy, *inversion of the uterus,* an extremely dangerous complication, may occur. After separation of the placenta, expulsion should occur quickly in order to prevent unnecessary blood loss. The uterus cannot contract properly before the placenta has been removed. In order to prevent blood loss, constant application of the hand to the uterine fundus *after* birth of the infant to detect first signs of placental detachment, vigorous massage after separation, and immediate delivery of the placenta will decrease the amount of blood loss.[4] Some obstetricians may follow this procedure and may ask the nurse's assistance in detecting the detachment of the placenta, in massage of the fundus, and expression of the placenta after delivery. This is especially true when anesthesia prevents the patient from bearing down to assist in this procedure. Figure 24-3 demonstrates the expression of the placenta.

The placenta is delivered by two methods which can be differentiated in Figure 24-4.[5] The first method, Schultz's mechanism, is said to occur in about 80 percent of deliveries. The placenta is turned inside out and is born with the fetal side presenting. The second method is called Duncan's mechanism and occurs in about 20 percent of the deliveries. In this method, the maternal side presents on delivery of the placenta.

It is estimated that even with efficient management of the third stage of

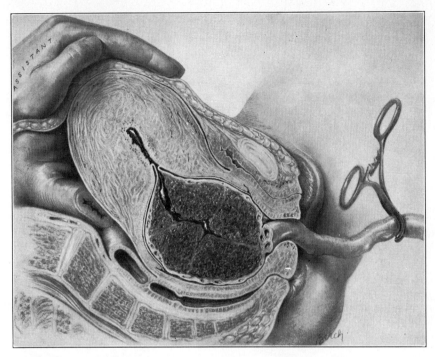

FIGURE 24-3
Expression of the placenta. The fundus should be firm before this procedure is carried out.
(From Louis M. Hellman and Jack A. Pritchard, Williams Obstetrics, 14th ed., Appleton-Century-Crofts, New York, 1971, p. 416. By permission of the publisher.)

labor, approximately 250 to 300 cc of blood are lost in the average patient. It is extremely important to estimate the amount of blood that is lost so that, if necessary, blood or intravenous fluids can be administered to the mother after delivery. It is important for the nurse who is caring for patients in the delivery room to be accurate in the estimation of blood loss. Knowing that the mother has lost an extra amount of blood will alert the nurse to assess the effect of the blood loss on the new mother. The patients' blood pressure and pulse should be taken frequently. The nurse must watch for other specific signs of hypovolemic shock, such as pale color, increase in respirations, euphoria, vertigo, restlessness, and air hunger. The nurse must also be prepared to administer blood or intravenous fluids immediately when ordered by the physician.

If the placenta does not separate promptly or if there is bleeding from the uterus, the obstetrician will proceed to remove the placenta manually. Figure 24-5 demonstrates this procedure.

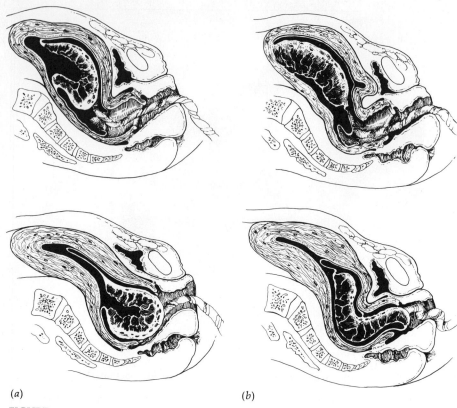

(a)   (b)

FIGURE 24-4
Two methods of placental delivery. (a) Schultz method. (b) Duncan method.
(From Ralph C. Benson, Handbook of Obstetrics and Gynecology, 4th ed., Lange Medical
Publications, Los Altos, Calif., 1971, pp. 134–135.)

A study of Figure 24-5 indicates that one disadvantage of manual removal of the placenta is introduction of infection into the uterine cavity. The nurse may need to assist the physician in changing gloves, drapes, etc., if the delivery field becomes contaminated.

Taylor indicates that if manual removal is necessary, the more time between the birth of the baby and the manual removal of the placenta, the greater the chances are of infection in the uterus.[6]

The physician inspects the placenta immediately after delivery to determine if any cotyledons have been retained. If placental fragments or entire cotyledons are retained, the chance of hemorrhage is increased because the uterus cannot contract completely. Retention of placental fragments is also conducive to infection. When the uterus attempts to contract but is unable

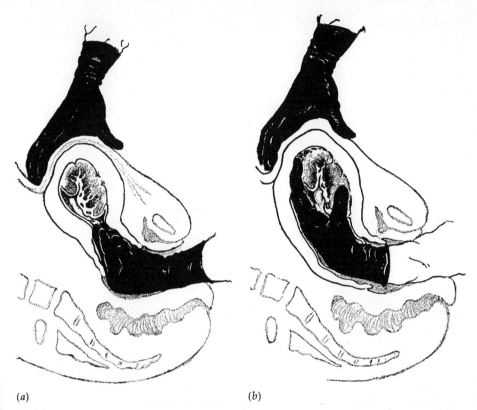

(a)   (b)

FIGURE 24-5
Manual removal of the placenta. (a) Method of introducing the internal hand and creat-
ing pressure on the fundus with the external hand. (b) Technique of separating the
placenta before it is removed.
*(From E. Stewart Taylor, Beck's Obstetrical Practice, 9th ed., The Williams & Wilkins
Company, Baltimore, 1971, p. 201. By permission of the publisher.)*

to do so because of the retained fragments, these contractions cause the
mother pain. If the fragments must be removed later, the procedure may
cause discomfort to the mother.

If the mother is experiencing pain during the placental expulsion, then
the nurse should provide support by holding the mother's hand. Coaching
the mother by speaking into her ear is helpful to reinforce the doctor's requests. The nurse can also support the mother by placing her hands gently
but firmly on the mother's shoulders.

Retained placental fragments are a cause of late postpartal hemorrhage
and often necessitate the mother returning to the hospital for dilatation and
curettage after she has been dismissed.

Nursing Tasks

CARE OF THE MOTHER

The nursing tasks involved in caring for the mother are as follows:

1 Support and assist the mother in expelling the placenta.
2 Assist with the delivery of the placenta if indicated.
3 Observe and estimate as accurately as possible blood loss.
4 Detect signs of uterine relaxation and hemorrhage by:
    a Taking the blood pressure and comparing it with previous readings.
    b Palpating the pulse and detecting a weak beat, increased rate, or other irregularity.
    c Measuring the height and degree of firmness of the fundus.
    d Apprising the physician of any change in the mother's condition and, if none, informing him that all vital signs are stable and the fundus is firm.

CARE OF THE INFANT

The nursing goals and tasks involved in caring for the infant are as follows:

1 Assess the status of the newborn in relation to his adaption to the extrauterine environment.
2 Assess the gross normality of the newborn infant.
3 Establish a patent airway.
4 Maintain adequate oxygenation.
5 Maintain body warmth.
6 Provide proper identification of the baby.
7 Prevent infection.

The reader is referred to Chapters 28 and 29 for detailed information regarding the tasks outlined above.

It should be emphasized that the nurse will have to set priorities, depending on the amount of assistance available and the problems that arise with either the mother or the baby. For example, let us say the nurse is checking the mother's vital signs to detect any sign of hemorrhage, and it is observed that the newborn's color is somewhat dusky. The nurse must immediately return to the newborn, identify the problem, and resuscitate the baby. After the baby's condition is stable the nurse must return to the assessment of the mother's situation.

At the same time if there is *any* indication that the mother is bleeding excessively, then the nurse must ask for assistance from another nurse or from the obstetrician. Setting priorities, especially when complications arise, is a complex situation and requires knowledge and judgment on the part of the nurse.

PREVENTION AND DETECTION OF HEMORRHAGE AND OTHER MATERNAL COMPLICATIONS

Nursing Knowledge Needed

The third stage of labor is dangerous for the mother because of the possibility of postpartum hemorrhage and resultant hypovolemic shock. Hemorrhage is said to occur if there is more than 500 cc of blood loss.[7] This amount of blood loss is fairly common even with the most skilled obstetric care. Every effort should be taken to avoid such an occurrence and to detect signs that might lead to hemorrhage before the hemorrhage occurs. Bleeding of 500 cc is encountered once in every 20 to 30 deliveries. Hemorrhages of 1,000 cc and over are encountered once in about every 75 cases, whereas a blood loss of 1,500 to 2,000 cc is only occasionally encountered. Based on this information, the nurse must constantly be aware of the status of bleeding in the new mother. Hemorrhage can be a result of *uterine atony, lacerations,* or *retained placental fragments.*

Hemorrhage in the delivery room and in the first hour postpartum is probably due to uterine atony, as this is the most common cause of hemorrhage at this time. If there is a blood loss of 1,000 cc, a blood transfusion may be given to prevent the possibility of infection, shock, acute kidney tubular necrosis, pituitary and/or adrenal necrosis.[8]

The large blood vessels within the muscle fibers of the uterus and especially those in the placental site are open and gaping. Therefore, the nurse should recognize the necessity for the uterus to contract and stay contracted. If there is only a slight degree of relaxation, the uterus may fill with blood, which will further prevent the uterus from contracting. More bleeding may occur. The nurse should ascertain the level of the fundus in relation to the umbilicus. If it is higher during the next check, the doctor should be apprised of this finding. The nurse and doctor would then collaborate as to the plan of action in order to prevent hemorrhage. Care must be taken that massage of the fundus is not done during repair of the episiotomy without consulting with the doctor. Upon the doctor's request, the nurse then proceeds to massage the fundus and expel the blood. *Care should be taken to avoid pushing hard on the fundus when it is not contracted.* The proper method of palpating the fundus is described in the following chapter, "The Fourth Stage of Labor."

It is important for the nurse to anticipate complications so that care can be planned and implemented. Considering the many tasks and priorities in the delivery room with a new baby, a new mother, and the necessity to help the family feel they have achieved success in their efforts, the nurse must be able to identify patients who are more likely to have postpartum bleeding. Never forget there are patients who hemorrhage for the first time. If the nurse knows those patients who may more likely hemorrhage for whatever reason, extra care and watchfulness for such a complication can be provided. This might require checking the fundus, pulse, and blood pressure more frequently than hospital routine requires. The nurse should be prepared to administer intravenous aqueous infusion with oxytocin during the third stage of labor, since this procedure may be ordered by the obstetrician if hemorrhage is suspected. Hellman indicates the usual dosage of oxytocin is 20 to 40 units per liter of infusion administered at 30 to 60 drops per minute.[9] Some of the predisposing factors to hemorrhage following the third stage of labor due to uterine atony in the new mother are as follows:

1 Any condition that entends the uterus beyond what is "normal" (large babies, hydramnious, twin pregnancy)
2 Premature separation of the placenta and placenta previa
3 Operative delivery, such as forceps extraction
4 Large amounts of medication late in labor or general anesthesia
5 Previous uterine atony after the third stage of labor in previous pregnancies
6 Prolonged first and second stages of labor
7 Very rapid labor
8 Labor induced and maintained with oxytocin
9 Older women of high parity
10 Preeclampsia and eclampsia[10]

To help prevent postpartum hemorrhage due to uterine atony, the nurse should be familiar with the various drugs used to assist the uterus in contracting. It is often the nurse who administers these drugs in the delivery room, and, therefore, the nurse must be alert for signs and symptoms of side effects. Table 24-1 lists the most commonly used drugs, their effects, advantages, disadvantages, and side effects. This information should be familiar to the nurse.

The use, especially the timing of administration, of these drugs varies from physician to physician and from hospital to hospital. At times, various combinations of these drugs are used, at other times no drugs are used.

It should be noted that oxytocin acts quickly, but does not last as long as ergonovine and methylergonovine. However, oxytocin avoids the problem of blood pressure elevation more common with ergonovine and methylergonovine.

One of these oxytocic drugs is usually given after the placenta is delivered or in some cases with the delivery of the anterior shoulder of the baby. The latter procedure requires skilled obstetric care as it may cause the placenta to be retained. However, excessive bleeding may be avoided when this procedure is carefully executed. The nurse must be aware of the different use of these drugs and should anticipate their use so that they are administered when the physician requests them. His plan of care depends on the proper timing of these drugs and the nurse should recognize that such timing is important in order to prevent unnecessary bleeding in the new mother. If the drugs are given too soon, it is possible that the placenta cannot escape from the uterus, thereby causing unnecessary difficulty. If they are given too late, the mother may loose unnecessary amounts of blood. Precautions must be taken so that patients who have elevated blood pressure are not given ergonovine or methylergonovine. Any of the side effects of these drugs should be watched for and reported to the physician immediately.

The second most frequent cause of hemorrhage is lacerations of the perineum, vagina, and cervix. Inspection of the cervix and vagina is done by the doctor to determine if there are any lacerations. If an episiotomy has been performed, this will usually prevent the possibility of tears in the pelvic floor. Since the nurse is often responsible for "cleaning up the patient" and placing a perineal pad on the patient before the patient leaves the delivery room, it is necessary to be aware of bleeding from lacerations and/or sutures. At this time, the lacerations will have been sutured and inspection of these sutures for bleeding and/or a hematoma should be done before allowing the patient to leave the delivery room. Lacerations are fairly common in primigravidas and precipitous births.

An episiotomy is often done to avoid lacerations in the perineum and rectal sphincter. An episiotomy heals more readily than a laceration. The nurse should be aware of why lacerations occur, as these cause additional trauma and pain to the mother in the postpartum period.

The causes for lacerations of the perineum include:

1 Rapid and sudden expulsion of the presenting part during delivery
2 Large size of the infant
3 Difficult forceps deliveries and breech extractions
4 Contraction of the pelvic outlet
5 Exaggerated lithotomy position
6 Friable maternal tissues

Since the nurse is responsible for positioning the patient on the delivery table, she should be aware of the problems that may occur if the patient is improperly positioned in the lithotomy position. Refer to Chapter 23 for the proper positioning of a patient.

The third cause of hemorrhage is retained placental fragments. The nurse must recognize the importance of inspecting the placenta to be sure that it has been completely removed. Retained placental fragments cause late postpartum hemorrhage and increase the chance of infection in the new mother. This type of hemorrhage causes a complication that interferes with

TABLE 24-1
DRUGS COMMONLY ADMINISTERED DURING THE THIRD STAGE OF LABOR

Name	Effects	Route	Disadvantages	Available dosage	Rate of action	Precautions	Side effects
Ergonovine (Ergotrate)	Produces uterine contractions of 3 or more hours, acts rapidly and sustained—no tendency to relaxation.	Orally, IM, IV	Given IV, BP increase of 20 mmHg or more in 22% of patients. Given IV, headache and vertigo in 30–50% of patients. Given IV, temporary chest pain, palpatation, dyspnea 5–10%. Cannot be given prior to placental expulsion.	1 cc, 0.2 mg	Rapid	Sensitivity with prolonged use	Nausea and vomiting; rarely transient hypertension.
Methyl-ergonovine (Methergine)	Produces stronger and longer contractions than ergonovine.	Orally, IM, IV	Given IV, BP increase of 20 mmHg or more in 10% of patients. Given IV, headache and vertigo in 30–50% of patients. Given IV, temporary chest pain, palpatation, dyspnea 5–10%. Cannot be	0.2 mg/cc (1/320 gr)	30–60 seconds after IV, 2–5 minutes after injection, 3–5 minutes after oral administration.	Administer 1 cc slowly over 60 seconds. Check BP frequently and at intervals of 1 hour after.	Nausea and vomiting, transient hypertension, dizziness, tachycardia. When administered as a dilute IV, infusion has little effect on BP or electrocardiogram.

Oxytocin (Pitocin and Syntocinon, a synthetic drug that has replaced posterior pituitary extract, Pituitrin, because of vasopressor effect)	Produces contraction of uterus like ergonovine for first 5–10 minutes, then normal rhythmic contraction of amplified degree and intermittent periods of relaxation. Avoids elevation of BP.	given prior to placental expulsion.	IV	10 units/cc	Few, except antidiuresis.	Acts quicker than ergonovine, but effect is not as lasting.	Not used by more than one route of administration because of inherent problem of controlling dosage. Has antidiuretic effect. Watch if patient is receiving fluids.

SOURCE: Developed from E. Stewart Taylor, *Beck's Obstetrical Practice*, 8th ed., Williams & Wilkins, Baltimore, 1966; Louis M. Hellman and Jack A. Pritchard, *Williams Obstetrics*, 14th ed., Appleton-Century-Crofts, New York, 1971; *Physicians' Desk Reference*, Litton Publications, Oradell, N.J., 1969; and Betty S. Bergerson, Elsie Krey, and Andres Goth (eds.), *Current Concepts in Clinical Nursing*, Mosby, St. Louis, 1969.

mothering activities and often causes a return to the hospital or the operating table.

Nursing Tasks Involved in Prevention of Hemorrhage

The nursing tasks involved in obtaining this goal are:

1 Identify previous predisposing factors from the patient's history which might indicate the possibility of hemorrhage.
2 Check the fundus frequently. This may entail constant check by maintaining the hand on the fundus to detect the slightest fundal change, or it may entail checking the fundus every few minutes.
3 Massage the uterus and expel clots of blood as necessary.
4 Check vital signs frequently, basing the time interval on previous assessment of the possibility of hemorrhage and other factors that indicate need for frequent check of vital signs, such as spinal anesthesia, maternal cardiac complications, and amount of medication and anesthetics received.
5 Administration of the oxytocic drug or drugs in the prescribed amount and at the appropriate time.
6 Complete reevaluation of the patient's signs of bleeding *before* leaving the delivery room, with an assessment of the type of care needed in the recovery room. If the patient indicates various predisposing signs of hemorrhage, arrangements for a constant attendant in the recovery room may be essential. If the patient is doing well, then frequent sequential checks must be arranged. These postpartum checks are described in detail in Chapter 25. Assessment of the state of the episiotomy should be done prior to leaving the delivery room.

NURSING GOAL: ESTABLISHING MOTHER-INFANT-FAMILY RELATIONSHIPS

Nursing Knowledge Needed

During the third stage of labor, the physician is busy facilitating the delivery of the placenta, determining if there is hemorrhage present, and establishing the respirations of the newborn infant. The nurse also is involved in tasks that assist this process, as has been described in the previous section. However, once the baby is born, the new mother may be intensively engaged in seeing her new baby and ascertaining what he is like. New mothers' behaviors, once their babies arrive, are as varied as are the women themselves. Some laugh, some cry, some are quite verbal and share their feelings, others are extremely quiet in their response to their babies. It is important for the nurse to recognize this individualism and not to insist that a mother behave

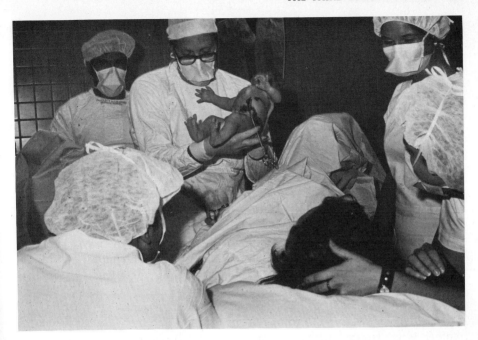

FIGURE 24-6
A successful delivery is promoted by the cooperative interaction of all members of the health team and the family. *(Courtesy of The University of Colorado Medical Center, Denver, Colorado)*

in a manner different from her pattern or her ability to behave at this point in time. Many factors seem to influence the way the new mother behaves toward her baby.

1 The mother's own personality and her way of responding to situations of excitement, stress, or joy
2 The mother's cultural background and the way she feels she should respond in this situation
3 The type of labor and delivery and the degree of fatigue, pain, or fear she has experienced during this process and whether or not she wanted to have a baby
4 Her marital status and whether she is keeping the baby
5 The baby; whether the baby "fits" the baby the mother wanted as to sex, size, and condition; whether she is aware of how newborn babies look, regarding color, size, vernix caseosa, blood
6 The tone and atmosphere of the delivery room staff and whether she feels comfortable, important, or accepted, regardless of her response
7 The presence or absence of her husband; if he is present, his response may in turn influence the mother's response
8 The amount of medication or type of anesthesia she has received

Discussion of whether the father should be present in the delivery room is widespread, and there are differing opinions about the value of this procedure. If the father is present, his needs should be considered so that he can participate in holding the baby and supporting his wife. If he is not, consideration should be given as to how he might be included in the birth of the baby from afar. Often women who have just delivered a baby prefer to let the father know of the baby's birth in a specific way. Some women will want the nurse to inform him immediately that all is well when the baby is born. Other women will want to wait until they can tell the father themselves. The nurse should have explored this with the couple *before* delivery so that the woman can inform the father in the desired manner.

Many psychologists indicate the importance of the mother establishing a relationship with the newborn baby immediately after birth. Dr. Bradley, who advocates *Husband-coached Childbirth,* and many of the physicians who propose psychoprophylactic methods of preparation for childbirth, indicate the importance of immediately seeing and holding the baby for the new mother and father.[13] Caplan indicates that if this initial reaction is delayed, often the establishment of a positive relationship between the mother and her baby is delayed. Maternal feelings are said to develop more readily when the mother is confronted with her baby immediately and is able to touch and hold her baby. Response to the newborn even initiates the *release* of oxytocin that stimulates the mother's uterus to contract. Indeed, then, nature intended for the mother to hold her baby immediately and the procedure, still seen too frequently, of not allowing the mother to touch and handle her baby is an unnecessary restriction in most situations.

Every effort should be made to allow the mother to see and hold her baby. The mother will need to establish the baby's identity very soon and respond to the baby's needs and desires. The sooner she can see him as an individual with a specific sex and personality, the better she can care for her baby. Touching the baby and holding him is extremely important, and she should not be denied this opportunity (Figure 24-7).

If the condition of the mother does not warrant immediate contact with her baby, arangements should be made as soon as the mother's condition allows. Many times obstetric staff has the idea that if the mother missed this experience, she will have to wait until "babies are brought out" according to hospital procedure and schedule. If the nurse believes that maternal-infant relationships are fostered and enhanced by early encounter between mother and baby, every effort will be made for the mother to see and hold her infant as soon as possible.

In making judgments about whether a mother should be allowed to hold her baby after delivery, the baby's condition should be evaluated and the judgment made on the basis of this condition. Normal newborn infants who are of adequate size, in good condition, and not depressed by too much

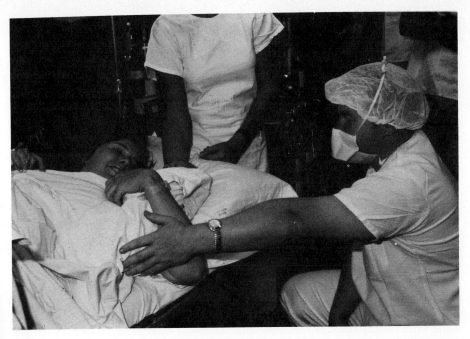

FIGURE 24-7
Interaction of the mother, father, and child as the mother leaves the delivery room. Positive interaction will encourage a satisfying relationship between the mother and her infant. (*Courtesy of The University of Colorado Medical Center, Denver, Colorado*)

maternal medication are not traumatized if the parents hold them or look to see if the baby is "all there."

However, babies who are small for gestational age, who are born prematurely, who have problems breathing, or who are listless because of medication may not be able to tolerate this procedure. When this is the case, certainly the safety of the newborn must take precedence. He may need to be transferred immediately to an intensive nursing unit. If the baby's condition prevents the mother from holding the baby, the nurse must see to it that the mother is brought to the baby or the baby is within seeing distance of the mother at the earliest time possible.

A frequent argument for not allowing fathers to be present in the delivery room or for not allowing the parents to be able to see and hold their baby immediately after delivery is that the baby has a defect. Parents must adjust and accept this situation. If parents wish to hold their baby who has a defect, they certainly should not be denied this privilege. A mother who saw her baby, with a cleft lip, for the first time several days after delivery explained with a sigh of relief on seeing her baby, "Oh it is not nearly as bad as I imagined!" How disconcerting to allow this mother to imagine a defect many times worse than the one present by delaying showing her the baby!

When there is a complication present in the newborn that threatens life, the parents should know what is happening to their child and should be able to see their infant and the efforts being made to assist him. Often the parents are shielded from knowing about the baby's condition and prevented from seeing the care the baby is receiving. This may be detrimental to the parents. If the parents see the concentrated care given their baby, they are often less upset; they feel everything possible is being done. If the staff is truthful and open about the condition of the baby, the parents learn to trust the staff.

Helping the mother feel she is close to her baby still needs to be accomplished. This can be accomplished in different ways. Some of the ways that closeness when apart may be accomplished include letting the mother know what is happening to her infant, telling her what his condition is at the moment, letting the mother know where the baby is going, and reporting his condition and what is happening to the baby as frequently as possible.

The birth of the baby gives the nurse an excellent opportunity to enhance the mother's and the father's level of achievement in the birth process. This need for achievement is great and can often forestall guilt feelings that come later when the mother feels that she was unable to cooperate to the degree she wanted to during labor and/or the birth of her baby. Positive accomplishments by the patient need to be reinforced by the nurse. The mother needs to feel successful. After all, having had a baby *is* an achievement! The following example, which emphasizes the patient's need to feel she has successfully given birth to her baby, might demonstrate this point more completely.

A nurse was talking with a newly delivered mother who had a severe cardiac complication. The purpose of the discussion was to help the new mother plan her postpartum activities to compensate for her cardiac condition in the care of her new baby and her other young child. Not much progress was being made, and the patient appeared very sad and finally started crying. The nurse asked the patient what was wrong. The patient replied, "I was a failure, I *couldn't* help but push when the baby was born! That doctor was so angry at me! I tried, really I did . . . !" The patient was feeling some guilt, and possibly her mothering activities would be hindered. The patient had done well, with her cardiac condition, to deliver the baby safely, and yet she was deeply concerned about being an uncooperative patient. The physician was tense because of the patient's condition and relayed his tension to the patient by strongly insisting that the patient not push, a necessity to this situation. Time was spent in exploring how difficult it would be not to push, that she was not to blame, that the doctor was expressing his concern for her, and that she had done well. Her labor nurse was asked to reinforce this. Patients seem to be very sensitive to their performance and need reassurance that they did well in light of their particular situation.

The procedure of allowing the mother to carry the baby from the delivery room walking or in her bed is an important one in establishing mother-infant relationships and in allowing the new mother to feel important, for she has indeed achieved a great task. This should be done when the condition of the mother and her infant allow such a procedure. Also, the desire of the patient should be considered. If the new mother does not desire to hold her baby at this time, this procedure should certainly not be forced upon her, but she should not be denied this privilege because of "hospital routine."

Some hospitals allow the mother and baby to occupy the same room during the first hour postpartum and allow the infant to remain with the mother at all times in a rooming-in situation. Skilled nursing care is done concurrently rather than separately in this situation.

Women who have already decided not to keep their babies often are not allowed to see and hold them. This should be an individual decision and should not be dictated by hospital policy. If the mother desires to see and hold the baby, she should not be denied this opportunity. After all, it is her baby and it may be important for her to see that the baby is normal and healthy. She must make her decision to relinquish the baby in light of all the facts and in light of her response to the baby. If the mother does not wish to see her baby, it should not be encouraged. This subject is complex and highly individual and should be planned with each person involved as well as some knowledge of how the patient is handling the situation of relinquishing her baby.

Nursing Tasks Involved

1 Assess the condition of the mother and the infant to determine if the mother can see and hold her baby.
2 Facilitate the mother's touching of her baby, the exploration of all parts, and encourage her to fondle the baby as desired in relation to the condition of the baby.
3 Dry the infant to prevent overexposure, providing warmed blankets, and a warmed crib.
4 Create an atmosphere that encourages the mother to feel comfortable in handling the baby.
5 Include the father in the birth of the baby if he is present. If the father is absent from the delivery room, inform him in the manner he and the mother wish.
6 Compliment the mother on the task she has just completed, encourage the physician to do so if he has not done so already, point out things the mother did well in order to enhance the patient's sense of self-esteem and well-being.
7 Foster continuity of the mother-infant relationship by allowing the infant to remain with the mother when possible, or inform the mother of the baby's condition, and what is being done for him.

PROMOTION OF SAFETY, COMFORT, AND RELAXATION IN THE NEW MOTHER

Nursing Knowledge Needed

The term labor is an appropriate one, since the pregnant woman has indeed labored. There has been a great expenditure of energy, physically and psychologically. She may have had a long labor that interfered with her normal sleep; she may have had times of discouragement, anxiety, pain, and fear. All of this as well as having had her food and fluids restricted may have decreased her energy stores, and she may be tense and fatigued, even though she is excited and happy. She may or may not become aware of uterine contractions and feel discomfort as the placenta is delivered. Her response to the entire birth process may be one of relief, or it may be one of excitement. Regardless of her reaction, the nurse needs to help the mother relax and become comfortable.

The type of anesthesia the patient had will influence the patient's needs and the nursing actions to meet this goal of promotion of comfort, relaxation, and safety. For example, if the patient has had a general anesthetic, the nurse's activities immediately after the baby is born would center around tasks that detect the patient's response to this anesthetic and help provide safety and adequate recovery. If on the other hand, the patient has had a regional anesthetic, such as a caudal or saddle block, the patient may not experience physical pain, but will have emotional responses that will need nursing support or intervention. If the patient has had a local anesthetic, she may be aware of uterine pain which may interfere with establishing a relationship with her newborn.

At times, the physician may administer a tranquilizer when the patient is extremely tense or a pain medication when pain is a problem. The nurse should make every effort to help the patient relax because it is essential that the mother is relaxed, rested, and fully restored from fatigue or anxiety as soon as possible so she can take on the mothering role. The nursing care which facilitates patient rest and relaxation is described in Chapter 25.

Various other needs of the new mother may have been interfered with because of the labor process. The new mother may be experiencing some degree of discomfort because of any or all of the following:

1 Lack of adequate food and fluids
2 Inadequate elimination as labor progressed
3 An uncomfortable position in stirrups, wet linens because of the obstetric preparation
4 Coolness because of the delivery room temperature
5 Interference with her need to be with her husband and family
6 Anxiety due to stress of labor and delivery

The nurse should take steps as soon as possible to relieve situations that cause discomfort. The nurse might provide ice chips or a drink of some sort that provides some calories, check the position of the stirrups and reposition them if there is any pressure on the popliteal space, and remove the patient from the stirrups as soon as possible. The nurse should provide dry linens, a clean gown, and a warm blanket when the patient is transferred from the delivery table.

To allay emotional discomfort that may be interfering with the patient's ability to relax, the nurse should assess the patient's reason for anxiety and take steps to help the mother relax. Perhaps an opportunity to communicate with her family will help her relax.

Special care should be taken to avoid trauma as the patient is removed from the stirrups and placed on a bed or stretcher. The type of care in taking the patient down from the delivery table depends on the type of anesthetic administered. If the patient has had none or only a local anesthetic, the nurse can help her move her legs. She may experience some difficulty if she has been in stirrups for a long time or if she has been improperly positioned. If the patient has had a regional anesthetic, such as a saddle or caudal block, she will not be able to move her legs. Her legs must be moved by the nurse. Care should be taken to move both legs at the same time, in the same way, and with adequate support. If one leg at a time is moved, then there will be stress on the ligaments that may cause pain and trauma in the future. If the patient has had a spinal anesthetic, special care should be taken to avoid an elevation of the patient from the vertical position. She should be carefully lifted or log-rolled from the delivery table and her head should not be elevated for 6 to 8 hours, or as ordered by the physician.

If the mother was anesthetized during delivery, she may need reassurance that she has given birth and that all is well with her and the baby. Her need for relaxation and sleep may be demonstrated by intermittent dozing. This should be allowed as much as possible, since this is her taking-in time. She will need extra food, sleep, rest, and attention so as to move into taking-on activities of mothering. The goal of providing comfort and rest is extremely important and should be begun as soon as possible.

Nursing Tasks Involved in Providing Rest, Relaxation, Comfort, and Safety

1 Assess the individual mother's needs. Is she excited, tense, anxious, fatigued?
2 Create an atmosphere conducive to rest.
3 Provide physical comfort by appropriate position, clean linens, blanket, or medication, if indicated.
4 Use caution in removing the patient from the stirrups of the delivery table to avoid discomfort or future trauma.

5 Provide fluids, as needed by the patient.

6 Provide an opportunity for the patient and her family to visit with each other as soon as possible.

PROVIDING CONTINUITY OF CARE THROUGH ADEQUATE REPORTING AND RECORDING

Since nursing care for the newly delivered mother at this time is usually divided between delivery room, recovery room, nursery, and postpartum areas, extra care must be taken to provide continuity of care. It is hoped that new ideas will bring changes which will provide nurses for patients rather than "area" nurses in the maternity units across the country. The frequent change of nurses necessitated by days off and change of shifts is made even worse when the patient must change nurses frequently during her short hospital stay.

Since the patient's care is likely to be ministered by a number of nurses within the same day or even within an 8-hour period, it is extremely important for the delivery area nurse to communicate appropriate and accurate information in writing and by an oral report which will help the nurse who will be caring for the patient after leaving the delivery room. The nurse who receives the new mother needs information concerning the patient's needs and previous problems that were encountered as well as the patient's preference in care.

Regardless of the various reports and charts that are unique to a particular delivery room setting, the delivery area nurse should recognize various areas of information that are important to the nurse who will be caring for the mother and the baby so that care can proceed without interruption. The knowledge the delivery area nurse should pass on to the nurse who cares for the patient immediately postpartum, regardless of *where* the patient is cared for, should include:

1 The patient's gravida and para, an assessment of fundal height and the consistency of the uterus, as well as the amount of blood loss during delivery. The estimate of blood loss should include the amount in the delivery room and a specific description of the amount lost on perineal pads, e.g., the number and the amount of saturation of the pads during a specific period of time.

2 The amount and type of drugs received by the patient that might affect her care, such as narcotics, tranquilizers, anesthetics (local, regional, or general), and oxytocics; unusual response or allergies to medication.

3 The type of episiotomy and if there were lacerations or unusual trauma.

4 The physician's orders for the patient.

5 The last time the patient voided.

6 The predisposing factors that indicate the possibility of postpartum hemorrhage.

7 The parents' response to the newborn and their desires regarding seeing and holding their baby.

8 Intravenous feedings and/or blood transfusions during labor and delivery or which may be currently running, amount remaining, orders to discontinue or continue.

9 Factors that indicate the possibility of infection, dehydration, or extreme fatigue or exhaustion in the patient.

10 Previous vital signs, especially when problems are anticipated.

11 The condition and sex of the baby.

The knowledge the delivery area nurse should pass on to the nursery nurse should include:

1 Condition of the infant at birth, Apgar score at 1 minute and at 5 minutes

2 Amount and type of anesthetic or analgesic the mother received

3 Type of resuscitation used for the infant

4 Sex of the baby, time of birth, and considerations such as spontaneous or forceps delivery, prolonged labor, meconium in the amniotic fluid, tachycardia, bradycardia, or arrhythmia during labor and delivery

5 Response of the mother and father to the newborn and plans made with them in regard to establishing a relationship with the baby

6 Condition of the mother

7 Method of feeding the infant

8 Type and amount of medication given to the infant

9 Bracelet information that identified the infant with his parents

10 Baby's pediatrician or general practitioner

Whether these are written or verbally reported may depend on several factors. Most hospitals require all of the above information to be written. In addition, the nurse should mention many of these factors verbally when they influence the care the nurse will give the patient. Some discussion of a plan of care is valuable as the nurse who has cared for the patient in labor and delivery may have identified various patient needs that only the nurse who cares for the patient later in her postpartal period can provide. Some of these needs would include the new mother's need for teaching and support in mothering activities.

This chapter deals with a very brief time in the patient's birth experience. However, nursing care during this time is very important to the new family, as it may help prevent a postpartum hemorrhage, which can result in death. More frequently, this is the time in which the mother may experience a delay in recovering from the birth experience and/or a delay in taking on the mothering role. The nurse who cares for the patient in this stage also can do much to enhance the patient's sense of achievement for her efforts in the birth process. In addition to assisting the newborn in adjusting to the extrauterine environment, the nurse can also help establish a positive family experience by providing opportunities for the mother and father to relate to their baby and begin building a relationship. Rather than being distracted by menial tasks, nursing care during the third stage of labor can become one of magnitude and importance and may be extremely satisfying to the nurse and helpful to the patient as the patient *begins* the all-important task of becoming a mother.

REFERENCES

1 Taylor, E. Stewart: *Beck's Obstetrical Practice,* 9th ed., Williams & Wilkins, Baltimore, 1971, p. 199.
2 Hellman, Louis M., and Jack A. Pritchard: *Williams Obstetrics,* 14th ed., Appleton-Century-Crofts, New York, 1971, p. 415.
3 Ibid., p. 416.
4 Calkins, L. A.: "Management of the Third Stage of Labor," *Journal of the American Medical Association,* 101:1128, 1933.
5 Fitzpatrick, Elise, Sharon Reeder, and Luigi Mastroianni, Jr.: *Maternal Nursing,* 12th ed., Lippincott, Philadelphia, 1971, p. 223.
6 Taylor: op. cit., pp. 201–202.
7 Fitzpatrick, et al.: op. cit., p. 493.
8 Taylor: op. cit., 202.
9 Hellman, et al.: op. cit., p. 42.
10 Ibid., p. 421.
11 *Physicians' Desk Reference,* Litton Publications, Oradell, N.J., 1969, pp. 823–824, 1083, 1406, 1407.
12 Bergerson, Betty S., Elsie Krey, and Andres Goth (eds.): *Current Concepts in Clinical Nursing,* Mosby, St. Louis, 1969, pp. 542–565.
13 Bradley, Robert A.: *Husband-coached Childbirth,* Harper & Row, New York, 1965.

BIBLIOGRAPHY

Bradley, Robert: "Father's Presence in Delivery Rooms," *Psychosomatics,* vol. 3, no. 6, November–December, 1962.
Calkins, L. A.: "Management of the Third Stage of Labor," *Journal of the American Medical Association,* 101:1128, 1933.

Caplan, Gerald: *Concepts of Mental Health Consultations, Their Application in Public Health Social Work*, Children's Bureau, New York, 1959.

Davis, M. E., and R. Rubin: *De Lee's Obstetrics for Nursing*, 17th ed., Saunders, Philadelphia, 1963.

Juzwiah, Marijo: "An Intimate Look at Husband Coached Childbirth," *Registered Nurse*, p. 45, December 1966.

Larson, Virginia: "Stress of the Childbearing Year," *American Journal of Public Health*, 56(1):32–36, January 1965.

Littlefield, Vivian: "An Investigation into the Effects of Supportive Nursing Care on Primiparous Patients during Labor and Delivery," an unpublished study presented to the graduate faculty of the University of Colorado School of Nursing, 1964.

———: "Maternal Satisfaction with the Birth Experience and Maternal-child Adjustment," an unpublished study presented to the graduate faculty of the University of Colorado School of Nursing, 1964.

Quilliga, E. J.: "Symposium on Physiology of Labor," *Clinical Obstetrics and Gynecology*, 11:13–191, 1968.

Rubin, Reva: "Attainment of the Maternal Role. 1. Processes," *Nursing Research*, 16(3):237–245, Summer 1967.

———: "Attainment of the Maternal Role. 2. Models and Referrants," *Nursing Research*, 16(4): 342–346, Fall 1967.

Wiedenbach, Ernestine: *Family-centered Maternity Nursing*, Putnam, New York, 1967.

25 | THE FOURTH STAGE OF LABOR

Joy Clausen

The fourth stage of labor marks the completion of the tasks associated with the first three stages of labor. Expressions of quiescence, of relief, of accomplishment, intermingled with excitement, radiate from the mother's face. Hopefully, labor and delivery has been a shared experience between the mother and the baby's father. He may manifest expressions similar to the mother's, both of them sensing that the baby's birth is, indeed, an accomplishment which heralds the beginning of new and different roles for all persons in the family unit.

The first critically important hour postpartum is defined as the fourth stage of labor. Just as the first three stages are particular delineated events in the birth process, the fourth stage of labor begins with the expulsion of the placenta and terminates the end of the next hour.

The mother, baby, and perhaps the father spend a portion of the fourth stage of labor in the delivery room. Their immediate needs and the nursing care involved during this delivery room stay were discussed in detail in the preceding chapter. This chapter will focus on the fourth stage of labor when the mother has been transferred from the delivery room to the recovery room and the baby is in the nursery.

Not all hospitals have obstetric recovery room facilities. However, nursing care is facilitated and patient care enhanced when a well-planned, well-equipped, and proficiently staffed recovery room is available for newly delivered mothers.

DYNAMICS ASSOCIATED WITH THE FOURTH STAGE OF LABOR

Psychosocial Dynamics

As the nurse responsible for the care of a newly delivered mother, you are the person who will initiate interaction between mother, father, and baby. This may be an easier task for the nurse if the family unit is one which has been traditionally defined by society as the norm of wife-mother, husband-father, and baby. But society is changing, and we find new and different social norms.

The family unit of today may consist of the mother of the baby; the father of the baby, who may not be the mother's husband according to the legal definition, or a man who is not the father of the baby; and the baby. It is sometimes difficult for nurses to assume the role of initiator of mother-father-baby interaction because of these new and different arrangements. Often it is necessary for the nurse to spend time working through personal feelings alone, as well as with significant others, in order to arrive at an operational definition of the term family unit.

Have the mother and father seen the baby yet? If the mother was under general anesthesia during delivery and/or if the father was not allowed in the delivery room, there is a possibility that they have not had an opportunity to see and hold the baby. Perhaps one or the other has seen the baby, but they have not been afforded the opportunity to *hold* and *fondle* the baby together. The sensitive, caring nurse can easily assess the mother's and father's needs in this area.

An important part of the question of whether or not the mother and father have seen the baby is, "Do they *want* to see the baby?" They may be utterly fatigued, unable to cope with holding and relating to the baby until they have replenished their own energies. They may want to see the baby but may feel apprehensive about holding such a new and little being.

The needs of the mother and father concerned with seeing and holding the baby can be assessed with ease if the nurse will *listen* to what they are saying and if a few, gentle questions are asked of them during the initial visit in the recovery room. "Would you like to hold your baby?" "Do you feel alert enough for the little one to visit for a short time?" "Would you like me to stay with you and help you learn to hold the baby?"

EMOTIONAL MANIFESTATIONS

The pregnant woman during the second and third stages of labor is "turned-in."[1] She is unto herself, working diligently on childbearing. The nurse may find that during the fourth stage of labor the mother is not really anxious to see or hold the baby. This may indicate several things, one of which may be that she has not yet transcended the turned-in phase. Then, too, she may be truly fatigued from the childbearing process. The fatigue, either by itself or in combination with the residual turned-in phase, affects the degree to which the mother can extend herself to her new baby. The father may choose to adhere to the mother's wishes regarding seeing and holding the baby. It is the astute, perceptive nurse who is able to comprehend and interpret what the mother and father are actually saying and act accordingly. In some instances, because of the nurse's assessment of their behavior, it is wise *not* to urge them to interact with the baby immediately, but instead to wait until such time that fatigue and the turned-in phase subside. When the mother and father indicate readiness, the baby should be taken to them, allowing them sufficient time to examine, to cuddle, to become acquainted.

There is a wide range of behavior displayed by mothers and fathers during the first hour after delivery. Many exhibit profound fatigue, just as one experiences after strenuous physical exercise. However, even though fatigue may be prevalent, a state of elation may be concomitantly present. A common statement by mothers during this time is, "I am *so* tired, yet I feel *so* awake and excited!"

A mother who has been given a general anesthetic during delivery will behave differently from one who has been awake. The former mother will need time to awaken fully, and as a consequence, there will be a greater time lag until she exhibits any particular behavior in relation to labor and delivery, toward the father, or toward the baby. She may find it difficult to believe that the delivery is over and that the baby has really been born.

It is not uncommon for the mother and father to relieve their tensions by such emotional outbursts as crying, laughing, shouting, talking constantly, embracing, and kissing lavishly. These emotions may be heightened when the baby is being cuddled between them. It is indeed satisfying for the nurse to witness these behaviors, not only from the standpoint that such behaviors aid in tension reduction for the mother and father, but also because the observed closeness between these people is at an intense *emotional* level. This is the beginning of an immensely important period of role transition for mother and father, a transition that takes time, fortitude, patience, and knowledge before it comes to fruition!

A common complaint of mothers after delivery of the baby and placenta is a feeling of chill. This chill often occurs while the mother is being prepared for transfer to the recovery room, while she is being transferred, or immediately after transfer. The mother actually shakes as a manifestation of the chill. The chill and overt shaking usually do not last over 15 minutes.

There are numerous hypotheses regarding cause of the chill, some of which include the following:[2, 3, 4, 5]

1 The mother's nervous reaction and exhaustion related to childbearing.
2 Muscular exertion during labor and delivery causes disequilibrium between the internal and external body temperature.
3 There is a sudden release of intraabdominal pressure after the uterus is emptied.
4 Lack of aseptic technique during labor predisposes to infection in the mother, giving rise to chills as one manifestation of the infection.
5 Postpartum chills probably represent minute, circulatory amniotic fluid embolism and are associated with scanty amniotic fluid volume.
6 Previous maternal sensitization to elements of fetal blood, as well as fetal/maternal transfusions at time of delivery, causes a reaction in the mother manifested by chills.

The chills are annoying, sometimes frightening, as well as embarrassing to the mother and father. Whether this reaction is emotional, physiological, or an interaction of the two, the nurse can be helpful by reassuring the mother and father that chills are not uncommon after delivery. Comfort measures should be supplied by the nurse and include warm blankets and gown, an increase in room temperature, and warm fluids by mouth, if not contraindicated.

Mothers often ask the same questions, over and over again, about their delivery and about the baby. The nurse should recognize this as normal behavior which is a necessary process in order that the mother is able to move out of the symbiotic relationship she had with the fetus during pregnancy.[6] The baby must be a separate person before the mother can become acquainted with him. This psychological separation of baby from mother is an important phase in the development of the maternal role and in the mother-child relationship yet to develop. The disengagement of the symbiotic mother-baby relationship of pregnancy is sometimes referred to as "cutting the psychological cord."

The fetus has now become a living, breathing baby. However, the mother and father do not necessarily experience an affective relationship with the baby immediately after birth. There is often a time lag of a few hours to a few days or weeks before the mother and father experience feelings of motherliness or fatherliness toward the baby. Mothers in particular, if questioned about when they first experienced a maternal feeling, can often identify almost the exact instance the feeling occurred. They will say that the feeling usually appeared suddenly and describe it as a feeling of warm protectiveness for the baby.[7]

It can be a frightening experience for a mother to experience lack of feeling for her baby, particularly when she believes that she *should*, in fact, have immediate motherly feelings when the baby is first placed in her arms. The same is true for the father. If a nurse assesses from the parents' behavior that this is a concern, it can be explained to them that there is sometimes a period of time before maternal and paternal feelings are experienced toward the baby. The optimum time for such anticipatory guidance, however, is before delivery. If parents know about the possibility of a time lag, then they will be more cognizant of their lack of feelings toward the baby, should this occur, and some of their concern might be allayed. The maternity nurse plays an integral role in helping the mother and father to anticipate and understand present and future parent-child relationships.

THE MOTHER-FATHER ROLE TRANSITION

William Shakespeare once wrote [8]

> All the world's a stage,
> And all the men and women merely players:
> They have their exits and their entrances;
> And one man in his time plays many parts.

We can apply Shakespeare's words to childbearing in that the man and woman are the players who have made entrance into parenthood, one of many parts, or roles, they will play during their lifetime.

Role refers to the *behavior* expected of one who occupies a certain status. Status is defined as the *position* of an individual in a group. [9]

The concept of role is not an isolated entity. It implies a set of reciprocal behaviors which includes one's own behavior, as well as the behavior of the others in a situation. An ascribed role is one which is assigned to a person according to a criterion that can be known in advance, such as sex and age. An achieved role is one which is secured through individual choice and competition. Likewise, there are ascribed statuses and achieved statuses. The person, as a man or woman, holds an ascribed status, whereas becoming a mother or father is an achieved status.

People occupy many different statuses and are expected to fill the roles appropriate to the statuses. For instance, the newly delivered mother may occupy the status of wife, woman friend, unmarried woman, secretary, nurse, mother, daughter, or any combination. She is expected to behave in accordance with the duties and privileges associated with these statuses; these are her roles. Likewise, the father may occupy the status of husband, man friend, unmarried man, lawyer, teacher, father, son, or any combination. His behavior, then, is also that which is expected of one who occupies these statuses. These are his roles.

The acquisition of a maternal or paternal role is a continuous, active process. Role training for these important roles begins in early childhood when the child plays house, helps mother clean, or watches father shave. There are countless incidents in family life from which children gradually form a mental picture of how women and men act, of how husbands and wives interact, and of how mothers and fathers treat their children.

Reva Rubin cites five operations involved in the attainment of the maternal role.[10] Although these operations are written from the context of attainment of the *maternal* role, they certainly are transferable to the attainment of the *paternal* role.

The operations include mimicry, role-play, fantasy, introjection-projection-rejection, and grief-work. These are classified into three phases: mimicry and role-play are forms of the *taking-on* phase; fantasy and introjection-projection-rejection are forms of the *taking-in* phase; and grief-work represents the *letting-go* phase, by which one relinquishes a former status or role.

The operations are sequential and cyclical during the prenatal period. The delivery of the baby marks the begining point of a cycle of operations during the postpartum period. The five operations are not entities which stand alone, for no single operation occurs independently of the others.

The operations can be conceptualized as outer circles in order of depth of role achievement, with the inner core depicted as role achievement. Figure 25-1 illustrates this conceptual framework.

Mimicry refers to the process by which a woman adopts behavior manifestations, such as affect of speech, gestures, and dress which are symbols of the status she wants to obtain. Role-play, although it is similar to mimicry, goes one step further in that it constitutes not only outward symbolism but also is an *acting out* of expected behavior of a person in a similar situation.

Fantasy may be an element of role-play, but the difference is that with pure fantasy, there is no acting out. The operation of fantasy initiates the movement from the taking-on phase to the taking-in phase. The other operation in the taking-in phase, introjection-projection-rejection, resembles mimicry. However, in mimicry, the role model is from without, whereas in introjection-projection-rejection, the operation begins with self (introjection). Then a role model is found outside of self (projection), and the behavior of the role model is matched with the behavior that the woman is experiencing. If the matching is appropriate and is a "fit," all is well, and she is able to add to her existing knowledge and behaviors. But if the "fit" is unsatisfactory, it is cast off (rejection) and other role models go through the same process until a "fit" is found.

Grief-work is the release of former identities associated with roles which are not compatible with what is anticipated in the new role. It is neither a taking-on nor taking-in operation. During the grief-work operation, former roles, pleasant and unpleasant, are reviewed through memory. This review tends to release some of the bonds associated with the former roles, hence, the former self.

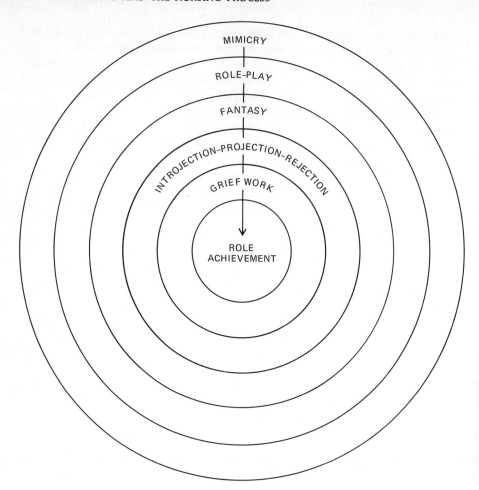

FIGURE 25-1
A conceptual framework of Reva Rubin's five operations involved in the attainment of the maternal role.

People are confronted many times during their lifetimes with role transitions. They are working much of their lives on expected behaviors (roles) ascribed to particular positions in society (statuses).

Portions of transition to the maternal and paternal roles are accomplished during a person's life even before the prenatal period. But it is during the fourth stage of labor that the maternal and paternal roles begin to become realities. The mother and father continue their work with the five operations during this time in order to actualize their identity as a mother and father. They continue to seek role models for their behaviors, and the maternity nurse is a person, close in time and space, to whom they can relate.

In the recovery room during the fourth stage of labor, the nurse may perceive that the mother and father are not comfortable holding the baby. This is an opportunity for the nurse to offer to demonstrate for the parents comfortable and safe methods by which they can hold and fondle the baby. In this way, the mother and father will be able to mimic and role play the nurse-model's behavior, which in turn will help them become more secure in their transition to the maternal and paternal role.

It is not uncommon for a nurse to hear parents exclaim while viewing and holding their baby for the first time something similar to, "Oh, she is the most beautiful, marvelous baby!" This description may not fit with anyone else's appraisal of the baby. The nurse should be cognizant of the fact that there is a possibility that these parents are continuing the fantasy developed about the baby during pregnancy. They may not be perceiving the baby as reality and may be projecting their intrapersonal fantasies about the baby onto the real baby. This information can be shared with other members of the nursing team as well as with the physician. By doing this, the parents can be observed throughout the postpartum period to ascertain whether or not they begin to perceive and respect the baby as a *real* person, rather than as a fantasy carried over from pregnancy.

Meeting the Mother's and Father's Physical Needs

Childbearing is a biological as well as a psychosocial event. The biological component affects the psychosocial, but is focused primarily on body functioning, be it the mother's, the father's, or the baby's. The psychosocial component, although it has profound effects on the biological, focuses on mother, father, and baby as feeling, thinking, behaving people. The parents and newly delivered baby should always be thought of as bio-psycho-social beings, even though for learning purposes it is sometimes necessary to concentrate study on either the biological or the psychological or the sociological component.

In most institutions, the newborn is transferred to the nursery after immediate care is given in the delivery room. Therefore, the physical care of the newborn during the immediate fourth stage of labor is discussed in detail in Part IV.

With what biological concerns of the mother and father should the nurse be concerned during the fourth stage of labor? *What* nursing care is offered, and *why*? *How* does the nurse care for a mother and father during the first critically important hour postpartum?

TRANSFER TO THE RECOVERY ROOM

The newly delivered mother is transferred from the delivery room to the recovery room after the baby has been transferred to the nursery and after the physician has repaired the episiotomy. If the mother has had a general anesthetic during delivery, she should be fully awake before the transfer so that she may be under constant surveillance by the anesthesiologist or nurse anesthetist, and/or doctor during the important recovery period.

The mother is moved via a transfer cart or in a bed from the delivery room to the recovery room. She may experience some nausea from this movement. This nausea is thought to be precipitated not only by the movement, but by anesthesia, medications, an empty stomach, emotions, or a combination of these factors. It is a wise nurse who places an emesis basin on the cart or bed during the transfer!

Under optimum conditions, the father has had opportunity, if he so desired, to be with the mother during labor *and delivery*. As a consequence, he is with the mother during the transfer. This is not always possible, however, because of time and circumstances surrounding the delivery and/or because of hospital policy. Nevertheless, the nurse can use ingenuity during the mother's transfer in order to include the father and baby, thus initiating interaction between members of the family unit.

In some hospitals, the baby is nestled in the mother's arms during the transfer. This technique enables the mother to be the person who first introduces baby to father. This appears to be a most satisfying experience for all concerned.

The nurse attends to the utmost safety precautions as soon as the mother is placed on the transfer cart or bed, before the actual transfer is begun. These precautions include a comfortable position and body alignment; appropriate blankets which provide privacy, warmth, and are not static; an emesis basin; and paper handkerchiefs. If an intravenous feeding is in place, the nurse must check for patency and possible infiltration. Safety straps are secured, and side rails are raised. The wheels of the cart or bed are locked as the mother moves from the delivery table to the transport vehicle. The wheels are unlocked during the transfer but are locked as soon as the movement of the cart or bed ceases.

If the baby is transferred with the mother, it works well if the mother lies on her side with the baby nestled in her arms. Maintenance of body heat is of critical importance for a newborn and is a body function which is not fully activated at this time. Therefore, the baby is wrapped securely in dry, warm blankets which will not create static electricity. Patency of the baby's airway must be ascertained and maintained before and during the transfer. An aspiration bulb syringe can be placed near the baby to be used if necessary. The baby's umbilical cord is checked immediately before movement of the vehicle in order to rule out bleeding.

The implementation of these safety precautions will help to assure the nurse that mother and baby are physically safe in an environment which protects their well-being. Hence, the nurse will find it most appropriate to step aside and allow mother, father, and baby privacy during these tender moments.

In some institutions, the nursery nurse is called after the visit and takes the baby to the nursery. In others, the nurse wheels the mother and baby, accompanied by the father, to the nursery and transfers the baby to the nursery nurses. Sometimes, as was mentioned previously, the baby is transferred to the nursery before the mother is out of the delivery room. These procedures are dictated by hospital policies, and differ widely. Whatever the case may be, the nurse who is responsible for the care of the mother during the fourth stage of labor is responsible for providing mother, father, and baby the opportunity to be together if they so desire as soon after delivery as possible.

Let the father help with the transfer if he shows the slightest willingness or desire to help! He is an integral part of the childbearing process, and a creative nurse will include him in every way possible. He can help steer the cumbersome cart or bed. He can help lift the mother or help her roll onto the recovery room bed. He can help rearrange furniture in the recovery room to make room for the transfer vehicle. He should realize that he is needed and important at this time.

THE NEED FOR REASSURANCE AND REST

Childbearing is often accompanied by an element of apprehension for both the mother and father. The environment is usually strange to them, and in addition, they observe a myriad of equipment in the recovery room. They may feel somewhat emotionally insecure during the first hour postpartum, and they may not know quite what to think about the new baby. The father may have heard the mother scream out during delivery, and may be wondering why this happened and what will happen now. The mother may experience episotomy discomfort, afterpains, nausea, or leg cramps and may not know why.

The mother and father need reassurance. Ernestine Wiedenbach defines reassurance most appropriately as "the presence of someone who knows what to do."[11] In addition to knowing *what* to do, the maternity nurse should know *how* to do it, *why* it is done, and *when* to do it. This, then, is the essence of reassurance that the mother and father need from the nurse.

Second to reassurance is the need of the mother and father for rest. This is often a difficult task to accomplish during this time because of the excitement inherent in the childbearing process. It is difficult for the parents to quiet down; there is so much to talk about and share with one another. Other things are also happening which deprive the mother and father of rest. The happenings may be positive, such as visiting with the baby, or they may be necessary, such as the nurse checking the mother's physical stability.

Reva Rubin identifies a phase of restoration, or regeneration, which begins immediately after a deep, spontaneous, therapeutic sleep.[12] If this sleep is interrupted, the restorative phase is delayed, and as a consequence, the mother may exhibit sleep hunger.

Although a deep, restorative sleep may not be possible during the first hour postpartum, the knowledgeable, efficient nurse will lay the groundwork in order that deep sleep will be attainable at a later time. This groundwork can be accomplished by expert patient observation for signs of uterine atony, deviations in vital signs, perineal hematomas, urinary retention, or other untoward conditions which unless they are resolved, will cause the mother sleep loss during a time when necessary deep sleep would have otherwise been acquired.

The mother should be encouraged to at least try to rest, if not sleep, during this first hour postpartum. The nurse can facilitate patient rest by careful scheduling of patient care. The mother should not be disturbed too frequently or unnecessarily, and care should be organized in order that a maximum amount be completed through brief contact during specific intervals.

Proper body alignment is a prerequisite to rest. Can the mother align herself comfortably, or does she need help? (She surely will need help if she has had a saddle block or caudal anesthesia!) Does she have sufficient pillows with which to prop her head, arms, legs, and back? (Check the physician's orders. Some physicians do not allow a pillow under the head after a saddle block.)

Is the mother warm enough, or too warm? (Newly delivered mothers often compain of cold feet.) Are the bed linens clean and smooth and secure, both under and over her? Is her perineal pad clean and in place? Has she had food and fluids, if allowed?

All of these measures are important for the comfort of the parturient. The absence or presence, as the case may be, of any one or a combination of those outlined above will not be conducive to rest. The nurse has the ultimate responsibility to the patient to help induce rest by aiding in her comfort.

Fathers become tired, too. The hours are often long during the time he gave support to the mother-to-be through labor, and sometimes delivery. Does he need a cup of tea or coffee, a sandwich, some milk or juice? What would be quick and nourishing for him from the unit kitchen? Where could he go close by for a quick snack?

Perhaps he would rather rest. Is there an easy chair and footstool for him, an extra pillow, and is the room temperature comfortable for him?

Rest can come only after the mother and father are reassured, only after they feel the nurse knows what to do, how to do it, why it is done, and when to do it. Comfort measures are only a part of reassurance. The mother and father continue to gain reassurance as they assess the competence by which the nurse cares for the mother during the postpartum checks.

PATIENT CHECKS DURING THE FIRST HOUR POSTPARTUM

The nurse is responsible for checking the mother's physical condition after she has been settled in the recovery room bed. The technique of the check should be organized in order that important observations are not deleted.

The patient checks include (1) palpation of the fundus of the uterus; (2) massage of the fundus and observation for bladder distention; (3) expression of clots and free blood from the uterus; (4) measurement of the fundus in relation to the umbilicus; (5) inspection of the perineum for discoloration and swelling; (6) inspection of the perineal pad and change, if necessary; (7) recording of blood pressure and pulse; and (8) offering food and fluids if allowed, and comfort and safety measures.

It is important that the checks be done according to specific time intervals so that the nurse is able to assess and compare the mother's condition on a sequential basis. The American College of Obstetricians and Gynecologists recommends that the postpartum patient be under constant observation by an experienced nurse, and that the mother be checked every 15 minutes during this hour for uterine atony, hemorrhage, deviations in blood pressure and pulse, and other complications.[13] The mother should be checked more often than every 15 minutes if there are any indications of deviations in her physical condition.

Explain the procedure to the patient! This is, indeed, a basic nursing skill, but it must be reinforced that the nurse take time, especially before the initial check, to explain to the mother and father what is involved in the nursing care about to be administered. The nursing care involved with palpation, massage, and expression of the uterus may be uncomfortable for the mother, and she should be prepared for this possibility. The nurse should also share with the mother the information that if she relaxes her abdominal muscles, this portion of the check will be expedited for both the mother and the nurse.

A basic nursing skill which is often neglected on maternity wards is that of providing the mother with privacy. Too often there is unnecessary exposure of the mother's body during the postpartum check because of lack of proper screening devices or draping procedures.

It is not a steadfast rule or procedure that the father leave the room while the nurse checks the mother. Certainly there are times when this is appropriate, but it is not the majority of the time. The father and mother are consulted regarding their desires in this situation. If they prefer that he remains in the room during the check, the nurse can again use creativity to provide privacy for the mother. For, instance, the nurse can have the mother

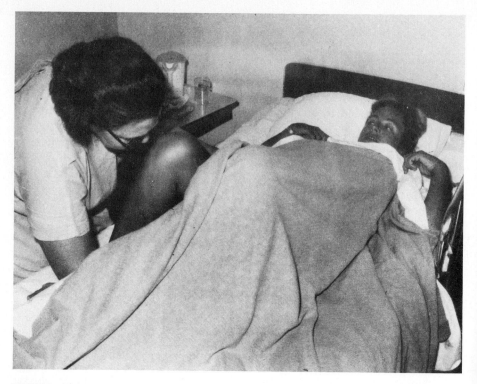

FIGURE 25-2
Providing the mother with privacy during the postpartum check by fashioning a tentlike structure from the bed linens.
(Courtesy of Abbott Hospital, Minneapolis, Minnesota.)

elevate and flex her legs so that the bed linens form a tentlike structure, as shown in Figure 25-2. The mother is asked to hold the bed linen taut by pulling the linen to her upper chest and neck. The nurse then approaches the mother from the side, and exposes the mother's abdominal and perineal area by lifting the loose linen flap formed by the mother's thigh and lower leg. The linens on the side facing where the father is sitting or standing are left intact, thus providing the mother with privacy.

Another method by which the mother can be afforded privacy without the father leaving the room is by the nurse approaching the mother from the side on which the father is sitting, thus using the nurse's body to shield the mother from exposure during the check.

More often than not, if the father remains in the room during the check, he will look out the window, read, or become otherwise engaged during this time. He usually senses the mother's need for privacy at this time and acts accordingly.

PALPATION, MASSAGE, EXPRESSION, AND MEASUREMENT OF THE UTERUS

If a nurse were to place in order of importance nursing care which involves contact with the hands during the first hour postpartum, palpation, massage, expression, and measurement of the fundus of the uterus would be paramount.

During the fourth stage of labor, the uterus continues to contract and relax. The uterus controls postpartum hemorrhage by contracting and compressing the patent blood vessels at the site where the placenta was implanted. Gradually, thrombosis develops within the sinuses. Therefore, the most immediate precaution to postpartum hemorrhage is sustained contraction of the uterus.[14]

Medication, such as Ergotrate, Syntocinon, Pitocin, or Methergine, is given to the mother intravenously or intramuscularly during the delivery of the baby's anterior shoulder, during the delivery of the placenta, or immediately after the placenta is delivered. These medications, known as oxytocics, stimulate uterine contractions, the effect of which may last several hours.

Oxytocics work well in prevention of uterine atony, the most common cause of postpartum hemorrhage. Nonetheless, the action of these, like other drugs, is contingent to a large degree on the overall physical condition of the patient. It must *not* be assumed that because sufficient doses of oxytocics were administered to the mother, constant surveillance of the condition of her uterus is not necessary. The tone of the uterus is dependent on many factors other than whether or not the mother has had oxytocics. These factors will be discussed later in this chapter.

Contraction of the uterus occurs when the mother hears the newborn baby's cry or when she can see or hold the baby. These contractions are brought about by the sympathetic nervous system which is activated by the mother's emotions.

In some hospitals, the baby is put to breast on the delivery table. This action also tends to cause the uterus to contract and is prophylactic to postpartum hemorrhage.

Under normal conditions, the postpartum checks are not lengthy procedures. As the nurse acquires competence in checking the mother, it will be found that these checks can be completed thoroughly and efficiently in just a few minutes without conveying haste to the mother and father.

Sufficient time is spent to ensure that the needs of the mother and father are met, and the nurse is fully cognizant of the mother's immediate condition. Conversely, the checks are not drawn out unnecessarily, depriving the mother of needed rest.

In preparation for the postpartum check, the perineal pad is released, and the mother's legs are spread and flexed. If spinal or caudal anesthesia was used, it may not be possible for the mother to flex her legs without help. The fundus of the uterus is palpated by placing the side of one hand on top of and slightly cupped under the fundus, while the other hand is placed suprapubically with the exertion of slight pressure as shown in Figure 25-3. Ideally, the fundus should lie on the midplane of the pelvis, at or below the umbilicus.

If the fundus is boggy, it is massaged until it contracts and becomes firm. Care must be taken not to overmassage or overstimulate the fundus. Unnecessary manual stimulation, in the absence of bleeding or increased size of the uterus, may cause overstimulation of the uterine muscles, which will result in undue muscle fatigue with consequent relaxation of the organ and possible hemorrhage.

The bladder area is observed at this time for signs of distention. If the mother has had intravenous therapy during labor and delivery, the bladder will tend to fill more rapidly because of hydration of body tissues. The palpation maneuver performed by the nurse facilitates observation of the bladder, but in addition to the maneuver outlined above, *limited* pressure is exerted on the fundus by the hand that is cupped above and slightly under the fundus.

In the event that the bladder is filling or full, a bladder bulge will be evident and feels and appears as a spongy, fluid-filled mass below the uterus and above the symphysis pubis. Figure 25-4 shows a full bladder postpartum. The nurse's left hand is palpating the fundus of the uterus, which is high in

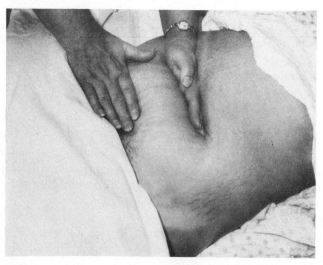

FIGURE 25-3
Hand maneuvers involved in palpation of the fundus of the uterus.
(*Courtesy of Abbott Hospital, Minneapolis, Minnesota.*)

the abdomen to the patient's right. The nurse's right hand is shown palpating the full bladder area. The mother will inform the nurse when she has the urge to urinate. However, patients, particularly those who have had a caudal or saddle block, often do not experience the urge to urinate during the first hour postpartum.

A full bladder inhibits contraction of the uterus by elevating the uterus high in the pelvis and displacing it from midline. The mother should be given the opportunity to void, and in the event she cannot, the nurse should follow doctor's orders regarding emptying of the bladder.

Expression of the fundus is done by utilizing the same hand maneuvers as those shown in Figure 25-3. In addition, during expression pressure is applied to the fundus with one hand while equal pressure is applied suprapubically with the other hand. Expression is done in sequential 3- to 5-second intervals, with several seconds' rest between, until the nurse is sure that clots and free blood held in the uterus have been expressed sufficiently.

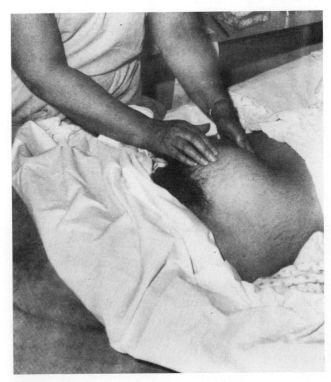

FIGURE 25-4
Palpation of a full bladder on a postpartum patient. The nurse's left hand indicates the fundus of the uterus, which has been displaced by the large full bladder underlying the nurse's right hand.
(Courtesy of Abbott Hospital, Minneapolis, Minnesota.)

After palpation, massage, and expression have been completed, the uterus usually stays firm for a period of time. However, there is always the possibility that it may not remain contracted. If there is any doubt in the nurse's mind regarding the tone of the uterus, or if during the check it is believed that bleeding and clotting is heavier than what it should be, the nurse should repeat the maneuvers more frequently than the suggested every 15 minutes.

A measurement of the height of the fundus is taken after the fundus is expressed, measuring from the top of the fundus to the umbilicus, using a measuring tape or in fingerbreadths as shown in Figure 25-5.

The fundus of the uterus tends to lie closer to the umbilicus in mothers who are multiparous than in those who are primiparous. Multiparas usually have larger uteruses than primiparas, due to repeated stretching of the muscle fibers with subsequent loss of muscle tone.

Some factors which effect the size, placement, and muscle tone of the uterus include presence of hydramnios antepartum, size of the baby, multiple births, uterine inertia during labor, length of labor, effects of oxytocics, and the amount of urine in the bladder.

INSPECTION OF THE PERINEUM

Perineal discomfort is a common complaint of mothers during the first hour postpartum, particularly after the period of time during which the anesthetic

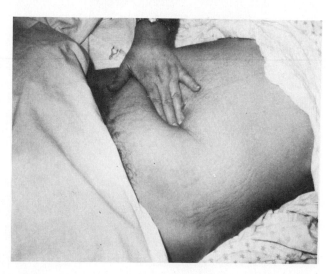

FIGURE 25-5
Measurement of the fundus of the uterus in fingerbreadths, from the top of the fundus to the umbilicus.
(*Courtesy of Abbott Hospital, Minneapolis, Minnesota.*)

loses its effect. Some physicians order an ice bag applied to the perineum for several hours postpartum. The cold lessens the edema in the episiotomy area and also tends to numb the area so that the mother's discomfort is not as pronounced.

While inspecting the perineal area during the postpartum check, the nurse may observe swelling or ecchymosis. This is indicative of the formation of a perineal or perineal-vaginal hematoma. If the hematoma continues to enlarge, the mother will complain that in addition to severe pain in the perineum, she is experiencing rectal pressure as though she needs to evacuate her bowels.

The nurse can make a positive nursing diagnosis of a hematoma by touching the area *very lightly* with a sterile gauze, or with the patient's perineal pad. If the swelling is more than edema, and is, in fact, the beginning of a hematoma, the mother will complain of extraordinary tenderness when touched. The doctor should be notified immediately. The hematoma should *not* be left unattended for it may continue to enlarge, causing the mother increasing pain. Even more important, hematomas can grow to the extent that the mother will exhibit signs of circulatory shock from extravasation.

The importance of the nurse's inspecting the mother's perineum during the first hour postpartum cannot be overemphasized.

PERINEAL CARE

It is not necessary to perform any particular type of perineal care during the first hour postpartum except to keep the area as clean and dry as possible. Regular change of perineal pads and linens under buttocks is required in order to keep the lochia from becoming dry and adhering to the mother's body. Often it is necessary for the nurse to wash the perineal area and buttocks with a mild soap and water to remove lochia not absorbed by the perineal pad. The perineal area approximate to the episiotomy should be washed first with a gentle, patting motion, taking care to wash from the vaginal and episiotomy area toward the rectum.

When checking the perineal pads for amount of lochia, the mother is rolled on her side so that the nurse can better determine the amount of bleeding. The lochia is prone to collect under the buttocks and sacral area, and is obscured from sight if the patient is not turned on her side during the check.

The lochia during the fourth stage of labor is rubra, neither dark red nor bright red. Normally, it has a fleshy odor, similar to that of fresh blood. This lochia consists of blood from the placental site, shreds of membranes, vernix, lanugo, decidua, and meconium.

Particular note is taken during the postpartum checks of the odor, consistency, and color of the lochia. Putrefactive bacteria cause foul-smelling lochia which is an indication of infection in the mother, and therefore possibly the baby. Lochia which contains strings of mucus also indicates infection. Size and consistency of lochial clots are observed and noted in the chart. If the nurse has any doubts as to whether or not the clots contain placental tissue, they should be saved for inspection by the doctor and this information reported to the doctor.

A constant, *bright red* trickle of lochia from the vagina in the presence of a well-contracted uterus is an indication of fresh bleeding. This is the result of cervical or vaginal laceration or both. The doctor is notified immediately so that the laceration can be repaired as soon as possible.

The nurse can keep a perineal pad count without a doctor's order so that the estimation of blood loss is more accurate. Notations are made in the mother's chart of how many pads were used, the degree of saturation of each pad, the size and character of clots, and the color of the lochia. The pads are kept in a covered container so that the nurse is able to compare blood loss between and during the postpartum checks.

BLOOD PRESSURE AND PULSE RECORDS

Blood pressure and pulse recording of patients in the hospital could be interpreted with more accuracy by nurses and physicians if base-line data were obtained on these patients before they entered the hospital. Obstetric personnel are more fortunate than those in other departments of the hospital in this respect, due to the fact that blood pressure and pulse rate base-line data on the mother can often be secured from the prenatal record.

The optimum postpartum blood pressure and pulse recording is that which most closely approximates the mother's blood pressure recording and pulse rate prenatally, provided these vital signs were within normal limits at that time. If the mother's blood pressure was elevated during pregnancy, it is not uncommon for it to quickly descend to within normal limits soon after the birth of the baby.

Excitement after delivery may cause elevated blood pressure and pulse in some mothers. An injection of Ergotrate may cause some women to experience elevated blood pressure and pulse rate. The combination of the general anesthesia, cyclopropane, and oxytocics administered during or after delivery have been cited as causative agents of elevated blood pressure and pulse in the postpartum patient.

Caudal and saddle block anesthesia have been identified as agents which lower vital signs through their effect on the sympathetic nervous system. Women who have been heavily sedated during labor and delivery exhibit lowered blood pressure recordings and pulse rates.

The irony which accompanies reliance upon blood pressure and pulse recordings as indicators of circulatory shock resulting from hemorrhage is that the blood pressure and pulse will show only moderate fluctuations even though the mother may be bleeding heavily. After a large amount of blood has been lost, and the circulatory system is no longer able to compensate for the decrease in blood volume, the pulse rate increases rapidly to the degree that it is difficult to count. The blood pressure drops abruptly, although this drop is very often observed several minutes *after* the *pulse rate increases.* For this reason, many physicians and experienced maternity nurses believe that the pulse rate is a more accurate indicator of the patient's condition than the blood pressure.

The mother's vital signs are influenced by her circadian rhythm, or biological clock. Research has shown that the blood pressure is highest between 4 and 6 P.M. and lowest between 1 and 6 A.M. The blood pressure begins to rise, with corresponding rise in pulse rate, early in the morning as the person approaches wakefulness. Considerations of circadian rhythm should be taken into account by the nurse in interpreting the mother's vital signs during the first hour postpartum, as well as through the entire postpartum course.

The pulse rate is usually slower during the postpartum period until the seventh to tenth postpartum day, at which time it returns to the normal rate. This decrease in rate is thought to be associated with the change in the mother's patterns of activity.

FLUIDS, FOOD, COMFORT AND SAFETY MEASURES

The offering of fluids and food during the fourth stage of labor is largely dictated by the physician's orders and by the mother's physical condition and needs. Some physicians order that fluids and food be withheld from the mother until all effects of caudal, saddle block, or of course, general anesthesia are gone.

Some women experience nausea at this time as a result of the movement of the bed or cart during transfer to the recovery room, anesthesia, medications, an empty stomach, or a combination thereof. Tea or a carbonated beverage and dry soda crackers or toast are usually tolerated well if the mother shows interest in trying food. It is surprising how many women want to try fluids and food right after delivery, even though nausea may be present! They are quick to attribute their nausea to hunger. Often the mother is correct in her assessment, but there are times when she is not. The nurse should anticipate these errors and place an emesis basin close by, in an inconspicuous but accessible location.

Encourage the mother to eat a small amount at first, to eat slowly, and to chew the food well. The degree of hunger and thirst experienced by mothers varies from those who are disinterested in food and fluids to those who are ravenous. The ability of the mother to tolerate food and fluids will depend in part on her degree of hunger and the *haste* with which she attempts to ingest the nourishment.

Comfort and safety measures instituted by the nurse for the newly delivered mother are similar to those for other postanesthesia patients. These were discussed at length earlier in this chapter in relation to the nurse's role in providing reassurance and rest. That the nurse's responsibility for the patient's comfort and safety is the basis for the nurse's existence can be deduced from the heritage of the nursing profession.

THE CESAREAN SECTION MOTHER AND FATHER

The psychosocial dynamics associated with the fourth stage of labor differ little between the cesarean section mother and father and those who have been delivered vaginally. The primary difference is that the cesarean section mother and father often experience a longer time lapse between delivery of the baby and expression of emotions. Then, too, the five operatives concerned with role attainment postpartum may not be manifest as soon. These delays can be attributed, in part, to the surgery, the anesthesia, and the subsequent time required to overcome the effects of both. The mother and father need facts and reassurance about the mother's and baby's conditions before they are able to cope with the emotional aspects and role transitions associated with childbearing.

Probably the greatest variances in the psychosocial dynamics between the cesarean section mother and father and the vaginally delivered mother and father are observable later in the postpartum period, during which time the mother and father address themselves to care of a high-risk baby, adjustment of the mother postoperatively, and inherent implications thereof.

The cesarean section mother spends the majority of the first hour postpartum in the postoperative recovery room. The time interval for patient checks may be more frequent than every 15 minutes and will depend on hospital policy set forth for immediate postoperative care. Concentrated attention is given to the mother for signs of abdominal incision bleeding, as well as vaginal bleeding.

The postpartum checks are conducted with the same maneuvers as those for a vaginally delivered mother. The nurse must be very gentle when palpating the fundus so that unnecessary stress is not placed on the abdominal incision. It is wise to check with the physician before expressing the uterus. There are several different opinions about expression of a cesarean section mother's uterus. Some believe it must be done, with gentleness of course, while others believe it should not be done as part of the postpartum check. Abdominal dressings often prohibit either accurate palpation or effective expression of the uterus.

Nursing care of the cesarean section mother during the first hour postpartum is otherwise like that of abdominal surgery patients.

Usually, the father is allowed to be with the mother, if only for a brief time. If possible, the baby should be brought to the mother, but these factors are contingent on the condition of the mother, the condition of the baby, and hospital policies.

SUMMARY

The first hour postpartum is of critical importance to the well-being of the newly delivered mother. The uterus continues to relax and contract just as it did during the first three stages of labor. Hence, this time is referred to as the fourth stage of labor.

The newly delivered mother is a bio-psycho-social being. As a consequence, nursing care is rendered which is appropriate to the integration of these three components.

Childbearing includes not only the mother and baby, but the father of the baby. The nurse is as cognizant of his needs during this time as she is of the needs of mother and baby.

REFERENCES

1 Rubin, Reva: "Puerperal Change," *Nursing Outlook*, 9(12):753–755, 1961.
2 Fitzpatrick, Elise, Sharon R. Reeder, and Luigi Mastroianni, Jr.: *Maternity Nursing*, 12th ed., Lippincott, Philadelphia, 1971, p. 302.
3 Hellman, Louis M., and Jack A. Pritchard: *Williams Obstetrics*, 14th ed., Appleton-Century-Crofts, New York, 1971, p. 471.
4 Jaameri, K. E. U., A. Jahkola, and J. Perttu: "On Shivering in Association with Normal Delivery," *Acta Obstetricia et Gynecologica Scandinavica*, 45(4):383–388, 1966.
5 Goodlin, R. C., L. P. O'Connell, and R. E. Gunther: "Childbirth Chills. Are They an Immunological Reaction?" *Lancet*, 2:79, 1967.
6 Caplan, Gerald: *Concepts of Mental Health and Consultation, Their Application in Public Health Social Work*, Children's Bureau, Washington, D. C., 1966, pp. 79–82.
7 Ibid., pp. 62–63.
8 Shakespeare, William: "As You Like It," Act II, Scene 7.
9 Horton, Paul B.: *Sociology and the Health Sciences*, McGraw-Hill, New York, 1965, p. 100.
10 Rubin, Reva: "Attainment of the Maternal Role," *Nursing Research*, 16(3):240–244, Summer 1967.
11 Wiedenbach, Ernestine: *Family-centered Maternity Nursing*, 2d ed., Putnam, New York, 1967, p. 307.
12 Rubin: "Puerperal Change," p. 754.
13 *Standards for Obstetric-Gynecologic Hospital Services*, The American College of Obstetricians and Gynecologists, Chicago, 1969, p. 42.
14 Wiedenbach: op. cit., p. 333.

PART IV

CHILDREARING AND THE NURSING PROCESS

Today's complex mobile society, in which man assumes many roles, moves at such a rapid pace that little time is allowed for childbearing and child-rearing in a relaxed manner.

The increasing demand for maternity beds and the spiraling cost of health care require that healthy newly delivered mothers and infants, no longer in need of medical care, leave the hospital setting within 48 to 72 hours after delivery. Although this practice promotes early uniting or reuniting of a family within the familiar environment of their home under more natural conditions than those found within a hospital, it does not foster extensive nursing care.

Although the nurse's exposure to the family in the hospital is extremely brief, the quality of nursing care is far more important than the quantity. It is imperative, therefore, that the nurse be able to quickly identify the needs of the new family, utilize appropriate measures for meeting these needs, and evaluate nursing intervention to determine its effectiveness.

In Chapter 26, Joseph and Peck provide a detailed description of postpartum needs of the family. The physical and emotional changes occurring, primarily in the mother, prescribe the nurse's course of action in facilitating a smooth period of readjustment.

Another member of the family experiencing rapid change is the neonate. Within a matter of minutes, he has been forced from a warm, wet environment, where his total bodily needs have been efficiently met by his mother, into a world not quite so wet or warm. Hopefully, his needs will continue to be met by his mother and other caring people.

The consumer's health needs, which includes those of the newborn, far exceed the amount of health care available. One approach to this problem is to expand the role of the nurse. If the nurse assumes more responsibility in assessing the newborn's needs and condition, the perinatologist can devote more time to the high-risk infant. For the nurse to assume this additional responsibility, theoretical knowledge, clinical expertise, and sound judgment are required.

The first 24 hours after birth are considered to be the most crucial period of the newborn's life. It is imperative that he be closely monitored so that his environment can be adjusted in relation to physiological change.

Early discharge from the hospital again demands effective use of the nurse's time. The nurse facilitates not only the newborn's adjustment to life and to his family but also his family's adjustment to him.

The process of family readjustment, continuing in the home setting, is assisted by the community health nurse. Ideally, it is the same nurse who gave support to the family during the antepartal period. The process is greatly enhanced by oral and written communication between the hospital maternity nurse and the community nurse throughout the maternity cycle.

Not all postpartum families request or accept the service of the community nurse, and not all of them need it. However, there is one family who could benefit from this support in many instances, and that is the single-parent family.

In Chapter 27, Worthy states that in over 24 percent of families there is only one parent—usually the mother. Her concern for herself and her infant are not unlike those of the two-parent family, but when no mate is present with whom problems and concerns can be shared, they increase in magnitude. In this situation, the community nurse can offer guidance and help.

UNIT A

THE IMPACT OF BIRTH ON THE FAMILY

26 | POSTPARTUM NEEDS OF THE FAMILY

Sharon Serena Joseph and Rana Limbo Peck

Every family member has a period of readjustment when the new baby arrives; however, the mother's readjustment is perhaps more extensive, since changes occur in her physical state, her habits, and her feelings. During the early puerperium the mother, especially the primipara, finds herself in a tremendous state of emotional flux, and the frontispiece of this book symbolically illustrates many of the emotional struggles occurring within her.

The mother senses that the time is near for her to regard the infant as a separate individual; but she hestitates and thinks, "not yet." Hence, her arms enfold the infant more firmly, uniting her body with that of the baby. Later the mother may feel capable of seeing the infant as an individual separate from herself, but then the desire to be one with her child may converge upon her again. "Not yet" may mean that the mother is not ready to give up the baby that was within her body, or it may mean that the mother is hesitant about accepting the overwhelming role of parenthood and the changes that this new role will require the mother and her family to make.

Whether or not a new mother is able to identify feelings similar to those just mentioned, the fact that the woman has recently given birth creates changes in her behavior and emotions. These same emotions, though not quite so extensive, may occur in the husband and siblings as well. This state of flux, which can be referred to as a developmental crisis, provides a unique opportunity for the hospital, clinic, or public health nurse to intervene. Howard J. Parad defines the crisis intervener as one who enters the problem situation and helps those involved mobilize their strengths in order to move out of the crisis or crisis-like state in a manner which is acceptable to those involved.[1] As an intervener, the nurse must possess a thorough understanding of the physical and psychological alterations taking place within the mother as well as an awareness of the dynamics involved in the changing family structure.

IN SEARCH OF SELF

Phases of the Maternal Role

Many deep emotional changes occur within the mother during the puerperium and have been described by Reva Rubin as the phases of taking-in, taking-hold, and letting-go.[2] An understanding of these phases and the variations within them will provide a theoretical base on which to plan nursing care.

TAKING-IN PHASE

This first phase may last from 2 to 3 days, during which time the mother's primary concern is with her own needs—sleep and food. To some extent, the woman reacts passively and initiates little activity on her own. The mother may find herself ravenously hungry, and the need to satisfy her own hunger may cause her to become apprehensive about her infant's oral intake.

The mother is often quite talkative during this phase and will talk at length about every detail of her labor and delivery experience, as seen in Figure 26-1. It is as if she is attempting to put everything together, to make it more meaningful to her, to absorb the experience and make it part of her inner self. She may repeat and interpret the recent events first to her husband and family and then to friends and to anyone who will listen.

This talkativeness is not to be taken lightly by the nurse. As an enthusiastic listener the nurse can help the mother interpret the events so that the whole experience becomes more meaningful to both mother and father. It is also an invaluable opportunity for the nurse to determine how the mother has perceived the labor and delivery experience and can provide important information for evaluating the future maternal-child relationship. The mother is very perceptive at this time and will sense whether the nurse is interested in her as a person or only in getting her temperature taken and recorded. A few minutes of listening and a few encouraging words can give the mother ego support which is greatly needed as she prepares to enter the second phase.

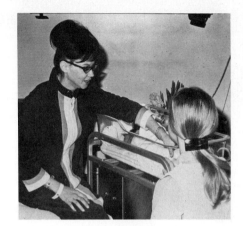

FIGURE 26-1
A nursing student listens to a mother re-
count her labor and delivery experience.
*(Courtesy of University of Colorado Medi-
cal Center, Denver, Colorado)*

TAKING-HOLD PHASE

About the third postpartum day, the mother begins the taking-hold phase in
which the emphasis is placed on the present. She becomes impatient and is
driven to organize herself and her life. She has progressed from the passive
individual to the one who is in command of the situation. Since the physical
changes are so overwhelming to her, she is relieved to know that she can
regain control of her body and that everything will return to the prepregnant
state.

It is during this time that she begins to take hold of her job of mothering the new infant, for once she has her own body and self under control,
she is able to move on to the infant. The mothering tasks become very important, taking priority over all else. If she has difficulty mastering a task,
she becomes intolerant of herself, feeling she is a failure, that she is inadequate, and that the baby is rejecting her.

The new mother is trying hard to be perfect, although she is often quite
unsure of herself. A task that appears simple to the nurse may seem monu-
mental to the mother; for as Rubin points out, the mother looks but does not
see. Common sense becomes most uncommon, and what looks simple becomes
difficult. The following situation illustrates this point. The nurse sees that a
mother is having difficulty diapering the baby and relieves the mother of her
frustration by diapering the baby neatly, quickly, and efficiently. In reality
what has happened is that the well-meaning nurse has made the mother feel
inadequate. The mother wonders if she will ever handle the baby as well as
the nurse, and because her security is threatened, she becomes frightened at
the prospect of caring for her infant.

The nurse should recognize the mother's fears and desires which are so
evident during this phase. The nurse's greatest contribution to the mother at
this time is staying with her while she diapers the baby, and complimenting

her on a job well done. The nurse must determine what has priority for the mother at the time—teaching or ego support.

A similar situation might occur during feeding. If the mother has difficulty getting the baby to nurse or to take the bottle, she is likely to interpret this as rejection of her by the infant; hence, she again feels inadequate in her mothering tasks. Successes at this time are important events in the development of a warm and healthy mother-child relationship.

The taking-hold phase lasts about 10 days. Once the mother has taken control of her own physical being and taken hold of the mothering tasks, she is able to extend her energies to her husband and other children. The nurse should recognize this course of events and help the husband understand what is happening to his wife who was once so loving and caring. He may feel left out and needs to understand that this is a temporary situation during which he will probably have to give more than he will receive. A few timely words to a husband can do much toward maintaining a satisfying marriage.

Since this is a time when the mother is taking hold of many things and is striving to master new tasks, teaching is an important and significant aspect of nursing care. Another point to remember is that the mother is curious about many things concerning herself and the baby and is willing to learn and to try new ways. It is perhaps unfortunate that many mothers are discharged from the hospital on the third postpartum day. This means that the hospital nurse never sees the mother during the taking-hold phase; hence, the best opportunities for teaching are missed. Many hospitals have organized teaching programs hoping that the new mothers will absorb some of the material presented. Such programs are of value and should be developed, but ideally the nurse would use physiological and psychological knowledge of the postpartum woman and teach to meet the individual needs. It would also warrant a nurse skilled in observation who can use creativity in presenting information to the patient without appearing perfect and omniscient. Since the patient usually requires little physical care, the nurse has more time for such individualized teaching.

LETTING-GO PHASE

The third phase of Reva Rubin's description of the restorative process is the letting-go phase. As the frontispiece of this book illustrates, the woman often has difficulty letting go of the infant as part of her body. The cutting of the umbilical cord is the first step in the infant's journey to independence, for once the cord is cut he depends on his own body to perform the life tasks of eating, breathing, and eliminating waste products.

The mother often feels a deep loss because what was once part of her body and her imagination is now reality and separate from her. The woman may quietly grieve over this loss. Many changes have taken place within her, and a new life awaits her; however, she must first accept the baby as a person with a personality of his own, and second, she must establish new norms for herself, her baby, and her family.

Conflicts of the Maternal Role

The arrival of the baby creates many conflicts within the mother even though she may have planned for this child for several months. Whether the pregnancy was planned or not, the presence of a helpless infant brings about changes in the mother's life-style. The following five conflicts were described by Ross Laboratories in a study on maternal attitudes.[3]

DEPENDENCY AND INDEPENDENCY

The mother's need to be dependent is very real during the early puerperium. It is as if she is at first overwhelmed with what she has done—delivered a baby. The new mother finds that a dependent role is safe and secure, but her situation demands that decisions be made. The attainment of maturity and independence is what she has strived for since childhood, and her new role reinforces the achievement of this goal. She is caught in conflict between doing what she knows is expected of her—making independent decisions for her baby—and doing what she feels more secure in doing—letting others make decisions for her and her baby. Ultimately she is forced to make these decisions, and she often feels she has inadequate experience on which to base these decisions. The teen-age mother, however, needs special consideration regarding this conflict, since she is also experiencing a dependent-independent conflict between adolescence and adulthood.

IDEALIZED AND REALISTIC ROLE

During pregnancy the mother may have daydreamed about what it would be like after the baby was born, seeing herself rocking and cuddling the infant, very content and satisfied with life. During the weeks following delivery, she comes to see her mothering role more realistically, and it includes getting up at night to feed the baby and changing and laundering the diapers as well as rocking the baby and cooing fondly over him. The reality of caring for a helpless infant is forced upon the mother who may feel guilty because she considers the baby a lot of work.

LOVE AND RESENTMENT OF INFANT

The infant has many needs for which he is dependent on the mother to fulfill, and since he does not know patience, he will vocally make his wants known. The mother retains many of the needs she had prior to the arrival of the baby, and conflict may arise as she tries to fulfill both her needs and her infant's. She sometimes finds her needs incompatible with the infant's, and although she loves her baby, she may resent his intrusion on her privacy. Many times the woman was treated as someone special while she was pregnant, and now that the baby has come, everyone's attention is on the infant. She may resent this fact and at the same time feel guilty because she has such feelings.

SELF-FULFILLMENT AND MOTHERHOOD

When a baby has come into the family, the woman finds that she is no longer just a woman and wife. She has become woman, wife, and mother which requires a change in her self-concept. Previous to the birth she may have seen herself as a school girl, a bride, a career girl. Some of these roles may now seem incompatible with her new role as mother; hence, conflict may arise. She may find it difficult to give up her career, and although many women continue to work following delivery, adequate arrangements must be made for the infant's care.

The mother and father can no longer do things on the spur of the moment, since an evening out will mean that they must arrange to have a baby-sitter. This can be a difficult adjustment for the new mother or for the mother whose children are older and have become more independent. She must give up part of her former role identity and establish a new role in which she can be happy. The mother can still be a creative person who works in the community, but she will have to consider the infant as she plans for her own self-fulfillment.

LOVE FOR HUSBAND AND INFANT

Previous to the baby's birth, the woman may have devoted much of her time to her husband, and now she finds her time must be divided between husband and baby. Both she and her husband may find this difficult to accept. The mother feels conflict within her because she wants to continue to give the same attention to her husband, but she finds the baby often interrupts and demands her attention.

Often the woman settles the conflict within her by becoming so involved with the infant that she forgets that her husband still needs much of the attention she gave him prior to the baby's arrival. The woman should be reminded that she remains first a wife and then a mother. A woman who is happily married will find that she is a happier mother.

Postpartum Blues

With all the physiological and psychological changes taking place within the mother, she is prone to postpartum depression, or "blues." The new mother may be unsure of herself in her new role; hence, too many helpful suggestions and words of advice may cause her to become tense and upset. She worries about obtaining the approval of her neighbor or her mother yet resents all their knowledgeable advice. She needs encouragement and acceptance from these people, and an occasional helpful hint may be welcomed. In anticipation of such frustration the nurse might suggest that the new mother listen and take what advice fits into her life-style and politely ignore the rest. The mother should be encouraged to relax with her infant and do things as she wishes. The baby will survive her mistakes, and together they will adjust.

If the mother finds that she is easily upset during the early puerperium, she should be reminded that this is normal and is due to the many changes occurring within her. The nurse should let her know that it is all right for her to cry if she feels like it. Many women feel that they are "going crazy" and are losing control of their emotions, since one minute they are happy and the next they are sad. The nurse should encourage her to talk about her feelings and above all let her know that these reactions are normal. Some women have a delayed postpartum depression which may occur as late as 3 to 4 weeks after delivery.

The Multiparous Mother

The mother having her second child may say that she feels so much more confident with this baby than she did with her first, as she is more secure in the mothering tasks. She may jokingly say that she will enjoy this baby because she learned from her first child. It is important for the nurse to remember that the woman who has other children will still pass through Rubin's three phases and still feels emotional conflicts following the delivery.

It is also appropriate for the maternal-child nurse to discuss with the mother how she plans to manage sibling rivalry that may arise when the new baby is brought home. A mother may say that there will be no problems; however, the nurse might remind her that the first child has received the parents' entire attention and, like most human beings, will find it difficult to share the limelight. The nurse should learn the ages of the other children and incorporate knowledge about the various age groups in conversations with the mother as the nurse helps to prepare her for eventual discharge. The task of discussing sibling rivalry with the postpartum mother is frequently overlooked; however, it can be of prime importance in attempting to maintain an intact, content family. These mothers often miss their older children very much while they are in the hospital, and it is frequently the first lengthy separation for both mother and child.

One woman was quite anxious to see her two-year-old child and could not wait to be discharged. On the day of discharge she was prepared to receive a warm welcome from her toddler. Instead of hugs and kisses she found the child wanted nothing to do with her. The mother was crushed and quite depressed. The child was upset with the mother because she had left him, and 2 days seemed an eternity to a child who had no concept of time. Since the child was hurt by his mother's absence, he was unsure whether he would accept her back so readily. The mother needed to be aware of how the child felt and to act appropriately. A woman in this situation can be encouraged to spend time with the older child each day—time that is his alone. A gift for the older child from the mother when she arrives home from the hospital often serves to remind him of his importance. This is just one of the many experiences that a woman may face when she returns to her other children. The arrival of a new baby causes change for every member of the family and is a time of developmental crisis for all involved.

Development of the Maternal-Child Relationship

Because it is the mother who is the primary source of socialization for the infant during the first year of life, it is advisable to have an understanding of how she initially establishes a relationship with her new baby; for it is she who conveys warmth, affection, distance, and rejection as she conducts her caretaking tasks, becoming the chief influence in the infant's life. Much has been written about the importance of a good mother-child relationship, a product of her adjustment to the new infant. It is of great importance for the maternal-child nurse to recognize the characteristics of a healthy and normal mother-infant relationship in contrast to one which deviates from the norm. The nurse's knowledgeable intervention at this time could be crucial in the lives of the new mother and growing child.

The pregnant woman's attitude toward the fetus, though not so much her attitude toward the pregnancy itself, has been found to correlate closely with her initial contribution to the mother-infant relationship.[4] The mother who has been very emotionally attached to the baby within her is more likely to remain that way after the birth. On the other hand, it is usual for someone who has viewed the fetus in an intellectual, detached way to be much less demonstrative and affectionate toward her newborn.

DEFINITION AND DESCRIPTION

One cannot adequately define a mother-child relationship solely by viewing the mother, for the system of interrelating is a circular one in which the mother responds to the baby on the basis of how she perceives his needs. Concurrently, through his activity, appearance, size, and actions the infant communicates to his mother, generating a response from her. In a healthy relationship this response is an effort by the mother to satisfy his needs primarily on the basis of the baby as an individual, and not according to the mother's own need for self-fulfillment.[5]

The first interaction between mother and baby is one of exploration and examination. When a mother is able to see her infant for the first time and the infant is nude, she will rapidly progress from poking with fingertips at the baby's extremities to encompassing the trunk with her palm.[6] The time required for the new mother's initial investigation varied from 4 to 8 minutes in the group studied, but a longer time is needed if separation after delivery has been prolonged. The description of maternal exploration is a species-specific behavior and important for a nurse to understand because the nurse is able to provide the mother with the opportunity and time to fulfill this needed release of initial maternal behavior.

Interest in the baby's eyes is demonstrated repeatedly by new mothers when they see or hold the baby for the first time. A statement such as, "Come on now, open your eyes," often heard from new mothers, reflects this intense interest in having eye-to-eye contact with the infant. Desire for the "en face"[7] position was demonstrated in all the mothers in the above study as they explored the infants, as shown in Figure 26-2.

In order to execute nursing care which is of optimum benefit to the new mother, it is helpful to assess how she and the baby interact. A new mother may appear very frightened and disturbed when her baby is brought to her. She may become much less fearful if her husband enters the room but may still be obviously upset by having relatives or friends view this initial encounter with her offspring. This mother often does not feel an immediate warm attachment to the baby, and her husband may warm up to the infant faster than she does. During pregnancy she may have viewed the fetus intellectually, without a strong emotional tie. Now that she is face to face with her "little stranger," she is unsure of herself and seems awkward when she finally handles the baby. She may at first feel more comfortable looking at the baby, rather than holding him.

Gerald Caplan, in his description of initial maternal behavior, has coined the term "maternal time-lag"[8] to identify the span of time required for a new mother to feel that the baby really belongs to her. The importance of understanding and assisting the mother becomes more obvious as ongoing care is given for this mother carries out tasks with less affection and fondling and has a difficult time with diapering, feeding, bathing, etc. The baby's needs are seen objectively rather than felt subjectively because the infant is not perceived as an extension of the mother, and, therefore, she cannot respond to his needs as quickly and assuredly. Breast-feeding may be more difficult, especially in finding a suitable position, since she cannot sense the baby's discomfort as she can her own. The nurse needs to be a role model, demonstrating a maternal figure. The mother handles intellectual information well, such as what toys to buy, how to dress the baby, or what temperature to keep the bedroom; however, the primary goal of nursing care for this mother involves being a strong mother figure, meeting first the mother's own needs as always, and then going on to being very affectionate toward the baby. That includes cooing, fondling, cuddling, talking—all demonstrating

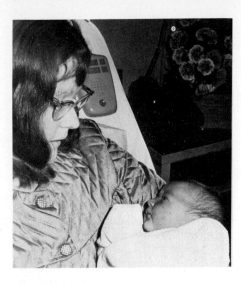

FIGURE 26-2
A new mother shows intense interest in
her baby's eyes.

maternal warmth. These mothers may never have been exposed to what
"mother love" entails; therefore, a well-prepared nurse can interpret the
verbal and nonverbal communication the mother gives and show her this
type of caring. The mother may feel guilty because she did not respond to
her infant with instant love. The nurse can relieve the mother's guilt by as-
suring her that the lag in maternal feelings is normal, whether she is a
primipara or multipara.

One views in contrast Caplan's description of the mother who during
her entire pregnancy has displayed a strong emotional attachment to the
fetus. She talks to the unborn child, calling him by a pet name. These mothers
usually name their babies early, talk incessantly about the joys of pregnancy,
and have a very close relationship with the baby soon after birth.

The frontispiece of this book illustrates the emotions of this mother as
she gazes fondly down at her child and the two figures become one. After
delivery the mother shows a great deal of warmth and affection toward her
baby, and as one views the mother and child, the feeling of oneness per-
vades. She is able to endow the new baby with a personality but does not
yet see him as an individual apart from herself. Normal behavior of the newborn such as regurgitating, dirty or wet diapers, and crying are all perceived
subjectively, as though they were happening to the mother herself. The
maternal time-lag is much shorter and may in some mothers appear to be
absent. It is difficult for this mother to "let go," but the acquisition of the
maternal role up to that point seems relatively easy, even natural. These
mothers cuddle their babies a great deal, deriving pleasure from the sharing
of warmth. Breast-feeding appears easy and natural, usually continues suc-

cessfully, and the nurse notices a certain look of contentment on the mother's face as she nurses.

The mother who maintains a very close relationship with her baby needs guidance in seeing the child as an individual. The nurse who says, "Look how he raises his head," or "Did you see how startled she was by the loud noise?" is pointing out individual characteristics. During the hospital stay, this mother may respond very poorly to intellectual information; however, she will seem receptive to instruction involving motor activities with the baby, such as diapering, bubbling, bathing, etc.

ASSESSMENT OF THE RELATIONSHIP

In evaluating the mother's relationship with her infant it is helpful if the nurse has more to depend upon than observational skills. Dr. Dane Prugh uses a series of questions when he interviews new mothers which can be employed, as well as Caplan's theory, as predictive tools in assessment of the mother-infant relationship.[9] The nurse may wish to use all or some of these questions to obtain a more realistic picture of the new mother's feelings now and prior to the birth of her baby. They may be used in any order after the first question.

1 How are you feeling? Do you have any concerns about the baby or about how the baby looks to you? This is a warm-up question, but it may produce some interesting information. It is a good idea to first ask the mother how *she* is feeling because practically everyone who enters the room will go to the baby first. Once she has given information about herself, then the question can be asked about the baby. Some of her concerns about the baby are small ones, such as milia or erythema toxicum, but she may also bring to the interviewer's attention the fact that the baby's eyes are draining or that his jaundice has increased a great deal since the evening before. This time can be used for explanations and reassurance.

2 What is the baby's name? When did you choose the name? After the mother tells the interviewer what the baby's name is, it is well to explore with her how she chose the name. One mother admitted very freely that her baby's first and middle names were chosen after people she disliked intensely. Or a mother may name a boy after her husband, who is abusive to her. In these cases, negative feelings may be projected toward the new infant because of the child's name, thereby creating a high-risk situation which should be carefully followed by the community health nurse. The parents who cannot agree on a name may be signaling that they cannot agree on other issues either,

and marital problems can be inferred. The time the infant's name was chosen is useful in determining the feelings the mother had toward the fetus. The emotional, attached mother as described by Caplan usually names her baby much earlier, while the unemotional, intellectual mother may still be trying to decide on a name the day she is discharged from the hospital.

3 How did you feel when you felt the baby move for the first time? Mothers who have established a strong relationship with the fetus and who will predictably relate well with the new infant say that they were excited, elated, and could not wait to have their husband feel the baby move in utero. A mother who is having a more difficult time relating to the baby may describe the baby's movements as painful or generally a nuisance, and many times she will go into detail about how the baby kept her awake at night and made it difficult for her to breathe.

4 Did you have a mental picture of the baby around the time when the baby moved or later in the pregnancy? Many mothers who have very positive responses to the other questions cannot remember having any mental image of the fetus. Others say they pictured the fetus as a tiny infant. Concern about the response to this question is elicited when the mother says she saw the fetus as, for example, a one-year-old. This mother may be fearful of her ability to care for the baby during his first year if for some reason she could not picture him as an infant.

5 When asking this next question, the interviewer should preface it with a statement similar to, "Most women having a baby for the first time think they will feel immediate maternal warmth, but it is completely normal not to feel this way for a while." Then the question can be asked, "How is it with you?" or "How has it been for you?" Phrasing the question in that way elicits a truer response than asking the woman if she feels like a mother, since everyone answers affirmatively to that question. By prefacing the suggested question with such a statement, the mother feels much more comfortable in admitting her real feelings. By asking this question, the nurse is able to see if the mother is experiencing a maternal time-lag, and it gives the nurse an opportunity to put the mother at ease regarding her feelings about the baby. It is surprising to watch the look of relief pass over many mothers' faces when they are told it is normal to have a lag in their maternal feelings. Clues may have been given prior to asking this question such as, "I just can't believe this baby is really mine," or "It seems impossible that I'm a mother." Dr. Prugh feels that the time-lag averages somewhere between 12 to 15 hours and 3 to 4 days; however, he and Caplan both acknowledge that it may last a period of months and still be normal.

Basic maternal behavior is best understood if the preceding types of new mothers are placed at opposite ends of a continuum. It is essential for the nurse to comprehend maternal behavior as constantly changing, with each mother a little different from the next. Viewing behavior on a continuum exemplifies this state of flux and demonstrates the variety of "normal." Most new mothers cannot be placed at one end of the continuum or the other, but rather fall somewhere in between, exhibiting behaviors from each end. The usefulness of the theory appears clearer as one plans and executes nursing care for a patient during the postpartum period. Even though either end of the continuum describes a healthy mother, the nurse is able to hasten the mother's progress to the goal of either "letting-go" or attainment of maternal feelings by realizing her approximate position on the continuum at the time.

The usefulness of the community health nurse cannot be overemphasized, since it is this nurse who will have contact with the mother long after her hospital stay. Besides being a resource person, role model, and health counselor, the community health nurse is in the best position to evaluate the new mother's progress in relation to role taking and attainment of maternal feelings. Since the maternal lag may normally last up to a month or 6 weeks, intervention can be planned if the lag is prolonged. And considering that the emotional separation between mother and infant may not occur until 7 months, ongoing care seems of utmost importance.

Nursing Intervention

Maternal behavior is learned, acquired through years of observation, personal experience, play acting, and development of a self-concept. Studies have repeatedly shown that response to motherhood is not an isolated event in a woman's life but directly correlates with her attitudes toward menstruation, pregnancy, breast-feeding, and sexual intercourse.[10] The mother whose maternal behavior comes more slowly may very well have negative feelings about one of the other areas which combine to compose her sexuality. Some women are completely at ease breast-feeding their babies with visitors gathered around the bed, and others are so modest they wish no one to observe the feeding. Being mindful of the variance in self-concepts enables a maternal-child nurse to put the mother at ease in such situations by pulling the curtain or asking visitors to wait in the lounge. The nurse's intervention at this point ultimately furthers the mother-infant relationship and the growth of maternal behavior. A mother's comfort and relaxed state provide a safe and secure environment for the infant, while the mother's anxiety is also communicated to the baby. An anxious mother usually has a more irritable baby who has difficulty feeding, especially at breast. It should be the goal of every maternal-child nurse to help a mother attain a feeling of comfort with her baby. In some instances this process takes longer than others, but it should always be uppermost in the nurse's mind. This feeling of comfort cannot be achieved without letting the mother try things for herself, but with anticipatory guidance from the nurse. Seeing that she can perform as a mother is a great reward for both patient and nurse and, finally, is a tremendous ego strengthener. There is a certain amount of safety and security associated with the hospital environment because of the presence of doctors, nursing personnel, technical equipment, and even the hospital routine. The mother who has not been helped during her hospital stay to gain a feeling of comfort and confidence with her new infant has not been given optimal care. The process does not end in the hospital, but it must have its beginnings there if there is to be stability in the family environment following hospitalization.

The maternal-child nurse has other unique responsibilities to the family, including involvement with them during hospitalization of the mother and infant. Parents at times can feel overwhelmed by all the medical people around them whom they feel are so knowledgeable. This is especially true when either mother or baby is ill. A medical problem during this period of developmental crisis in the family is easily misinterpreted by the individuals involved. The parents at times view the situation as worse than it is, or they do not have an understanding of the facts and the probable outcome. At this point the nurse should be available to the parents as a source of strength and a resource person. A doctor's explanation is often filled with medical terminology that should be clarified. The nurse is in the position to realize that parents seldom grasp the meaning the first time they are informed of their baby's illness, however minor the illness is. They hear only that something is wrong, and immediately fear and anxiety block out whatever follows. It is not unusual to approach parents to whom the pediatrician has just given a careful description of their infant's heart murmur and hear one of them ask, "I think he said our baby has a heart murmur. What is a heart murmur anyway?"

If the baby's illness requires that he be transferred to an intensive care area or forbids him to be brought to the mother's room, the involvement continues as the nurse accompanies the parents to visit the baby. The nurse's presence and continued support at this time help alleviate some of the parents' anxiety and is an act of nursing care which is greatly appreciated.

The nurse should communicate an attitude of caring, characterized by a free and easy environment with as few rules as possible. New mothers are especially sensitive to criticism, and guidance by a nurse who has communicated this sense of caring to the mother will be accepted without hurt feelings and tears. The maternity unit is no place for a stern and rigid nurse. Harshness and criticism are confusing and upsetting when the mother knows she is doing her best. When teaching is done with love and understanding, an entirely different attitude is conveyed to the mother; therefore, when ego strength is weak, as it often is during this time of passivity and dependency, it is important to emphasize the positive in what the mother is capable of doing.

THE CHANGING BODY

Anatomic Alterations

Physiological changes occur throughout the pregnancy, labor, delivery, and the puerperium. The nurse should assume the responsibility of keeping the mother informed of the processes which are taking place within her body and of making her aware of their physiological importance.

THE UTERUS

Following the delivery of the placenta, the uterus, which now weighs 2 pounds, normally contracts into a hard mass about the size of a grapefruit and should be palpated in the midline halfway between the umbilicus and the symphysis pubis. Within the next 12 hours the uterus rises to the level of the umbilicus or slightly below, after which time it rapidly begins to decrease in size. On the fifth postpartum day, it should be approximately 4 to 5 fingerbreadths below the umbilicus and should weigh about 1 pound.

By the tenth postpartum day, the uterus has descended into the true pelvis and is no longer palpable abdominally. By 6 weeks the uterus has fully involuted and weighs about 2 ounces, which is slightly more than its nulliparous weight. This process of involution is accomplished by autolysis, an enzymatic breakdown of cells, the products of which are removed by the circulating blood and eliminated through the urine.[11] This process may be less rapid when the uterus has been markedly overdistended as in the cases of polyhydramnios, multiple gestation, a large baby, or in the grand multipara.

During the early postpartum days, the endometrium is also undergoing rapid change. The lining, exclusive of the placental site, resembles a large desquamating wound which is restored by the end of the third week. The placental site heals less rapidly, requiring up to 6 weeks and leaving no permanent scar tissue at the site.

THE CERVIX

Following the third stage of labor, the overdistended cervix appears soft and flabby; unlike the endometrium, the cervix begins a simultaneous process of healing and regeneration. During the first 2 days postpartum, two fingers can be readily inserted into the cervix, but by the end of the first week it scarcely accommodates one finger. Anatomically, the internal cervical os returns to its tightly closed state and the external os remains slightly open, but because of the delivery process itself, the cervix never regains its nulliparous appearance.

THE VAGINA

The vagina, which is greatly distended during the birth process, becomes relaxed and edematous following delivery. It slowly diminishes in size but never regains its pregravid state, with rugae beginning to reappear around the third week. Most women are unaware of any change in size or tonicity of the vagina following labor and delivery; however, occasionally a mother will complain of dyspareunia (painful intercourse) which is usually caused by a tender perineal scar secondary to the episiotomy repair.

THE ABDOMINAL WALL

After delivery, the muscles of the abdominal wall are soft and flabby, but if tone has been maintained during pregnancy, the abdominal muscles usually return to their normal state by the end of 6 weeks. Unfortunately, poor muscle control prenatally requires additional time for regaining muscle tone, and a slight protuberance of the abdomen may be evident for as long as 3 to 12 months; in fact, the muscles may never return to their prepregnant state.

Stretch marks, or striae gravidarum, are caused by a rupture of the elastic fibers in the skin, as shown in Figure 26-3. These marks appear as brownish or pinkish streaks on the abdomen and breasts and less frequently on the hips and thighs. Gradually the striae become silvery white but never completely fade, a fact which often causes the mother some distress since she may not feel comfortable in a two-piece bathing suit.

The rectus muscles, which are divided by a narrow muscular sheath, may show a marked separation, or diastasis. This condition prevents adequate support of the abdominal organs but is lessened by attention to proper exercise, diet, rest, and posture during pregnancy. Diastasis of the rectus muscles can be felt quite easily during a postpartum fundus check as the rectus muscles are prominent and displaced laterally, and the fundus can be palpated just through the abdominal wall.

THE BREASTS AND LACTATION

The breast is composed of 15 to 24 lobes separated from one another by fatty tissue. These lobes are divided into lobules, each lobule containing a certain number of acini, or alveoli, as illustrated in Figure 26-4. To understand milk production, it is necessary to be aware of the structure of an alveolar cell. The constituents of breast milk are manufactured in the lining of the alveolar cell, the epithelial layer. After this process, the myoepithelial cells in the walls of the alveoli contract, forcing the milk from the alveoli

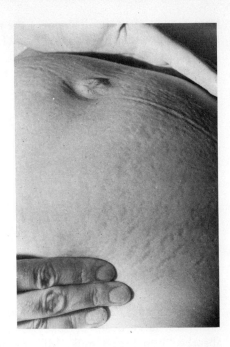

FIGURE 26-3
Striae gravidarum as seen in the post-partum patient. (*Courtesy of The University of Colorado Medical Center, Denver, Colorado*)

into small ducts. These ducts connect with larger ones called lactiferous ducts, which have orifices on the surface of the nipple.

The mechanism of milk production and ejection (called let-down) is determined hormonally. During pregnancy, the circulating estrogen, progesterone, and chorionic somatomammotropin (CST) have been preparing the breast for lactation. The estrogen primarily affects the ducts; the progesterone affects the alveoli.[12] The exact role of CST is still unknown at this time.

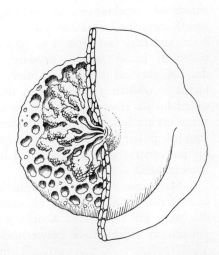

FIGURE 26-4
A cross section of the lactating breast.
(*Courtesy of Elizabeth Riska Townsley.*)

Immediately after the delivery of the placenta, these hormone levels diminish, thereby activating the anterior lobe of the pituitary to release prolactin, which acts on the epithelial cells of the alveoli, stimulating them to produce milk. This process, which takes from 2 to 4 days, is enhanced by the sucking stimulus of the baby.

Sucking also triggers the release of oxytocin by the posterior lobe of the pituitary, thereby initiating the let-down reflex. The oxytocin causes contraction of the myoepithelial cells as well as the uterine myometrial cells. The truly amazing part of this reflex is that once a woman is conditioned to nursing, the cry or thought of a baby is sufficient to activate let-down of the milk.

Breast milk is bluish white in color and appears to be very watery. It is high in both lactose and fat, low in protein and phosphate.[13] The composition is reversed in its precursor, colostrum, which is normally found in the alveoli during the latter phase of pregnancy. Colostrum, a yellowish fluid, which is high in antibodies, is an excellent food for the baby during the 2 to 3 days before the milk comes in. Breast milk is quite often mixed with colostrum for a week or longer.

Drugs such as antibiotics, sulfonamides, bromides, iodides, certain cathartics, large doses of salicylates, certain anticoagulants, and alcohol are absorbed into breast milk. Milk of magnesia and mineral oil are safe laxatives, heparin may be used as an anticoagulant, but tetracycline and oral anticoagulants are definitely contraindicated for a nursing mother.

THE LOCHIA

During the early weeks of the puerperium there is a vaginal discharge varying in amount and color called lochia. Lochia rubra occurs during the first 2 to 4 days of the puerperium and consists of blood from the placental site, shreds of membranes and decidua, vernix, lanugo, and meconium. By the fourth day, the lochia has turned a brownish or dark red color, has a fleshy odor, and may last from 4 to 10 days. Lochia serosa, as it is called, is composed of blood, wound exudate, leukocytes and erythrocytes, shreds of decidua, cervical mucus, and many microorganisms. After the tenth day, the lochia is whitish yellow due to the increased number of leukocytes and is called lochia alba. Lochia may last anywhere from 3 to 6 weeks. If lochia rubra occurs following the appearance of lochia alba, it is usually a warning sign of possible postpartum complication. Rest and medication to cause uterine contractions are indicated in an attempt to avoid a late postpartum hemorrhage.

Many mothers worry about clots, and the nurse should inform the mother that small clots are not unusual, but large clots or any tissue in the discharge are considered abnormal and should be reported. At times it is difficult to differentiate between clots and tissue. Tissue is stringy, has a whitish cast to it, and may look like hamburger meat; a clot is red, dissolves on crumbling, and on gross examination has the appearance of liver. If there is any question, the specimen should be saved for observation by the physician. If the lochia remains red beyond 4 days, it indicates slow involution of the uterus which could be caused by retained placental fragments. Early ambulation causes the uterus to involute more quickly, and the duration of lochia rubra is therefore shortened. A strong, offensive odor is an indication of infection and should be reported to the physician and noted on the patient's chart.

The nurse is responsible for checking the color, amount, and odor of the lochia. This is usually done about every 4 hours during the first day following delivery and at least once a day throughout the remainder of the mother's hospital stay. It is helpful to the mother if she understands the color changes of the vaginal discharge and how long she can expect it to last. It is also wise to caution her about the odor of the lochia so that she may report any abnormalities to her physician should they arise during the weeks following her discharge from the hospital.

Lochia contains large amounts of bacteria which may not cause problems for one mother but may be highly infectious to another; therefore, clean technique is of utmost importance when caring for these patients.

Clinical Manifestations

BODY TEMPERATURE

Definitions of what constitutes a temperature elevation vary. A postpartum patient is described as febrile if her temperature exceeds 38°C (100.4°F) in any two consecutive 24-hour periods excluding the first 24 hours;[14] however, temperatures between 37.5°C and 38°C may be indicative of a beginning infection. A temperature that is defined as an elevation by a particular physician or hospital should be rechecked at least every 4 hours until it has remained in the normal range for two successive 4-hour periods.

Slight temperature elevation in the postpartum patient is common, and it is important for the nurse to understand this in order to assess and report changes in body temperature knowledgeably. The most common reason for a temperature rise during the first 24 hours is dehydration. Since labor is such hard work, a laboring patient may perspire profusely; the loss of fluid, along with the fact that oral fluids are often restricted and intravenous fluids sometimes omitted, may lead to dehydration and a slight increase in temperature. This elevation responds to an increase in fluids, sometimes as much as 4,000 cc in a 24-hour period. A patient is usually unaware of her temperature elevation and may need constant encouragement to take sufficient oral fluids. She may prefer juices or coffee to water, and these preferences should be honored by the nurse in the plan of care. One must be careful, however, of water intoxication due to the overzealous administration of fluids.

In rare instances, a temperature elevation in the first 24 hours is not due to dehydration but to a previously existing infection. This viral or bacterial infection can usually be distinguished from dehydration. The patient with an infection experiences chills, temperature spikes, and a feeling of general malaise; the dehydrated patient commonly exhibits a flushed face, dry skin or mucous membranes, and is unaware of any temperature elevation. The two most common causes of a sudden increase in temperature after the first day are endometritis (puerperal fever) and urinary tract infection.

An elevation in temperature on the third or fourth day postpartum was once considered to be due to breast engorgement. This concept of "milk fever" has been shown to be a fallacy, for most of these temperature elevations are secondary to an infectious process. In rare instances, however, extreme engorgement may lead to a sudden, short-lived temperature spike not lasting more than 12 hours. Special attention should be paid to the comfort of a patient with a fever. As the fever decreases, the patient may experience diaphoresis. A blanket or sponge bath is comforting, and she may appreciate a cool cloth for her face during the elevation.

THE PULSE

Bradycardia is common in the early puerperium. The heart rate usually averages between 60 and 70 but may drop to 50 or even lower on the first or second day. In a woman who is nervous or who has lost a large amount of blood, this drop in pulse may not be as dramatic. The bradycardia is not as evident if there is early ambulation, except in the early morning before arising. By the seventh to the tenth day, the pulse has returned to normal. A sudden spike in pulse taken while the woman is resting may be indicative of an early infection.

UTERINE AFTERPAINS

The uterus of a primipara generally maintains a state of tonic contraction unless blood clots or placental fragments remain in the uterine cavity. When these conditions exist, the uterus actively contracts in an effort to remove them. The uterus loses some of its tonicity if it has been unduly stretched. Rather than maintaining a state of sustained contraction, the muscles relax and contract at intervals in an attempt to return to normal. This cycle is interpreted as waves of pain, commonly referred to as afterpains. Mothers who breast-feed feel these pains more strongly, since the oxytocin released as the baby nurses also stimulates contraction of the uterus.

These afterpains may last as long as 7 days but usually diminish in intensity after the third day. The nurse must remember that many women require an analgesic for this pain. Having the mother lie on her abdomen often eases the discomfort, and the nurse should encourage the mother to empty her bladder. A full bladder elevates the uterus high in the pelvis which necessitates stronger uterine contractions in order for the uterus to return to its normal position and size. It is important for the nurse to be sympathetic as the mother may be quite uncomfortable while the pains persist.

THE BOWELS

Early ambulation has helped the problem of constipation during the puerperium but has not eliminated it. Several contributing factors to the new mother's difficulties with elimination are the relaxed abdominal and intestinal muscles, the cleansing enema before delivery, and lack of solid food during labor.

The fluid imbalance which may occur as the lactating breasts demand more fluids and the body eliminates much fluid is another cause of constipation, and therefore the postpartum mother should be encouraged to have an adequate fluid intake. If proper muscle tone has been maintained during pregnancy, the possibility of developing postpartum constipation is lessened.

A painful episiotomy and/or sore hemorrhoids hinder evacuation by preventing a woman from bearing down to aid in elimination. A topical anesthetic spray, sitz baths, ice packs, analgesics, or ointments may help to relieve some of the perineal discomfort. A laxative may be ordered routinely or as needed; however, a mild laxative should be given by the evening of the second day if the patient has not yet had a bowel movement. Some doctors order small enemas or suppositories if there has been no bowel movement by the morning of the third day.

THE URINE

There is an increased amount of body fluids during pregnancy, and when the delivery is over, diuresis ensues in the body's effort to return to its nonpregnant metabolic state. This diuresis usually occurs during the second to fifth postpartum days, and there may be as much as 3,000 cc of urine excreted in a 24-hour period. It is not unusual to find sugar in the urine caused by the lactose being produced by the mammary glands as they are preparing for milk let-down. This is most noticeable during establishment of lactation and when the mother is weaning. Proteinuria is often present due to breakdown of the cells of the uterus during the process of involution. The proteinuria usually disappears by the third day, but may continue in trace amounts until involution is complete.

It is sometimes difficult for the mother to urinate following delivery, but she should void within 4 to 8 hours after the birth. There are certain factors contributing to the mother's difficulty with voiding during the first 12 hours:

1 Trauma to the bladder due to the pressure in labor of the fetal head against it
2 Edema of the urethra and vulva due to the birth process
3 Increase in the amount of urine in the bladder due to the normal diuresis
4 The decrease in intraabdominal pressure immediately postpartum secondary to the distention of the pregnant abdominal wall
5 Possible decrease in the sensitivity of the bladder for several hours, depending on the kind of anesthesia the mother has received

What effect does a distended bladder have on the mother? It can prevent the uterus from contracting properly, thus increasing the chances of a postpartum hemorrhage. If the nurse notices that the bleeding is heavier than normal, the mother should be encouraged to void in an effort to decrease the amount of bleeding. A distended bladder may cause the mother to void small amounts, often less than 100 cc, which indicates that she is not emptying her bladder, and residual urine can cause infection.

Bladder distention can be detected in several ways. The mother may complain of feeling full, or she may be distended and be totally unaware of the problem. If the uterus is displaced above the umbilicus and deviated to the right or left, this is usually indicative of a full bladder. A soft puffiness just above the symphysis is also a sign of a full bladder. It is the nurse's responsibility to make pertinent observations and report the findings to the physician.

There are several techniques of preventing overdistention of the bladder. Once again early ambulation is encouraged, since it is easier for the mother to void if she is able to get up to the bathroom. Many women find it difficult or impossible to void on a bedpan or in a reclining position (in the case of a woman who has had spinal anesthesia). If she is unable to void, the nurse should encourage fluids. A warm sitz bath and/or shower, pouring warm water over the symphysis and labia, having the mother concentrate on voiding, or encouraging her to blow bubbles through a straw in a glass of water may serve as stimulants which aid in emptying the bladder.

If these measures are unsuccessful, the physician may order the mother to be catheterized. The catheter will rarely remain in the bladder longer than it is necessary to empty it of urine. If the mother has been voiding small amounts, less than 100 cc, the physician may order the nurse to catheterize the patient for residual urine immediately after voiding. If there is more than 150 cc of residual urine, he may request that the catheter remain in place for 24 hours. Usually after 24 hours, the edema of the urethra and vulva decrease enough so that the mother does not have difficulty voiding. When the catheter is removed, culture and sensitivity should be obtained, and the nurse should encourage the mother to drink fluids and to void within 6 to 8 hours following the removal of the catheter. The amount voided should be recorded on the patient's hospital record, as well as the position of the uterus following the voiding.

THE CIRCULATION

An increase in blood fibrinogen has been noticed during the first postpartum week which may be a contributing factor in the development of thrombophlebitis. Early ambulation helps to decrease the possibility of thrombophlebitis by preventing venous stasis.

There is an increase in the number of leukocytes, especially if the labor has been long. The white blood cell count may be as high as 30,000 at the end of the first week, but this does not necessarily indicate an infection.[15] The leukocytosis demonstrates that the body has mobilized its defense system against possible infection and aids in the many repairs taking place within the body.

The hemoglobin or hematocrit is checked on the third postpartum day and should not differ significantly from the value during early labor. If the difference is marked, it usually indicates a considerable blood loss. The mother who is anemic may require additional time during the day for rest and sleep, and she may be given iron either orally or parenterally prior to discharge from the hospital.

During pregnancy, the body carries approximately 2 additional liters of blood which are eliminated by the renal system and by diaphoresis within the first 2 weeks postpartum. The diaphoresis occurs frequently during the night and categorically has been called "night sweats." Heavy sweating may continue for as long as 3 weeks; therefore, daily bathing, frequent clothing changes, and protection from chilling are essential.

Circulation to the lower extremities is often sluggish during pregnancy because of the pressure of the uterus, preventing adequate drainage of the pelvic vessels. Following delivery it is important to promote good circulation which can be done partially through proper positioning. The mother who is supine or in an extreme Fowler's position decreases the flow of blood to the legs. The best position to enhance circulation to all areas of the body is to elevate the head of the bed to about a 45° angle and to elevate the knees slightly, thus allowing a free flow of blood to and from the lower extremities.[16] When the mother is sitting on the side of the bed, her feet should not be dangling, since this constricts the popliteal arteries and veins. She should have her feet resting flatly on a chair, preventing constriction of any of the major vessels, and crossing of the legs should be discouraged. These suggestions are especially beneficial to the mother who has difficulty with varicosities. The physician in such cases may recommend that the patient wrap her legs in elastic bandages or wear elastic hose. The legs should be rewrapped at least twice a day and whenever necessary. Usually the superficial varicosities will improve noticeably within the first few days postpartum as a result of the marked decrease in total blood volume, but the larger veins may never return to their normal size.

THE PERINEUM

Sutures used in repair of the episiotomy dissolve in about 3 weeks, and care of the perineum during this time centers mainly on cleanliness. Mothers should be taught to dry their perineal area from front to back, blotting rather than wiping, since improper cleansing may cause contamination of the urinary meatus and a resulting urinary tract infection. Taking frequent sitz baths in the hospital and using a bathtub at home are good practices to keep the area clean and to promote healing; however, a separate washcloth should be used for the perineum. Doctors will sometimes prescribe ice packs to be applied to the perineum during the first 12 to 24 hours to prevent or decrease edema, which is the primary cause of initial discomfort. After this time, a patient finds the warm or hot sitz bath more soothing and comforting than the ice packs. A perineal heat lamp may be ordered, but dry heat may cause a pulling or drawing of the sutures. Therefore, moist heat is preferable.

Lacerations of the perineum extending back to or including the rectal sphincter cause added discomfort. The same suggestions that were described above for general episiotomy care are employed. Topical anesthetics, ointment, and analgesics also aid in reducing the pain of a laceration or troublesome episiotomy.

OVULATION AND MENSTRUATION

If the mother is not nursing, menstruation will usually return within 6 to 12 weeks following delivery. The menses may not recur for as long as 18 months in the nursing mother but usually return in approximately 4 months. Ovulation occurs in 6 to 8 weeks in the nonlactating mother and in approximately 11 weeks in the lactating mother. The nursing mother should be made aware that breast-feeding is not to be considered a form of contraception, since she may ovulate without first menstruating.

The first menstrual period following delivery may be heavy and last longer than a normal menses, and it is not unusual for small clots to be passed. Some women have irregular periods for a few months as the body continues to attempt to regain its nonpregnant normal state. It is the responsibility of the nurse to inform the mother of these facts so that she will not become alarmed when any of the abovementioned events occur.

SPECIAL NEEDS

A mother's need for sleep during the early puerperium has been described as sleep hunger. Immediately after delivery she may be elated and wide awake, but soon she becomes extremely tired and needs rest. This overwhelming need to rest may descend upon the postpartum patient at any time. A wise nurse senses this need and allows time for morning and/or afternoon naps. It may be necessary for the nurse to alter hospital routines, such as temperature taking or a sitz bath, somewhat if a mother is in the midst of this deep sleep.

The appetites of new mothers vary tremendously. Some crave food almost immediately after delivery and continue to eat large meals while others prefer smaller portions. Snacks between meals are usually welcomed, especially by nursing mothers. The nurse should keep in mind individual differences and varying nutritional requirements in caring for the postpartum patient.

The need for increased fluids has been discussed previously. A mother may not feel thirsty; therefore, an explanation of why fluids are important will usually motivate her to drink adequate amounts.

THE ART OF FEEDING

Whether a mother chooses to breast- or bottle-feed, she will undoubtedly find herself eager for the feeding instruction and guidance given to her by the nurse. Many women believe that babies naturally know how to eat and that regardless of how a mother elects to feed her infant he will accept the food with only a minimal amount of effort on her part. Experience has shown this to be a fallacy, for certain learned skills are required for feeding to be successful. Feeding is a primary caretaking responsibility executed by the mother in the care of her newborn infant, and for this reason it is an area that should not be taken lightly by the nurse. Success in feeding brings delight and a feeling of accomplishment to the new mother, while failure at getting the baby to eat may bring about depression or a feeling of rejection, thus upsetting the desired pattern of events during the postpartum period.

The mother should select the method of feeding that seems best for her, giving special consideration to her husband's feelings; however, the nurse's responsibility to the mother includes antenatal and postnatal education on certain facts about both breast- and bottle-feeding. It is the purpose of this section to help the nurse become aware of the hows and whys of feeding so that, in turn, the nurse can serve as a resource person to the new mother, giving her needed guidance in whatever method of feeding she has selected for herself and her new infant.

Breast-feeding

A recent study conducted at the University of Colorado Medical Center[17] showed that of the clinic population which the center serves, 34 percent of new mothers chose to nurse their babies in the immediate postpartum period. Follow-up at 1 month indicated that only one-half of those women were still nursing, and of that group, slightly over half of them had nursed babies before. It is worthwhile to note that of the mothers who had stopped nursing, one-third had done so at the ill-considered advice of a physician. Antenatal instruction and rooming-in were not found to influence whether a mother continued nursing or not, although 69 percent of the breast-feeding mothers chose rooming-in.

In contrast, 43 consecutive patients seen in a private practice had a success rate which was much higher than that found in the clinic population. Of the 80 percent who chose to nurse, 94 percent were still nursing at 1 month. The patients who had stopped did so at the advice of a pediatrician. From this study, one concludes that a higher socioeconomic level and more education seem to correlate positively with successful nursing; however, an understanding of breast-feeding and its problems by both physician and nurse is certain to raise the success rate of the poorer, less educated women.

Some mothers are hesitant to breast-feed because they feel they will be constantly tied down to the baby with little free time for themselves and their husbands. Others have been told that breast-feeding is superior because it brings the mother and baby closer emotionally and makes the infant feel more secure. The facts are that a nursing mother can and should go out with her husband, leaving the baby at home. And the chief benefits of breast-feeding in most instances are physiological, rather than psychological, for a mother who bottle-feeds can certainly feel as close to her infant as one who breast-feeds.

Although it is estimated that between 75 to 90 percent of the babies born in the United States are bottle-fed, there seems to be a trend toward breast-feeding by younger mothers. They select the more natural way of feeding but are sometimes disillusioned to find that this natural way takes a great deal of patience and skill.

Many breast-feeding mothers throughout the country have received needed help from a group of women who belong to an organization called La Leche League. The term "la leche" is taken from the Spanish language and simply means "the milk." This organization was established in Illinois in 1956 by a group of women who nursed their babies successfully and wanted other women to have equally rewarding experiences.[18] La Leche League is found in most large cities, and breast-feeding mothers should be made aware of the group. The league provides a list of telephone numbers of women who have nursed their infants and are willing to help others with common problems arising during the nursing experience. They also have meetings for expectant mothers where they discuss breast-feeding and teach the women how to prepare for nursing.

BENEFITS TO THE MOTHER

There are well-known and documented physiological benefits to the breast-feeding mother. In studies conducted on women of various cultures throughout the world it has been shown that mothers who nurse have a markedly decreased chance of developing breast cancer. In Western culture breast-feeding has been on the decline in the last few generations while during the same time mammary cancer is on the rise. In a study done in Boston on 473 women with breast cancer, it was concluded that there is an increased incidence of developing breast cancer in women who nursed less than 3 months.[19] This study does not establish cause and effect, but it does point out an association between breast cancer and nursing. The reason may be a function of suppression of ovarian hormones. This is substantiated by the fact that both pregnancy and lactation suppress ovarian function and the incidence of breast cancer is decreased in multiparous women and mothers who have breast-fed.

New mothers who do not wish to nurse are given diethylstilbestrol to suppress lactation. The incidence of thrombophlebitis, although quite low, is four to ten times higher in these women than in their nursing counterparts.[20] Laboratory studies on mothers who have received this medication show a substantial increase in blood coagulability.

Postpartum uterine involution is more rapid in mothers who breast-feed. Therefore, delayed postpartum hemorrhage is also less common, and there is less chance of uterine perforations with the insertion of an intrauterine device for contraception at the routine 6-week postpartum examination.

Though breast-feeding should never be depended upon as a means of contraception, lactation has been shown to suppress ovulation for 75 days postpartum in almost 100 percent of mothers who do not supplement their infants with bottle or solid food. Thus, breast-feeding, for a short time, is probably preferred to contraceptive hormones which produce hypercoagulability if given soon after delivery. These oral hormones also lessen the milk supply, at times causing the entire supply to dry up.

BENEFITS TO THE BABY

Dr. J. David Baum suggests several benefits to the breast-fed baby,[21] some of which are listed below. The colostrum and breast milk provide antibody protection against several types of viruses, including all three varieties of polio, and the Coxsackie Type B which causes newborn myocarditis and aseptic meningitis. The oral polio vaccine exhibits a high failure rate when given to infants who are being breast-fed.

Breast-fed babies show a marked decrease in respiratory infections and gastroenteritis. Lysozyme, an enzyme with antiseptic qualities that destroys foreign protein, is thought to play a significant part in the destruction of invasive organisms in the gastrointestinal tract. Especially important here is its attack on *Escherichia coli* organisms, the chief cause of gram negative sepsis of the newborn. Breast milk, with its high lactose content and poor buffering quality, keeps the pH of the stomach lower. Since *E. coli* may grow at a pH of 7.1, the increased acidity caused by breast milk inhibits its growth and possible resulting infection.[22] Along with lysozyme, secretory IgA, an immuno-globulin, is resistant to enzyme breakdown and gives the gastrointestinal tract additional resistance to invading microorganisms.

Allergic disorders such as infantile eczema, asthma, and hay fever are much less common in breast-fed babies. The mechanics by which the body uses breast milk to protect against these allergies is not fully understood; however, it is known that cow's milk is highly allergenic, and antibodies to cow's milk are found in high concentrations in the formula-fed infants soon after birth.

Neonatal tetany is not seen in wholly breast-fed babies.[23] This condition is caused by the high phosphorus level in prepared formulas. There is an inverse relationship between serum phosphate and serum calcium; therefore, as the infant ingests more and more phosphorous, the calcium level drops, causing symptoms of tetany. Artificial feeding also provides the infant with a high concentration of fatty acids, which may contribute to the condition by binding calcium in the gastrointestinal tract.

The sodium and solute concentration in formulas is much higher than in breast milk. In some cases, the solute load is too great, and overloading of the kidneys occurs.

It is observed that quite often obese infants become obese adults or at least have a problem maintaining a desired weight. Since the weight gain of a breast-fed infant is less than that of a bottle-fed one, obesity becomes an important consideration when evaluating the two types of infant feeding. It is sometimes difficult for parents to see the thinner baby as healthier than the chubby cherub because for many years it was maintained that a fat baby was a healthy one. Only recently has this statement been challenged, bring-ing with it the need for explanation and encouragement by the nurse to the mother whose baby is breast-fed and not gaining weight as rapidly as his bottle-fed counterpart.

Malocclusion is an improper placement of the teeth and may involve teeth, bone, and muscle tissues. Because of the forward tongue thrust used by the bottle-fed baby to control the flow of milk into his mouth, the likelihood of malocclusion is greater than in breast-fed infants.[24] Figure 26-5 illustrates the pressure exerted on the anterior gum by thrusting the tongue forward.

It was originally proposed that sudden infant death syndrome (crib death) was a result of an anaphylactic reaction to aspirated cow's milk protein in an already sensitized infant. Although this theory is not substantiated,[25] sudden infant death is rarely seen in a solely breast-fed baby.

HELPING THE MOTHER BEGIN

During the first 2 to 3 days postpartum, the mother's breasts secrete colos-trum. The nurse should remind the mother that the yellowish secretion pro-vides nourishment and maternal immunities for the infant, and that sucking

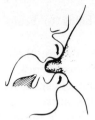

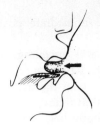

Notice how lips clamp "C" shape in nipple areolar concave junction fitting "like a glove". Cheek muscles contract.

Tongue thrusts forward to grasp nipple and areola.

BREAST

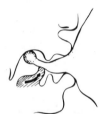

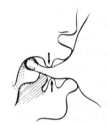

Nipple moves against hard palate as tongue whips <u>backward</u> bringing areola into mouth. NEGATIVE pressure is created by tongue and cheeks against nipple. <u>Suction effect</u> is created.

Gums compress areola squeezing milk into <u>back of throat</u> where <u>suction</u> occurs against nipple. Milk flows against hard palate from high pressure system to negative pressure at back throat.

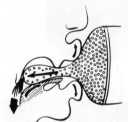

BOTTLE

Large rubber nipple strikes soft palate (with gagging) and displaces proper tongue action. Tongue moves <u>forward</u> with "anterior tongue thrust" against gums to control milk overflow into esophagus. Lips flange "O" shape. Compression does not occur. Cheek muscles relax.

FIGURE 26-5
Sucking mechanism at the breast and bottle.
(Reproduced from Richard M. Applebaum, "The Modern Management of Successful Breast Feeding," Pediatric Clinics of North America, 17:203, 1970. By permission of the publisher.)

during the immediate postpartum period helps to bring in the milk more quickly.

Help and encouragement are essential during these early days if the mother is to have a successful breast-feeding experience. The nurse should be available to help the mother during all feedings, especially the first one. In a rooming-in situation, it is not difficult for the nurse to arrange to be nearby when the baby begins to feed. A demand schedule means that not all babies will be feeding at the same time; hence, the nurse can give individualized help to the mother.

Before the mother begins to nurse, she should make sure that her hands are clean. It is not necessary for the mother to wash her nipples before each feeding because, as was previously stated, breast milk contains an antiseptic. If the infant is crying hard when he is brought to the mother, she should first calm the baby by holding him firmly and closely and by talking gently to him. An upset baby who is put to breast does not realize the nipple is in his mouth and will continue to cry loudly which tends to upset the mother and frustrate the infant. Once the baby is calm, he will be able to grasp the nipple and begin sucking.

There are several positions which the mother may assume while breast-feeding. She should be familiar with the different positions so that she may decide upon those most suitable for her and the baby. The one used most frequently is the sitting position shown in Figure 26-6. The mother sits in the

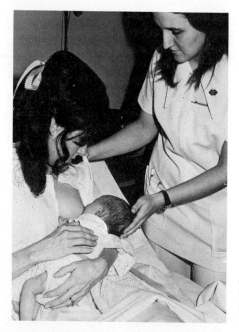

FIGURE 26-6
Proper positioning is important for successful nursing. (*Courtesy of The University of Colorado Medical Center, Denver, Colorado*)

bed or a chair, and holding the infant securely, she places the infant's arm underneath her arm, thereby aligning the baby's mouth with the mother's nipple. To get the baby to turn toward the breast, the mother strokes the cheek close to her, causing the infant to root for the nipple.

Many mothers find that a side-lying position is especially convenient during the night feedings or when a period of rest and relaxation is needed. Figure 26-7 illustrates two variations of this position. She may lie on her side with head and shoulder supported by pillows. The baby is placed close enough to her so that the nipple touches the baby's lips and he is able to grasp it easily. At other times the mother may want to rest her weight on her elbow as she gets the baby into position.

While the mother is learning the art of nursing, she may find it necessary to grasp the breast with index and middle fingers and guide the nipple into the baby's mouth, as shown in Figure 26-8. If the baby is slow to take hold, the nurse might suggest that the mother express a few drops of colostrum or milk onto the baby's lips which often entices him to grasp the nipple.

The proper placement of the nipple is on top of the baby's tongue with as much of the areolar area as possible in his mouth. A common misconception is that all of the areola must be in the baby's mouth in order for him to

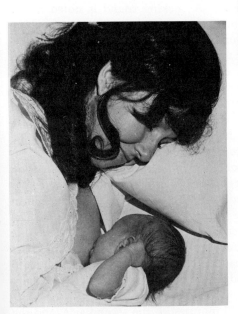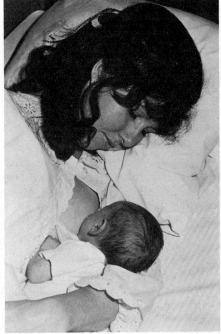

FIGURE 26-7
This mother demonstrates two side-lying positions for nursing. (*Courtesy of The University of Colorado Medical Center, Denver, Colorado*)

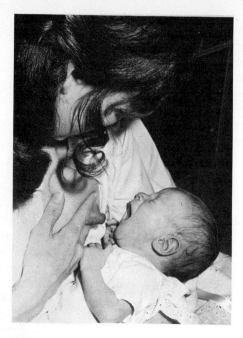

FIGURE 26-8
Compression of the areolar area facilitates
the baby's initial grasp on the nipple.
*(Courtesy of The University of Colorado
Medical Center, Denver, Colorado)*

nurse or suck properly. The nurse can tell if the baby is sucking correctly
by observing him carefully as he nurses. A clicking sound is noted as the
infant swallows, but other sucking noises are probably indicative of an improper grasp on the nipple. Also, the nurse can observe the areola being drawn
in as the baby sucks, indicating proper mouth positioning.

During the early days of nursing, the mother should be cautioned not to
feed too long at any one feeding as her nipples will become sore. It is recommended that she nurse from 3 to 5 minutes at every feeding during the first
day, from 5 to 7 minutes during the second day, and from 7 to 10 minutes
during the third day. In a week she should be able to nurse 10 minutes on
the first side and 20 minutes on the second side.

The mother should nurse from both breasts at each feeding, alternating
the side on which she begins. A suggestion to help the mother remember
which side to start on at the next feeding is to have her put a safety pin in
the bra strap on the side on which she will begin to nurse the next time. The
baby should nurse on both breasts because he sucks hardest on the first side
and he gets about 90 percent of the milk in that breast during the first 5 to
10 minutes of nursing. Using both breasts provides the necessary stimulus to
keep up a sufficient amount of milk production in the breasts. This is especially
important during the early weeks of nursing.

Not all babies want to nurse for 20 minutes on the second side, and the
mother should be reassured that the baby takes as much as he needs. Some
infants begin suckling quite easily at the first feeding, and others require more

help in getting started. The mother may feel that it is so easy when the nurse gets the baby started but quite difficult when she is trying to get him to suck by herself. The nurse can remind the mother that both she and the baby are learning to nurse and that once they begin working as a team, she will have no problems getting him to suck.

The newborn is very sleepy and often drifts off to sleep soon after he starts to nurse. Once he gets a little food in his stomach he feels warm and comfortable next to his mother and promptly goes to sleep. In a short while he will awaken and demand to eat again. Such situations can be avoided if the mother is taught how to keep the baby awake during the feeding. When the mother is ready to nurse, she can loosen the blankets around the baby so that he is not quite so warm and drowsy during the feeding. If this does not work, she may try any of the following: rub the soles of the baby's feet, stroke his abdomen, loosen or remove his shirt, or change his position. If the mother has difficulty keeping the baby awake, a nurse should be available to help her with the baby, and ease the mother's frustration.

The procedure of alternate massage[26] is suggested for use in the early nursing experience when the baby is sleepy in order to empty the breasts as completely as possible. Very often, a new baby begins sucking with vigor, and then it is noticed that after a minute or so the infant starts taking long, slow, rhythmic sucks. When these long, slow sucks become short and fast, or if the infant takes rest periods too frequently, alternating massage of the breast with the sucking will stimulate more milk to be released from the ducts. The shorter, more rapid sucking of the infant indicates the milk is flowing less freely, creating negative pressure, which contributes to nipple soreness.

The massage should begin only after the character of the sucking changes, otherwise the milk will flow too quickly and cause choking. The breast is massaged from the back and middle portion near the axillary area toward the nipple. After several massages the infant will begin taking long, slow sucks again as the milk flows freely. The position of the fingers can be rotated to stimulate as much of the breast tissue as possible.

When the baby is finished nursing, the mother should not pull him off the breast but should learn to release the suction on the nipple by gently squeezing the infant's cheeks or by putting her finger into the side of the baby's mouth and releasing the suction, as shown in Figure 26-9. If she tries to remove the baby without first breaking the suction, the infant will continue to suck as she is pulling him away, causing the mother discomfort and quite possibly sore nipples.

COMMON PROBLEMS OF BREAST-FEEDING

Engorgement

About the third day, when the milk begins to come in, engorgement may cause some problems for the mother. Hopefully she will be in the hospital

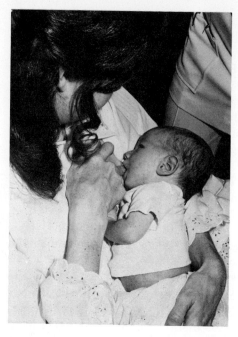

FIGURE 26-9
The mother releases the baby's suction on
the nipple by inserting her finger into the
corner of his mouth. (*Courtesy of The
University of Colorado Medical Center,
Denver, Colorado*)

when this occurs so that she may receive guidance from the nurse. Engorgement is a process of swelling and hardening of the breast tissue brought about by milk being released into the ducts with an increase in blood and lymph supply to the breast. It usually reaches a peak between the third and fifth postpartum days and lasts about 48 hours. The condition is usually more marked in a primigravida or in the multigravida who has not nursed previously.

The degree of discomfort from this noninflammatory process varies with each individual; however, most women experience at least mild swelling and tenderness. The severity is lessened by frequent nursing which keeps the breasts emptied and clears the ducts for the passage of the milk. Engorgement usually begins at the top or outer aspect of the breast and extends into the axillary area where a small nodule may be palpated. This stage is often referred to as the milk "coming in." An extremely engorged breast shows induration extending into the areolar and nipple areas, a condition which needs immediate attention to facilitate the baby's nursing. The breast may show red striations and appear shiny as a result of the overstretching of the skin. If engorgement is allowed to progress to this point, emptying of the breast (the primary treatment) becomes quite difficult.

Besides emptying of the breast, treatment includes a good supportive bra, heat or ice packs, and perhaps a mild analgesic. If it is difficult for the baby to grasp the nipple and areola because of extensive engorgement, hot packs, manual expression (Figure 26-10), or a hand breast pump may be utilized to obtain a small amount of milk from the breast prior to nursing, thereby softening the tissue. Occasionally a nipple shield is used for a short time at the beginning of the feeding which will draw out the nipple so that when the shield is removed, the infant will be able to suck directly from the breast. If ice packs are used between feedings to decrease swelling and relieve the pain, then hot packs will usually be needed to stimulate let-down at feeding time. A mother who is in pain may be tense and irritable. The nurse can help her relax by administering an analgesic about one-half hour prior to the feeding which enables her to be more patient and optimistic when the baby is ready to nurse. The mother needs to be reminded that this is a temporary condition.

Once the milk is in, some mothers complain that it comes out too quickly, causing the baby to choke. If this occurs, the nurse can suggest that the mother express the fast flowing milk into a cup until the stream slows down. Once some of the tension is relieved, the mother should have no problem getting the baby to nurse with ease.

The mother is often concerned with how frequently she should nurse her baby. During the early days, she may find it necessary to feed the infant as often as every 2 hours; however, once the milk supply is well established (approximately 2 to 4 weeks) and the baby has adjusted to his home, it is suggested that she try to feed no oftener than every 3 hours. The baby will get into the habit of nursing every 2 hours if the mother lets him, and then her life becomes one continuous feeding session.

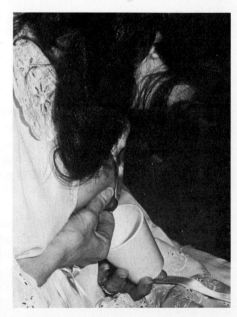

FIGURE 26-10
Milk can be manually expressed from the breast by compression of thumb and index finger behind the areola. Pressure is exerted backward rather than forward on the breast. (Courtesy of The University of Colorado Medical Center, Denver, Colorado)

Worries of the Nursing Mother

"Will the baby smother while I am nursing?" The woman who has large breasts will find it necessary to push down on some of the breast tissue with her finger to facilitate the baby's breathing. She should be reminded that the baby will instinctively stop sucking if he is unable to breathe.

"Is the baby getting enough milk?" Mothers may often be overly concerned with how many ounces the baby takes at a feeding. Often the hospital nurse will weigh the baby prior to the feeding and then following the feeding. The nurse announces to the mother that the baby took 2 ounces and is doing well or that he only took 1 ounce and this is not enough. Such procedures only make the mother more apprehensive about how much the baby gets. The nurse can be helpful by telling the mother that if the baby is voiding six or more times a day and if the urine is pale in color, then he is getting enough fluid. Another way of telling if the baby is getting a sufficient amount of milk is if he does not demand to feed for 2 to 3 hours between nursings. The nursing mother needs to be encouraged to relax and not to worry so much about time and ounces.

"My milk is too watery." This is another common concern of nursing mothers. Breast milk is bluish white and appears watery like skim milk; the mother should be reassured that this is the proper appearance of the milk.

"My baby has a bowel movement every time I nurse him, and he has diarrhea." Breast-fed babies often have an explosive bowel movement with each feeding and others will go as long as 5 days or even longer without a bowel movement. Breast milk is high in water content which helps prevent constipation. The stool from a nursing baby is loose and varies from a bright yellow-gold to a brownish-green; unlike stools from the bottle-fed baby, it has no strong odor.

"Can I eat spices or chocolate when I am nursing?" This is another frequent misconception about breast-feeding. Occasionally some babies will react to the abovementioned foods by having loose stools and gastric distress. In general, the baby will have no problems if the mother eats spices and chocolate in moderation. If she notices that a particular food seems to be causing the baby some distress, she should eat the food again and observe the infant's reaction to it. If it causes him gastrointestinal distress, it would be wise for her to avoid that particular food while she is nursing.

"Can I diet while I am nursing a baby?" Crash diets are not recommended for anyone and especially not for a nursing mother; however, there is no reason why a woman cannot lose weight and nurse at the same time. The only real food requirement for nursing is extra fluids. She should be encouraged to increase her daily fluid intake to 3 quarts per day. Many physicians recommend that the nursing mother continue to take vitamins while breast-feeding, and as with all mothers good food habits are stressed.

"How can I breast-feed if my baby is sick or premature?" When a mother wishes to obtain breast milk for a premature or ill infant who is not able to nurse, an electric breast pump provides a rapid and complete emptying of the breasts. The milk can be saved and brought to the hospital for the baby. The nurse should be familar with the availability and workings of an electric pump, which can be bought or rented from a hospital supply house. An alternative method is to manually express the breast milk.

Sore and Cracked Nipples

Some soreness of the nipple area is a frequent occurrence in a nursing mother; the degree of tenderness, however, is dependent on many things, most of which the knowledgeable maternity nurse can alleviate. A conscientious woman who has prepared her breasts antepartally is less likely to experience soreness after delivery, but the preparation is not a guarantee that she will be able to nurse without discomfort. Since the skin of blondes and redheads is more sensitive than that of dark-skinned women, they usually experience more soreness of nipples. A sore nipple carefully examined may appear to have small fissures or cracks on the surface of the skin. Proper steps to promote healing should be taken so that breast-feeding may continue. Some helpful hints the nurse should give to the mother as soon after delivery as possible, if the instruction has not been done antenatally, are discussed below. The preferential treatment of sore or cracked nipples involves healing them *before* they inhibit or temporarily stop the breast-feeding experience.

Nursing mothers should be instructed to clean the nipple area with plain water only, omitting soap and astringents such as alcohol, tincture of benzoin, or witch hazel. The cleansing need only be done once a day and is not necessary before each feeding. If mothers are concerned that the breast will be unclean for the baby, they can be reassured by the knowledge that the lysozyme in breast milk is an antiseptic. For an especially sensitive nipple, the nurse may suggest the use of a cotton ball instead of a cloth for cleaning the area.

An excellent method of preventing or reducing nipple soreness and cracking is air drying of the nipples for 10 to 15 minutes after each feeding. The mother might leave the flaps of her nursing bra open, or insert small tea strainers, with the handles removed, inside the cups of her bra to promote free circulation of air with the flaps closed. Plastic-covered pads or plastic-lined bra cups are to be avoided, for moisture that is retained inside the bra next to the nipple increases the chances of skin breakdown and slows healing and toughening of the skin.

Most doctors recommend that a vitamin or pure lanolin ointment be applied to the nipples after they have been air dried to promote healing and toughening of the skin. If an ointment is used after nursing, it should be gently but completely rubbed in so that air is allowed to reach the nipples. The ointment used should be one which is harmless to the baby so that unnecessary cleansing of the breast can be avoided.

To minimize soreness it is usually recommended that nursing time be increased gradually, as mentioned in the previous section. Mothers who overdo by letting the baby nurse as long as he wishes right from the beginning usually become quite uncomfortable by the second day. Since it is the frequency of the feedings, not the length of time of sucking at each feeding, that determines milk supply and the time of the first let-down, one is justified in suggesting to the mother that she limit the length of the initial feedings.

Some mothers change positions for each feeding, thereby putting the greatest pressure of the baby's suck on different areas of the nipple. She might lie down, sit on the edge of her bed, sit in a rocking chair, place the baby on a pillow in her lap, or hold the baby's head with her hand rather than cradling it in her arm. These are all variances which the mother may wish to try before leaving the hospital while the nurse can help and give suggestions.

Engorgement frequently leads to sore nipples; therefore, prevention of severe engorgement should be a prime concern of the nurse caring for a nursing mother. An extremely swollen breast causes the baby to grasp the nipple area improperly because he is not able to draw a large amount of the areolar area into his mouth. So instead of compressing and sucking, he merely chews on that part of the breast which is available to him—the nipple.

Treatments with a sun lamp or gooseneck lamp with a 20-watt bulb are both recommended for sore or cracked nipples. An ultraviolet bulb may be purchased and used in any ordinary lamp socket or stand, thereby giving the healing warmth of a sun lamp without purchasing the expensive equipment. Mothers who use an ultraviolet light must shield their eyes, and expose their skin no longer than ½ minute the first day, 1 minute the next 2 days, and 2 minutes the fourth and fifth days. If there is any sign of reddening of the skin, the mother should be instructed to go back to ½ to 1 minute and begin working up again. She should be positioned about 4 feet from the lamp, and the treatment should only be done once a day. Using an ordinary light bulb, the mother may sit closer to it (about 18 inches) and she does not need to shield her eyes. The exposure time can be lengthened to 5 to 10 minutes at a time which can be repeated several times a day. Treatment with dry heat as mentioned above can be initiated when nipple soreness is noticed; but if the skin has broken down and is bleeding from the fissures, treatment is essential.

If the soreness is quite uncomfortable for the mother, nursing less frequently will not decrease her discomfort because then the baby will be nursing from an overfull breast. It is better to limit nursing time to 10 minutes on each side rather than to nurse less often. The baby should start on the side that is less sore to stimulate milk ejection; once let-down has occurred he can be changed to the other side. If both breasts are equally tender, application of a hot cloth or towel to the breasts just prior to nursing will trigger milk ejection, after which the baby can be put to breast. If the soreness or cracking is so severe that feeding must be discontinued on one side, the milk from that breast can be manually expressed for 24 to 48 hours, and the baby can nurse from the other side. The hand expression should be used along with air drying, light, ointment, etc.

Sore or cracked nipples can be a major problem for a mother who is intolerant of pain or one who has been led to believe that nursing a baby is a simple procedure. It is, therefore, the responsibility of the nurse to constantly remind the mother that this soreness is temporary and that her discomfort will subside. So often a mother will say, "If I have to go through this every time I nurse, I'm not going to be able to do it." All the suggestions presented previously must be combined with sympathy, understanding, and encouragement from the nurse to help the mother through this particular time in her nursing experience.

Blistered Nipples

A nipple which is blistered is usually indicative of improper sucking by the baby. It most often is caused by the infant grasping only the nipple, and not the areolar area. The nipple remains at the front of the baby's mouth, where the action of his tongue and gums causes blistering. These blisters may bleed when they are broken which is not harmful to the baby but may frighten the mother. Prevention here is certainly preferable to cure. A mother may not realize the baby is not sucking properly unless the nurse observes the feeding and points this out to her. Ultraviolet light and resting the nipple for 24 to 48 hours are the preferred methods of treatment.

Anxiety or Overexertion

Anxiety, upset, or emotional trauma influence milk ejection; therefore, a mother who is not able to relax prior to nursing may find that her milk will not let-down. If at all possible, she should be encouraged to lie down while nursing and concentrate on relaxation of her entire body. If lying down is not possible, perhaps she could put her feet up and read a magazine. Because of the close relationship between thoughts of the mind and actions of the body, her main goal must be gearing her thoughts toward something other than the cause of her upset. If the emotional upset is continual over a period of time, the doctor may prescribe an oxytocic nasal spray to aid in let-down. The nasal spray is also useful when overexertion or lack of rest inhibits milk injection.

Mastitis

Mastitis frequently presents itself as soreness in a particular area of the breast, usually accompanied by induration and erythema. A nursing mother with these symptoms should consult her doctor. Often she will be able to continue nursing as long as treatment of the infection has begun. A breast abscess which requires incision and drainage will not interfere with nursing once it is healed. The mother can continue nursing on the unaffected breast and hand express the milk from the abscessed one.

The Baby Who Will Not Suck

An infant who refuses to suck at the breast or who thrusts his tongue toward the roof of his mouth presents a special problem. These babies will almost always suck beautifully from a bottle nipple; therefore, it is imperative not to supplement them with an artificial nipple. Besides causing the baby to become accustomed to it, the mother loses all confidence when she sees her baby refuse her breast and gulp down milk from a bottle. Supplements may be given with a spoon, cup, or an eye dropper. The eye dropper is preferred in this situation because milk can be dribbled down over the breast into the baby's mouth, hopefully helping him to begin sucking from the breast. Another suggestion is to express some colostrum from the breast.

Inadequate Milk Supply

The mother who says she does not have enough milk for her baby probably is not nursing often enough. This complaint is frequently heard at about 6 weeks and then again at 3 months, both times that babies have growth spurts. The nurse should inform the mother of this and also remind her that the oftener the baby nurses, the more milk she will have. If she would feed the baby frequently (every 2 hours or even more often) during her waking hours, she will find that her supply will increase. *The milk supply is directly related to the frequency of nursing—the more often the baby nurses, the more milk is produced.* The supply and demand concept is sometimes hard to remember when a baby is awakening every hour to 2 hours to be fed; therefore, the community health nurse can give encouragement to the mother during these frustrating times.

SPECIAL CONSIDERATIONS

Weaning

It is not unusual for a new mother to ask the nurse how long she should continue to nurse the baby. There is no definite cutoff point—it is entirely up to the mother to decide when she would like to wean the baby. Some women nurse as little as 6 weeks and others will nurse for over a year.

When the mother has decided to wean the baby, the easiest and most comfortable way to do so is gradually. The nurse might suggest that the mother eliminate one breast-feeding a day and cup or bottle-feed at that time. In a few days, the mother may again eliminate another nursing and feed the baby twice by cup or bottle. She should continue in this manner until her milk has dried up. La Leche League suggests that the mother wean the baby when the infant seems to be less interested in the breast.[27] They also suggest that the mother not offer the child the breast unless he wants it; this allows the child to wean himself. If the baby is recovering from an illness, if he is teething, or if there has been an emotional upset in the family, weaning should be delayed. The baby's life should be calm and happy when the weaning is begun so that he has only one new situation with which to contend.

Supplemental Feeding

Supplementary or complementary feedings are defined here as formula, water, or glucose water given after breast-feeding, or in place of a breast-feeding once the mother's milk is well established. Many hospitals use the supplementary bottle following a breast-feeding until the mother's breasts fill with milk. The idea of the supplementary feeding is to keep the baby hydrated and satisfied; however, if the mother's colostrum supply is adequate and the baby appears satisfied after breast-feeding, the bottle should not be forced upon him. It may be that the greatest harm done by feeding a baby supplements with a bottle is teaching the mother a psychological dependence on the bottle, undermining confidence in her ability to breast-feed. Varying opinions exist as to the appropriateness of ever supplementing through a bottle nipple, since the milk flows easier from such a nipple and the infant's suck is weakened. In an infant whose suck is weak and who is not nursing well, it is preferable to supplement using a spoon, cup, or eye dropper so that his suck will be stronger when he does nurse. In discussing supplementary feedings, the nurse should encourage the mother to spend some evenings out with her husband and to leave a bottle at home for the baby. She may wish to manually express the milk from her breasts into a bottle or to mix an artificial feeding. After lactation is well established, her milk supply will not be noticeably lessened by giving the baby an occasional bottle. Some mothers feel tied to their babies, thinking that they either cannot go out or must take the baby along. A word of encouragement from the nurse to take an evening off can go a long way in easing the mother's anxiety.

Nursing Twins

Mothers who wish to breast-feed twins should be given some hints from the nurse before time for discharge. After she gets home she will be doubly busy and will appreciate having the art of nursing well under way. A modified demand schedule might be suggested to her so that her entire day is not spent feeding, meaning when one twin is awake and ready to eat, she awakens the other and feeds him at the same time. The milk supply will be adequate because of the supply and demand principle of breast milk. When she nurses both of them at once, the new mother will need to sit up, holding the twins in her lap, as shown in Figure 26-11, or at her sides with their bodies on pillows. She can experiment with them in her lap with them facing the same direction, or with both of them facing toward her. The mother may choose to breast-feed twin A and bottle-feed twin B at one feeding, and at the next feeding breast-feed twin B and bottle-feed twin A.

The Working Mother

It is very possible to have a full-time job and still breast-feed. Often mothers will mention to the nurse while they are in the hospital that they plan to stop nursing and go back to work in 6 weeks. If they do wish to continue to nurse longer than that and must go back to work, they can come home to feed the baby once during the day; if that is not possible, they can hand express the milk at work and save it for the baby-sitter to give to the baby during the next day. Hand-expressed milk can be stored in a freezer for as long as 1 month and in a deep freeze for 3 months.

Leaking Breasts

It is common for the second breast to leak as the baby nurses on the first side because of the milk letting-down in both breasts at the same time. In order to keep the mother's clothes dry a washcloth may be inserted into her bra on the second side. Most new mothers who breast-feed will have some leaking of the

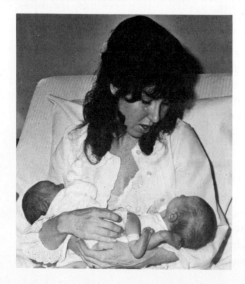

FIGURE 26-11
This mother demonstrates one way of positioning twins while nursing. (*Courtesy of The University of Colorado Medical Center, Denver, Colorado*)

breasts between feedings for at least the first few weeks until lactation is well established. Nursing pads are available which can be inserted into the bra to absorb the leakage; however, they do prevent air from circulating freely due to the plastic coating. For this reason cotton handkerchiefs or other lightweight fabric is preferable. If let-down occurs unexpectedly while out in public, the new mother should be instructed to very unobtrusively press her forearms against her breasts for a few seconds until the tingling sensation stops.

Bottle-feeding

If the mother chooses to bottle-feed her baby, the nurse should support this decision and help her learn the art of formula feeding. One of the first things a bottle-feeding mother asks about is sterilization. Many pediatricians still believe that sterilizing is necessary; however, the current trend is toward a clean technique rather than a sterile one. The mother should be instructed to wash the bottles and nipples, and they can be washed with the rest of the dishes. A bottle brush should be used for cleaning whether the bottles are washed in a dishwasher or by hand, as milk which is dried in the bottom of the bottle or in the nipple provides an excellent medium for growth of bacteria.

The kind of formula used will vary and most pediatricians have a preference. Some mothers will use the prepared formulas and others the evaporated milk formula. If the woman has been instructed to use a prepared formula, she will find that it comes in three forms: powdered milk, concentrated liquid, and ready-to-use. The powdered milk is the cheapest but most difficult to prepare as many women have difficulty getting the powder to dissolve in the water. The nurse might suggest that she use hot water in preparing the bottle, and some mothers find that they need a beater to remove the lumps from the milk. If she chooses the concentrated liquid form, this is prepared by adding equal amounts of milk and water. She should be advised to buy this by the carton as it is cheaper than buying one can at a time. The ready-to-use formula is the most expensive and needs no preparation. Once a can of milk has been opened, it should be stored in the refrigerator and used within 24 hours.

In the past, mothers made enough formula to last 24 hours; however, the current trend is to prepare one bottle at a time to decrease the incidence of bacterial growth in the milk. Warm water can be used to mix with the milk to bring it to room temperature so that heating the bottle will be unnecessary.

Some pediatricians are beginning to recommend that the mother start feeding her baby milk with 2 percent butterfat after the first month. This milk has less animal fat and is high in protein. They have suggested that the high carbohydrate content in the prepared formulas causes the baby to become hungry more frequently; hence, he eats more and gains weight rapidly, thus generating new fat cells.[28]

How much the baby takes varies from feeding to feeding and from infant to infant. If the baby is fed on demand, he will be hungry at the time of the feeding and will take what he needs. As with the breast-feeding mother, the woman who is bottle-feeding should try to keep the baby awake so that he does not take just enough to satisfy him for a brief time and then fall asleep. He is getting enough if he goes from 3 to 4 hours between feedings.

When the mother is ready to feed the baby, she should assume a comfortable position and try to be as relaxed as possible. Since this is the time when the baby gets to know his mother and feels warmth and security within his life, propping the bottle should be discouraged. Propping is also dangerous to the infant, because he may choke on the milk when his mother is not near enough to help him. The bottle should be held so that no air is in the nipple when the baby is sucking, and the nipple should be completely filled with milk. A baby may take about 20 minutes to eat, and the mother should plan for this time as she arranges her daily schedule.

Bubbling the Infant

Both breast- and bottle-fed babies will need to be bubbled during, following, and sometimes prior to the feeding. The baby who has been quite fussy before the feeding may need to be bubbled first, since he swallows a lot of air when he is crying. Air in the stomach often causes the baby to feel full before he has taken much milk. The air displaces the milk, thereby filling the stomach and sometimes causing the baby to regurgitate.

A mother may bubble the baby quite frequently during the feeding; however, she should be aware that each time the baby takes hold of the nipple, he swallows a mouthful of air before the seal is complete. It is sufficient to bubble the newborn infant about every ounce and the older baby about every 2 ounces. The breast-fed baby can be bubbled when changing breasts. The mother should learn to know her baby, and if he seems to need bubbling more frequently, she should do so. The baby is bubbled at the end of the feeding to rid the stomach of air which could cause gas pains or regurgitation.

The baby may be bubbled by having the mother put him over her shoulder and gently rub his back, as pictured in Figure 26-12. It is not necessary to pat the baby vigorously, since this often causes him to spit up that which he has just eaten. Another position which is good for bubbling is for the mother to set the infant on her lap, placing her hand under the baby's jaw to support his head, and lean the baby forward as she gently rubs his back. The nurse can suggest that the mother try both methods so that she can provide some variety for the infant. Some infants will burp quickly, and others require a longer period of time and greater patience on the part of the mother.

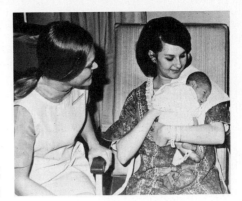

FIGURE 26-12
The most common position for bubbling an infant. *(Courtesy of The University of Colorado Medical Center, Denver, Colorado)*

Pacifiers

All babies have a strong sucking need, and it seems appropriate to discuss pacifiers briefly. Many women prenatally object to them; however, they find that when the baby is taken home and is fussy for no explainable reason, a pacifier settles him by fulfilling his sucking need. This urge to suck, which is felt by the infant as an uncomfortable sensation in his mouth,[29] usually disappears by 4 to 5 months of age; therefore, a mother should be encouraged to allow the infant to wean himself from the pacifier at that age if he has lost interest in it. The nurse should reassure a mother who feels guilty about using a pacifier that her infant's need to suck is normal and natural and that a pacifier is preferable to his thumb.

The Nuk Sauger pacifier is ideal, since it is shaped like the nipple on the mother's breast as the baby sucks (Figure 26-13), and orthodontists feel it lessens the chance of malocclusion later in life. Occasionally a baby will refuse this kind of pacifier, and the mother should not hesitate to try one of the other varieties readily available in most drugstores and supermarkets.

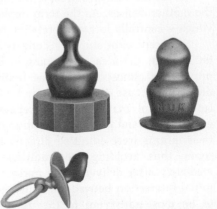

FIGURE 26-13
The Nuk Sauger primary exerciser. Two views of the Nuk Sauger Bottle Nipple. *(Courtesy of Rocky Mountain Dental Products Co.)*

ENVIRONMENT

Establishment of a suitable environment plays an essential part in fostering the beginning of healthy family interrelationships (see Figure 26–14). In order for this environment to be favorable for the family, it must be planned according to a philosophy of maternity care geared to the needs of the family and the individual mother and infant. This basic philosophy must be one of freedom and direction with a minimum of strictness and regimentation. The success or failure of the environment being a positive phase during this developmental crisis is dependent on each nurse's own commitment to family-centered maternity care. The nurse must assimilate the philosophy and in some cases pass it on to other personnel in order to maintain the tone of the entire unit. To develop such a philosophy a sound understanding of the physical and psychological changes occurring within the mother and the family at the time of the baby's arrival is essential.

Availability of the Baby

In order for the family concept to be continuous, it is obvious that the baby must be available to the mother whenever she wishes. This means that the maternity unit should be set up in one of two ways: (1) a central nursery regarded by the staff as being a place where the baby is kept when the mother does not wish him at her bedside or (2) rooming-in.

A rooming-in unit is designed with the baby's crib always at the mother's bedside or with a nursery adjacent to the mother's room available. In some units the baby is with the mother 24 hours a day, and she is the primary caretaker at all times. In other instances, rooming-in is modified so that the baby is kept in the adjacent nursery during the night. In either setup, if the mother is in need of rest or is unable to care for the baby for a period of time, ideally she should be able to return the baby to a nursery.

With the central nursery, the baby is taken to and from the nursery as the mother desires. As the term implies, there is one nursery for all the babies which is centrally located in relation to the mothers' rooms.

A recent pilot study[30] done at the University of Colorado Medical Center brought the idea of rooming-in back to its initially defined function—to provide an atmosphere for the family to remain together from the time of delivery. Because of studies done by Klaus and Kennell[31] showing the harmful effects of maternal-infant separation, it was decided to manipulate the environment and prevent separation completely. Newly delivered mothers and their infants were admitted directly to the rooming-in unit from the delivery room, thus avoiding the traditional separation of parents and baby immediately after delivery. The nurse was able to observe and be a part of the initial interaction between parents and infant, an experience which was found to be most satisfying to the nurses involved in the study. Time-honored

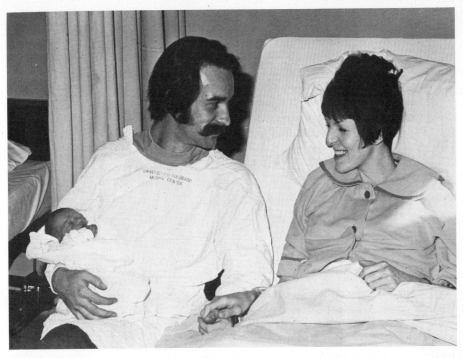

FIGURE 26-14
The father is welcome in a family-centered maternity unit. (*Courtesy of The University of Colorado Medical Center, Denver, Colorado*)

routines such as immediate application of silver nitrate to the infant's eyes, delayed first feeding, emptying of the stomach with a mucous trap, total body bathing, and observation of the infant while in an incubator were dispensed with in order to duplicate the naturalness and flexibility of a home delivery. The positive response of the parents and the excellent condition of the infants may lead the nurse to reevaluate the hospital-imposed separation of the family following delivery.

Availability of the Nurse

Besides the availability of the baby, the success of a family-centered program is also dependent on the availability of the nurse. Ideally the nurse responsible for the mother's care should also be responsible for the baby's care, for the two should be regarded as one unit. This negates the traditional titles of "postpartum nurse" and "nursery nurse" and develops the term "maternal-child nurse." This expands the nurse's role far beyond the one of custodial caretaker; it initiates creativity and purposefulness in planning and executing care. Separation of the two nursing roles leads to anxiety and frustration within the parents because the questions concerning their baby must often be referred to someone else. The separation of the two roles also leads to conflicts between the postpartum and nursery nurses, as each feels his role to be more important. The lack of communication between the two areas is also a source of difficulty in providing optimal patient care; however, when division of the two roles is unavoidable, it is each individual nurse's responsibility to be aware of both mother and baby, keeping a direct line of communication open to the nurse in the other area.

When the family-centered concept is practiced, the nurse has the opportunity to observe early mother-child and family interactions, intervene when appropriate, and be involved in teaching. This expands the nurse's role far beyond the one of custodial caretaker and enables her to be creative and purposeful in planning and executing care.

Visiting Policies

Visiting policies are an important part of postpartum care, and even though it is a controversial issue, it is one which needs to be considered carefully. First there is concern about infection being passed from visitors to the baby. Current theory reveals that clean technique by all those coming in contact with the baby is adequate for protection of the infant. This involves washing hands thoroughly, and placing a cover gown over street clothes; it does not include wearing a mask. Most hospitals limit the number of visitors coming into the mother's room at any one time, and usually a restriction is placed on who can be in the room when the baby is with the mother. These restrictions need to be periodically and realistically evaluated so that unnecessary restrictions are not placed on the family for the benefit of the hospital routine and nursing personnel.

The mother's rest must be considered when establishing visiting policies. It has been mentioned that she requires a great deal of sleep during the early puerperium; therefore, it may be wise at times to be aware of the mother's fatigue and intervene by suggesting that visitors leave. The nurse should realize that it may be difficult for the mother to make that suggestion herself when she is being visited by close relatives or friends.

The more progressive institutions now allow grandparents and great-grandparents to hold and feed the baby during the hospital stay; however, in the mobile society of today in which married children are often far away from parents, the mother may wish to have as visitors a best friend, sister, or other close relative. One wonders why these people are kept from the mother at a time when it is important for her to share such a great event in her life with others to whom she is close. Another logical question may be why a grandparent is regarded as cleaner than a friend.

Siblings are not to be forgotten in establishing visiting policies. A flexible unit should provide opportunity for the mother to visit her other children, such as having a lounge area next to the maternity unit for that purpose.

Included in this same idea is the importance of allowing siblings to see the new baby, as in Figure 26-15. Touching or close contact with the infant by the sibling is not suggested; however, the mother can stay with the older child as the nurse shows the new baby to him.

Demand Feeding

Adherence to a strict feeding schedule promotes the idea to mothers and nurses that babies are fed by the clock rather than according to their own hunger needs. The infant has needs in his own right, one of which is to take in food when his stomach is ready for it. Hunger needs vary according to body size, activity, output, and the type of feeding (whether by breast or bottle). The mother who tries to feed an infant who is not hungry, but who is due to eat by the clock, finds herself frustrated and anxious as she perceives the baby's disinterest as rejection of her. This is a prime example of a baby's negative contribution to the mother-infant relationship, which could be a positive contribution if he were ready to eat. When a mother feels rejected, confidence in her mothering tasks is weakened, and depression is often the outcome. This feeling of rejection is heightened if the baby is being breast-

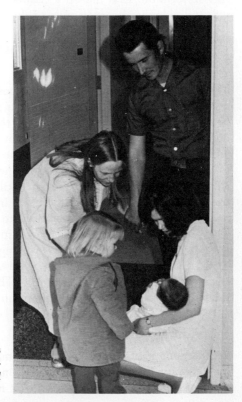

FIGURE 26-15
Proud parents share in three-year-old Tina's first encounter with her new sister. (*Courtesy of The University of Colorado Medical Center, Denver, Colorado*)

fed. Demand feeding, therefore, is regarded as essential to provide an environment that gives the mother the best possible chance to have a successful feeding experience.

Demand feeding allows the nurse to spend more time with each mother, since most of the babies will be eating at different times. It also portrays an idea of flexibility and individual needs which were previously mentioned as important concepts in family-centered care.

Routines and Willingness to Change

Hospital routines interfere with administration of individualized nursing care. The day begins with checking temperature at 6 A.M., doctors' rounds at 7 A.M., and breakfast at 8 A.M. By this time the groggy mother is encouraged by the nurse to take her bath in order to be ready for the infant's morning feeding, which is usually about 10 A.M. It would seem that these regimented schedules meet the needs of nurses and doctors, but not the mother. Many mothers complain about the lack of sleep while they are in the hospital. During the day when a mother is beginning her restorative process, which requires added sleep, hospital routine consistently interrupts and interferes with this restoration. It is indeed a challenge for the maternal-child nurse to provide individualized care in spite of the hospital-imposed routines.

GUIDANCE AND EVALUATION DURING THE PUERPERIUM

Teaching of the parents during the postpartum period is a task that should not be overlooked by the nurse. Instruction given during the antenatal period needs reinforcement, and many times the actual birth of the baby precipitates questions and problems that were not foreseen. The situations for learning are easily found on the postpartum unit; however, how and when to do the teaching has long been a problem. The mother is in the hospital for such a short time that the nurse must be skillful and creative in teaching without overloading the mother with too much information.

There are several considerations to be made before any teaching is done. The woman should be physically comfortable, have some motivation to learn, and the place selected for the teaching situation should be calm and quiet. The teacher should not present a threat to the mother and should also be relaxed and comfortable in that role. The atmosphere should be one in which the mother feels free to ask questions and discuss her feelings.

Individualized Teaching

Because pregnancy and birth are normal events and the postpartum mother has few physical needs, the nurse has more time to spend doing individualized teaching (see Figure 26-16). The nurse needs to assess where the mother and/

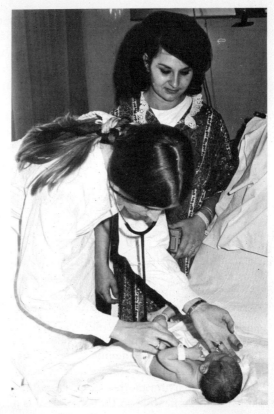

FIGURE 26-16
A child health associate performs the discharge physical examination and teaching at the mother's bedside. (*Courtesy of The University of Colorado Medical Center, Denver, Colorado*)

or the family are in the developmental crisis of pregnancy and delivery. For instance, a woman who has had four babies may need counseling in how to manage that many children at home; whereas the greatest need of the primipara who has never held a small baby is learning to feel comfortable with her infant. Likewise, the new father who expresses anxiety that the baby might break may need a nurse nearby when he first holds his infant. Parents who have not had a baby for several years will probably require the same support and assistance that the first-time parents need.

The emphasis in many hospitals is on the techniques of bathing, formula preparation, bubbling, etc. Techniques are an important part of teaching, but until the parents feel comfortable in holding the baby, they probably will not comprehend much of what is taught to them about tub bathing the infant. That is why the main focal point of teaching with these parents should be in helping them rely on their own observational abilities and their common sense. A mother who continues to use soap daily on her baby's dry, flaky skin needs teaching which stresses observation of the baby over routine. If a mother is assisted in thinking through the symptoms of illness in a new baby, she will probably remember them better than if a nurse were to present them to her in a lecture.

In contrast to the first-time mother is the multiparous woman who has recently had an infant and seems very comfortable in caring for the new baby. She may not be interested in attending a bath class but is deeply concerned about how the other children in the family will accept the new baby. This may require a nurse to sit down and discuss possible and realistic ways to introduce the infant to the other family members.

Group Teaching

Teaching may be done through a lecture during which a nurse gives information to a group of mothers in a group situation in which there is a give-and-take between the mothers, as pictured in Figure 26-17. Ideally the group sessions are conducted by a nurse who is able to guide the discussion and present information where appropriate. This is not an easy task, since the group will probably meet just once and for a short time. The mothers will probably have sore perineums and will not want to sit for any length of time. It takes a skilled nurse to create an exciting group discussion and to realize that the postpartum mother is undergoing a great deal of stress. The teaching plan should be flexible so that the nurse is able to work with the mother when she is receptive to learning. Though there are many problems involved with group teaching, it is recommended that the nurse experiment with the method. A group situation along with individualized teaching can do much in preparing the mother to return to her home environment with confidence in herself and her mothering tasks.

Postpartum Exercises

During the early puerperium the mother should be made aware of the value of exercising and getting her weight back to her prepregnant state. It frequently happens that a woman never quite loses the weight gained in pregnancy or gets her abdominal muscles back in shape; hence, with each succeeding pregnancy she finds herself adding a few extra pounds and her muscles becoming more and more relaxed. For this reason it is advisable to have the mother begin selected exercises while she is still in the hospital, and she should be encouraged to continue them at home. Now is the time for her to tone and tighten her stretched muscles and to lose whatever weight she has gained during pregnancy.

Our society has become somewhat obsessed with weight, and the current

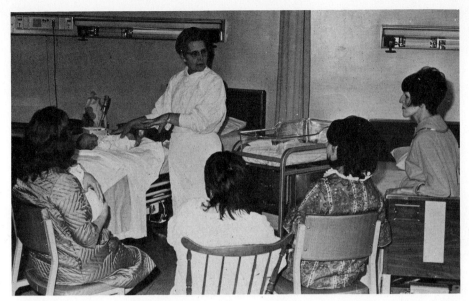

FIGURE 26-17
The nurse guides a group of mothers in a discussion on infant care. *(Courtesy of The University of Colorado Medical Center, Denver, Colorado)*

trend favors slender women. Obesity is a common occurrence, and this is an excellent time to work on preventing such a problem. To encourage the overall health of the woman, it is advisable to take this opportunity to show her how to get her weight and muscle tone back to normal. A woman's figure influences her self-image and feeling of general well-being.

The mother will have many demands on her time after she goes home, so it is not wise to give her too many exercises. It is better to select a more realistic regimen for the mother to achieve and maintain. Several drug companies publish pamphlets on postpartum exercises, and the nurse might review them and select one for use on the postpartum unit. Many hospitals have prepared mimeographed sheets on postpartum exercises which they hand out to the mothers, and sometimes the physical therapist gives the instruction. It is helpful to give the mother written material so that she will have something to refresh her memory when at home. It is the nurse's responsibility to be knowledgeable about the exercises and to teach them as appropriate.

The following exercises are very basic and can be easily taught. There are many others, but these have been found to be beneficial to the postpartum mother during the early days after delivery. They require regular daily practice if success is to be the outcome. It is wise to remind the woman that exercising will not decrease her weight, but it will tone the muscles. A sensible diet plus exercise should be recommended to the mother who wants to regain her figure.

1 Deep abdominal breathing used to strengthen the diaphragm (Figure 26-18a). Begin on the first postpartum day. Take a deep breath, raising abdominal wall, and exhale slowly. To insure exercise is being done correctly, place one hand on the chest and one on the abdomen. When inhaling, the hand on the abdomen should be raised and the hand on the chest should remain stationary. Repeat exercise 5 times.

2 Head and shoulder raising. On the second postpartum day lie flat without a pillow and raise head until the chin is touching the chest. On the third postpartum day raise both head and shoulders off the bed and lower them slowly (Figure 26-18b). Increase gradually until able to do 10. This is an early exercise which helps to tone the abdominal muscles.

3 Leg raising (Figure 26-18c). This exercise may be begun on the seventh postpartum day. Lying down on the floor with no pillow under the head, point toe and slowly raise one leg keeping the knee straight. Lower the leg slowly. Gradually increase to 10 times each leg. On the ninth postpartum day, slowly raise both legs together. This is an excellent exercise for strengthening abdominal muscles.

4 Pelvic tilt (Figure 26-18d). Lie flat on the floor with knees bent, inhale, and while exhaling flatten the back hard against the floor so that there is no space between the back and the floor. While doing this, tighten abdominal muscles and the muscles of the buttocks.

5 Kegal exercise. This exercise is used to strengthen and tone the muscles of the pelvic floor. The mother should be instructed to do this daily for the rest of her life. Exercise can be done lying on the floor with ankles crossed or sitting in a chair with knees apart and feet flat on the floor. Tighten the muscles around the anus as if to control a bowel movement and then tighten the muscles around the vagina and urethra as if to stop urine in midstream. Now hold these muscles tightly to the count of 6 and then relax. This exercise can be done on the first postpartum day; it also increases the circulation to the perineal region, hence promoting faster healing of the episiotomy.

6 Situps (Figure 26-18e). In 2 weeks, the mother may begin situps, slowly increasing the number until she is able to do at least 10. Lie flat on back with hands on hips. Slowly raise head, shoulder, and trunk until attaining a sitting position. This is another good exercise for toning and strengthening abdominal muscles.

After 2 weeks the mother may do almost any exercise she chooses. It is wise to remind her that if she notices that the lochia turns bright red after she has been exercising, she should stop for a few days until the bleeding is no longer bright red. If the mother does these six exercises faithfully and follows a careful diet, she will find that she is able to regain her figure quickly.

Evaluation of Learning

In an effort to evaluate the learning that has taken place in the hospital, the nurse can arrange time to sit down and talk with the mother about how she feels regarding herself, the baby, and the events that have just taken place. If a bath demonstration has been given, the nurse may wish the mother to bathe the infant again when the nurse is available to check on the learning and answer any additional questions. It is extremely important that the mother be made to feel comfortable while doing this. In some hospitals, the nurse may have a mother who has had other children give the bath demonstration while the nurse guides the group discussion. Some mothers would enjoy doing this, and others would feel very threatened by talking before a group. The nurse should be flexible enough to try a variety of teaching methods.

Information should be obtained as to the kind of help the mother will have at home. This help might be a mother, mother-in-law, sister or other close relative, next door neighbor, or a hired person. Those mothers who will be left alone at home should be given a telephone number to call, either that of the postpartum unit or the community health nurse. The establishment of a warm, friendly relationship with the mother in the hospital becomes even more important as discharge day nears. The mother who has become close to a nurse or nurses will be much more likely to call if she experiences any difficulty than will the mother who felt alone and without aid in the hospital.

Follow-up on the teaching that has been done is also a necessary function of the community health nurse. This nurse is the person most able to evaluate the learning that has taken place since the visiting nurse is able to see the mother in her home. The hospital nurse can begin a teaching program, and the public health nurse can add to and follow up on it. Such a system requires good communication between staff and agency. It is the hospital nurse's responsibility to initiate the public health referral if none has been made and to communicate exactly what the mother has been taught, how the woman reacted to it, and the nurse's evaluation of what has occurred during the hospital stay. In a family-centered maternity program, no one nurse can do all things for the patient, but via effective communication, excellent nursing care can be carried out.

In summary, teaching is the focal point of nursing on the postpartum unit, whether it is done formally or informally. It provides a continuous challenge for the nurse and offers an opportunity to be creative.

The Cesarean-section Mother

The cesarean-section mother provides the nurse with another good opportunity for teaching, since she is hospitalized longer and has more time to develop a relationship with the nurse. During the early days following surgery, the

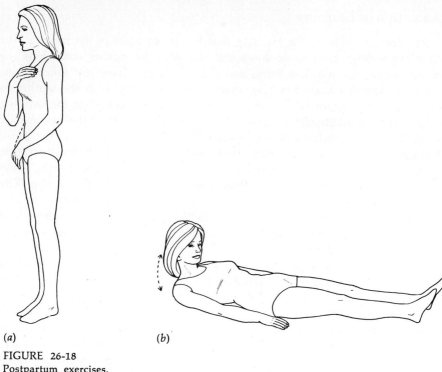

(a)   (b)

FIGURE 26-18
Postpartum exercises.
(Courtesy of Elizabeth Riska Townsley.)

mother's main concern will be with her physical well-being. She will need medication to ease her discomfort and more physical care than the routine postpartum mother. This woman tends to recover quickly and by the end of the first or second day she is beginning to take an interest in the infant.

If the mother had general anesthesia for her surgery, there may be a greater lag in maternal feelings than in the mother who had the cesarean section under a regional block. The mother who is awake and able to see the baby immediately after birth usually feels that she has been an active participant in the delivery; whereas the mother who has been put to sleep for the surgery may find that emotionally she is not as involved with the infant during the early puerperium. The mother whose cesarean section is planned and without a long labor may demonstrate a shorter maternal lag than the one who has an emergency section and no chance to psychologically prepare for the delivery. All these things must be taken into consideration as the nurse plans the patient's care and teaching.

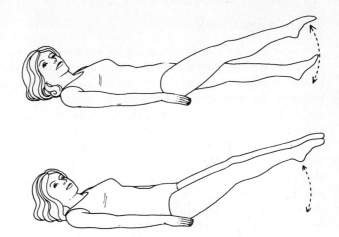

(c)

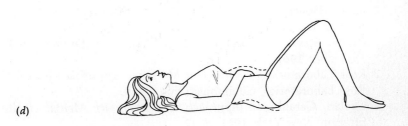

(d)

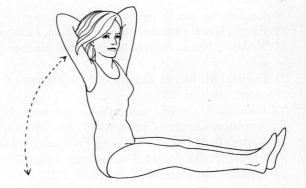

(e)

The 6-Week Check

The new mother should return to be examined by her doctor about 6 weeks postpartum. The purpose of this visit is to ensure that the puerperium has progressed normally, and it is important because it may be the last medical contact with the mother unless she has a problem or until she becomes pregnant again. This check consists of a thorough pelvic and breast examination, measurement of blood pressure and weight, a urinalysis, and sometimes a hematocrit and rubella immunization. The visit provides the doctor with information he needs to assess the mother's progress through the puerperium and also enables the woman to ask questions and bring to the doctor's attention any special concern. The 6-week examination is an excellent time to instruct the woman in breast self-examination if she is not already familiar with the procedure, and she should also be reminded of the importance of annual or semiannual Papanicolaou smears, the test for cervical cancer.

REFERENCES

1 Parad, Howard J. (ed.): *Crisis Intervention: Selected Readings*, Family Service Association of America, New York, 1965, p. 2.
2 Rubin, Reva: "Puerperal Change," *Nursing Outlook*, 9(12):753–755, December 1961.
3 Ross Laboratories: *A Study in Maternal Attitudes*, Medical Department, Ross Laboratories, Columbus, Ohio, 1959.
4 Caplan, Gerald: *An Approach to Community Mental Health*, Grune & Stratton, New York, 1961, p. 90.
5 Ibid., p. 103.
6 Klaus, Marshall, John Kennell, et al.: "Human Maternal Behavior at the First Contact with Her Young," *Pediatrics*, 46:188, August 1970.
7 Ibid., p. 190.
8 Caplan: op. cit., p. 90.
9 Prugh, Dane: personal communication, January 21, 1972.
10 Newton, Niles: *Maternal Emotions*, Hoeber-Harper, New York, 1955, p. 62.
11 Garrey, M. M., et al.: *Obstetrics Illustrated*, Williams & Wilkins, Baltimore, 1969, p. 287.
12 Hellman, Louis M., and Jack A. Pritchard: *Williams Obstetrics*, 14th ed., Appleton-Century-Crofts, New York, 1970, p. 470.
13 Kagan, B. M., et al.: "Feeding Premature Infants—Comparison of Various Milks," *Pediatrics*, 15:376, January–June, 1955.
14 Hellman and Pritchard: op. cit., p. 471.
15 Ibid., p. 473.

16 Smith, Christine: *Maternal-Child Nursing*, Saunders, Philadelphia, 1963, p. 174.

17 Bowes, Watson A., Jr., Sharon Joseph, and Rana Peck: unpublished data, 1971.

18 La Leche League International: *The Womanly Art of Breastfeeding*, 13th ed., Interstate Printers and Publishers, Danville, Ill., 1971, p. 151.

19 Moore, Francis D., et al.: "Carcinoma of the Breast," *New England Journal of Medicine*, 277:294, 1967.

20 Daniel, D. G., H. Campbell, and A. C. Turnbull: "Puerperal Thromboembolism and Suppression of Lactation," *Lancet*, 2:288–289, 1967.

21 Baum, J. David: "Nutritional Value of Human Milk," *Obstetrics and Gynecology*, 37(1):126–129, January 1971.

22 Bullen, Catherine, and A. T. Willis: "Resistance of the Breast-fed Infant to Gastroenteritis," *British Medical Journal*, p. 342, August 7, 1971.

23 Baum, J. David, et al.: "Hypocalcaemic Fits in Neonates," *Lancet*, 1:598, March 16, 1968.

24 Graber, T. M.: *Orthodontics, Principles and Practice*, 2d ed., Saunders, Philadelphia, 1966, p. 316.

25 Valdes-Dapena, Marie A.: "Sudden and Unexpected Death in Infancy: A Review of the World Literature 1954–1966," *Pediatrics*, 39:133, January 1967.

26 Iffrig, Sister M. C.: "Nursing Care and Success in Breast Feeding," *The Nursing Clinics of North America*, 3:347–349, June 1968.

27 La Leche League International: op. cit., p. 131.

28 Lubchenco, Lula O.: personal communication, February 19, 1972.

29 Fraiberg, Selma H.: *The Magic Years*, Scribner, New York, 1959, p. 70.

30 Andresen, Mary, Lula O. Lubchenco, and Rana Peck: unpublished data, August 1971.

31 Klaus, Marshall, and John Kennell: "Mothers Separated from Their Newborn Infants," *Pediatric Clinics of North America*, 17(4):1035, November 1970.

BIBLIOGRAPHY

Andresen, Mary, L. O. Lubchenco, and R. Peck: unpublished data, August 1971.

Applebaum, Richard M.: *Abreast of the Times*, Copyright Richard M. Applebaum, 1969.

———: "The Modern Management of Successful Breast Feeding," *Pediatric Clinics of North America*, 17(1):203–225, February 1970.

———: "The Physician and a Common Sense Approach to Breast Feeding," *Southern Medical Journal*, 63(7):793–799, July 1970.

Baum, J. David: "Nutritional Value of Human Milk," *Obstetrics and Gynecology*, 37(1):126–129, January 1971.

———, L. Cooper, and P. A. Davies: "Hypocalcaemic Fits in Neonates," *Lancet*, 1:598–599, March 16, 1968.

Benson, Ralph C.: *Handbook of Obstetrics and Gynecology*, 4th ed., Lange, Los Altos, Calif., 1971.

Birch, William G.: *A Doctor Discusses Pregnancy*, Budlong, Chicago, Ill., 1969.

Bowes, Watson A., Jr., S. Joseph, and R. Peck: unpublished data, 1971.

Brown, James W., and James W. Thornton, Jr.: *College Teaching: Perspectives and Guidelines*, McGraw-Hill, New York, 1963.

Bryant, Richard D., and Anna E. Overland: *Woodward and Gardner's Obstetrics Management and Nursing*, 7th ed., Davis, Philadelphia, 1964.

Bullen, Catherine L., and A. T. Willis: "Resistance of the Breast-fed Infant to Gastroenteritis," *British Medical Journal*, pp. 338–343, August 7, 1971.

Caplan, Gerald: *An Approach to Community Mental Health*, Grune & Stratton, New York, 1961.

Countryman, Betty A.: "Hospital Care of the Breast-fed Newborn," *American Journal of Nursing*, 71(12):2365–2367, December 1971.

Daniel, D. G., H. Campbell, and A. C. Turnbull: "Puerperal Thromboembolism and Suppression of Lactation," *Lancet*, 2:287–289, 1967.

Davis, M. Edward, and Reva Rubin: *Obstetrics for Nurses*, 17th ed., Saunders, Philadelphia, 1962.

Egli, G. E., N. S. Egli, and Michael Newton: "The Influence of Number of Breast Feedings on Milk Production," *Pediatrics*, 27(2):314–317, February 1961.

Fitzpatrick, Elise, Sharon Reeder, and Luigi Mastroianni, Jr.: *Maternity Nursing*, 12th ed., Lippincott, Philadelphia, 1971.

Fraiberg, Selma H.: *The Magic Years*, Scribner, New York, 1959.

Garrey, M. M., et al.: *Obstetrics Illustrated*, Williams & Wilkins, Baltimore, 1969.

Graber, T. M.: *Orthodontics, Principles and Practice*, 2d ed., Saunders, Philadelphia, 1966.

Greenhill, J. P.: *Obstetrics*, 13th ed., Saunders, Philadelphia, 1965.

Haire, Doris, and John Haire: *Implementing Family-centered Maternity Care with a Central Nursery*, Childbirth Education Association of New Jersey, Hillside, N.J., 1968.

Hellman, Louis M., and Jack A. Pritchard: *Williams Obstetrics*, 14th ed., Appleton-Century-Crofts, New York, 1971.

Iffrig, Sister M. C.: "Nursing Care and Success in Breast Feeding," *The Nursing Clinics of North America*, 3:345–354, June 1968.

Ingalls, A. Joy, and M. Constance Salerno: *Maternal and Child Health Nursing*, 2d ed., Mosby, St. Louis, 1971.

Iorio, Josephine: *Principles of Obstetrics and Gynecology for Nurses*, 2d ed., Mosby, St. Louis, 1971.

Kagan, B. M., et al.: "Feeding Premature Infants—Comparison of Various Milks," *Pediatrics*, 15:373–381, January–June 1955.

Klaus, Marshall, and John Kennell: "Mothers Separated from Their Newborn Infants," *Pediatric Clinics of North America*, 17(4):1015–1035, November 1970.

———— and ————, et al.: "Human Maternal Behavior at the First Contact with Her Young," *Pediatrics*, 46(2):187–192, August 1970.

La Leche League International: *The Womanly Art of Breastfeeding*, 13th ed., Interstate Printers and Publishers, Danville, Ill., 1971.

Lesser, Marion, and Vera Keane: *Nurse-Patient Relationships in a Hospital Maternity Service*, Mosby, St. Louis, 1956.

Lubchenco, Lula O.: personal communication, February 19, 1972.

McLennan, Charles E.: *Synopsis of Obstetrics*, 7th ed., Mosby, St. Louis, 1966.

Moore, Francis D., et al.: "Carcinoma of the Breast," *New England Journal of Medicine*, 277:293–296, 1967.

Newton, Michael, and Niles Newton: "Postpartum Engorgement of the Breast," *American Journal of Obstetrics and Gynecology*, 61(3):644–667, March 1951.

Newton, Niles: *The Family Book of Child Care*, Harper & Row, New York, 1957.

————: *Maternal Emotions*, Hoeber-Harper, New York, 1955.

———— and Michael Newton: "Mothers' Reactions to Their Newborn Babies," *Journal of the American Medical Association*, 181(1):206–210, July 21, 1962.

Parad, Howard J. (ed.): *Crisis Intervention: Selected Readings*, Family Service Association of America, New York, 1965.

Peplau, Hildegard: "Anxiety in the Mother-Infant Relationship," *Nursing World*, 134:11, 33–34, May 1960.

Prugh, Dane: personal communication, January 21, 1972.

Redman, Barbara Klug: *The Process of Patient Teaching*, Mosby, St. Louis, 1968.

Reed, Constance: *Rapid Post Natal Figure Recovery*, Ortho Pharmaceutical Corp., Rantan, N.J., 1968.

Ross Laboratories: "A Study in Maternal Attitudes," Medical Department, Ross Laboratories, Columbus, Ohio, 1959.

Rubin, Reva: "Attainment of the Maternal Role, 1. Processes," *Nursing Research*, 16(3):237–245, Summer 1967.

————: "Attainment of the Maternal Role, 2. Models and Referrants," *Nursing Research*, 16(4):342–346, Fall 1967.

————: "Basic Maternal Behavior," *Nursing Outlook*, 9(11):683–686, November 1961.

————: "Maternal Touch," *Nursing Outlook*, 11(11):828–831, November 1963.

————: "Puerperal Change," *Nursing Outlook*, 9(12):753–755, December 1961.

Sawin, Clark T.: *The Hormones: Endocrine Physiology*, Little, Brown, Boston, 1969.

Smith, Christine Spahn: *Maternal-Child Nursing*, Saunders, Philadelphia, 1963.

Spock, Benjamin: *Baby and Child Care*, Pocket Books, division of Simon & Schuster, New York, 1957.

Stewart, Bernice C.: *Best-fed Babies*, The Association for Childbirth Education, Seattle, Wash., 1965.

Stuart, Harold C., and Dane G. Prugh (eds.): *The Healthy Child*, Harvard, Cambridge, Mass., 1960.

Taylor, E. Stewart: *Beck's Obstetrical Practice*, 9th ed., Williams & Wilkins, Baltimore, 1971.

Valdes-Dapena, Marie A.: "Sudden and Unexpected Death in Infancy: A Review of the World Literature 1954–1966," *Pediatrics*, 39:123–138, January 1967.

Warner, Marie Pichel: *A Doctor Discusses Breast Feeding*, Budlong, Chicago, 1970.

27 | SIGNIFICANT OTHERS IN CHILDREARING

Elizabeth J. Worthy

In previous chapters the impact of the birth of an infant on the family and the tasks and relationships of the primary family unit have been studied. The focus has now shifted to those infants for whom the primary family cannot provide full care or whose parents (or parent) elect to place them with other members of their family, other family units, or in group care. The societal content within which alternate care for infants and young children has developed, the needs and the resources available to the primary family, factors which enter into the choice of a placement for a child, and the nursing function in alternate care situations will be explored in this chapter.

There are two major thrusts to family life: (1) the basic biological nature and needs of its members and (2) the requirements of the society in which it exists and which it subserves by preparing its offspring to live within it.[1] The dependency of the young child and the time which must elapse before he can take care of his own needs make it imperative that he be raised in a favorable environment and by people to whom his welfare is as important as their own. "His dependency and his prolonged attachment to them (family and extra-family members) provide major motivation and directions for his development into a member of society."[2] All that he experiences later is perceived and understood according to foundations established during these early years.

Many pressures are exerted on the family in present-day society. Margaret Mead summed them up two decades ago when she stated, "We now expect a family to achieve, alone, what no society has ever expected an individual family to achieve unaided. In effect, we call upon an individual family to do what a whole clan used to do."[3] The developing family as seen by Mead is founded on a somewhat narrow base. Economic pressures, job security, emotional immaturity, and mobility are only a few of the threats which can seriously undermine family stability.

In reviewing trends in the development and restructuring of the American family, Talcott Parsons has pointed out that the family has now become a more differentiated unit and that its functions in relationship to other units have become more specialized.[4] The loss of functions to some other units has already occurred. These include the school and peer group, the mass media, business units, and many other social institutions. Parsons has also described the comparative "isolation" of the nuclear family, emotionally, economically, and geographically. He did not see the restructuring of the family as a general tendency toward dissolution. Rather, he believed that, as the role and function of the primary family unit became more highly differentiated from other units in society, its main functions would emerge, thus resulting in greater stability. In his opinion the role differentiation of both parents and children becomes a focal point. The "shift in balance of the sex roles," as viewed by Parsons, leads to the wife-mother taking over more of the managerial functions within the family, including that of the management of childrearing. The husband-father then assumes more of the "chairman of the board" functions and maintains, through his occupational role, the field of extra-family relations, rather than being the supreme authority in his own home. The mother, having longer and more intimate contact with their child, increases the emotional intensity and dependency of the parent-child unit and reduces the amount of conformance to a final authority expected from him. The child is regarded more as an individual who has some part in decision making and who is led rather than forced to higher levels of growth.[5] The high degree of emotional intensity, the relative isolation of the primary unit, and the comparative lack of extra-family contacts can provide difficulty for the child when he is first exposed to extra-family groups, whether in preschool or grade school situations.

Typically a family develops through predictable sequences of growth stages. "Before one family unit has completed its cycle, its grown children have been launched to start out on theirs. Most twentieth century families have the privilege of seeing a second, third, or even fourth life cycle spin off as children marry and rear their children who grow up marry and have children, who in turn marry and repeat the family life cycle pattern while older members of the family are still living."[6] Family life cycles have altered considerably during this century. Because of improved health care, and social and economic conditions, Albrecht[7] has predicted that five, or even six, contemporaneous generations of families may be likely in the future.

Reuben Hill's study of three-generation families has confirmed ongoing interaction in a continual flow from one generation to the next.[8] He found sharing of activities, visiting, and help exchanges among the three generations; the most frequent interaction was between adjacent generations. Each generation turned to the kinship network for help in solving problems, the middle generation being the "lineage bridge" between older and younger generations. The elderly might have problems with illness or household management; the parent generation may need emotional gratification; and the married children generation may require help with finances or child care. This degree of interdependence was advanced by "heavy involvement" of the middle generation, who give more assistance up and down the generation ladder than they receive. The three-generation family received less help from health, religious, social, or welfare agencies, compared with that which they received from their own family members. In 1 year alone, over 3,780 instances of different kinds of help (in illness, with finances, in child care, and in household and emotional crises) were reported. In each generation, members consistently reported receiving more help than they gave to others. The popular picture of the modern family as a small susceptible nucleus which is not sustained by other thoughtful relatives is reflected by research. Observation and experience evidences a modified extended family within a sound network of generational involvement.

The evidence alluded to above, while not taking all possible points of view into consideration, permits us to review some aspects of the societal context in which alternate care for infants and growing children has become necessary. Families have become smaller and their functions more specialized; although more family members are living longer, and a rich network of relationships between generations is possible, there are many threats to family development and stability. Some of these are discussed below.

THREATS TO FAMILY STABILITY AND THE MAINTENANCE OF AN INTERRELATIONAL NETWORK

The Single-parent Family

There are a growing number of single parent families in which the parent, invariably the mother, seeks to raise young children alone. Of 23,399,000 women in the United States who had been married, 5,802,000 were reported to be divorced, widowed, or separated in 1969.[9] Comparable figures for one county in the state of Washington indicated that 68.1 percent of the women had children under eighteen years of age, while 10.7 percent had children under six years of age. Of necessity many of these women will join the labor force if they do not wish or are ineligible for public assistance. The personal and family problems of the single parent are multiple. According to Goode, contemporary American society has failed to define a role for her; what she may or may not do within the family setting is not prescribed. Lacking such prescriptions, Goode concludes that many participants in marital dissolution could be expected to undergo considerable personal disorganization.[10] The above factors could also affect the young child's ability to cope with this crisis situation and his adaptation to a new way of life. At this point both parents could be unavailable to give support to the child—the father geographically, the mother emotionally. The position of either or both parents in the extended family is also altered. The supportive network of relationships may no longer be available to them. One or both may move to another area or withdraw from relatives, friends, and neighbors, alienating themselves from a society in which there is no formal position for them.

The Impact of Poverty, Mobility, and Marital Discord

The impact of these three factors on the family unit has been well documented. Working women in the poverty group, white or nonwhite, single or wed, carry many burdens, such as discrimination (racial, economic, or sex), inadequate preparation for work or for marriage, lower wages, and a higher probability of marital disruption. They may be able to cope with many of these burdens but may be overwhelmed by the cumulative effects of chronic economic dependency: periodic or continuous unemployment, debts, inadequate housing, poor standards of housekeeping, resultant malnutrition, apathy, and inability to profit from experience. The low-income families are often repeaters in the poverty cycle (the genetically disadvantaged) and may be considered, by their more affluent neighbors, to be the troublemakers in their communities.

The *mobility*, either forced or habitual, of many families in cities or rural areas weakens the interacting network of the extended family and again leaves the family or single parent alienated from society and from the supports which, inadequate as they may be, could be available to them. Much time and energy needs to be expended by individuals and groups in order to learn how to work with or within a system of care, be it social, economic, or health care. Families who are on the move soon give up as each system presents its complexities, time after time. The causes of *marital discord* have been described by many authors. Moses sums them up as stemming from the facts that (1) the original choice of a partner may have been largely a compromise for one or both partners; (2) the needs of both, which may act as motivation of behavior, are constantly changing; (3) the demands of one partner on another may be inconsistent, contradictory, incompatible, or out of touch with reality;

and (4) communication is frequently inadequate between partners who may have had little opportunity to learn how the other partner thinks or perceives.[11]

Infants born into such families may fail to thrive physically, emotionally, or intellectually if the interacting climate is unstable. They may be unplanned, unwanted, neglected, or even abused. One should hasten to say that higher income groups, especially those who have limited psychosocial resources, are not exempt from such problems.

The Working Mother

In March 1970, 4.6 million mothers in the national labor force had children under six years of age, and at that time women comprised 38 percent of the national labor force.[12] Women supposedly achieve their goals in family life by being competent wives and mothers. Economic, societal, and personal pressures can make this goal difficult to achieve. Some women become disillusioned with the tasks of motherhood and housekeeping for which they may have little aptitude, and they may need to get away from what they consider to be a "humdrum" existence. Others wish to compete with men in occupations hitherto considered reserved for men only, while others seek to work in occupations or professions for which they are already highly skilled. It is obvious that not all women who work are in the lower-income groups. In many instances a desire for a higher standard of living is supported by two wage earners in a family. All married women, ill- or well-prepared, are at a serious work disadvantage when compared with men and single women. They may not have access to the basic support systems for child care, housekeeping, illness care, or preventive health and social services. Such services are often inconveniently located and run impersonally, and many women are reluctant to use them, even if available. The extended family network may be absent or fragile in texture—mothers tend to work too hard and for too long in order that they might "break even," financially.

It appears that many family units can and do provide for at least some of the intra- and extra-family needs of their young children through utilization of some available resources. It is also evident that the so-called multiproblem family, within which factors such as poverty, mobility, and marital discord threaten the stability of the family unit, may not be able to make such provision. To whom shall they turn? How can and does the community attempt to supplement or, in some instances, replace the extended family? What specific measures can be adopted in order to protect vulnerable infants and young children from the damaging effects of early inadequate environments, whether these be in their natural homes, the homes of relatives or sitters, or in a group setting? How can we preserve the positive features of a warm and challenging home setting in which there is a working mother and supplement her care?

ALTERNATE CARE FOR YOUNG CHILDREN
Problems and Resources

Until very recently no official planning or allocation of resources has been offered, at any level, to assist with the development of alternate care programs for infants and children under three years of age. In fact, such programs were discouraged, although the need for "suitable" placement for infants has been present for many years. Parents could not, and have not, waited for official sanction.

Findings from a national study revealed that over 45 percent of the mothers surveyed who worked full time had found placements for their children under three years old at home with father, siblings over sixteen years of age (27.5 percent), or with nonrelatives in the home (17.8 percent). Placement in the home of a relative was also high (22 percent). The corresponding figures for those mothers who worked part time were: care in the home with relatives, 36.4 percent (almost 4 percent of these relatives were under sixteen years of age); care in the home by nonrelatives, 8.8 percent; and placement in the home of a relative, 9.4 percent. The 4.1 million mothers who were working or looking for work in 1968 (the number increased to approximately 4.6 million women in 1970) had almost 2 million children under three years of age. Mothers without husbands were more likely to be working than those with husbands; 27 percent of the mothers in the labor force with husbands had children under six years old, but 51 percent of the mothers in the labor force without husbands had children under six years old. Thirty-two percent of nonwhite (as opposed to 17 percent of white) working mothers provided the main source of income for their families. Many mothers of children under three years old chose part-time rather than full-time work. Mothers in all socioeconomic groups have felt and expressed guilt feelings about leaving their young children at a time when they are considered to be highly vulnerable to adverse factors in their environment.[13] Conversely, to quote Robinson, "Many mothers can function more happily as mothers and as individuals when they are away from home part of the day; many children, too, can profit from the brief time in the care of others."[14]

The depth of satisfaction which mothers experience when they obtain care for children outside the home varies greatly. Mothers of young children and those who lead a busy and overburdened life caring for older children seem more likely to be dissatisfied. When the children are cared for in their own homes by relatives or baby-sitters, mothers have been found to be more satisfied. They also appear to be more satisfied if they expect relatively little of an unpaid neighbor or a grandparent. In the national study the relatively small number of mothers working full time who placed their young children in the homes of nonrelatives or in group day care arrangements or who looked after them themselves at work were more satisfied with group day care, even though their expectations of this service were higher.

In one small unpublished study of 41 mothers whose infants were born in a university hospital setting in a metropolitan area, the investigator studied the types of substitute care which mothers used in the early weeks and months of life.[15] His findings included the fact that 37 percent of full-time working mothers were leaving their infants with others for a large part of the week. Over half the infants had been left overnight in the care of others, 15 percent before the age of two months. The mothers all experienced difficulties in making such arrangements and also in arranging temporary baby-sitting services. They were more satisfied with care in the home. When the infants were out of the home for 6 to 8 hours in the care of others, 30 percent of the mothers expressed dissatisfaction with such provisions. Poor quality of care and higher cost were the main reasons for their dissatisfaction. Dissatisfaction increased to 50 percent if only low-income mothers were considered. The investigator also found that 35 percent of the mothers who were most affected by this lack of "good" alternate care placements would have returned to work if satisfactory arrangements could have been made. In this study, low-income mothers were the most dissatisfied, presumably because they were even less able to pay for "good" care, if it existed. This dissatisfaction may also have kept them from entering training programs through which they could increase their incomes and thus be able to afford "better" care, if it existed.

A survey of 516 urban families was carried out in North Carolina in 1965.[16] Approximately half these families were nonwhite. Highly pertinent questions were asked. How many infants experienced supplemental mothering during part of the day, in or out of their homes? Who supplied the care? What age was the infant when this care was provided? How satisfied was the mother? What was the potential demand for such services? What were the other preferences? The answers were equally pertinent to our discussion.

More than half of the white children and almost half of the nonwhite children were under six months of age when someone other than the mother had begun to care for them regularly. Two-thirds of these white infants were placed in settings away from their homes. For nonwhite infants, 30 percent were experiencing supplementary care—18 percent in their own homes and 14 percent away from home. Sixteen percent of the total sample were in daytime care outside their own homes. Two-thirds of these white infants were in day care homes, while half the nonwhite infants were in the homes of relatives.

Most of the mothers were satisfied with the arrangements they had made. There were more dissatisfactions among nonwhite mothers and among mothers whose infants were in care away from home. The sample included mothers from low-, middle-, and high-income groups, and the study indicated that 90 percent of the low-income infants and 83 percent of the middle-income infants were being cared for by relatives or sitters in their own homes, while only 50 percent of the high-income group had their children cared for in their own homes, and 26 percent had arranged for care outside the home.

Also, most of the mothers in this sample indicated that they would be working regularly if dependable sources of care were available. Most expressed a preference for care of children in their own homes. There was a marked preference for a nursery center for group care among both white and nonwhite families, but only one-third of the white mothers and fewer of the nonwhite mothers gave this as their first choice.

Many federal training programs, such as the Manpower Development and Training Act, the Job Corps for Women, the Work Incentive Program, and the training programs under the Economic Opportunity Act, provide opportunities for unskilled women to obtain training so that they may work to support their families. Some of these programs also supplied group care programs for the children of their trainees who were under contract. The Report of the President's Commission on the Status of Women has emphasized that more women would be joining the labor force and would be remaining in it.[17] Women's liberation movements all over the United States have stressed the need for supplemental care for children so that women could be free to seek work if they should wish to do so and that they be placed in a position of equality with men in relation to access to the basic support systems for child care mentioned previously. Employers are increasingly turning to the provision of day care programs as a means of attracting and keeping women employees.

Young infants who require more permanent placement outside the home because of total parental inability to provide care and protection for them include the infants of unwed teen-agers without resources, of abusive or emotionally disturbed parents, and of rejective parents of unplanned or handicapped infants. Parents such as these provide society with the responsibility for many infants, whose numbers are gradually decreasing, but for whom the initial placement from the hospital nursery is still a serious consideration.

It was estimated in 1967 that nearly 6 percent of the total births in any year (about 245,000) are to unwed mothers, and of these almost 60 percent are nonwhite.[18] Adoption or foster care is still considered to be the first choice of most infants. Homes are not as readily available for the nonwhite infants, however, largely because of societal and cultural pressures within the black culture and of the slow development of interracial adoptions. In many communities, agencies exist to identify all such infants, preferably before birth, to provide parental counseling for the natural parents and their families, and to actively recruit adoptive and foster parents. Social and economic support similar to that which natural parents require will prevent many of these infants from being placed in institutional care. But there are still a proportion, the "hard to place" or "unadoptable," among them, for whom group care in institutions is inevitable, either on a temporary or more permanent basis. This group has been estimated at several hundred thousand and includes those over two years of age, the nonwhite, and the handicapped, who may require special care.

For the unwed teen-ager who wishes to keep her infant, special programs have been developed to aid her to remain within an educational setting during pregnancy and following the birth of her infant. This has created a new demand for infant care during school hours. More than 200 such educational programs have received federal support, and according to Caldwell, of 67 infant care programs recently surveyed, one-third were concerned with the needs of the school age parents.[19]

The need for acceptable facilities for child care in a variety of situations has been illustrated. Communities all over the country are often unable or unwilling to help the mothers of young children to make arrangements for care which will be in the best interests of children and families. However, an increasing number of communities are being forced to become aware of the situation as parents and professionals become increasingly vocal about needs and problems.

Informal Sources

It is evident that many informal sources of care for children exist. Grandparents, aunts and uncles, siblings, high school students, unemployed adults of both sexes, some with interest in or aptitude for child care, are available to parents. Communes provide care for the children of their members—a "multiple parenting" situation. Neighborhood groups in some areas cooperate to provide care for individual infants and children or for groups. That parents use these sources is clear, but reported dissatisfactions indicate that informal sources are considered insufficient to meet the needs for quality care of young children in a community.

Members of the modified extended family continue to operate within an interrelational network despite threats to existence of the family. However, because informal sources are too few in number and threats to family stability high, there has been, for many years, a need for communities to help supply alternate sources of supplemental care through formal channels.

Formal Sources

Formal resources are many and varied, and considerable confusion has existed among parents and professionals alike because of the wide range of programs offered, the wide age span of the children requiring care, the overlaps and gaps in the services provided, the terminology used to describe the resource, the quality of the services provided, the number available within a given community at a given moment, and the costs to the community. State or federal standards regulating the operation of such resources, "recommended" standards, and statements of principles of care also vary considerably. They may require only that zoning, fire safety, and sanitation requirements be met, or they may include highly complex, educational, social, or health regulations, many of which cannot be measured quantitatively.

The formal sources of alternate care for infants and young children usually include:

1 *Institutional care*, either in large (up to 300 infants) or small (10 to 15) institutions.
2 *Foster family care*, typically of four to six children, under six years of age (and including one or two infants) in a private home.
3 *Family day care home*, also including up to six children and one or two infants (in a private home). The infants include the foster mother's own children.
4 *Group day care home*, including up to 12 children, in a private home and requiring additional employees. Infants are not usually placed in these settings.
5 *Group day care* of over 12 children in a hall, school, church, or other building planned and used for this specific purpose.
6 *Adoptive care* in a private family, arranged preferably through a social agency in order to protect both groups of parents and children alike and to provide the adoptive parents with all the responsibilities and joys of the primary family unit.
7 *The expansion and use of homemaker services* to provide help for families with infants and young children, in their own homes.
8 *Parent-Child Centers*, a component of Head Start, recently launched (1967) in a number of cities throughout the United States and aimed at preserving links between mother and child. Several of these centers offer infant care programs.

MAKING THE CHOICE FOR INFANT CARE

The choice of a program of care for an infant will be based on a number of considerations.

Fostering Childrearing Capacities of the Primary Family

Most parents want to do what is best for their infants but may lack the knowledge, skill, or personal, social, and extra-family resources to be able to do so. Professionals must know whether the family needs only support in specific areas of daily living or in planning for tomorrow or if, at the other end of the spectrum, placement outside the home on a temporary (crisis-oriented) or permanent basis has to be considered for the safety and welfare of the infant. Parents need to feel that they play a large part in such decisions. The use of homemaker services (still underdeveloped) may be expanded in families in which the basic need is for teaching principles of child care in the home. These persons could fill this need for a number of young men and women who are inadequately prepared for family life and could relieve them of some of the anxieties related to child care in the family routine through helping to preserve family unity and integrity.

Parental Involvement in the Placement of the Infant

This will range from the young teen-age unwed mother's relinquishment of her infant in a hospital ward, through a wide variety of situations in which temporary or long-term placement is required in order to assist one or both parents to deal with a crisis, or to intervene in a long-term problem situation. These situations might threaten the life of the infant or the existence of the family unit.

The Availability and Acceptability of a Source of Care to the Parents

Geographically, economically, culturally, or emotionally, either on a long- or short-term basis, the proximity to, knowledge of, and involvement of parents in the program have been proved to be essential to its success in many instances. The mother, especially, needs to have close ties with the director and the facility in order to have input into the program on behalf of her infant and to receive reports of progress or specific activities—educational, social, or health—in which he is involved. In those instances in which the community, through one of its social agencies, takes over total responsibility for care, even temporarily, the professional has the same responsibility for close contact and involvement.

The Type and Scope of Services Offered by the Resource Selected by the Family

Parents and professionals alike need to have information about the goals and scope of the programs offered, especially if they will include infant stimulation programs which are liable to enrich his daily life and which could be transferable into his own home, when possible. Powell describes these programs as "arranging circumstances in the environment that reinforce a child's strengths and skills . . . and capitalize on readiness to learn new tasks and skills."[20] Health and developmental screening programs and nutritional and social services may also be available to the infant and his parents as well as basic care.

Age and Developmental Level of the Infant at the Time of Placement

His ability to make such a transfer will depend on the support and information provided for the parent or primary caretaker and the gentle easing of the infant into the care situation during the transition period. In discussing group care of infants, Provence reassures all concerned about the ability of the normal infant to make this transition and to continue to develop normally if the caretaker can provide for him in a manner in which his development is supported rather than interfered with. [21]

The Stability of the Arrangements for Care

The importance of consistency of care has been alluded to. The haphazard nature of many informal child care situations has also been reported. It should be possible to plan group care for an infant so that changes in caretaking and learning environment are kept to a minimum.

The Ability of the Primary Family to Adjust to Placement of the Child

Long-term goals for the placement of the child in the home again (or in a setting approximating a home, should he be in an institution and should it be deemed necessary and desirable by parent and professional) must be kept constantly in sight.

The Changes in Professional Attitudes toward Placement of Infants and Young Children

Concern has long been expressed about childrearing in group situations in the United States. This concern was early associated with studies of institutionalized infants who demonstrated severe distortion of physical, emotional, and cognitive development. [22, 23, 24, 25, 26] Concern has also been expressed by Ribble about the rights of infants—the infant's need and right for personalized mothering care in the early weeks and months of life. [27] However, it is evident that the preservation of the nuclear family unit is not always possible. Alternate resources may have to be found for infants without families, sometimes on a permanent basis. In other situations in which only temporary help is needed, or when day care can be provided, a support system which will assist family members to retain as much parental responsibility as they can tolerate at a given point may be all that is required. The conclusion has persisted, however, that care for infants and young children within the family is always superior to that in any institution or care situation outside the home, however well organized this may be. [28] Professional attitudes are beginning to change. Mavans et al., writing about group care in *Early Child Care: The New Perspective*, reminds professionals that:

1 Many mothers make "casual" and "shifting" arrangements for the care of their young children for a variety of reasons. (This, it must be said, is often necessary as so few resources exist in some communities.)
2 The number of foster homes often lags behind the demand. Infants may be shifted from one to another, with little long-term planning and often as a matter of dire necessity. It is very hard to supervise such arrangements.
3 The patterns of childrearing observed in some segments of the country tend to perpetuate some physical, emotional, and intellectual handicaps from one generation to another; opportunities can and do exist to break into this cycle of events and help infants to grow and develop into sturdy children and adults, freed from some of these deficits.
4 A number of other countries continue to use and to be enthusiastic about group care for infants.[29]

Robinson, in discussing the changing attitudes of professionals, sums up his thinking in relation to day care as, "what was at issue was 'deprivation of stimulation' and 'deprivation of (generalized) mothering' and that separation from the mother for a portion of the day would not lead to the dire results formerly predicted."[30]

In a discussion on group care in the United States, Whittaker says that recent governmental statements seem to indicate that the federal government may be shifting its policy, as expounded at the First White House Conference on Children in 1909 and reiterated at every such conference since, that "the home is the highest and finest product of civilization and that children should not be separated from their parents by reasons of poverty alone," to the present (1971) proposed welfare regulations that "the home is the highest and finest product of civilization for some children and that children may be separated from their parents (at least for day care) for reasons of poverty, alone."[31] He points out that it is essential that we separate the question of effectiveness of group care for young children, as an alternative to the nuclear family, and the separation of certain groups of young children from their families solely because they are poor. Evidence has certainly been growing that poverty homes are often poorly suited to the needs of young children and that the relationship of some young children to their own mother does not necessarily enhance their intellectual and social growth.

Caldwell has reminded us that there has been much wariness about planning definitive programs for young infants within what she terms a "developmental milieu." There has been an implicit assumption in many communities that any setting which preserves life through its ability to meet basic needs for shelter, food, and protection from hazards was adequate for the care of young infants. Caldwell has examined some of the basic assumptions relative to the provision of short-term care for infants and concludes that from the scientific and lay literature and from the practices in health and welfare agencies one could infer that the optimal learning environment of the young child was (a) in his own home, (b) within the context of a warm and loving relationship, (c) with his mother or a close mother figure, and (d) under conditions which provide for a wide variety of input, both social and cognitive. However, she questions whether one should support the first factor so enthusiastically if (b), (c), and (d) could reasonably be obtained outside the home.[32] Many professionals are trying to keep an open mind about infant care programs and are attempting to evaluate the quality of the mothering experiences which the infant receives rather than the amount of time he spends outside the home.

A report prepared for the Child Development/Day Care Workshop in Warrenton, Virginia, in July 1970 states:

> Much of the movement in rethinking child care services for infants and toddlers came from three sources: research showing the crucial importance of the experiences in the first three years of life for later development; research on the effects of an enriched environment during those early years; and a long and serious look at the effects of Headstart and similar programs, where two conclusions were drawn: (a) programs must begin before children are three years old, and (b) most important of all, parents must be involved in the programs. *Only when the entire family unit is strengthened will there be important and lasting changes in the child.* Parents want and need good child care programs. Parents care about the welfare of their children. They must be helped to achieve this [italics supplied].[33]

GROUP CARE FOR CHILDREN

Economics

The willingness of this nation to pay for the quality child care programs which have been and will be devised by parents and professionals has been questioned many times. These programs, if they be of the quality required, will demand long-term commitment to the goals of care, to the recruitment and training of personnel to staff such activities, and to funds to support them so that they can be of major benefit to those who need them most. Costs of group care programs vary tremendously according to the type and level of program, the quality of care offered, and the area of the country in which they are located. Family day care costs have been estimated at about $2,000 per child per year without considering capital investment in home and equipment. Day care now being offered is likely to be in the range of $1,000 to $2,000 per year per child. This is dangerously low—acceptable costs are more likely to be in the range of $2,400 per year per child under three years old; again, this is without including capital investments and without the addition of research activities, which have pushed the cost of some programs up to $8,000 per year per child. Public assistance programs offer $5.00 per day per child on an average; i.e., approximately $1,200 per year per child. If the infant is to receive a program which will enhance his growth and development rather than provide for custodial care, the high cost is inevitable. All parents are not able to contribute toward the costs of care. Capital expenditure for space, equipment, program materials, staff salaries and inservice training, and health and social work service (often donated) will all add to the costs. It is small wonder that housing in church basements, poorly prepared personnel, restricted programs, low salaries, donated services, and low prestige are the rule rather than the exception in child care services. Infant care centers, mostly experimental in nature, have fared better because of strict licensing arrangements but have faced the same financial problems and the transient nature of the services provided, as money runs out.

Licensing Standards

Standards for group care services are published by each state, and mandatory licensing is the rule rather than the exception, although in some areas the regulations are not rigorously enforced. National professional organizations have also published recommended standards, i.e., The American Public Health Association (1967), The Child Welfare League for America (1969). The American Academy of Pediatrics (1971) (the latter relating specifically to the health care of infants under three years old) and the former Children's Bureau (1967).[34, 35, 36]

The Day Care and Child Development Council of America, Inc. has prepared a statement of principles relating to the development of a locally controlled, publicly supported, and universally available child care system (1971).[37] Community-coordinated child care (4C) programs have been developed in approximately 150 communities in an effort to coordinate child care programs and provide maximum use of available funds, staffing, and facilities. This program emphasizes local efforts and citizen participation in child care.

The Needs of Infants

The needs of infants in group care have been variously described; Huntington and Provence summed them up succinctly in 1970:[38]

> The infant must have his health and nutritional needs met in addition to clothing and shelter. He needs an adult's assistance in providing for his

physical comfort, in managing his bodily activity, in protecting him from hazards to health and safety, and in caring for him when he is sick or injured.

The infant needs to be able to form an attachment to one major caretaker; someone who cares for him and he for her. This should not compete with maternal care when this is available, but be supplementary to it. In the fulfillment of his basic physical needs, both mother and caretaker can deepen their attachment to this specific infant. Other persons may well care for him and will of necessity do so, but mother or principal caretaker are around to assist him to form attachments to these other persons in his life.

The infant needs lots of company, people who will interact with him in a loving, caring manner and who will respond to his behavior by talking to him, playing with him, caressing him, feeding him, bathing him, or dressing him. To quote Huntington and Provence, "Language is one of the least expensive and most accessible tools we have for interacting with children and supporting their increasingly complex understanding of the world."[38]

The infant needs new and challenging activities and experiences within his physical and social environment so that he remains active and interested in it and revels in its variety.

The infant needs to be able to learn through constant personal exploration of his life space. The more he learns, the more he is stimulated, and the more he continues to learn.

The infant needs some order and predictability in his physical and social world. Routine periods for sleep, rest, feeding, and quiet periods are a balancing force for a rich and stimulating learning environment.

The infant needs adults to set limits for him, to know what is acceptable social and physical behavior and what is not and to deal with resulting frustrations in such a manner that learning continues to take place.

The infant needs to be able to develop a happy, confident self-image because of the quality of people and of experiences to which he is exposed. The sturdy personality of the toddler and preschool child who has successfully handled early developmental tasks reflects the attainment of trust and personal autonomy as he relates to others. He needs to feel that others love and respect him for what he is. His ability to model the behavior of others allows him to pick up many of their attitudes and values. These become a part of him; some of this can be taught but most of it is caught in these early years.[39]

Characteristics of the Environment

With these needs of infants in mind, what are the salient features of the environment in which the infant in group care can grow and develop?

A group care environment should be a stimulating, learning environment in settings both indoor and outdoor. Warmth, comfort, bright colors, and soft and rough textures should be available, and the environment should be free from physical hazards and contain the necessary services (care, protection, food) and equipment, all of which will ensure the continuing growth and development of the young child.

A group care environment should offer a "relatively high frequency of adult contact, utilizing a relatively small number of adults."[40] These adults are carefully screened for personal and health characteristics, preferably prepared in early childhood education, education, basic nurturing, and health care (including dental care) and are provided with stimulating inservice training programs.

A group care environment should offer a carefully planned daily program which will meet the needs of infants at various levels of development. The program should include activities, rest, a balanced nutritional intake provided at appropriate intervals, sleep periods, quiet periods, listening or singing to music, opportunities for indoor and outdoor play, and for practice of newly acquired physical, intellectual and social skills.

A group care environment should maintain close contacts with the community through parent (or mother) meetings or classes in order to facilitate ideas about infant development, behavior, or problems; informal personal discussion with parents; the use of volunteer caretaking or social or health services; excursions into the community; an active public relations program to allow the community access to the center through the use of articles, pictures, and other media; and home visiting by staff.

The Health Program

The main thrust of a health program would be directed toward the control of infection; the prevention of accidents and other environmental hazards; the promotion of health through screening, immunization programs, developmental testing, nutritional assessment, and parent and staff education; and the recognition and referral of developmental deviance or disease in infants to appropriate sources. The following questions might well be asked of an adequate health care program for infants:

1 Has the infant had a pre-entry medical examination? Was his mother or principal caretaker present? Are his health records complete? Is his immunization schedule up to date? Does he have a private physician, attend a public clinic, or does he need to be referred for medical or nursing supervision? Have other disciplines been involved in his care at any time?

2 Has an assessment of the infant's health and developmental status been carried out since he was placed in group care? By whom? When?

How often has it been repeated? What tools and techniques were employed? What were the major problems identified? What priorities were set? Where are the records filed?

3 What long-term and short-term goals of health care were established for this young infant in group care? Was a plan of care devised? To whom was this plan communicated? When and how was the plan implemented? What family and community resources were explored and utilized?

4 What was the outcome of this plan of care? What criteria for evaluation were established? How was the promotion of health and the treatment of illness related to other activities and programs in the group care setting?

NURSING FUNCTION

The nursing function in group care settings is closely related to the answers to the preceding questions. Nursing can and does play a prominent role in the prevention, identification, treatment and care, and referral to other resources of many young children in group care.

Although the infant care center is required by state regulation in many states to be under general medical supervision, this is often limited to advisement regarding standards of medical care to be observed, preadmission medical examination of specific children, and incenter clinics set up for the prevention and early identification of disease.

Each infant should be under the health supervision of a physician or public clinic, and parents are encouraged to obtain such supervision.

The infant care center is also required to obtain the services of a registered nurse, or in some instances, a licensed practical nurse who undertakes the major responsibility for the development and maintenance of a health program.

The Health Program

1 Consultation to the director and staff on matters relating to the health of the children is provided by health professionals, such as the nurse (and social worker, dental staff, and nutritionist, when available). The health program should be the outcome of discussions between these groups and the parents, and all parents must be made aware of the program in order for it to be effective.

2 Written policies and procedures regarding standing orders for minor acute illnesses, first aid, major medical emergencies, and the inability of most agencies to administer medication must be available to director and staff. These are developed by the nurse and center staff in consultation with a physician.

3 All persons in contact with the children must be in good health and

free from communicable disease. Regular checks are necessary in order to ensure that this is accomplished.

4 Regular monitoring of the physical, social, and emotional environment in which the child is receiving care must be considered.

5 General health supervision, including evidence of the pre-entry medical examination to exclude previous illness or disability; an assessment of the child's present health; the status of the immunization program and its regular updating for each infant; the screening of developmental progress; and conferences with the parents and agency staff to provide for their ongoing input are all regular features of the health program. Identification of the specific health needs of each infant or group of infants and the development of plans to meet these needs would follow. Evaluating the effects of these plans and their implementation is a major responsibility of the nurse, director, and parent together. The nurse plays a prominent role in teaching the agency staff to:

a Recognize acceptable standards of health in an infant

b Carry out a simple health examination on a regular basis

c Identify a child who is sick or in need of care (physical, emotional, nutritional, dental, social, etc.); recognize developmental deviance

d Provide for sickness care where this is required

e Maintain safety standards and carry out first aid measures efficiently

f Perform hand-washing and cleansing and placement procedures related to the direct care of a young infant and his environment, based on accurate knowledge and understanding of his needs

g Report and record all information clearly

h Ensure that the nutritional status of each child is adequate and that his nutritional intake in the center is sufficient for his growth and development

i Provide for childrearing activities such as toilet training, bathing, feeding, intellectual and social stimulation, and mothering activities so that close links with his regimen at home are preserved.

Setting up group training sessions for both staff and parents, which cover any or all of the points raised above has been found to be most effective. Focusing on a health or social problem identified by the staff and then moving on to other pertinent areas provides the nurse with an entrance point into the system at a time when interest is high.

The nurse, as a citizen, also plays an important part in the identification of the need for child care programs in a community, of working actively with citizen groups toward the development of a variety of such programs, in order to meet the wide variety of needs. Contacts with agencies and planning groups should also enable the nurse to help monitor quality of care as well as quantity.

While the needs and resources described above are still far from reaching a meeting point, group care for infants at all income levels is growing. The low status and poor quality of some present services are improving. The financial support is beginning to emerge. In an article written for *Saturday Review* in February 1971, Bettye M. Caldwell provides strong direction for the future:[41]

> At this moment in history, when we are on the threshold of embarking on a nationwide program of social intervention offered through comprehensive child care, we let ourselves prattle about such things as cost per child, physical facilities, or even community control. And when we begin to think big about what kinds of children we want to have in the next generation, about which human characteristics will stand them in good stead in a world changing too rapidly, we fall back on generalities such as care and protection. Yet any social institution that can shape behavior and help instill values and competencies and life-styles should also shape policy. Early child care is a powerful instrument for influencing patterns of development and the quality of life for children and adults. Because of its power, those who give it direction must not think or act with timidity.

REFERENCES

1 Lidz, Theodore: "The Family as the Developmental Setting," in Anthony E. James and Cyrille Koupernik, *The Child in His Family*, Wiley, New York, 1970, pp. 19–39.
2 Ibid., p. 24.
3 Mead, Margaret: "What Is Happening to the American Family?" in *New Emphasis on Cultural Factors*, Family Service Association of America, New York, 1947.
4 Parsons, Talcott: *Family Socialization and Interaction Process*, The Free Press, Glencoe, Ill., 1955, pp. 3–33.
5 Ibid., p. 215.
6 Duvall, Evelyn: *Family Development*, 4th ed., Lippincott, Philadelphia, 1970, pp. 106–132.
7 Albrecht, Ruth: "Intergeneration Parent Patterns," *Journal of Home Economics*, 46:31, January 1954.
8 Hill, Reuben: *Family Development in Three Generations*, Schenkman, Cambridge, Mass., 1970, chap. 4.
9 *Child Care: We Care*, League of Women Voters, U.S. Department of Labor, Employment Standards, Administration Women's Bureau, Washington, D.C., 1971.

10 Goode, William J.: *After Divorce*, The Free Press, Glencoe, Ill., 1956, p. 186.

11 Moses, Harold: "A Note on Marital Discord," *Child and Family*, 5(3): 54–56, Summer 1966.

12 *Child Care: We Care*, op. cit.

13 Low, Seth, and G. Spindler: *Child Care Arrangements of Working Mothers in the United States*, Children's Bureau Publication #461, Washington, D.C., 1968.

14 Robinson, Halbert B.: unpublished paper, 1971.

15 Rowles, Roger: "A Study of Caretakers of Young Babies Born at University Hospital," unpublished research project, University of Washington, 1969.

16 Keister, Mary Elizabeth: *Patterns of Daytime Care of Infants under Three Years of Age* (summary report), Guilford County, N.C., 1965.

17 *American Women*, Report of the President's Commission on the Status of Women, Superintendent of Documents, Washington, D.C., 1963.

18 American Academy of Pediatrics: *Adoption of Children*, American Academy of Pediatrics, Evanston, Ill., 1967.

19 Caldwell, Bettye: "What Does Research Teach Us about Children under Three?" *Children Today*, 1(1):6–11, January 1972.

20 Barnard, Kathryn, and M. L. Powell: *Teaching the Mentally Retarded Child: A Family Care Approach*, Mosby, New York, 1972.

21 Provence, Sally: *Guide for the Care of Infants in Groups*, Child Welfare League of America, New York, 1967.

22 Bakwin, H.: "Emotional Deprivation in Infants," *Journal of Pediatrics*, 35:512–521, 1949.

23 Bowlby, John: *Maternal Care and Mental Health*, World Health Organization, Geneva, 1952.

24 Bowlby, John: "The Nature of the Child's Tie to His Mother," *International Journal of Psycho-Analysis*, 38:350–373, 1958.

25 Provence, Sally, and Rose C. Lipton: *Infants in Institutions*, International Universities Press, New York, 1960, pp. 9–52.

26 Spitz, Rene A.: "Hospitalism: An Enquiry into the Genesis of Psychiatric Conditions in Early Childhood," in Ruth S. Eissler, et al., *The Psychoanalytic Study of the Child*, vol. I, International Universities Press, New York, 1945, pp. 53–74.

27 Ribble, Margaret A.: *The Rights of Infants*, Columbia, New York, 1943.

28 Wolins, Martin: "Some Theory and Practice in Child Care: A Cross Cultural View," *Child Welfare*, 42:369–377, 1963.

29 Mavans, Allen E., et al.: "The Children's Hospital in Washington, D.C.," in Laura L. Dittman (ed.), *Early Child Care: The New Perspectives*, Atherton, New York, 1968.

30 Robinson: op. cit.

31 Whittaker, James: *Group Care in America: Review and Preview,* unpublished paper, 1971.

32 Caldwell, Bettye M.: "What Is the Optimal Learning Environment for the Young Child?" *American Journal of Orthopsychiatry,* pp. 8–21, January 1967.

33 Huntington, Dorothy, and Sally Provence (co-chairmen): *Child Development/Day Care Workshop,* Airlie House, Warrenton, Virginia, July 23–30, 1970. (Guiding Principles of Early Child Care, years 1–12.)

34 American Public Health Association Committee on Child Health: *Health Supervision of Young Children,* 3d ed., American Public Health Association, New York, 1960.

35 Child Welfare League of America: *Standards for Day Care Services,* Child Welfare League of America, New York, 1964.

36 American Academy of Pediatrics: *Standards for Day Care Centers for Infants and Children under Three Years,* American Academy of Pediatrics, Evanston, Ill., 1971.

37 Day Care and Child Development Council of America: *Statement of Principles,* 1971.

38 Huntington and Provence: op. cit.

39 Ibid.

40 Caldwell, Bettye M., and Julius B. Richmond: "The Children's Center in Syracuse, New York," in Laura L. Dittman (ed.), *Early Child Care: New Perspectives,* Atherton, New York, 1968, p. 342.

41 Caldwell, Bettye: "A Timid Giant Grows Bolder," *Saturday Review,* pp. 47–53 and 65–66, February 20, 1971.

BIBLIOGRAPHY

American Academy of Pediatrics: *Standards of Child Health Care,* American Academy of Pediatrics, Evanston, Ill., 1967.

Care of Children in Day Care Centers, World Health Organization, Geneva, 1964.

Care of Well Children in Day Care Centers and Institutions, World Health Organization, Technical Report Series #256, World Health Organization, Geneva, 1963.

Class, Morris E.: "Licensing for Child Care—A Preventive Welfare Service," *Children,* September–October 1968.

Deprivation of Maternal Care: A Reassessment of Its Effects, World Health Organization, Geneva, 1962.

Dittman, Laura: *Children in Day Care with Focus on Health,* U.S. Department of Health, Education and Welfare, Children's Bureau, Washington, D.C., 1967.

———— (ed.): *Early Child Care: The New Perspectives*, Atherton, New York, 1968.

Hazelkorn, Florence (ed.): *Mothers at Risk*, Adelphi University School of Social Work Publications, Garden City, N. Y., 1966.

Hille, Helen M.: *Food for Groups of Young Children Cared for during the Day*, U.S. Department of Health, Education and Welfare, Children's Bureau, Washington, D.C., 1969.

Murphy, Lois B.: "Children under Three: Finding Ways to Stimulate Development," *Children*, pp. 46–52, March–April 1969.

————: *Nutrition and Feeding: Infants and Children under Three in Group Day Care*, U.S. Department of Health, Education and Welfare, Washington, D.C., 1971.

Provence, Sally: "Children under Three: Finding Ways to Stimulate Development, II," *Children*, pp. 53–62, March–April 1969.

————: "Guide for the Care of Infants in Groups," Child Welfare League of America, New York, 1967.

U.S. Department of Health, Education, and Welfare: *Children Today*, vol. I, January–February 1972. (Formerly entitled *Children*; entire issue devoted to day care for children.)

Walters, James, and Nick Stinnet: "Parent and Child Relationships, A Decade of Research," *Journal of Marriage and the Family*, vol. 33, no. 1, February 1971.

Yarrow, Leon J.: "Maternal Deprivation: Toward an Empirical and Conceptual Reevaluation," *Psychological Bulletin*, 58:459–490, 1961.

UNIT B
THE NEWBORN

28 | THE PHYSIOLOGICAL
BASIS OF
NEONATAL NURSING

Rose S. LeRoux and Shirley Stratton Yee

The effects of the complex interplay of genetic endowment, intrauterine environmental factors, obstetric-pediatric management, and nursing care are manifest in the status of the newborn infant at birth. The major part of the development of the infant has gone on in utero unperceived by direct clinical observation and largely inaccessible to treatment. Much research has been generated by this perplexing state. Current scientific research focuses on both fetal and neonatal physiology. Although there are many interesting studies available on the subject, there appears to be little absolute agreement among scientists regarding many facets of fetal and neonatal physiology. Some of the facts which have been previously discovered are now interpreted differently. When it was known that babies grew at different rates in utero, the terms *small for gestational age* and *low birth weight* replaced the blanket term *premature*. Because of the changing concepts regarding the fetus and the neonate, nurses who wish to become proficient in their care would do well to consult the most current research studies available on this subject. The basic

The authors gratefully acknowledge the assistance of Barbara F. Brockway, Ph.D., Associate Professor of Physiology, University of Colorado School of Nursing, in the preparation of this chapter.

tenets of infant care persist. They are to provide the newborn infant with protection from harm, adequate food, a stable environment, and bodily contact in which love and security are communicated.

The neonatal period is arbitrarily designated as that time from birth to 28 days of life. It is during this period, especially during the first 24 hours, that the infant is at high mortality and morbidity risk. To provide optimal care to the neonate during this period, the maternity nurse should possess a considerable amount of theoretical knowledge, clinical expertise, and superior judgment. Careful monitoring of the condition of the neonate, manipulation of his environment as necessary, and assisting in the infant's transition from intrauterine to a stable extrauterine environment are all part of the nursing role. The nurse must assist the parents in taking on new roles and must recognize potential problems in this area. Early discharge of infants and their mothers from hospitals often precludes the identification of high-risk mother-infant relationships as well as any potential physical problems with the infant. Nurses who work with mothers and their newborn infants would do well to follow them from birth through the first month of life, both in the hospital and in the home setting. It is obvious that it would be in the best interest of the infant to begin care of the potential mother in the preconceptual period.

Most infants are normal when they are born and proceed through the transitional period with a minimum amount of difficulty. Most of the organ systems are prepared to adapt and function in the extrauterine environment. However, many organ systems are not *quite* physiologically mature at birth. Therefore, a neonate does not at birth function physiologically like an adult or even like an older child. The neonatal period is characterized by a considerable amount of instability of many systems; however, each organ system will continue to develop according to its own timetable in an orderly fashion. In order to understand the neonate's behavior the nurse must realize that the observed behavior depends in a large part on an intact and functional physiological mechanism and its relative maturational stages. The term "normal" should not mislead the nurse who cares for newborn infants into assuming that they need any less attention than those infants labeled "high risk." The nurse should sharpen the ability to examine and observe newborn infants for the accumulation of many and varied insignificant signs which may indicate impending difficulties. Neonatal nursing practice is based on strong theoretical and empirical knowledge derived from direct observation and care of neonates.

The field of neonatal physiology is complex and challenging. This chapter does not purport to cover the subject in depth. Information important to nursing has been extrapolated at the risk of oversimplification. It is strongly recommended that the reader consult current physiology and pediatric texts for more complete information on the subject.

CARE OF THE NEONATE IMMEDIATELY FOLLOWING DELIVERY

The birth of an infant marks the *beginning* of extrauterine existence and the *continuation* of a process of growth and development which began with the fertilization of the ovum by the sperm. At birth, the infant loses the metabolic support of the placenta. Through his own breathing, he must inhale oxygen, perfuse vital gases through his cardiovascular system, and exhale carbon dioxide. Negotiating successfully from intrauterine to extrauterine life is a major challenge to the neonate. Although most of the neonate's organ systems are prepared to adapt to extrauterine life, they will not reach a state of mature functioning for varying periods of time after birth. This relative immaturity makes it difficult for the newborn infant to adapt to unusually stressful environmental conditions.

A considerable amount of clinical expertise is required of the medical-nursing team in the delivery room. There are times when both mother and infant may be having acute problems, and the delivery room team must rapidly institute appropriate treatment to each simultaneously. Time is frequently the critical variable affecting a favorable outcome. Therefore, hospitals which assume the responsibility for delivering mothers should provide for expert obstetric and pediatric management. The articulation of obstetrics and pediatrics is nowhere more dramatically illustrated than in the delivery room.

The Establishment of Respirations

The priorities of delivery room care in regard to the baby are to establish respirations, to monitor the cardiovascular system, and to provide temperature regulation and support. Failure to breathe for only 2 to 4 minutes may cause death in an adult. In contrast, an infant can tolerate much longer periods of anoxia. However, the extent of brain impairment which results from failure to breathe within a few minutes of birth may be greater than is presently documented. The long-term effects of anoxia can only be hypothesized since few follow-up studies are available. Existing evidence supports the proposition that the *prompt onset of breathing should be considered essential* to the neonate's subsequent mental and physical development. Animal studies have indicated that there may be several factors which contribute to the neonate's apparent resistance to the life-threatening effects of anoxia. These factors are the infant's low body temperature, low and variable energy metabolism, low cerebral metabolism, and the amount of blood glucose available. The ability to resist the harmful effects of anoxia are lost shortly after birth. A healthy infant whose mother has not received large amounts of analgesia or anesthesia during labor and delivery should breathe within a few seconds or, at the most, a few minutes after birth. Many infants breathe as soon as the head is delivered.

Physical-sensory and *biochemical* factors appear to stimulate the onset of respiration, but the exact cause remains a subject for research. Among the physical-sensory factors are the rapid expansion of the chest following the compression which has occurred during passage of the infant through the birth canal, the stimulation of the infant's tactile receptors through handling during and immediately following delivery, the abrupt change from a fluid to air environment, and the change from a higher to lower temperature. A powerful effort is required to open alveoli in the lungs, for the surface tension of the alveolar fluid must be overcome. *Surfactant* which is present in the normal lung assists in overcoming the surface tension. Care should be taken to avoid administration of oxygen at extremely high pressures, for studies have shown that high pressure oxygen can severely damage the alveolar cells which produce surfactant.

The biochemical changes occur simultaneously with the physical-sensory changes. When the umbilical cord stops pulsating anoxia results from the interruption of the oxygen supplied by the placenta. Carbon dioxide accumulates in the blood, lowering the pH to a point at which the respiratory centers of the medulla are stimulated and breathing should result. Although the initial expiration of the neonate should clear the airway of accumulated amniotic fluid and permit inspiration, it is wise to suction mucus and fluid from the infant's mouth as soon as the head is delivered. This procedure prevents aspiration of this material if the infant gasps with his first breath. A small, soft rubber bulb syringe is usually used for this purpose. A soft catheter attached to a De Lee mucus trap or a mechanical suction machine may also be used. Care must be taken not to traumatize the delicate tissues of the infant's oropharynx. If a large amount of mucus is present, the physician may hold the infant in a head down position to facilitate drainage from the infant's oropharynx.

Efforts to stimulate crying in the newborn infant are usually limited to gentle rubbing of the infant's back. Slapping the soles of the infant's feet, alternate hot and cold tubbing of the infant, and other such methods are considered dangerous and ineffectual. They only delay the institution of appropriate resuscitation measures.

Every delivery room should be equipped with resuscitation equipment. Personnel who deal with the establishment of respiration in the neonate should be knowledgeable about the procedures proposed by the American Academy of Pediatrics regarding resuscitation of the infant. If a pediatrician is not regularly available in the delivery room, those persons who are available should be trained in resuscitation techniques. Routine procedures should be delayed until respirations are established and maintained in the neonate.

The quality and rate of respirations are extremely variable during the newborn period and are largely diaphragmatic in character. Shallow, slow, and labored breathing is not normal and may require emergency treatment. It is important for the nurse to observe the normal synchronous movements of the infant's thorax and abdomen during respiration to detect early signs of respiratory difficulty. In some newborn infants there may be a few alveoli which do not expand completely for more than a week. Usually these findings are within normal limits.

Changes in the Cardiovascular System

At birth changes occur in the cardiovascular system which result in altered pathways of blood flow and variations in blood volume, pressure, and chemical composition. The clamping of the cord eliminates the supply of oxygenated blood from the placenta. Thereafter the infant must obtain oxygen from the lungs. To accomplish oxygenation of the blood by the lungs several alterations in the anatomic structure of the circulatory system must occur. These changes are brought about by complex biochemical factors in the blood as well as alterations in blood volume and pressure within specific blood vessels. It is beyond the scope of this chapter to discuss the biochemical alterations that precipitate the circulatory changes, but a brief explanation of the structural alterations will be given.

Following delivery the supply of oxygen from the placenta is removed by the interruption of blood flow through the umbilical cord. The resultant lack of oxygen is one of the factors leading to the first insufflation of the lungs, as has been previously discussed. After the initial inspiration the resistance to blood flow through the lungs is greatly decreased. Blood flowing through the pulmonary arteries increases the pressure in these vessels. The increased pressure is a precipating factor in the closure of the *ductus arteriosus*. It is probable that the increased oxygen content of the circulating blood in the pulmonary arteries also contributes to the closure. The closure of the ductus arteriosus accompanied by the closure of the *foramen ovale* and the obliteration of the umbilical vessels leads to the establishment of the adult pattern of circulation in which the unoxygenated blood is separated from the oxygenated blood. There is a short interim during which the infant retains some of the fetal patterns of circulation. Figure 28-1 shows the normal pathways of circulation in the fetus, neonate, and adult.

Table 28-1 illustrates that these circulatory changes are not instantaneous with the first respiration. The ductus arteriosus remains partially patent for 24 to 48 hours, after which it closes functionally. In most infants it remains closed and is obliterated anatomically at about 3 months. However, in cases of neonatal hypoxia the ductus arteriosus may reopen, causing an increased right-to-left shunt. It is probable that some cyanotic episodes in neonates are related to this phenomenon. The flap of the foramen ovale is pushed shut against the atrial septum as soon as the pressure of the blood in the left atrium exceeds that in the right. It is now believed that there is some shunting of blood through the foramen ovale for about the first week following delivery. After this period the foramen ovale remains functionally closed

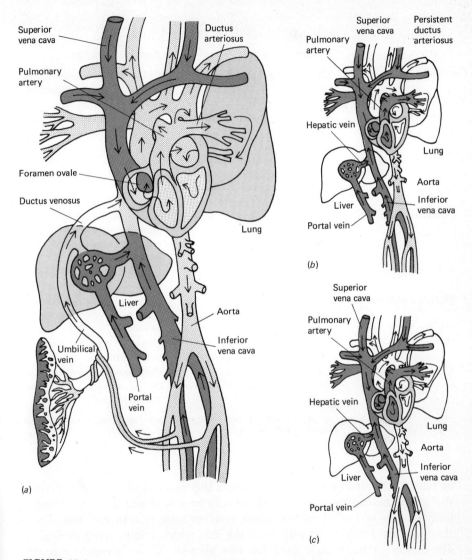

FIGURE 28-1

(*a*) Fetal circulation. (*b*) Immediate postdelivery circulation. (*c*) Normal circulation. (*From Ralph C. Benson, Handbook of Obstetrics and Gynecology, 4th ed., Lange, Los Altos, Calif., 1971, pp. 74–75. By permission of the publisher.*)

in the normal person, although it may be anatomically patent to some degree in a few adults.

An important but controversial factor in the hemodynamics of the newborn is the time of clamping of the umbilical cord. The infant receives an additional 50 to 100 cc of blood if clamping is delayed until the cord ceases

TABLE 28-1
CHANGES IN THE CIRCULATORY MECHANISM AT BIRTH

Structure	Prenatal function	Postnatal function
Umbilical vein	Carries oxygenated blood from placenta to liver and heart.	Obliterated to become ligamentum teres (round ligament of liver).
Ductus venosus	Carries oxygenated blood from umbilical vein to inferior vena cava.	Obliterated to become ligamentum venosum.
Inferior vena cava	Carries oxygenated blood from umbilical vein and ductus venosus and mixed blood from body and liver.	Carries only unoxygenated blood from body.
Foramen ovale	Connects right and left atria.	Functional closure by 3 months, although probe patency without symptoms may be retained by some adults.
Pulmonary arteries	Carry some mixed blood to lungs.	Carry unoxygenated blood to lungs.
Ductus arteriosus	Shunts mixed blood from pulmonary artery to aorta.	Generally occluded by 4 months and becomes ligamentum arteriosum.
Aorta	Receives mixed blood from heart and pulmonary arteries.	Carries oxygenated blood from left ventricle.
Umbilical arteries	Carry oxygenated and unoxygenated blood to the placenta.	Obliterated to become the vesical ligaments on the anterior abdominal wall.

SOURCE: C. Henry Kempe et al., *Current Pediatric Diagnosis and Treatment*, Lange, Los Altos, Calif., 1970, p. 21. Used by permission of the publishers.

to pulsate. According to some physicians this extra blood makes available to the infant an increased amount of iron to be stored and utilized during the first months of life when the infant receives little iron in his food. During this time the infant must rely upon the iron which was received during fetal life to satisfy his body's need for this element. Other physicians contend that the advantages of the extra blood have not been clearly proven. In addition, research studies have demonstrated that the increased amount of blood in an infant who is already polycythemic and vulnerable to respiratory distress may produce mild pulmonary edema. Some investigators have noted that the incidence of pulmonary rales and transient cyanosis is more consistently associated with late clamping of the cord.[1] At present the trend seems to be toward early rather than late clamping of the cord. The advantages of the increased iron supply to the infant are considered by many physicians to be less important than the risk of inducing respiratory distress. While there is no undue hurry to clamp the cord, the baby is no longer held below the level of the mother's body to induce more blood flow into the circulation nor is the cord stripped, as was previously done.

Temperature Regulation and Support

Proper temperature regulation of the newborn infant has been shown clearly to increase the infant's chances for survival.[2, 3, 4] It is well known that wide variations in temperature can cause death in man. An adult generally is able to control the temperature of his environment, adjust himself to it, or remove himself from it. He is able to raise his body heat production by shivering which may increase the metabolic rate of the body by 180 percent over basal levels. He can lower his body temperature by sweating.

By contrast a newborn infant has difficulty in adapting to even moderate variations in temperature. He has relatively poor resources to resist the effects of both heat and cold. This inadaptability is due in part to the fact that the mechanisms of sweating and shivering are not well developed in the neonate. The sweat and sebaceous glands which are present have little homeothermic function until a month or so following birth. Added to this liability is the newborn's large surface area in relation to body mass and the meager amount of subcutaneous fat which results in poor insulation. The blood vessels therefore lie relatively close to the surface of the skin and are sensitive to environmental temperature. The environmental temperature influences blood temperature, which affects the regulatory centers for temperature control located in the hypothalamus. These factors all contribute to the relative instability of body temperature characteristic of the neonatal period.

At present much research is being done regarding the contributions made by various organs and tissues to heat production in the neonate. There is little agreement among investigators. Brown fat, which has a high mitochondrial content, a rich nerve and blood supply, and a high metabolic rate in vitro is thought by some researchers to aid in temperature control in the neonate exposed to cold much as it does in the hibernating animal. The *in vivo* contribution of brown adipose tissue to thermal homeostasis in the newborn infant is not presently known. The largest amounts of this fat are found in the intrascapular region of the neonate's body; some is also found in the thorax and perirenal areas.

Research studies have demonstrated that when the neonate is exposed to temperatures lower than his neutral temperature range, he makes an effort to increase his metabolism and raise his body temperature by crying, by increased skeletal muscle activity, and by increased respiratory rate. The *neutral temperature range* is defined as that set of environmental conditions in which oxygen consumption is at a minimum.

Increased respiratory rate (leading to increased oxygen intake) as a response to cold is a phenomenon occurring only in the neonate and may be referred to as metabolic or chemical *thermogenesis*. The demand for additional oxygen occurs in response to increased catabolic cell activity during which heat and other forms of energy are released. If the demand for oxygen by the body tissues exceeds the supply over a period of time, the risk of neonatal acidosis increases. In the absence of sufficient oxygen the neonate's cells perform relatively more anaerobic catabolism (e.g., the Embden-Meyerhof pathway of glycolysis) the by-product of which is an increase in blood acids (e.g., lactate). In addition the neonate may become extremely fatigued from breathing rapidly and working hard to obtain additional oxygen. If acidosis develops because of the preceding circumstances, the neonate must be warmed, given oxygen, and treated for acidosis immediately. Judicious monitoring of the neonate's temperature is required to prevent such complications from occurring. Chilling the neonate should be avoided under all circumstances. All procedures, including those of an emergency nature such as resuscitation, should be performed on the neonate in a warm area, such as a heated crib or incubator.

The prevention of loss of heat from the body is as important as heat production. The infant loses 27 percent of his body heat through evaporation of water from the skin and from the exhalation of water vapor from his lungs. To avoid heat loss through the evaporation of amniotic fluid from the skin the newborn infant should be swaddled in a warm, absorbent blanket and dried. Three per cent of body heat is lost by the infant through urine, feces, and warming inspired air. Because 70 per cent of body heat is lost through radiation, conduction, and convection, a warmed incubator, heated bed, or radiant heat shield should be provided immediately following birth. To derive maximum benefit from a radiant heat shield the baby should remain uncovered after drying. Such devices should be checked regularly for safety.

To maintain ideal body temperature in the newborn infant, the environmental temperature must be carefully monitored to prevent fluctuations. In addition to controlling the environmental temperature of the neonate, the nurse must observe him carefully and frequently. The nurse must discriminate whether crying, restlessness, and increased respirations in the neonate are due to the infant being cold or to other factors.

Essential Care in the Delivery Room

THE APGAR SCORING SYSTEM

The Apar scoring system provides a systematic and reliable appraisal of the condition of an infant at birth. It is best to use an automatic timer to remind the nurse to take and record the infant's scores promptly at 1 minute and 5 minutes of age. The infant's Apgar score provides valuable information about the infant's condition at birth and has proved to be a reliable predictive instrument. Follow-up studies indicate there is a high positive correlation between infants who have a low Apgar score at 5 minutes of age and subsequent mortality or neurological morbidity in those infants.[5]

The Apgar scoring system is based on the following five signs which are ranked in order of importance. Each sign is evaluated as illustrated in Table 28-2 and given a score of 0, 1, or 2 according to the degree it is present or absent. The maximum score an infant can receive is 10. Few newborn infants receive scores of 10, as *acrocyanosis* due to vasomotor instability is very common in the newborn infant. The *heart rate* is determined by auscultation of the apical pulse. If the heart rate is below 100 the doctor should be notified immediately. *Respiratory effort* and *muscle tone* are evaluated as described in the chart. *Reflex irritability* refers to the infant's response when he is disturbed by light slapping of the foot, oral suctioning, or insertion of a catheter into the nares. A healthy infant will respond to such irritation by grimacing, crying vigorously, or resisting. In approximately 15 percent of newborn infants the body will be completely pink by 5 minutes of age. In the other 85 percent the hands and feet remain bluish for some period of time. A score of 8 to 10 for a newborn infant is considered good; a score of 5 to 7 is considered moderately depressed; a score of 4 or less indicates a severely depressed infant and resuscitation may be indicated.

THE UMBILICAL CORD

After the umbilical cord has been clamped and cut, it should be examined for the presence of three vessels; two arteries and one vein. A single umbilical artery has been associated with congenital anomalies and is considered a congenital vascular malformation. The nurse should make certain that the clamps are secure and that there is no bleeding from the stump. The stump should remain uncovered to facilitate drying and healing.

TABLE 28-2
INFANT EVALUATION AT BIRTH

Points	*0*	*1*	*2*
1. Heart rate	Absent	Slow ($<$ 100)	$>$ 100
2. Respiratory effort	Absent	Slow, irregular	Good, crying
3. Muscle tone	Limp	Some flexion of extremities	Active motion
4. Response to catheter in nostril (tested after oropharynx is clear)	No response	Grimace	Cough or sneeze
5. Color	Blue or pale	Body pink; extremities blue	Completely pink

SOURCE: C. Henry Kempe et al., *Current Pediatric Diagnosis and Therapy*, Lange, Los Altos, Calif., 1970, as adapted from Virginia Apgar et al., "Evaluation of the Newborn Infant—Second Report," *Journal of the American Medical Association*, 168:1985–1988, 1958. Used by permission of the publishers.

PROPHYLAXIS AGAINST OPHTHALMIA NEONATORUM

A *1 percent silver nitrate solution* is recommended as prophylaxis against gonorrheal ophthalmia by the National Society for the Prevention of Blindness. The silver nitrate solution should be instilled so that it will cover all parts of the conjunctival sac and remain in contact with the sac for 15 seconds. To prevent chemical conjunctivitis, the silver nitrate solution should be thoroughly rinsed away with normal saline solution. Antibiotic ointments are not recommended as prophylactic agents because there are certain strains of gonococci which are resistant to them and there is concern about infants developing a sensitivity to them.[6]

INFANT IDENTIFICATION

When the newborn infant's condition is physiologically stable, the infant should be identified properly. This should be done while the infant is still in the delivery room with the mother. From a legal as well as a moral standpoint, proper identification is an extremely important procedure. Various procedures are used for this purpose. A recommended practice is to secure two identical identification bands to the infant's wrist and ankle. The bands should state the sex of the infant, the mother's full name and hospital admission number, and the date and time of birth. The mother should have a corresponding wrist band. The infant's footprints are generally recorded on the baby's hospital record which also contains the mother's right index fingerprint. It is important that prints be recorded carefully, since they are of no value unless they are very clear and legible.[7]

OTHER OBSERVATIONS

Although a thorough physical examination is usually deferred until the newborn infant has recovered from the birth experience, several important observations are generally made in the delivery room. Color, gross malformations, and unusual body configurations or facies (commonly associated with congenital syndromes) can be readily observed. *Choanal atresia* (obstruction of the posterior nares), which has been associated with many breathing problems of infants, can be ruled out by holding a hand across the infant's mouth to test if he can breath through his nose. Some physicians recommend passing a soft tube through the mouth into the stomach to rule out esophageal atresia. If aspiration of the gastric contents yields over 20 to 25 ml of fluid, an upper intestinal obstruction may be suspected. This procedure is not without hazard, since accidental irritation of the larynx can cause laryngospasm. Palpating the vertebral column carefully may rule out spina bifida occulta. The amount and color of amniotic fluid associated with delivery, the size of the placenta, and the amount of vernix on the infant should also be recorded.[8]

If the condition of the mother and infant warrants it and the mother so desires, she should be allowed to hold her infant while still in the delivery room. If the father is present, he should be included in these initial family interactions which facilitate taking on new family roles. Some mothers wish to nurse their infants in the delivery room. Nursing is a sound physiological practice which stimulates the pituitary gland to secrete oxytocin, causing the uterus to contract with a resultant decrease in uterine bleeding. Nursing has additional psychological benefits for both mother and infant. Therefore, if the condition of the mother and infant justifies it, the mother's request to nurse her infant in the delivery room should be honored.

CARE OF THE NEONATE IN THE NURSERY

Care of the Neonate in the Transitional or Observation Nursery

The neonate is transferred as soon as possible from the delivery room to a transitional or observation nursery if one is available. Infants who are high risk or obviously distressed should be transferred directly to an intensive care unit. Priorities for care of the neonate in the transitional nursery should be established. Such priorities are added to those already begun in the delivery room, namely, maintaining respirations and a patent airway, supporting the cardiovascular system, and regulating temperature control. That the first day of life is a critical one for most neonates is reflected in statistics regarding infant mortality rates. Of the total number of infant deaths occurring during the first year, the largest percentage occurs during the first 24 hours after birth; of these deaths, the great majority occur during the first hour after birth.

In light of this, arbitrary priorities for care have been set because the neonate is more vulnerable to certain conditions at particular times during his development (e.g., hemorrhagic disease). Prophylactic intervention at these crucial times prevents the development of serious problems. Although certain physiological mechanisms of the neonate have been selected for consideration, this does not imply that all physiological systems are not developing simultaneously (although at different rates). Nor does it imply that the emotional needs of the neonate are any less vital than his physiological needs. Underscoring all the care that is given by the nurse to the newborn infant are the infant's basic emotional needs for love, comfort, security, and protection from harm.

The priorities for transitional nursery care are to obtain base line data regarding vital signs and measurements, to assign the infant a mortality risk rating, to provide an environment which will facilitate transition through the birth recovery period, to provide prophylaxis against neonatal bleeding tendencies, and to observe the neonate carefully for the onset of illness. A method for charting some of this information is shown in Figure 28-2.

	Date
UNIVERSITY OF COLORADO MEDICAL CENTER	Ward
Colorado General Hospital	Name
	Hosp. No.
NURSES ADMISSION RECORD	Address

DATE: TIME OF DELIV.:   TYPE DELIV.:   CREDE:

PRENATAL CARE: MOTHER'S BLOOD TYPE:

RESUSCITATION:

COMPLICATIONS/COMMENTS:

                                           CALCULATED GEST. AGE:

ADMIT TIME TO NSY.:   CLINICAL EST. OF GEST. AGE:

ADMIT DATE TO NSY.:   SOLE CREASES:

COLOR: BREAST TISSUE:

CRY: EARS:

RESPIRATIONS: HAIR:

SUCTION(DE LEE) AMOUNT: VERNIX:

KIND: GENITALIA:

ACTIVITY: DESQUAMATION:

BIRTH WEIGHT: RESTING:

LENGTH: RECOIL:

HEAD CIRCUMFERENCE: PEDS CALLED:

RECTAL TEMPERATURE: CODING:

ANOMALIES/REMARKS:

                                           SIGNATURE:

FIRST FEEDING TIME: TYPE: AMOUNT:

  MODE: REGURGITATION: LAVAGE:

COMMENTS:

                                           SIGNATURE:

TRANSFER TO PLACE: DATE: TIME:

FIGURE 28-2

Nurses' admission record for newborn infants.

(Unpublished nursing record used at University of Colorado Medical Center. By permission of Sally Bolosky, Head Nurse, Newborn Nursery, University of Colorado Medical Center.)

Upon admission to the transitional nursery the infant should be placed in an incubator or warmed bed. Information regarding the antepartal history, the labor and delivery experience, and other relevant information should be recorded on the infant's chart. *Vital signs* should be checked frequently, since they are extremely variable in the neonate. Several consecutive determinations are necessary to establish a base line by which to compare later readings. Preferably the heart and respiratory rates should be taken when the infant is quiet, for they will increase markedly when the infant is crying. In any case, the state of the infant when vital signs were taken should be noted when the rates are recorded. The first temperature should be taken rectally to determine patency of the anus. All subsequent temperatures should be axillary recordings in order to prevent irritation of the rectum and the possibility of frequent stooling. Particular attention should be paid to the fact that *infants with infections often run subnormal or erratic temperatures*. Other signs such as poor feeding, vomiting, diarrhea, or lethargy are much more reliable indications of infection than is temperature.

Accurate measurements of the infant are essential for a number of reasons. They are used to help determine gestational age, as evidence of intrauterine growth retardation, to establish a base line against which to measure later growth of the infant, and to help identify high-risk infants. Measurements of weight, length, and head circumference are usually made in the transitional nursery after the infant has reached a relatively stable condition. These measurements are recorded on forms, as shown in Figure 28-3. Assuming that the infant is over 5 pounds, the absolute size of the infant is not as important as the *percentiles* within which each of his measurements fall. Weight, height, and head circumference lying in different percentiles increase the probability that the infant has suffered from some intrauterine growth retardation. Other reasons for disproportionate measurements include excess edema, abnormalities in the growth of the head, or any number of genetically induced syndromes.

The neonate should be evaluated according to the criteria outlined on a chart similar to that shown in Table 28-3. The estimation of gestational age, vital signs, measurements, and the general condition of the infant are all considered when assigning the infant a mortality risk rating. Figure 28-4 illustrates a mortality risk chart. The mortality risk rating determines whether or not the infant will remain in the transitional nursery or be transferred to an intensive care unit. The birth recovery period is characterized by rapidly changing physiological and behavioral characteristics. The infant's rating may change from low risk to high risk at any time during this period. The nurse who cares for neonates must be able to interpret the infant's behavior and symptomatology accurately and refer to a physician for treatment when indicated. The whole nursing process of observation, evaluation, intervention, and reevaluation should continue throughout the neonate's entire hospital stay and is not confined to only one period.

TABLE 28-3
CLINICAL ESTIMATION OF GESTATIONAL AGE: A GUIDE

Physical findings	Est ga		Weeks gestation																		
	24	25	26	27	28	29	30	31	32	33	34	35	36	37	38	39	40	41	42	43	44
Examination first hours																					
Vernix	Appears						Covers body									Decrease in amount			No vernix		
Breast tissue					None							1 - 2 mm		4 mm				7 mm or more			
Nipples				Barely visible						Well defined, raised areola							Well defined flat areola				
Sole creases				None				1, Anterior transverse			2, Anterior transverse			Anterior ⅔ sole			Creases involving heel				
Ear cartilage				Pinna soft, stays folded							Returns slowly from folding			Thin cartilage, springs back			Firm, remains erect from head				
Ear form				Flat, shapeless							Beginning incurving of periphery			Partial incurving upper pinna			Well defined incurving all of upper pinna				
Genitalia Testes and scrotum			Undescended					Testes high in canal, few rugae			Testes lower, few rugae			Testes lower, more rugae		Testes descended, pendulous scrotum, rugae complete					
Labia and clitoris				Labia majora widely separated, prominent clitoris							Labia majora nearly cover labia minora						Labia minora & clitoris covered				
Hair (appears on head @ 20 wks)			Eyebrow & lashes							Fine, woolly hair							Hair silky, single strands				
Lanugo (appears @ 20 wks)		Lanugo over entire body			Vanishes from face							Slight lanugo over shoulders					No lanugo				
Skin texture					Thin							Smooth, medium thickness				Desquamation					
Skin color and opacity				Translucent, plethoric, numerous venules (abdomen)										Pink, few large vessels overall				Pale pink, no vessels seen			
Skull firmness				Soft to 1 inch from anterior fontanel										Springy at edges of fontanel, center firm		Bones hard, sutures easily displaced			Bones hard, cannot be displaced		
Posture Resting	Lateral decubitus					Hypotonia		Slight increase in tone, lower extremity			Frog-like						Total flexion				
Recoil				Absent				Slight, lower extremities			None upper extremities Good lower extremities			Slow upper extremities					Good upper extremities		

Later examination

		24	25	26	27	28	29	30	31	32	33	34	35	36	37	38	39	40	41	42	43	44
Tone	Heel to ear				No resistance					Slight resistance			Difficult		Almost impossible				Impossible			
	Scarf maneuver					No resistance								Minimal resistance	Fair resistance					Difficulty			
	Neck extensors				Absent					Slight			Fair					Good				
	Neck flexors					Absent								Minimal					Fair			
Reflexes	Moro			Barely apparent			Complete, exhaustible				Good, complete			No adduction					Complete with adduction				
	Pupils to light												React									
	Grasp			Feeble				Fair			Solid, involves arms								May pick infant up				
	Rooting			Minimal with reinforcement			Good with reinforcement										Good						
	Crossed extension				Slight withdrawal					Withdrawal				Withdrawal & extension				Withdrawal, extension, adduction				
	Automatic walk						Absent							Minimal					Fair, toes	Good, heels			
	Trunk elevation						Absent						Slight				Good	Present				
	Glabellar tap				Absent						Appears						Present					
	Head turns to light					Absent						Appears					Present					
Clinical estimate, Ga																						
Calculated Ga		24	25	26	27	28	29	30	31	32	33	34	35	36	37	38	39	40	41	42	43	44
													Weeks gestation										

SOURCE: C. Henry Kempe et al., *Current Pediatric Diagnosis and Therapy*, Lange, Los Altos, Calif., 1970, p. 42, as adapted from Lula O. Lubchenco et al., "Assessment of Gestational Age and Development at Birth," *Pediatric Clinics of North America*, 17:125–145, 1970.

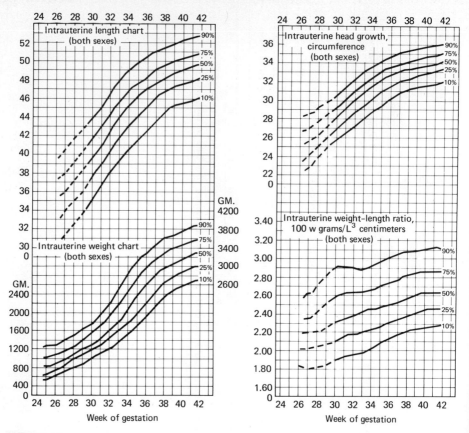

FIGURE 28-3

Colorado intrauterine growth charts. Percentiles of intrauterine growth in weight, length, head circumference, and weight/length ratio.

(From Lula O. Lubchenco et al., "Intrauterine Growth in Length and Head Circumference as Estimated from Live Births at Gestational Ages from 26 to 42 Weeks," Pediatrics, 37: 404, 1966.)

PROPHYLAXIS AGAINST HEMORRHAGIC DISEASE OF THE NEWBORN

All newborn infants demonstrate a moderate deficiency in the vitamin K dependent coagulation factors.[9, 10, 11] Most vitamin K absorbed in the body is formed by the action of bacterial flora in the colon. However, this flora is usually absent in the colon at birth. It may take the newborn infant several days to establish a normal flora. Therefore, production by the liver of coagulation factors, such as PTC, prothrombin, proconvertin, and Stuart Prower factor, which depend on vitamin K, is impaired. During this time the infant

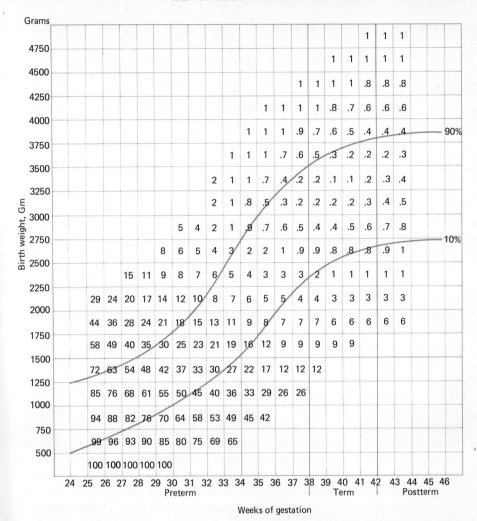

FIGURE 28-4
Neonatal classification and neonatal mortality risk by birth weight and gestational age. (*From Lula O. Lubchenco, "Neonatal Mortality Rate: Its Relationship to Birth Weight and Gestation Age," Journal of Pediatrics, in press.*)

may develop bleeding problems, such as ecchymoses, bleeding at the site of an injection of medication, bleeding around the umbilical cord, or excessive bleeding at circumcision. This problem, referred to as hemorrhagic disease of the newborn, can be prevented by a single intramuscular injection of water-soluble vitamin K. The usual dose is 1.0 mg, which may be administered to the infant in the delivery room or in the transitional nursery.

NEONATAL BEHAVIOR DURING THE BIRTH RECOVERY PERIOD

Although neonates recover from the birth experience at varying rates, Desmond has identified certain behavioral and physiological patterns which most neonates seem to go through before they reach a stage of relative stability. Desmond describes three overlapping stages characteristic of the birth recovery period. During the *first stage*, which may last for about 30 minutes, the infant may appear alert and active. There is a decrease in body temperature accompanied by an increase in motor activity, respiratory rate, and heart rate. There may be flaring of the *alae nasi*, grunting, and intercostal retractions which may be outward signs of the infant's efforts to accommodate for his lowered temperature. Bowel sounds are usually not heard. The infant may have large amounts of mucus which may cause him to drool or vomit. During the *second stage*, which may last from 30 minutes to 2 hours, the infant falls asleep and the respiratory and heart rates slow. During the *third stage*, however, the infant awakens, and the nurse may observe a return of the initial behavior. The heart rate increases; there may be large amounts of mucus, which affect respirations, and there may be periods of apnea. Rapid color changes may be noted which indicate vasomotor instability. Meconium may be passed during this stage. As mentioned previously, vital signs concerning the neonate's heart rate, respirations, and color should be taken and recorded at 15- or 30-minute intervals.[12]

Plethora may occur in the baby at about 6 hours following delivery. At this time the infant's skin appears quite red and may turn to a purplish-red when crying. In addition the skin may appear tight and shiny. This phenomenon is a result of the migration of fluid from the blood vessels into the extracellular spaces, resulting in a concentration of red blood cells within the vessels. Occasionally the hemoconcentration will reach a level at which the hematocrit is 80 percent. Unless the baby develops symptoms of respiratory distress or cardiac decompensation, no treatment is required, as the hematocrit will spontaneously return to the normal neonatal level of about 60 percent in 12 to 24 hours.[13]

Within 6 to 8 hours following delivery, the condition of most neonates tends to stabilize; the infant may then be bathed and dressed. A healthy newborn infant may be fed when he first appears hungry; this period usually coincides with the completion of the birth recovery period. The first feeding should consist of 5 percent glucose in water. The neonate may take very little of the first feeding or he may take several ounces. The nurse should observe and record the infant's ability to suck, the amount of mucus and regurgitation associated with the feeding, and the infant's tolerance for the feeding. When the neonate's vital signs are stable, his color is pink, and there are no apparent problems, the infant is transferred into a regular nursery or a rooming-in facility for the remainder of the hospital stay.

Continuing Care of the Neonate

Meticulous attention should be given to the neonate throughout his hospital stay. It is important that the *reasons* for procedures are clearly understood by the personnel who are to carry out these procedures. Even though actual techniques may vary from hospital to hospital, the underlying principles, based on the neonate's physiological and emotional requirements, should be consistent and provide the rationale for the care given. There also should be sufficient staff to carry out the care prescribed. The nurse who carries out the daily activities of feeding, diapering, and keeping the infant clean is in an optimal position for detecting subtle changes in the neonate's condition, appearance, and behavior. Maintaining a patent airway in the neonate is always of primary importance. The nurse should give special attention to proper and firm positioning of the infant on his side after feeding to prevent aspiration of feeding and mucus into the trachea. The nurse should report to the physician promptly any changes which are not in the normal range.

The priorities for care in the regular nursery are to prevent infection, to provide adequate food and fluids, to detect early signs of hyperbilirubinemia, to identify illness, to recognize congenital defects that were not previously noted, and to facilitate positive mother-infant relationships. This may be accomplished by daily systematic observation and examination of the neonate based on knowledge of his physiology and characteristics. A convenient way to chart these observations is through the use of a checklist similar to that shown in Table 28-4. The nurse can interpret the infant's behavior to the mother and assist her as she endeavors to understand and care for her infant. In the following section the priorities for care in the regular nursery will be discussed in relation to the systems which influence them most obviously. As previously stated all systems work together; a malfunction in one will affect another to some degree. Since the range of normality is fairly wide during the neonatal period, the infant's *normal characteristics* will be presented in chart form along with headings designating their usual manifestations and variations. This will permit the reader to readily note the parameters of normality.

PREVENTION OF INFECTION

The infant's ability to produce his own immunoglobulins depends on his genetic inheritance.[14] The infant's own immunologic system does not form these immunoglobulins in any significant amount until later in infancy. Therefore, during the first few months of life the infant must depend upon the passive immunity he has inherited from his mother. The infant's resistance to certain infections depends in large part on his mother's own experience with disease and with active and passive acquired immunity as well

TABLE 28-4
CHECKLIST OF SIGNIFICANT OBSERVATIONS IN NEWBORN INFANTS

Healthy findings	Neurological findings
Body temperature	Convulsions
Incubator temperature	Rigid
Weight	Opisthotonos
Respiratory rate	Twitching
Pulse rate	Irritable
Demanding	Hyperactive
Hungry	Tires easily
Sucks well	Less active
Gavages well, but slowly	Lethargic
Resisted gavage	Weak cry
Weight gain	Shrill cry
Good cry	Moro reflex poor or absent
Active	
Color stable	*Cardiovascular findings*
	Pallor
Gastrointestinal findings	Plethora
Gavaged poorly	Cyanosis, circumoral
Sucked poorly	Cyanosis, circumocular
Gagged	Cyanosis, extremities
Drooled	Cyanosis, generalized
Regurgitated	Bleeding (specify area)
Hiccups	
Mucus on gavage tube	*Respiratory findings*
Mucus, other	Oxygen flow (liters/min)
Abdominal distention	Oxygen concentration
Abnormal stool	Shallow respirations
Sore buttocks	Labored respirations
Weight loss	Deep respirations

as the particular antigens with which he comes into contact. Therefore, immunity is a highly individual matter. Some maternal antibodies are transported across the placenta during the last weeks of pregnancy. These antibodies can protect the neonate during the first few months of life from some of the childhood diseases. However, the antibodies inherited against pertussis are inadequate to protect the neonate from this disease, which is very serious during infancy. Immunizations against pertussis as well as diphtheria and tetanus should be started between one and two months of age. The infant is much more vulnerable to infection than is an adult or even an older child. A wide variety of organisms which may cause minor problems in an older child may cause septicemia in an infant. Septicemia is more common during

TABLE 28-4
CHECKLIST OF SIGNIFICANT OBSERVATIONS IN NEWBORN INFANTS (*Continued*)

Irregular respirations	Umbilical redness
Rest periods, < 10 sec	Umbilical oozing
Rest periods, 10–30 sec	Alcohol to cord
Apnea, > 30 sec	Pustular rash
Intercostal retractions	Other rash (specify)
Xiphoid retractions	Abscess
See-saw respirations	Eye discharge
Dilated alae nasi	Skin dry or peeling
Grunting	Skin irritated (specify area)
Cough	*Other*
Sneeze	
Stuffy nose	
Skin findings	
Mottled	
Harlequin syndrome	
Jaundice	
Petechiae (specify area)	
Ecchymoses (specify area)	
Edema	
Dehydration	
Sclerema	

NOTE: The severity of the sign is indicated by +, ++, or +++. If the symptom is present only before or after eating, the abbreviation ac or pc is used. This checklist is used by nurses instead of routine nurses' notes, each column used for one period of observation. The signs observed in the infant are checked, the time and date noted, and the item initialed. If situations other than those listed are present, detailed descriptions are written in the regular nurses' notes. A 24-hour summary of nursing observations is given to the physician at morning rounds. This and the physicians' examinations provide the data on which a decision is made concerning illness.
SOURCE: C. Henry Kempe et al.: *Current Pediatric Diagnosis and Treatment*, Lange, Los Altos, Calif., 1970, p. 49, as adapted from Lula O. Lubchenco, *Pediatric Clinics of North America*, 8:471, 1961.

infancy than at any other time. Viral infections such as herpes simplex, Coxsackie virus, and cytomegalic inclusion disease have grave consequences for the neonate and are associated with a very high mortality and morbidity rate.

Although nursery personnel can do little to alter the neonate's inherited immunity, efforts to prevent infection can be concentrated in four general areas:[15]

1 Infants whose history indicates they have high potential for infection should be *isolated* from other infants. This would include infants born of mothers whose membranes were ruptured for 24 hours or more,

infants born outside the delivery room or under unsterile conditions, and infants born of mothers suspected of having infectious disease. It is thought that many cases of neonatal herpes are acquired by the infant as he passes through an infected maternal genital tract.

2 Nursery personnel should be required to have regular physical examinations, including a chest x ray. They should be aware of the serious consequences to newborn infants of even a mild infection. Policy should be so established that all illnesses are reported and personnel will refrain from coming to work until they are completely well. No penalty or loss of pay should be feared from this action. Nursery personnel should also be aware of the threat to their own well-being by certain diseases of newborn infants. A pregnant nursery worker exposed to neonatal rubella is a case in point.

3 Meticulous attention to handwashing will reduce the possibility of transmission of common infectious pathogens from infant to infant. All persons should wash their hands for *3 minutes* before handling an infant. This initial scrub should include the hands and the arms up to the area above the elbows. A *1-minute* scrub between babies is required. Hands should be washed scrupulously before and after handling any infant or any object considered contaminated.

4 All formulas and linen should be sterilized. Other nursery equipment should be regularly disinfected.

PROVISION OF FOOD AND FLUID

Glucose Regulation

As soon as glucose feedings are tolerated well and there are no serious problems with regurgitation or with mucus, breast-feeding or full strength formula feeding is begun. The normal healthy infant should be permitted to regulate the volume and frequency of his feedings, provided that his calorie, electrolyte, and fluid requirements are met. Milk supplies calcium and phosphorous which the newborn infant needs for the formation of the bony matrix. If the milk is not fortified with vitamin D, the infant should receive a vitamin D supplement to aid calcium absorption. Vitamin D appears to inhibit the destruction of citrate ions which are necessary to form calcium citrate. In this way vitamin D increases the solubility of calcium and aids in calcium ion absorption. Vitamin C, which is required for proper formation of intercellular matrix of connective tissues—e.g., bone, cartilage, tendons—should also be given daily, as it is poorly supplied by milk and not stored in the body.[16]

The healthy term infant is able to ingest his nourishment by sucking and may average 2 to 4 ounces of milk per feeding. In general, the healthy neonate is able to digest, absorb, and metabolize milk fairly well. However, as with other factors in his environment, his nutritional and fluid intake should be carefully regulated. The infant's early feeding experiences have strong emotional, cultural, and social overtones. Many of the infant's later attitudes toward food and what it symbolizes can be traced back to his early experience with feeding. The newborn infant is very sensitive to the feelings of those who feed him toward himself as well as food in general. The foundations for feeding problems are laid early in infancy.

Food tends to pass rather rapidly through the neonate's stomach. Gastric emptying time varies from infant to infant as well as with the type of feeding given. More undigested protein may pass through the infant's stomach than an older child. When the infant's chyme reaches the small intestine, the undigested proteins are handled by protein-digesting enzymes. These enzymes break down the proteins to amino acids which can then be absorbed to provide body protein for the infant. This assumes that the infant's diet provides an adequate supply of protein.

Although the neonate readily assimilates disaccharides and monosaccharides, he has little ability to handle long-chain polysaccharides, e.g., cornstarch. This is due to a deficiency of pancreatic amylase in the neonate.

Glucose regulation and a tendency toward hypoglycemia in the neonate depend on a number of interacting factors. Immature liver function in the neonate results in low and unstable glucose concentration in the blood. The factors which may predispose the neonate to hypoglycemia include the infant's high metabolic rate, a relatively long period before the first feedings, and immature liver function. Because the liver cannot perform gluconeogenesis well, glucose stores in the liver are insufficient to keep blood levels of glucose high enough to meet the energy requirements of the infant. If feeding is unduly delayed, the infant becomes hypoglycemic and shows signs of hunger.

Most newborns have a drop in blood glucose levels during the first few hours after delivery. Usually this condition goes unnoticed, but some infants will exhibit signs of hypoglycemia, such as tremors, twitching, limpness, or lethargy. These infants should have blood glucose determinations made and, if found to be hypoglycemic (having a glucose level of less than 30 mg per 100 ml), should be given glucose orally or intraveneously. The method chosen will depend on the physical condition of the newborn and the degree of hypoglycemia that is present. Prolonged periods of hypoglycemia can cause brain damage in the infant since neurons mainly oxidize glucose as a source of energy.

The neonate absorbs fat slowly from the gastrointestinal tract. The exact cause of this is not known. Because of this slow absorption, it is recommended that infants do not receive formulas with high fat content. Such feedings fail to be absorbed and are merely lost to the body by way of the stools. Currently research is being conducted to discover if there is a possible link between the high incidence of heart disease in the United States and the fact that the great majority of infants in this country are fed cow's milk (which has a higher fat content than breast milk).

Fluid Balance

Regurgitation during or after a feeding is very common among infants. This is partly due to the labile musculature of the gastrointestinal system which causes reverse peristalsis at times. It is also due to the fact the infant tends to swallow air while sucking. The nurse should be sure that milk fills the entire nipple of the bottle so that the infant will not swallow additional amounts of air while feeding. The nurse should also "bubble" the infant before placing him in the crib. The nurse must discriminate between regurgitation and vomiting in the neonate.

The neonate passes stools frequently; they are softer and more liquid than those of an older child. The nurse must also differentiate between the infant's passing frequent stools and having diarrhea. Since it is often difficult to estimate the amount of fluid and valuable electrolytes lost through vomiting and diarrhea, these conditions present serious problems to the neonate if they develop. The nurse should weigh the baby daily and record the amount and character of each stool passed, the number of voidings, and the number of times and amount the infant vomits. A physician should be notified immediately if the amount of fluid lost seems excessive. Early recognition and treatment of this developing condition is of paramount importance.

In health, the neonate is able to regulate a normal fluid load well even though his renal and endocrine systems are immature and his gastrointestinal system labile. In the face of illness such as infection, vomiting, and diarrhea, however, the infant rapidly gets into difficulty. The neonate has several disadvantages in regard to balancing the volume and composition of his body fluids. The infant exchanges fluids seven times as fast, in relation to body weight, as does an adult and loses more water proportionately. There is a tendency toward acidosis in the infant because his metabolic rate is two times that of an adult in relation to body mass. Diarrhea can quickly exacerbate this predisposition.

The functional development of the neonate's kidneys is not complete until the end of the first month of life. The neonate concentrates urine to only one and one-half times the osmolality of the plasma instead of the normal three to four times, as in the adult. Because of this renal immaturity the infant does not excrete toxins as efficiently and reabsorb the substances he needs as fully as an adult. The influence of the infant's immature endoctrine system is also felt. In time of need—e.g., during diarrhea, vomiting, or infection—the neonate is unable to conserve the water he needs. This is because of the immature functions of both the hypothalamic antidiuretic centers and the distal tubule cells. The neonate is also unable to conserve sodium and other electrolytes when he needs them because of the immature function of the adrenal cortex and renal distal tubule cells.

PHYSIOLOGIC JAUNDICE

Jaundice that occurs on the second or third postdelivery day in a neonate who exhibits no other signs of illness is termed *physiologic jaundice*. This jaundice is a result of the cumulative effects of the hemolysis which is occurring and the immature functioning of the baby's liver. In approximately 50 percent of neonates the liver function is able to keep pace with the breakdown of red cells resulting in no clinical jaundice and little or no increase in serum bilirubin levels. In the remaining infants, most will show a rise in serum bilirubin above the normal level of less than 1 mg per 100 ml of blood. Many of these will demonstrate clinical jaundice.

Two main factors lead to the development of physiologic jaundice: (1) the polycythemia present in the normal newborn and (2) the relative inability of the newborn liver cells to conjugate bilirubin. As hemolysis occurs in the reticuloendothelial system, iron and protein released from the red cells are recirculated in the body for reuse. The toxic substance resulting from hemoglobin destruction is bilirubin which must be conjugated by the liver into a form in which it can be excreted from the body. To be transported to the liver, the bilirubin must be bound to albumin because any free unconjugated bilirubin in the blood is potentially able to bind to brain cells, causing severe brain damage known as *kernicterus*. It is not known why the neonate's brain cells are particularly susceptible to this type of damage. In the liver bilirubin is conjugated (bound to glucuronic acid) and excreted into the bile. From there it passes into the small intestine and out of the body.

Jaundice in the newborn is often difficult to detect but is extremely important to note as soon as it appears. *Any jaundice occurring within 24 hours after delivery must be reported at once.* Infants should be carefully examined in daylight at least once a day to determine the presence of jaundice. Blanching the skin of the chest or forehead is one way of detecting jaundice when it is not readily apparent in the sclerae or nailbeds. Jaundice in the neonate should never be treated lightly even though it is of the so-called "physiological" variety. In the presence of other disease or physiological handicaps, the baby may develop kernicterus at blood levels of bilirubin lower than 17 mg per 100 ml. It is necessary to distinguish between true jaundice and the yellow staining of the skin, nails, and vernix due to passage of meconium by the baby during labor and delivery.

Phototherapy is considered useful by some physicians in the treatment of physiological jaundice in selected neonates. The precise reasons for the effectiveness of light in reducing jaundice are not understood at the present time. In addition, the practice has not been in use long enough to be thoroughly evaluated.

Two major problems with this therapy are the possibility of retinal

TABLE 28-5
NORMAL RANGE FOR MEASUREMENTS AND VITAL SIGNS

Characteristic measurements and vital signs	Usual manifestation	Normal variations	Comment
Weight	3,400 Gm (7½ lb)	2,500 Gm (5½ lb)–4,100 Gm (9 lb)	Babies above 4,100 Gm (9 lb) or under 2,500 Gm (5½ lb) are often high risk.
Length	50 cm (20 in.)	45–55 cm (18–22 in.)	Difficult to measure accurately.
Head circumference	34–36 cm (13½–14½ in.)	32–38 cm (12½–15 in.)	Extremes in size may indicate presence of pathology such as microcephaly, hydrocephaly, or increased intracranial pressure.
Chest circumference	2 cm (¾ in.) less than head circumference	7 cm (2¾ in.) less to 5 cm (2 in.) more than head circumference	Greater variation may indicate head or chest pathology.
Heart rate	120–140 beats/minute	100–160 beats/minute; may be irregular, especially when crying	Rate is influenced by physical activity, crying, state of wakefulness, body temperature, disease, or other defect.
Respiratory rate	30–40/minute	20–60/minute; tends to be irregular	Same things influence respiratory rate which influence heart rate. Some normal babies may have short (10–20 sec) "resting" periods between respirations.
Temperature	36.5°C (97.7°F)–37°C (98.6°F) (axillary)	35.7°C (96°F)–37.2°C (99°F) (axillary)	Axillary temperatures are accurate if properly done. This method avoids irritation of rectum. May run subnormal temperature even with an infection.
Blood pressure	60/20–90/60	60/20–90/60	Blood pressure readings are rarely obtained in neonates.

damage and the questionable toxic effect of photochemical products in the body. When phototherapy is ordered the baby is placed unclothed, except for a diaper, in direct daylight or under cool blue fluorescent lamps. The candle-power to be used in the fluorescent lamps is under debate at this time. The infant's eyes should be covered to protect them from the light, however; care must be taken to prevent corneal damage from the bandage.

Characteristics of the Newborn Infant

Tables 28-5 through 28-10 provide information about the characteristics of the newborn infant and the range of normality of those characteristics. The usual manifestation and normal variation of each characteristic is listed, followed by explanatory comments. When indicated, a brief narrative illuminates the information contained in the tables. Table 28-5 shows the range of normal in measurements and vital signs for the neonate. The significance of obtaining accurate data on the size and vital signs of the infant has been discussed in a previous section of this chapter.

GENERAL APPEARANCE

Figure 28–5 depicts a typical newborn infant. Note that the head is disproportionately large for the body, comprising one-fourth of the total body length. The center of the baby's body is at the umbilicus rather than at the symphysis pubis as in the adult. The torso appears long and the extremities short. The flexed position in which the baby maintains the extremities contributes to their apparent shortness. The hands are tightly clenched. The neck appears

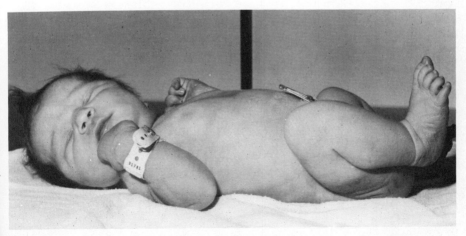

FIGURE 28-5
A normal newborn infant at rest. (Courtesy of The University of Colorado Medical Center, Denver, Colorado)

TABLE 28-6
CHARACTERISTICS OF NEONATE'S SKIN

Characteristics of skin	Usual manifestation	Normal variations	Comment
Color	Generally pink. May have occasional cyanosis around mouth or of hands and feet.	Mottling when unclothed. Harlequin color change. May be ruddy for several hours after birth.	Jaundice and pallor are not considered normal. "Physiological" jaundice may occur at 3–5 days of age. *Jaundice occurring within 24 hours of birth is abnormal.*
Consistency and hydration	Soft. Normal turgor. Medium thickness. Subcutaneous fat present.	May feel puffy. Amount of subcutaneous fat varies.	Thickness of skin indicates degree of maturity. Poor turgor indicates dehydration.
Condition	Intact and smooth. May have some dryness and peeling.	Petechiae over presenting part only. Ecchymoses from forceps. Mongolian spots on back or buttocks. Milia on face particularly on nose. Telangiectases on nape of neck and/or eyelids.	Rashes are abnormal except for erythema toxicum neonatorum. May have pigmented nevi or tufts of hair.
Vernix caseosa	Whitish, greasy material covering body.	May be thicker on some babies than on others. Tends to collect in body creases.	Markedly decreased amount or absence of vernix indicates postmaturity. Excessive amount indicates prematurity.
Lanugo	Fine, downy hair on face and shoulders.	May be absent.	A large amount of lanugo is indicative of prematurity.
Edema	Present, but not apparent.	Often presenting part and eyelids will be obviously edematous.	Obvious, generalized edema is abnormal. Baby will lose 6–10 percent of his birth weight within 3–5 days of birth.

short because the chin rests upon the chest. The baby has a prominent abdomen, sloping shoulders, narrow hips, and a rounded chest. The infant tends to remain in a flexed position resembling that maintained in utero.

Throughout the newborn period, the infant should be carefully observed for *symmetry of body parts* and the *positions* he assumes at rest. Asymmetries and unusual positions indicate that he should be thoroughly examined for the presence of fractures, paralyses, or other orthopedic defects. Often these asymmetries are within the normal range. They are frequently due to odd positions maintained in utero or unusual presentations during delivery. If the body part can be passively rotated into a normal position with no limitation of motion at the joint, the malposition will usually correct spontaneously as the infant grows. Following a breech delivery, the legs are often flexed on the abdomen for a period of time. It is important for the nurse to be aware of the normality of many of the rather odd positions and proportions of the newborn infant so that the appearance can be explained to the mother.

SKIN

Table 28-6 describes the major characteristics of the neonate's skin. During the first hours following delivery the infant's skin becomes progressively more plethoric because of the hemoconcentration which occurs at that time. As this decreases the infant becomes more pink but still may become quite red when crying. The ruddy appearance is largely due to the dilation of the superficial blood vessels lying close to the surface of the skin. The residual cyanosis of the hands and feet is most likely caused by sluggish peripheral circulation, as is the mottling which occurs when the infant is chilled. Illustration (A) of the color plate demonstrates a moderately plethoric infant with some cyanosis of the hand.

Harlequin color change is an example of vasomotor instability which causes the blood vessels on one side of the newborn's body to dilate while those on the opposite side constrict. This results in a very odd appearance, for there is a sharp line down the center of his body, dividing the reddish half from the blanched half. Harlequin color change appears and disappears spontaneously and is of no known medical significance. *Pallor* in a newborn is always a grave sign, signifying anemia secondary to internal hemorrhage, erythroblastosis fetalis, or shock due to sepsis or anoxia.

Generalized cyanosis usually indicates an increased need for oxygen. This may be a temporary condition which requires only a few hours of an oxygen-enriched environment, or it may be indicative of serious disease. Nursing responsibilities in dealing with cyanotic infants include careful recordings of when and under what circumstances cyanosis occurred as well as the maintenance of a patent airway and the proper concentration of oxygen in the incubator.

At birth the full-term infant's skin is normally smooth, well hydrated, soft to touch, and covered with varying amounts of lanugo and vernix caseosa. *Desquamation* is common in the first days following delivery. *Rashes* are usually abnormal except for the transient appearance of an urticarial type of rash which has been designated *erythema toxicum neonatorum*. The cause of this rash has not been determined and it disappears without treatment. Illustration (B) of the color plate shows an infant with erythema toxicum neonatorum and lanugo on the back. Lanugo is fine, downy hair found over the back and shoulders of some infants. *Mongolian spots* which appear as bluish-black areas over the lower back and buttocks are commonly found in nonwhite newborns. These tend to fade during the first years of life. Telangiectases (capillary hemangiomas) also seem to disappear after infancy, although it is likely that they do not actually become obliterated, but rather the skin becomes thicker making them less apparent. *Milia*, which are obstructed sebaceous glands appearing as small white papillae over the nose and chin, are illustrated in Figure 28-6. Milia will disappear spontaneously within several weeks.

During early infancy the outer layer of the skin is not an efficient barrier

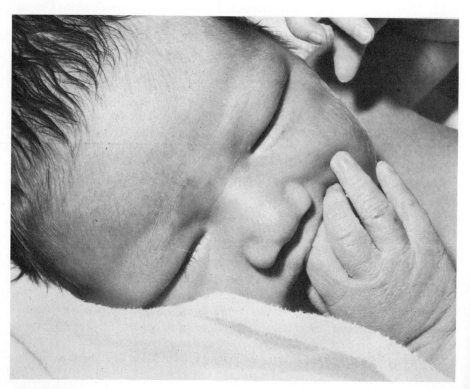

FIGURE 28-6
Milia evident on the nose of a newborn infant.

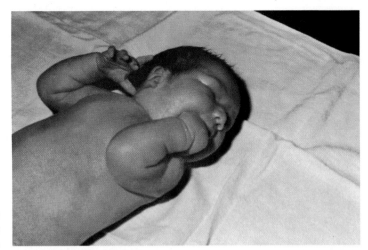

(A) Moderately plethoric infant with acrocyanosis.

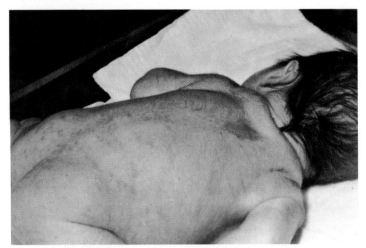

(B) Newborn with erythema toxicum neonatorum and lanugo.

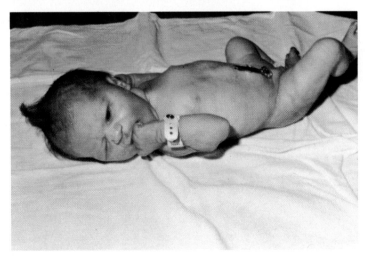

(C) Infant awake and alert.

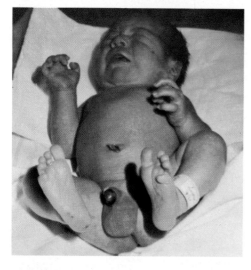

(D) Newborn infant crying.
Note healing umbilical cord
and recent circumcision.

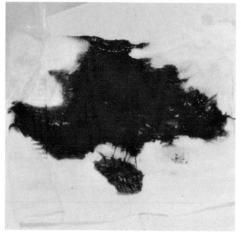

(E)

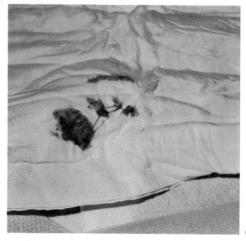

(F)

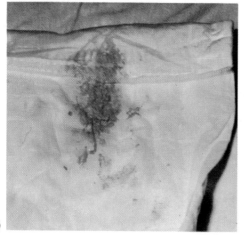

(G)

(E) Typical meconium stool.
(F) Typical transitional stool.
(G) Normal infant stool.

to pathogens. In addition the infant is prone to develop rashes or blisters from trauma that ordinarily would not produce these conditions in an older person. The reasons for the infant's skin sensitivity are not clearly delineated. However, the fact remains that special care must be taken to prevent skin trauma when cleansing an infant. Some pediatricians recommend that cotton dipped in sterile oil or in a nontoxic bacteriostatic agent be used to clean off the blood and vernix from the infant when he is initially bathed. Thereafter cotton balls moistened with warm water may be used for daily cleaning. Gauze is not recommended, since it tends to irritate the skin. Complete baths are not given while the infant is in the nursery, but all the body creases should be cleaned frequently to remove collections of material where bacteria may flourish.[17] Care of the umbilical stump is discussed later in the chapter.

BODY SEGMENTS

The appearance and characteristics of the neonate's body segments are described in Table 28-7.

The common asymmetries of the head are *cephalhematoma* and *caput succedaneum*. Cephalhematoma is caused by trauma to the head during birth which results in subperiosteal bleeding. It appears several hours after birth and will resorb by two months of age. Usually no treatment is required. Caput succedaneum is edema of the vertex of the head and is caused by pressure on the scalp during labor. It, too, will disappear spontaneously but in a much shorter time than cephalhematoma. The *fontanels* should be palpated frequently during the infant's stay in the nursery to assure that they are flat. Pulsation of fontanels may be normal. Bulging or tenseness indicates increased intracranial pressure and should be reported immediately. A depressed fontanel may indicate dehydration. The posterior fontanel is much smaller than the anterior fontanel and may not be palpable during the first hours after birth because of the overriding of the sutures during delivery. It closes any time from birth to two months of age. The anterior fontanel remains open for at least 3 months and may be palpable for as long as 18 months after birth; however, it usually closes between 10 and 14 months.

The eyes, ears, nose, and mouth should be examined for asymmetries, malformations, and placement on the face in relation to each other. In addition to looking at the parts separately, the face as a whole should be carefully observed. Many genetically determined syndromes present with distinctive *facies*. Some of the syndromes are quite obvious, but others can be overlooked unless the proportions of the face are compared to the size of the head and body.

When picked up, the neonate will usually open his eyes; at this time they may be examined for hemorrhages, opacities of the lens, and discharges. If the baby is rotated laterally he will develop a *nystagmus* which does not persist after he is replaced in his crib. *Epicanthal folds* can be found in normal

TABLE 28-7
CHARACTERISTICS OF NEONATE'S BODY SEGMENTS

Characteristics of body segments	Usual manifestation	Normal variations	Comment
Head	Usually molded if vaginal delivery, round if cesarean section. Anterior and posterior fontanels and sutures palpable. Fine, silky hair covers scalp.	Less molding occurs if baby is not first-born or if head has not been engaged long. Size of fontanels and amount of overlapping of sutures varies considerably.	Asymmetries should be noted and evaluated.
Eyes	Dark or slate blue color. Open when awake and not crying. No tears. Equal pupils which react to light. Focuses briefly on face.	Lids may be edematous. Conjunctival hemorrhages may be apparent. Occasional uncoordinated movements normal. Some newborns will produce tears.	Note epicanthal folds, placement of eyes in relation to each other, discharges, persistent uncoordinated movements.
Nose	In midline. Seems flattened. Little nasal bridge. Breathes easily through nose.	May seem deformed due to passage through birth canal. Some mucus present in nares.	Test for patency of nares. Baby should breathe easily with mouth closed. Note nasal discharge.
Mouth	Lips pink. Tongue does not protrude. Sucking initiated when lips touched. Scant saliva.	Epstein's pearls present on gum margins. May have transient circumoral cyanosis. Transient 7th nerve paralysis shown by asymmetrical mouth movements when crying.	Distinguish between Epstein's pearls and thrush. Note abnormalities, i.e., excessive salivation, protruding tongue, high arched palate, lip notches. A short frenum is considered insignificant. Note cleft lip or palate.
Ears	Well-formed. Cartilage present. Stand out from skull. Placed so that at least part of ear lies above a line drawn from outer canthus of eye to external occipital protuberance.	Preauricular papillomas may be present. Amount of cartilage varies.	Look for branchial clefts, low placement, malformations. Lessened amount of cartilage indicates prematurity.
Neck	Short, straight, head moves freely side to side.		Note webbing, torticollis, masses, restriction of motion, distended veins.
Chest	Almost circular. Symmetrical movements with respirations. Breast tissue present in both sexes.	Milky secretion may be evident from nipples.	Observe for retractions, fracture of clavicle, asymmetry of placement of nipples, and chest expansion.

Abdomen	Rounded and prominent. Respirations are largely diaphragmatic. Umbilical stump dry within several hours of birth. Femoral pulses present, equal.	Umbilical hernia may be present and is usually insignificant.	Must make a distinction between a normally prominent abdomen and a distended one. A scaphoid abdomen is abnormal. Diminished abdominal breathing indicates intrathoracic disease. Compare appearance of chest and abdomen. Observe for signs of inguinal hernia. Note signs of bleeding or infection in umbilical stump.
Genitalia	In both sexes, genitalia tend to appear large in relation to rest of baby.	May have increased pigmentation in dark-skinned races. Edema present in breech deliveries.	Examine genitalia carefully for signs of genital ambiguity or other abnormalities.
Female	Labiae appear large, particularly labia minora.	Mucoid or bloody discharge from vagina may be present.	Keep clean by wiping front to back.
Male	Scrotum pendulous. Rugae cover sac. Testes descended. Tight prepuce which is adherent to glans. Meatal opening in center of glans penis.	Size of scrotum and penis varies widely. Testes may be in canal or retract into canal if baby is chilled.	Check for epi- or hypospadius, phimosis, hydrocele. If circumcised, watch for signs of bleeding and infection. If uncircumcised, do not retract foreskin.
Extremities	Generally flexed but can be put through full range of motion passively. Fists clenched. Legs bowed. Plantar fat pad makes feet appear flat.	May retain in utero position when sleeping. Feet may turn in but can be passively turned out.	Observe for gross abnormalities, limitation of movement in any joint, fractures, paralysis. Check for dislocated hip. Count fingers and toes. Note webbing or absence of digits. Note size and shape of hands and feet. Check for simian creases.
Back	Spine straight, easily flexed. When prone, baby can lift head momentarily. Shoulders, scapulae, iliac crests on same plane with each other.	Some asymmetries may be normal if due to unusual fetal position and can be passively corrected.	Check for spina bifida occulta, pilonidal sinus.
Anus	Patent. Proven by passage of meconium on rectal thermometer.	If frequent rectal temperatures have been taken, anus may be irritated.	Note fissures, bleeding. Once patency is determined, take axillary temperatures.

Caucasian babies; however, other signs of mongolism should be ruled out before concluding that these are normal.

Keratin cysts commonly known as *Epstein's pearls* appear as white blebs along the gum margins and at the junction of the hard and soft palates. They are a normal manifestation in the newborn infant and can be seen at birth. *Thrush*, which is an infection of the mucous membranes of the mouth usually caused by *Candida albicans*, may appear on the third or fourth day after delivery. The white patches of thrush appear on the tongue and cheeks as well as the gums. This disease should be reported promptly so treatment can be instituted. The production of *saliva is scant* during the first weeks of life. If a baby has a large amount of oral mucus the cause should be determined before he is fed. *Tracheoesophageal fistula* is a common cause of this symptom. In addition, a baby with large amounts of mucus needs careful watching to assure that he maintains a patent airway.

The baby's neck should flex, extend, and rotate easily. If limitation of motion is noted, *torticollis*, a shortening of the sternocleidomastoid muscle, may be suspected. The shortening is caused by rupture of the muscle during a difficult delivery or the presence of a tumor in the muscle.

The excessive amount of *breast tissue* found in newborn infants, as well as the occasional secretion of a milklike substance, is produced by the influence of maternal hormones which crossed the placenta. This phenomenon occurs in both sexes and gradually recedes by one month of age.

An abdomen which is unusually flat is called a *scaphoid abdomen*. A common cause of this condition is the presence of a *diaphragmatic hernia* which allows much of the abdominal contents to lie in the thorax. Severe respiratory distress often accompanies this anomaly.

Frequent inspection of the *umbilical stump* is necessary to note bleeding or signs of infection. Seventy percent alcohol is applied daily to prevent the growth of bacteria. In addition, drying of the stump is hastened by leaving it exposed to the air. By the second or third day the stump should be sufficiently dry so that the clamps may be removed. Alcohol applications should be continued until the cord drops off. Since this does not occur until the end of the first week, the mother should be instructed on proper care of the stump.

There is presently some question concerning the advisability of circumcising all male babies. Circumcision is no longer considered a "routine" procedure. Each baby should be evaluated individually and consent from the mother is obtained before the procedure is done. The pros and cons of the procedure should be explained to the mother so that she can make an informed decision. Unless the prepuce is so tight that it obstructs the passage of urine, there is no medical indication for circumcision. However, there are very sound reasons from a physiological standpoint for delaying the procedure until after the first week of life. These reasons include the danger of infection, the bleeding tendencies of the neonate, and the risk of removing too much foreskin if the procedure is not performed carefully.

NEUROMUSCULAR ENDOWMENT

At birth the normal baby has an intact and fully functioning neuromuscular system. The status of this system is manifested in the muscle tone and strength exhibited by the baby, the spontaneous movements, as well as the responses to various external stimuli, the type and quality of the reflexes, the functioning of the senses, and the overall behavior patterns. The initial physical examination will cover most of these areas; however, continuous evaluation of these items is necessary to assure that the baby is well and stays well.

Early signs of illness appear in the form of relatively small deviations from the normal behavior patterns of the infant. The nurse who handles the baby from day to day is usually the first person to notice these changes. Doctors rely upon the nurse's observations of the baby's behavior during feeding, sleeping, and diaper changes to alert them to the possibility that a given infant is becoming ill or has a previously undetected defect. Changes in behavior point to pathology not only in the central nervous system but in other systems as well.

In evaluating the *muscle tone* of the baby the nurse should check for the *recoil* response in the extremities. If normal recoil is present, the arm or leg will immediately return to the flexed position after being passively extended by the examiner. Another method of determining muscle tone is for the examiner to rapidly move the hand or foot back and forth. The baby will alternately let the part flop and resist flopping during this maneuver. Equal amounts of flopping and resistance to flopping is the normal pattern. When suspended ventrally the baby will not sag into an inverted U position but will exhibit some attempts to lift his head and legs. Likewise in daily handling the infant is not entirely limp as he is moved about.

A degree of hyper- or hypotonia may be normal for a given baby just as there are normal variations in the recoil response, joint motility, and resistance to flopping. The difficulty lies in deciding when a given baby's response is normal and when it is not. An obviously flaccid or spastic baby is easily recognized, but it takes familiarity with a number of babies to develop a "feel" for the more subtle manifestations of hyper- or hypotonia. For this reason the baby's general muscle tone should be evaluated every time the baby is handled.

Reflexes

Table 28-8 lists the common neurological reflexes which are normally present at birth. The normal healthy infant will exhibit all of the *reflexes* listed

TABLE 28-8
COMMON NEUROLOGICAL REFLEXES AT BIRTH

Characteristic reflexes	Usual manifestation	Normal variations	Comment
Yawning Stretching Sneezing Burping Hiccoughing	Present in normal newborn.	May be temporarily diminished by central nervous system depression due to maternal medication present in baby's system, anoxia, or infection.	These activities of the baby need to be brought to the mother's attention as mothers are often surprised and frightened if they are not prepared for this behavior.
Rooting	Present. Elicited by softly stroking either cheek, corners of mouth, or upper or lower lip.	Strongest in hungry infant. May disappear after infant has been fed.	If weak or absent, indicative of prematurity, neurological defect.
Sucking	Present. Elicited by placing firm object in baby's mouth.	Normal baby will suck when stimulated in this manner.	Suck should be vigorous with good suction produced. Poor sucking has same causes as poor rooting.
Swallowing	Present. When sucking, infant will swallow any liquid obtained.	May cough, gag, or vomit.	
Moro	Present. Elicited by sudden movement of head and neck causing retroflexion. Response consists of abduction, extension, and adduction of arms with extension of fingers followed by vigorous cry.	If baby is deeply asleep may not respond well. Leg movements may follow arm movement pattern.	Note absence, incompleteness or asymmetry of Moro reflex. Note changes in Moro from day to day. Note nature of cry (absent, weak, high pitched, excessive).
Tonic neck	Not always apparent in newborns. Elicited spontaneously when baby is supine if baby turns head to side or can be precipitated by manually turning head to side. Response consists of extension of arm toward which head is turned and flexion of opposite arm.	Response most prominent between two and four months. Response not sustained in newborn.	Note if response is asymmetrical (stronger on one side than the other). If response is complete, easy to elicit, and sustained in newborn it may indicate central nervous system damage.
Traction response	Present. Pull baby up by wrists. Head will lag but as reaches upright position head and chest will be in line	General muscle tone and condition of baby will affect response.	Head control improves as muscle strength increases.

	momentarily, then head will fall forward. He will re-erect head spontaneously or with slight stimulus.	Observe general muscle tone as baby is suspended.
Incurvature of trunk	Present. Suspend ventrally and stroke sides alternately. Baby should turn pelvis to side stimulated.	
Grasping, palmar	Present. Press finger into baby's palm. He should grasp strongly enough to be lifted momentarily from bed.	
Plantar	Present. Prompt flexing of toes upon application of pressure to ball of foot.	
Positive supporting reaction	Present. Lift baby vertically. He will usually flex legs. Touch soles to bed and he will extend legs, then trunk and head.	
Placing	Present. Hold baby vertically with one leg out of the way. Move other leg to touch edge of table. Baby will flex knee and try to place foot on table.	
Stepping	Present. Hold vertically. Tilt forward and to one side with feet touching hard surface. Will alternate feet as if walking.	

in Table 28-8 and many others not mentioned. There is some confusion among writers regarding the terminology used in discussing reflexes as well as disagreement concerning the age of appearance and disappearance of a given reflex and the proper manifestation of the reflex. With some reflexes, such as sucking and rooting, the presence or absence is the more important aspect; with others, such as the tonic neck or Moro reflex, the important characteristic is the pattern of the response. In evaluating reflexes the length of time the response is maintained can be important as well as whether or not the response is obligatory.

Since many factors influence the baby's response to external stimuli, a poor performance at one time is not diagnostic of central nervous system damage. In judging the response, the state of the baby (whether awake, fatigued, sleeping, hungry, or satiated) should be considered as well as the environmental temperature, other stimuli, amount of clothing on the baby, and any disturbing procedures done to the baby prior to the testing. Additional factors to consider are the existence of other congenital defects or birth injuries, the presence of jaundice, other symptoms of illness, and the time and amount of medication given to the mother prior to the infant's birth.

A poor performance at one observation period may increase the nurse's

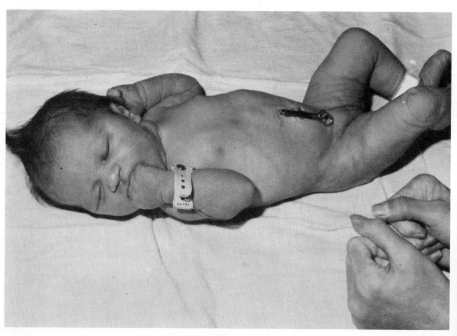

FIGURE 28-7
Baby at rest prior to testing for Moro reflex.

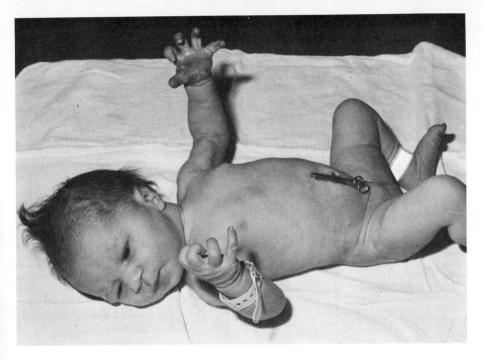

FIGURE 28-8
First stage in Moro response. Note abduction of arms and fanning of fingers.

"index of suspicion," but this should be followed by several examinations to determine a pattern of response for this particular baby. The gross abnormalities will be picked up readily, but subtle ones can escape notice for a considerable length of time. The nurse should know what reflexes the baby exhibited at his initial examination so that she can properly evaluate what she sees. If a reflex previously present is lost or diminished, this may be a significant fact to note. The state of the baby at the time the change in response was discovered should be recorded along with the response itself. Figures 28-7, 28-8, and 28-9 show the sequence of a Moro reaction. Figures 28-10 through 28-14 show typical reflex responses.

Senses

Table 28-9 describes how the neonate functions in regard to his basic senses. Although it is difficult to determine what the baby can see and hear, research over the past few years has led investigators to the conclusion that both these senses are better developed in the neonate than was previously

TABLE 28-9
CHARACTERISTIC SENSES AT BIRTH

Characteristics of senses	Usual manifestation	Common variations	Comment
Vision	Present. Baby blinks to bright light, tap on bridge of nose, or light touch of eyelid. Pupillary light reflex present. Fixates briefly on close objects.	May close lids to bright light or turn toward source of light.	It is normal for baby not to blink to a threatening movement.
Hearing	Present. Blinks to sound.	May respond to sound with eye movements, brief cessation of activity, startle reaction, or crying.	Routine testing of the hearing sense of newborns is performed in many nurseries. If the baby does not pass, he is usually referred for testing later. However, failure of hearing tests at this age is not diagnostic of deafness.
Touch	Present. Withdraws from painful stimuli including pressure and extremes of temperature.		
Taste	Present. Will have facial grimacing or make sucking motions to the four basic tastes.	May protrude tongue to try to get rid of substance.	Not necessary to test for taste or smell unless infant having trouble sucking.
Smell	Present.	Sense of smell may be stronger in infant than in adult but is hard to test for.	
Kinesthetic	Present.		See responses to change of position listed under reflexes.

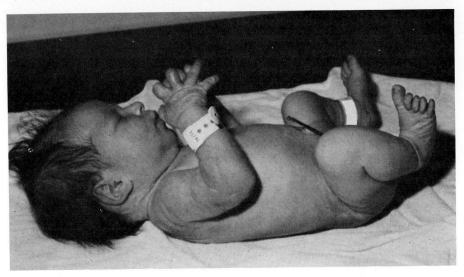

FIGURE 28-9
Second stage in Moro response. Note adduction of arms and flexion of legs.

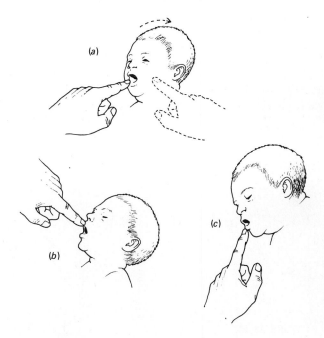

FIGURE 28-10
Rooting or reaction des points cardinoux.
(From Jerome Hellmuth (ed.), The Exceptional Child, vol.
I of The Normal Infant, Special Child Publications, Seattle,
Wash., 1967, p. 87.)

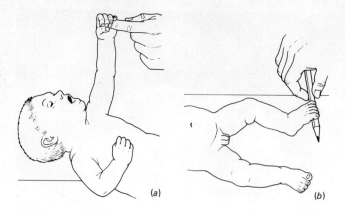

FIGURE 28-11
Grasp reflexes.
(From Jerome Hellmuth (ed.), The Exceptional Child, vol. I of The Normal Infant, Special Child Publications, Seattle, Wash., 1967, p. 88.)

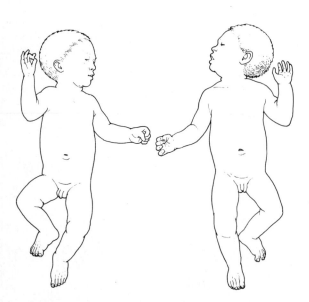

FIGURE 28-12
Tonic neck reflex.
(From Jerome Hellmuth (ed.), The Exceptional Child, vol. I of The Normal Infant, Special Child Publications, Seattle, Wash., 1967, p. 100.)

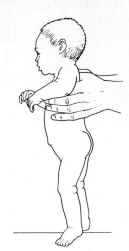

FIGURE 28-13
Reflexes in vertical suspension; positive
supporting reaction.
(From Jerome Hellmuth (ed.), The Exceptional Child, vol. I of The Normal Infant,
Special Child Publications, Seattle, Wash.,
1967, p. 108.)

thought. It is now felt that the baby has acute hearing after the middle ear
and eustachian tubes have been cleared of amniotic fluid. A baby's response
to loud noises consists of a startle, crying, or blinking, but the infant will
not turn toward the sound. These responses are the basis for the testing of
newborn infants' hearing, which is being done in many nurseries. Although
a failure to pass a hearing test in the newborn nursery is not diagnostic of
deafness, all babies failing such tests should be referred for later testing.

In regard to vision, it is believed that the baby can fixate on an object
perhaps with both eyes but certainly with one. The peripheral vision is well

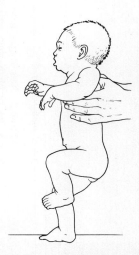

FIGURE 28-14
Reflexes in vertical suspension; the stepping
reaction.
(From Jerome Hellmuth (ed.), The Exceptional Child, vol. I of The Normal Infant,
Special Child Publications, Seattle, Wash.,
1967, p. 109.)

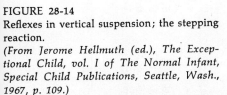

TABLE 28-10
NORMAL RANGE OF BEHAVIOR AT BIRTH

Characteristic behavior	Usual manifestation	Common variations	Comment
Activity	Goes through three stages in recovery from shock of birth, then settles into a pattern peculiar to the individual baby.	Ranges from deep sleep to intense activity during crying.	Need to distinguish between normal activity and the extremes of irritability or lethargy. Wide variation in normality.
Awake, not crying	Jerky movements. Symmetrical in arms, alternating in legs.	May be jittery or tremulous. Jaw and ankle clonus common.	Need to distinguish between normal "jitteriness" and convulsive twitching.
Awake, crying	Vigorous movements of all extremities accompanied by loud crying.	May have color changes during crying. Veins on forehead may stand out. May produce tears.	Watch for symmetry of movements. Character (sound quality) and frequency of crying should be noted. Any odd-sounding cries should be reported.
Sleeping	Sleeps quietly and when deeply asleep, is hard to arouse. Spends about 19–22 hours a day sleeping.	May twitch or jerk during sleep. Some babies sleep as little as 16 hours a day.	
Feeding	Sucks vigorously when nipple placed in mouth. Takes 2 to 4 ounces at a time.	May regurgitate mucus during early feedings. May vomit mucus, blood, or amniotic fluid.	Some vomiting and regurgitation is normal, but there is a narrow line between normality and pathology.
Voiding	Voids at birth or within 2 to 3 hours.	May not void for 12 hours.	If infant doesn't void by 24 hours, notify doctor. Observe force of urinary stream, color, and odor of urine.
Stooling	Meconium passed during first 24 hours after birth.	May not pass meconium for 48 hours after birth.	Meconium passed before or during birth is suggestive of fetal distress. Note time and amount of meconium expelled.

developed, and the infant has some ability to discriminate colors and patterns. Transient strabismus and nystagmus are normal in the newborn period.

Behavior

As Table 28-10 illustrates, the normal range of behavior for infants is very wide. At one end of the spectrum lie those infants who are placid, rarely cry, respond to stimuli in a muted fashion, and seem relatively indifferent to their environment. At the other end of the scale are those infants who are awake and crying much of the time. They tend to eat rapidly, regurgitate after feeding, and have frequent stools. They seem to be very alert to their environment and are easily disturbed by noises or handling. In between these extremes lie the majority of newborn infants. It is important for the nurse to observe and record the behavior pattern of each infant so changes can be readily identified. The information obtained can be used by the physician in the diagnosis of disease and by the nurse in helping the mother to become acquainted with her baby. Illustrations (C) and (D) of the color plate depict babies in various states of activity.

The urine of the neonate is scant in amount and pale yellow in color with a low specific gravity and a typical urine odor. Since one of the signs of some inborn errors of metabolism is a peculiar odor to the urine, it is necessary to note the odor as well as the color of each baby's urine. One of the inborn errors of metabolism, phenylketonuria, can now be detected by a blood test done on the baby after he has had 24 hours of a milk diet. This test is being routinely done on all babies before discharge. The infant voids frequently so the nurse usually has an opportunity to observe the force of the urinary stream. If the baby is noted to dribble urine more or less constantly and never exhibits a forceful stream, the possibility exists that there is an obstruction of the urinary tract. Occasionally babies will have a pinkish stain on their diaper which is caused by the presence of uric acid crystals in their urine. This condition will clear spontaneously.

The initial stool passed by the baby is a sticky, greenish-black, odorless substance. (See illustration (E) in the color plate.) It consists of the accumulation of secretions in the gastrointestinal tract, called *meconium*. As illustration (F) shows, after the baby begins to take milk, his stool goes through a *transitional stage* during which it is yellowish-green. When all of the meconium has been expelled the baby's stool is soft and yellow. A normal infant stool is shown in illustration (G). The physician should be notified if the stool deviates from the pattern described. Blood in the stool should be tested to determine whether it is of maternal or fetal origin. Passage of meconium in large amounts indicates the gastrointestinal tract is patent. It is possible for the baby to have a complete or partial obstruction in the upper part of the tract and still pass some meconium. Therefore, it is necessary to record the amount of meconium expelled as well as the fact that it was passed.

REFERENCES

1 Yao, A. C., et al.: "Expiratory Grunting in the Late Clamped Normal Neonate," *Pediatrics*, 48:865–870, 1971.
2 Hey, E. N., and Bridget O'Connell: "Oxygen Consumption and Heat Balance in the Cot-nursed Baby," *Archives of Disease in Childhood*, 45:335–343, 1970.
3 Hey, E. N., and G. Katz: "The Optimum Thermal Environment for Naked Babies," *Archives of Disease in Childhood*, 45:328–334, 1970.
4 Adamson, Karlis: "The Role of Thermal Factors in Fetal and Neonatal Life," *Pediatric Clinics of North America*, 13:599–619, 1966.
5 Apgar, Virginia: "The Newborn (Apgar) Scoring System: Reflections and Advice," *Pediatric Clinics of North America*, 13:645–650, 1966.
6 *Standards and Recommendations for Hospital Care of Newborn Infants*, 5th ed., Committee on Fetus and Newborn, American Academy of Pediatrics, Evanston, Ill., 1971, pp. 103–104.
7 Ibid., p. 104.
8. Kempe, C. Henry, et al.: *Current Pediatric Diagnosis and Treatment*, Lange, Los Altos, Calif., 1970, pp. 40–41.
9 Hathaway, William E.: "Coagulation Problems in the Newborn Infant," *Pediatric Clinics of North America*, 17:929–942, 1970.
10 Guyton, Arthur C.: *Textbook of Medical Physiology*, 3d ed., Saunders, Philadelphia, 1966, p. 1177.
11 Kempe: op. cit., p. 60.
12 Desmond, M. M., et al.: "The Transitional Care Nursery," *Pediatric Clinics of North America*, 13:651–668, 1966.
13 Kempe: op. cit., p. 43.
14 Guyton: op. cit., p. 1179.
15 *Standards and Recommendations for Hospital Care of Newborn Infants*, pp. 10, 40–42, and 47–54.
16 Guyton: op. cit., pp. 1179 and 1100.
17 Gellis, Sydney S., and Benjamin M. Kagan: *Current Pediatric Therapy—4*, Saunders, Philadelphia, 1970, p. 655.

BIBLIOGRAPHY

Adamson, Karlis: "The Role of Thermal Factors in Fetal and Neonatal Life," *Pediatric Clinics of North America*, 13:599–619, 1966.
Apgar, Virginia, et al.: "Evaluation of the Newborn Infant—Second Report," *Journal of the American Medical Association*, 168:1985–1988, 1958.
Barness, Lewis A.: *Manual of Pediatric Physical Diagnosis*, 3d ed., Year Book, Chicago, 1966.

Barnett, Henry: *Pediatrics*, 14th ed., Appleton-Century-Crofts, New York, 1968.

Benson, Ralph C.: *Handbook of Obstetrics and Gynecology*, 4th ed., Lange, Los Altos, Calif., 1971.

Desmond, M. M., A. J. Rudolph, and R. Phitaksphraiwan: "The Transitional Care Nursery," *Pediatric Clinics of North America*, 13:651–668, 1966.

Fink, H. William: "The Newborn at First Glance," *Hospital Topics*, 44:99–101, 1966.

Fitzpatrick, Elise, Sharon Reeder, and Luigi Mastroianni: *Maternity Nursing*, 12th ed., Lippincott, Philadelphia, 1971.

Gellis, Sydney S., and Benjamin M. Kagan: *Current Pediatric Therapy—4*, Saunders, Philadelphia, 1970.

Guyton, Arthur C.: *Textbook of Medical Physiology*, 3d ed., Saunders, Philadelphia, 1966.

Haynes, Una: *A Developmental Approach to Casefinding*, Children's Bureau, Washington, D.C., 1967.

Hellmuth, Jerome (ed.): *The Exceptional Infant*, vol. I of *The Normal Infant*, Special Child Publications, Seattle, Wash., 1967.

Hey, E. N., and G. Katz: "The Optimum Thermal Environment for Naked Babies," *Archives of Disease in Childhood*, 45:328–334, 1970.

———, and Bridget O'Connell: "Oxygen Consumption and Heat Balance in the Cot-nursed Baby," *Archives of Disease in Childhood*, 45:335–343, 1970.

Hymovich, Debra P.: *Nursing of Children: A Guide for Study*, Saunders, Philadelphia, 1969.

Kempe, C. Henry, et al.: *Current Pediatric Diagnosis and Treatment*, Lange, Los Altos, Calif., 1970.

———: *Current Pediatric Diagnosis and Treatment*, Lange, Los Altos, Calif., 1972.

Lanzkowsky, Philip, et al.: "Phototherapy—A Note of Caution," *Pediatrics*, 48:969–971, 1971.

Marlow, Dorothy R.: *Textbook of Pediatric Nursing*, 2d ed., Saunders, Philadelphia, 1965.

McKilligan, Helen R.: *The First Day of Life: Principles of Neonatal Nursing*, Springer, New York, 1970.

Nelson, Waldo E., et al.: *Textbook of Pediatrics*, 9th ed., Saunders, Philadelphia, 1969.

Quinn, Norman J.: "Diagnostic Catheter Examinations of the Newborn," *Clinical Pediatrics*, 10:251–256, 1971.

Standards and Recommendations for Hospital Care of Newborn Infants, 5th ed., American Academy of Pediatrics, Committee on Fetus and Newborn, Evanston, Ill., 1971.

Stuart, Harold C., and Dane G. Prugh (eds.): *The Healthy Child*, Harvard, Cambridge, Mass., 1970.

Watson, Ernest H., and George H. Lowery: *Growth and Development of Children*, 5th ed., Year Book, Chicago, 1967.

Whipple, Dorothy V.: *Dynamics of Development: Euthenic Pediatrics*, McGraw-Hill, New York, 1966.

Yao, A. C., et al.: "Expiratory Grunting in the Late Clamped Normal Neonate," *Pediatrics*, 48:865–870, 1971.

29 | PHYSICAL EXAMINATION OF THE NEWBORN

Ann Noordenbos Smith

Physical examination skills have become increasingly important to the nurse as new and extended nursing responsibilities are assumed in the nursery as well as in various community settings. Nurses are being called upon to make initial physical examinations of infants, hospital discharge examinations, and routine follow-up examinations. Public health nurses frequently perform physical examinations of infants in the home setting. In some areas of the country these examinations may follow home delivery. An increasing number of public health nurses are including physical examination as an integral part of a complete infant health evaluation in a well-baby clinic or a child health conference.

This chapter will focus on methods and techniques of examination of the infant. Details of specific findings or normal variations of findings in the newborn and early infancy period are described elsewhere in this text.

GENERAL CONSIDERATIONS

Before beginning the examination the nurse carefully reviews the antenatal history, including the health of the mother during pregnancy, medical supervision, diet, infections or other illnesses, complications of pregnancy, Rh typing and serology, and any drugs taken. Information regarding the birth history includes duration of the pregnancy, birth weight and length, gestational age, kind and duration of labor, type of delivery, sedation and anesthesia, resuscitation required, and Apgar score. The infant's body temperature, weight, respiratory rate, pulse rate, cry, color, and feeding activity are also evaluated. Such information from the infant's and mother's medical histories gives the examiner valuable clues as to where abnormality or pathology may be detected.

A systematic, orderly method is of extreme importance in performing a physical examination. Approaches to the infant may be modified according to varying circumstances; however, even modifications of the nurse's technique of the examination should be done in an orderly sequence so that no part of the examination will be missed.

The basic methods of examination include inspection, palpation, percussion, and auscultation—in that order. The nurse should develop a rigid routine of looking first, then touching, tapping (where appropriate) and then listening.

The system of examination described in this chapter begins with general observation of the infant, proceeds to examination of the skin, feet, lower extremities, genitalia, abdomen, chest, anus, back, neck, upper extremities, head, face, eyes, ears, mouth, and throat and is completed with a basic neurological evaluation. This particular system has the advantage of performing the most uncomfortable parts of the examination (evaluation of the ears, mouth and throat, and elicitation of the startle reflex) last.

The examiner should modify the system of examination according to the situation and the particular infant. For example, in approaching a sleeping infant, it may be best to begin by examining the abdomen and chest. If the infant is crying at the time of examination, one may wish to defer careful examination of the abdomen or the eyes until later. If the examining room is cool, as happens in some well-baby clinics, the nurse may wish to examine the infant's head and extremities first, and then proceed to the parts of the examination which require the infant to be exposed. After becoming familiar and knowledgeable with a systematic method of examination, the nurse then can adapt it to suit the particular circumstances.

The nurse's principal objective while carrying out the examination is to recognize and differentiate normal and abnormal findings, much in the same manner in which any patient is appraised for signs and symptoms pertaining to his condition. Skilled examination requires both broad and specific knowledge of the range of normal physical and behavioral findings of the normal infant. Findings which are dependent upon age or normal physiological processes must be differentiated from those indicating pathology. Abnormalities needing medical attention or correction must be differentiated from those which are self-limited or self-correcting.

Instruments needed for the basic physical examination include:

1 Stethoscope with diaphragm and bell. Of all the nurse's instruments, the stethoscope in particular should become a personal instrument. The ear pieces should be large enough and should fit the ears. Familiarity with one's own stethoscope reduces the possibility of mistaking extraneous sounds for physiological or pathological sounds.

2 Otoscope, preferably with a diagnostic head attachment. Batteries should be replaced frequently. The otoscope light should always be white and bright. Any dimness or suggestion of yellow indicates the batteries or bulb should be changed.

3 Ophthalmoscope. Most ophthalmoscopes are a standard size and fit handles which are interchangeable for otoscopes and ophthalmoscopes.

4 Tongue blade.

5 Measuring tape.

6 Small rattle or other noisemaker.

7 Flashlight or penlight.

Many nurses find it convenient to purchase their own instruments because of the advantage of using a familiar instrument and being able to maintain their instruments in a clean and working condition.

Infants are best examined on a table or in the crib and in an area where good lighting is assured. A pacifier may be used to help quiet the infant during the examination. The examiner's hands should be clean and warm and are washed after examination of areas of the body contaminated by urine and feces before moving to clean areas.

Afterward, a detailed recording is made of the examination, including all pertinent positive and negative findings. This record should be of such quality as to provide valuable base-line data for any other health professionals who may subsequently examine or have responsibility for the infant. A standard checklist for recording the examination is recommended. Adhering to a standardized system of recording the examination, even though the examination may have been performed in a different order, makes it easier for others to identify specific information more efficiently.

General appearance	Neck
Skin	Thorax
Lymph nodes	Lungs
Head	Heart
Face	Abdomen
Eyes	Genitalia
Nose	Anus
Mouth	Extremities
Throat	Spine and back
Ears	Neurological exam

THE EXAMINATION
General Observations

Careful observation of the infant before beginning the actual examination will provide valuable general impressions which can later be confirmed or modified. General size in relation to age is noted; any gross abnormality may be observed. Whether the infant has extra subcutaneous tissue is also noted. The infant's state of consciousness is evaluated—whether he is awake, irritable, alert, drowsy, lethargic, listless, or asleep. General activity, breathing, movement of extremities, and head and eye movements are observed. The infant's position at rest is studied, including whether his extremities are extended or flexed and any symmetry or asymmetry of position and body parts.

A general impression of skin color is gained. Is the infant ruddy or pale? Is the pigmentation of the skin uniform? Is the infant jaundiced or cyanotic? Does color change in relation to respirations and activity? Respirations are evaluated as to their depth, rate, and degree of regularity. Any change in behavior or activity during the examination is observed. If the infant begins to cry, the quality and pitch of the cry are noted. Crying should be stimulated if it does not occur spontaneously.

While undressing the infant fully in order to perform the examination, evaluation of response to stimulation and of muscle tone is made. Is the infant hypotonic or floppy? Is he jittery? Are his arms held in tight flexion? Does he startle easily?

Skin

Particular note of the skin is made at the outset of the examination and as each area of the body is examined. Basic morphology of lesions is observed and described whenever possible. Color, consistency, and hydration are noted. Mongolian spots, hemangiomas, presence and amount of vernix caseosa, lanugo, desquamation, macules, or papules are noted. Pallor, beefy red skin, presence of jaundice or cyanosis should be described. The skin is palpated to detect and evaluate any scaling, striae, turgor, edema, or ecchymosis. Skin turgor may be checked over the back of the lower leg or thigh or on the abdomen by grasping the skin between thumb and index finger and allowing the skin to return to its former position and noting whether the skin springs back or a fold persists for several seconds after being released.

Feet and Legs

With the infant in a supine position, color and temperature of the feet are compared, then each foot is examined separately. The toes are counted.

Extra digits, webbing, or abnormal spacing between the first and second toe are noted, and length of the toenails and color of the nailbeds are determined.

The Babinski reflex is elicited by stroking the plantar surface of the foot firmly with a sharp object such as the edge of a tongue blade. Grasp reflex of the toes may be elicited by stroking the bottom of the foot at the base of the toes.

Alignment of the foot and leg is noted. The feet at birth are usually held in varus or valgus attitude but can be straightened without forceful manual stretching. Range of motion of the ankle is determined to check for tight heel cords. Flexion and extension of the ankle should have a range of about 130 degrees.

The presence of ankle clonus is checked by stabilizing the leg with the foot held up from the table. With the examiner's thumbs on the distal part of the soles of the feet, the feet are dorsiflexed rapidly three to four times. One or two continued movements are normal; continued rapid clonic movement is abnormal.

The Achilles deep tendon reflex may be tested by dorsiflexing the foot and tapping the back of the heel with the flat of the finger and noting whether there is an ankle jerk due to plantar flexion of the foot. This reflex is often difficult to obtain in the newborn.

The resting position of the legs is noted. The legs are aligned and examined for bowing or internal or medial torsion of the tibia and knock-knee. A mild degree of bowing or medial rotation is considered normal in the newborn. The muscle mass of the legs is palpated for asymmetry or atrophy. Recoil of the lower extremities is tested by extending and then releasing the legs. Both legs return promptly to the flexed position in the full-term infant.

The patellar deep tendon reflex can be obtained in the newborn by tapping the patella with the flat of the finger. Range of motion of the knee is checked. The legs should fully flex on to the thigh, and the knees should not hyperextend.

Medial skin folds are inspected for symmetry on the anterior and posterior thigh. The presence of extra folds or asymmetry of folds may indicate hip dislocation.

Further investigation for congenital dislocation of the hip (Barlow's two-stage maneuver) is done by flexing the hips and knees, abducting the hips, and applying pressure forward with the examiner's fingers behind the great trochanter. When hip instability exists, a "clunk" is felt and often seen or heard as the femoral head snaps over the posterior acetabular rim into the socket. The hips are then flexed and slightly abducted, and pressure is applied to the upper medial thigh. If a "clunk" is detected, the hip can be dislocated backward.

Range of motion of the hip is examined and should be about 160 to 170 degrees in flexion and extension. The thighs flexed at the hip should abduct to an angle of about 160 degrees between the thighs. Limited abduction of one or both hips may indicate the presence of hip dysplasia.

Genitalia

Female genitalia is inspected structurally for the presence of labia majora, labia minora, clitoris, and vaginal orifice. In the newborn the external genitalia are often turgescent, the clitoris and labia minora are prominent, and a hymenal tag may be noted at the vaginal orifice. Any adhesion of the labia minora with occlusion of the vaginal orifice should be detected. Vaginal discharge, if present, is examined. The urethral meatus is difficult to visualize in the newborn; however, voiding should be observed, including the character (gushing or dribbling) of the stream.

In examination of the male genitalia the position of the urethral orifice is noted. The meatal opening should appear as a slit instead of round. In the uncircumcised male during early infancy adhesions may be present between the prepuce and the glans of the penis which prevent retraction of the prepuce so that the meatal opening cannot be visualized. This condition is not abnormal unless urinary flow is obstructed or signs of infection are evident.

The scrotum is inspected for symmetry and size. In newborn infants the scrotum may be small and firm or fairly loose, relaxed, and pendulous. Placing the thumb and index finger of one hand over the inguinal canal, the testes are palpated separately between thumb and finger with the other hand. The testes, measuring about 1 cm, and the spermatic cords are the only contents palpable in the scrotum. The presence of any other masses, tenseness, or bulging is abnormal. Stimulation of the cremasteric reflex by stroking the inner aspect of the thigh will cause the testis to rise in the scrotum or into the inguinal canal.

The inguinal area is examined for bulges, which may indicate the presence of hernia, and for lymph nodes. The presence and quality of femoral pulses are checked with the fingertips held firmly along the inguinal ligament.

Abdomen

Inspection of the abdomen precedes palpation, percussion, and auscultation. Abdominal breathing is noted, and respirations are counted. Degree of symmetry or asymmetry of the abdomen is observed. Any fullness, distention, or localized bulging of the abdomen, which may indicate hernia, diastasis recti, or weakness of abdominal musculature, is determined. The condition and turgor of the skin and presence or absence of superficial abdominal veins are determined. The umbilical cord should be carefully inspected for the presence of abnormal redness, wetness of the stump, or odor.

The abdomen is palpated in a systematic manner in order to detect any abnormality in the abdominal musculature or tenderness, organ enlargement, or abdominal mass.

Superficial palpation is performed with the flat surface of the fingers or fingertips, beginning in any one of the quadrants and proceeding in a clockwise manner until the entire abdomen is examined. Any weakness or herniation of the abdominal musculature is recorded as well as whether the abdomen is soft or hard or if tenderness is present. Tenderness is difficult to evaluate in the infant and may be correlated only with irritability or crying during the examination.

The edge or border of the liver may be palpable in the normal newborn. Palpating lightly with the fingertips from right lower to upper quadrant, the liver edge may be detected 1 to 2 cm below the right rib margin. The eleventh and twelfth floating ribs may be mistaken for superficial masses. The tip of the spleen may be felt at times in the normal newborn as a superficial mass in the lateral portion of the left upper quadrant.

After palpating the abdomen lightly, the four quadrants are palpated more deeply with the flat surface of the fingers. The kidneys may be felt immediately after birth. Masses may represent tumors, cysts, or structural abnormalities; all masses should be considered abnormal until adequately explained.

The abdomen is percussed by placing the finger of one hand firmly against the abdominal wall and using the index or middle finger of the other hand as a percussion hammer. All areas of the abdomen are quickly percussed to determine whether increased tympany or resonance is present. Distention of the abdomen and an increase in resonance indicate the presence of gas in the abdomen; distention of the abdomen with little resonance suggests fluid or solid masses in the abdomen.

Auscultation of the abdomen for peristalsis is done by placing the stethoscope firmly over the abdomen and listening carefully for metallic tinkling sounds. The sounds are of low intensity and occur with an approximate frequency of two to five per minute.

Chest

Inspection of the chest precedes palpation, percussion, and auscultation. Shape and size; the presence of gross anomalies, tumors, or fractures; a depressed sternum or any asymmetry of the chest; and breathing movements and rate are evaluated. Particular note is made of intercostal spaces and supra- and substernal areas to detect signs of labored breathing or retractions.

The breasts are inspected for presence of breast tissue, enlargement, signs of infection, development of the nipples and areola, and the presence of any supernumerary nipples, which may appear below the nipple line or in the axillary region.

The chest is examined for bulging or visible heart beat.

The entire chest is palpated with the flat surface of the fingers or finger-tips. The clavicles are examined for tenderness or the presence of crepitance or a bony mass which may indicate fracture. The presence or absence of breast engorgement is confirmed. Location of the apex beat gives information about heart size and location. Any abnormal vibratory thrills are recorded. Examination for lymph nodes in the axillary areas, rarely found in the normal new-born, is performed by gently palpating the chest wall in the axilla with the fingertips.

Percussion of the chest of the newborn infant usually reveals little information because of the difficulty of localizing the vibrations.

The chest is auscultated to determine the rate, rhythm, and quality of heart sounds. Auscultation is best performed with a stethoscope that can be fitted snugly against the chest. A small bell stethoscope is best for localizing specific sounds.

Auscultation of the heart includes listening over the entire precordium, below the left axilla, and posteriorly below the scapula. Special attention is paid to the areas where cardiac valve sounds are best heard—at the apex (mitral), at the second interspace to the left of the sternum (pulmonary), at the second interspace to the right of the sternum (aortic), and at the junction of xiphoid and the sternum (tricuspid). The first heart sound is due to closure of the mitral and tricuspid valves. The second heart sound is due to aortic and pulmonic valve closure.

Attention is given to listening to one thing at a time. First the rate and then the rhythm are determined. Differentiation is made between the first and second heart sounds, and these sounds are compared at the various listening posts; they should be sharp and clear. Extra sounds, sound of poor quality, or murmurs accompanying these heart sounds are considered abnormal.

The entire chest is then auscultated for breath sounds in a systematic manner, comparing one side of the thorax to the other. The type of breath sound, the presence of any extraneous sounds, rales, rhonchi, and wheezes are noted. A considerable amount of experience in determining the wide range of breath sounds is necessary before confidence in such evaluation is established. Turning the infant to a prone position, the posterior thorax is examined in a similar manner.

Back and Spine

With the infant in a prone position the entire posterior surface of his body is observed and palpated.

The presence of hair is checked. Hair is sometimes seen over the shoulders and back of the newborn, especially premature infants, but it disappears by three months of age. Tufts of hair anywhere over the spine, especially over the sacrum, may mark the site of a spina bifida occulta or spina bifida.

Any masses over the spine or abnormal curvatures of the spine should be noted. The size, shape, and symmetry of the scapulae are determined.

The buttocks and anus are inspected. Presence and character of stool are recorded, and any excoriation or fissure of the anal mucosa should be detected. If a pilonidal dimple is present in the coccygeal area, it should be carefully examined for the presence of infection, which may accompany a pilonidal cyst or sinus.

Neck

Examination of the neck begins while the infant is in a prone position. The neck is inspected for position (torticollis, opisthotonus), swellings, and edema. Webbing of the neck is difficult to determine in the infant and may appear as an extra skin fold on the back of the neck. If the infant lifts his head while in the prone position, this is observed. Motion of the neck is determined by gently rotating the infant's head from side to side and from flexion to extension. The neck is palpated for presence of lymph nodes and masses, and the sternocleidomastoid muscles are also palpated for masses. With the infant in a supine position the trachea is palpated to detect any deviation from the midline.

Arms and Hands

The upper extremities are inspected for congenital anomalies, including absence or defects of parts or all of the extremity. Are the extremities unusually long and thin? Are they broad and short? The position of the arms and hands at rest is observed. Does the infant flex his arms? The full-term newborn will exhibit flexion of the upper extremities with hands held in a grasping or clenched position. The arms are extended by the examiner beside the body; when released, there is prompt flexion at the elbow.

Fingers are checked for the following: clubbing; color and temperature, as well as any difference in color or temperature between the extremities; webbing or the presence of extra digits; length of the fingernails; any unusual shortness or curvature of the little fingers; presence of a simian crease on the palm of the hand. The grasp reflex is elicited by pressing the palmar surface of the hand with the examiner's index finger.

Range of motion of the wrist, elbow, and shoulder is recorded. Flexion of the hand at the wrist is about 110 degrees, and extension is 80 degrees; range of motion at the elbow is about 170 degrees. The shoulder abducts from the trunk about 120 degrees. The entire arm is palpated for any masses or fracture.

The biceps tendon reflex is sometimes difficult to elicit in the newborn. The examiner places the index finger of one hand on the tendon of the biceps muscle in the elbow area. The examiner's ring finger is on the wrist and the middle finger is underneath the arm. Using the index finger of the other hand, the examiner taps the finger which covers the tendon of the biceps. A short contraction can be observed and felt.

Head

The entire occiput is inspected. The shape of the head is examined for asymmetry due to edema, hematoma, molding, presence and character of hair, and condition of the scalp.

The infant's head is next palpated, and particular attention is given to the sutures and fontanels. The sutures are normally felt as ridges immediately after birth and any overriding of the sutures should be noted. Within a day the suture lines may be felt as depressions in the normal infant. The anterior and posterior fontanels are palpated and measured, and the presence of any other fontanel should be noticed. Tension of the anterior fontanel, whether it is depressed or bulging, is determined while the infant is in a sitting position. The normal anterior fontanel can be expected to be slightly depressed when the infant is sitting. Slight pulsations of the anterior fontanel are also normal. Edema of the scalp or cephalhematoma should be detected by palpation.

Measurement of head circumference is done by placing the measuring tape just above the infant's eyebrows and, posteriorly, over the most prominent part of the occiput.

FACE

Examination of the face begins with observation for symmetry between the left and right sides and between symmetrical parts. When the infant grimaces or cries it is noticed whether the facial contortions are symmetrical. The skin is inspected for edema, uneven pigmentation, hair, ecchymosis, or lesions. Spacing of the eyes is examined to detect hypotelorism or hypertelorism. Facial expressions of blandness, alertness, fussing, or crying are observed.

EYES

Examination of the eyes may be difficult in the newborn period because of the tendency for the infant to keep his eyes shut or because of periorbital edema. It is usually not helpful to attempt to forcibly hold the eye open. Gentle rocking of the head frequently causes the infant to open his eyes.

The structure of the eyelid and eye is inspected for the following abnormalities: bulging or sunken eyes; any drooping, edema, or inflammation of the eyelids; discharge from the eye; conjunctival edema; vascular infection; and scleral hemorrhage. The color of the sclerae should be noted.

The blink reflex may be stimulated by shining a bright light in the eyes. The cornea should be bright and shiny when illuminated by the examiner's light. Any haziness or dullness is abnormal. The color of the iris is noted, as is the shape (round, oval, or irregular) and the size (normal, constricted, or dilated) of the pupil.

The reaction of the pupils to light can be tested by shading one eye with the hand for a moment and checking whether the pupillary response is absent, discernible, or normal.

Whether the eyes are centered or deviated to the left or right and whether nystagmus is present should be recorded.

To use the ophthalmoscope, dim the lights in the room, set the opthalmoscope at 0 or −1, and direct the ophthalmoscope light at the pupil; a small red-orange circular spot should appear. This is the red reflex, caused by the light shining on the retina, and it indicates that opacities of the lens or other obstructions are not present.

NOSE

The nose is inspected for abnormality of shape, unusual flattening, flaring of the nares, patency, or nasal discharge. If sneezing occurs, it should be noted.

EARS

The ears are inspected for size, shape, position, and anomaly. An imaginary line is drawn between the lateral canthus of the eye and the most prominent point of the posterior occiput; the top of the ear should fall above this line.

Hearing is tested by sounding a bell or rattle near the infant's head. Blinking of the eyes, momentary cessation of activity, or startle activity indicates a positive response.

Otoscopic examination of the newborn often yields little information at birth because of the presence of vernix and debris in the canal, but the eardrum usually is visualized after a few days.

The otoscope is held between thumb and first finger with the other fingers resting on the infant's head. With the examiner's other hand the ear is pulled back and downward to straighten the canal, and the 3-mm speculum is introduced gently.

The condition of the canal is first inspected; then the color and landmarks of the tympanic membrane or eardrum are determined. The color of the normal drum is gray to bluish-white and translucent or opalescent. The landmarks of the normal tympanic membrane are caused by the position of the membrane in relation to the bones of the middle ear, particularly the malleus. Infection or other abnormality causes the landmarks to become distorted or absent.

The following landmarks are observed on the normal eardrum:

1 The umbo or point of maximum convexity of the drum, which appears as a white spot at about the center of the eardrum.

2 The long process or handle of the malleus, which appears as a small white streak running up and forward from the umbo.

3 The short process of the malleus, which is a small white process at the upper end of the malleus.

4 The light reflex, which is sharply defined cone-shaped reflection from the otoscope light, with the apex at the umbo and the base in the anterior inferior portion of the drum.

MOUTH AND THROAT

An adequate source of light (flashlight or penlight) and a small tongue blade are required for examination of the mouth and throat. First the lips are inspected for anomalies, such as harelip, and for dryness and lesions. The buccal mucosa, gums, and palate are examined, and note is made whether the palate has an unusually high arch and whether a cleft of the hard or soft palate exists.

It may be necessary to palpate the palate with the finger to ascertain whether a submucous cleft palate is present. Bohn's nodules and Epstein's pearls, small retention cysts on the midline of the palate or on the gums, may be detected. The tongue is examined for size and mobility. Generally, if the frenulum can be visualized or if the tip of the tongue is observed extending over the lower gum margin, significant tongue-tie is not present.

While using the tongue blade to hold the tongue on the floor of the mouth, the throat is then examined. The light and tongue blade are employed simultaneously so that when the infant gags the examiner is prepared to view the uvula and pharynx. Presence of the gag reflex and position of the uvula are observed, including bifurcation of the uvula if present.

Neurological Evaluation

The neurological evaluation is usually performed as an integral part of the basic physical examination, although the response of the infant to specific stimuli may be evaluated at the completion of the exam.

During the general observation, certain assessments are made which are most significant in the neurological appraisal. Eye and respiration movement and resting posture and motor activity have been evaluated. Movement of the arms and legs is observed throughout the exam as to whether the arms and legs are in flexion or extension postures and whether unequal movement of one extremity, jerking, or tremors occur. Facial expression is evaluated. The shape and size of the pupils and reaction of pupils to light has been tested. The upper and lower extremities have been moved through their full range of motion and resistance to this movement evaluated. Achilles, knee-jerk, and biceps tendon reflexes as well as palmar and plantar grasp and the Babinski reflex have been tested.

In addition, the rooting reflex is elicited by gently stroking the corners of the mouth and upper and lower lips in the midline. A positive response occurs when the infant opens his mouth or turns his head to the side of the stimulus. The sucking reflex is obtained by placing a finger or pacifier in the baby's mouth and noting the strength of the mouth movements and sucking response.

Grasping the infant's hands and arms, the examiner gently pulls the infant to a sitting position so that the degree of head lag can be observed. It is noted whether the infant's head is in alignment with his body when he reaches the vertical position. The degree of head control present with the infant in a sitting position is observed.

Incurvation of the trunk reflex is obtained by holding the infant in a prone position over the examiner's hand. By stroking the infant's back parallel to the spine the examiner detects presence or absence of movement of the pelvis toward the stimulated side.

The automatic walking reflex may also be tested. If the infant is held on a forward incline, allowing one foot to touch the table, the infant will right himself with that leg and flex the opposite leg. The opposite action occurs when the other foot touches the table.

The Moro, or startle, reflex is elicited by a loud noise such as clapping near the baby's ear, by striking the table on which the infant is lying, or by lifting the head of the bassinet a few inches and dropping it. The infant's arms, hands, and cry are noted. A complete Moro reflex consists of abduction of the arms at the shoulder, extension of the forearm at the elbow, and extension of the fingers followed by an adduction of the arm at the shoulder. Asymmetrical response, jerkiness or tremor, or slow or weak response are considered abnormal. A vigorous cry should follow the startle.

SUMMARY

Developing skill in physical examination is becoming increasingly necessary for the nurse, partly because of changing patterns of practice in maternal and child health. Nurses are assuming greater responsibility for evaluating the health status of infants, and the physical examination is one of the basic criteria on which the nurse bases a clinical judgment.

A broad knowledge of normal physical and developmental variations in the newborn infant is required, as well as knowledge of pathological signs and symptoms. When performing the physical examination, the nurse must maintain a high level of suspicion, and all unusual or unexplained findings must be brought to the attention of a physician or other qualified expert and pursued until a satisfactory explanation of the condition is found.

The importance of thoroughness and of developing a rigid system of examination is stressed. Most signs and symptoms of an abnormal or pathological state are missed, not because of the obscure or esoteric nature of physical findings but because of failure on the part of the examiner to observe and examine the patient carefully and failure to pursue vigorously suspicious or unexplained findings.

Every infant examined by the nurse is unique and must be evaluated in relation to his particular antenatal, natal, and neonatal history. The system of examination should be adapted to the individual infant and to the specific situation.

BIBLIOGRAPHY

Barness, Lewis A.: *Manual of Pediatric Physical Diagnosis*, Year Book, Chicago, 1966.

Brazie, J. V., and Lula O. Lubchenco: "Newborn and Premature Infant," in C. Henry Kempe, Henry K. Silver, and Donough O'Brien (eds.), *Current Pediatric Diagnosis and Treatment*, Lange, Los Altos, Calif., 1970.

Green, Morris, and Julius B. Richmond: *Pediatric Diagnosis*, Saunders, Philadelphia, 1966.

Judge, Richard D., and George D. Zuidema: *Physical Diagnosis: A Physiologic Approach to the Clinical Examination*, Little, Brown, Boston, 1968.

Lloyd-Roberts, G. C.: *Orthopedics in Infancy and Childhood*, Butterworth, London, 1971.

Prechtl, Heinz, and David Beintema: *The Neurological Examination of the Newborn Infant*, The Spastics Society Medical Education and Information Unit, published in association with William Heinemann Medical Books Ltd., London, 1964.

Silver, Henry K., C. Henry Kempe, and Henry B. Bruyn: *Handbook of Pediatrics*, Lange, Los Altos, Calif., 1971.

PART V

COMPLICATIONS OF CHILDBEARING AND CHILDREARING

From 1964 to 1970 the infant mortality rate in the United States dropped from 26.4 to 19.8 per 1,000 live births (Nation Standard Health Statistics). While these figures are encouraging, they do not lend themselves to complacency. In perinatal care, the main objective is an intact mother and infant—mere survival is a poor second.

The human wastage resulting from a high-risk pregnancy, predisposing to the delivery of a high-risk infant, may be minimal, partial, or complete. Contributory factors are multiple, complex, and interrelated.

Some maternal conditions affecting the newborn are the standard of living (socioeconomic and educational status), age of the mother (under fifteen or over thirty-five), unwanted pregnancy, lack of antenatal care, previous preterm deliveries; pre-existing disease (diabetes, hypertensive cardiovascular disease, renal disease), prenatal conditions (Rh isoimmunization), toxemia, vaginal bleeding, multiple pregnancy, abnormal presentation, acute infection, drug addiction, preterm and post-term delivery, premature rupture of membranes, and poly- or oligohydramnios.

High-risk infants are usually considered to be those born preterm or post-term (under 37 or over 42 weeks gestation) or those who are inappropriate for gestational age (large or small); those born with birth defects, such as brain damage from a difficult delivery causing hypoxia or hemorrhage, respiratory distress, hyperbilirubinemia, metabolic disturbance, or bleeding problems; those born as multiple births; and those with congenital or acquired infection.

The significance of a high-risk pregnancy has far-reaching effects. The tremendous psychological and socioeconomic stress created by the birth of a high-risk infant cannot be minimized because the impact is felt by both the family and society.

The health of a pregnant woman is not determined at the time she conceives; it is predetermined at the time of her conception. Therefore, it is imperative that preventive health measures be continuously emphasized. To resolve a problem of this magnitude, a joint effort and multidisciplinary approach is necessary. The Maternal-Infant Project, federally funded, has contributed greatly toward improved mother-infant care, which in turn has helped to reduce infant mortality. Equal educational and employment opportunity would probably help still more.

In the meantime, additional effort is being made to reduce infant mortality and morbidity by establishing centers throughout the country for care of high-risk newborns. Ideally the high-risk mother's antepartal care, delivery, and postpartum care will be provided at the same facility.

It is essential that these highly specialized centers be well staffed by personnel with theoretical knowledge, clinical expertise, and superior judgment. The demand for well-qualified nurses in this highly specialized area, however, far exceeds the supply. One means of meeting this demand would be to offer an elective in high-risk newborn nursing care on the basic level in schools of nursing. For additional preparation, interested graduate students might choose to become clinical specialists in this area. These qualifications are essential for the dynamic, exacting, therapeutic approach used to identify pregnant women at risk, fetuses in jeopardy, and high-risk mothers and infants. Those identified as such are closely monitored, aggressively treated, and thoroughly evaluated.

UNIT A

COMPLICATIONS OF CHILDBEARING

30 | PSYCHOLOGICAL AND SOCIOECONOMIC IMPLICATIONS

Barbara Cabela

Complications which occur in or result from any phase of the maternity cycle, whether they affect the pregnant woman, new mother, or the infant, have an impact on everyone closely involved with the family unit. In the home, in the clinic, and in the hospital the nurse is in a strategic position to care and to help; therefore, it is essential to be knowledgeable about the various complications; to be aware of the usual physical, psychological, and socioeconomic sequelae; and to be able to employ skills of observation, interpretation, intervention, and evaluation. In many instances no other member of the health team has as much knowledge of the total situation or as great an opportunity to provide care as does the nurse.

Before considering the effects of complications of childbearing upon the infant and family, it is necessary to briefly review the effects of an uncomplicated pregnancy and a healthy intact baby. Even though these more usual and desirable conditions prevail, the couple may very quickly be aware that all things did not happen as planned or feelings occur as anticipated prior to

The author wishes to acknowledge the impact of Florence G. Blake's guidance and support in helping this nurse expand and practice her philosophy of nursing care.

the pregnancy. The pregnant woman may resent the change in her body. The attractive, valued figure disappears. The new mother who eagerly anticipated motherhood may not feel motherly following delivery. Although she chose to terminate her career, at least temporarily, she may long for the stimulation and satisfaction experienced as a member of the working world. The expectant father may resent his wife's wish to decrease the number of social activities. The new father may feel responsible for the pain experienced by his wife during labor and delivery. Both parents are often concerned over increasing expenses. The infant may only faintly resemble the idealized baby pictured in the parents' minds prior to delivery. Usually these are minor or temporary problems or disappointments coped with readily by most parents. If their relationship is healthy, they are able to express their feelings, and they are able to resolve differences. Consideration of the above, however, should make one begin to think about the potential for the disturbing impact which the complicated pregnancy or the deviant infant has on the family unit.

COPING WITH STRESS AND CRISIS

The Concept of Coping

Regardless of the nature of the problem and whether it affects the parents, the infant, or both, one major goal of the nurse as well as other members of the health team is to help the family unit cope with the stress or crisis. The concept of coping is sometimes used to describe any adjustment behavior, whether it is maladaptive, maintains equilibrium, or is growth-producing. The use of defense mechanisms such as repression, denial, reaction formation, and rationalization represents an attempt to diminish the recognition or impact of experiences which may be distressing to the individual. They allow him to avoid dealing fully with unpleasant situations or unacceptable ideas. Although in some instances these mechanisms may be essential for the person to continue functioning, they are, objectively, less healthy ways of handling stress or crisis situations than the positive coping behavior described by some authors. This indicates that the term coping is not compatible with maladaptive behavior.

Coping, as used in this chapter, may be defined as adaptive behavior which is reality-oriented, purposeful, and under the control of the individual. It is an active and thoughtful approach used by the person to deal with stress of crisis.[1] Coping behavior is a positive process by which the person maintains his equilibrium or grows under disturbing conditions and masters new problem situations. It does not include the mechanisms of defense nor does it have a negative adjustment connotation. The ability to cope is related to past experiences and present resources.

The Nature of Stress and Crisis

Much research has been done on the physical and psychological aspects of stress and crisis. Although a variety of approaches have been used to study stress and crisis and some scientists have emphasized the physical while others concentrated on the psychological, there are some helpful similarities in the research which may be used to provide a framework for understanding what takes place and how to help those affected by the complications of childbearing.

There is difficulty differentiating between stress and crisis in the literature, as the two tend to overlap. Lazarus states that "stress conveys the idea that the person or animal is beset by powerful pressures which greatly tax the adaptive resources of the biological or psychological system."[2] According to Parad and Caplan, "a crisis is a period of disequilibrium overpowering the individual's homeostatic mechanisms."[3] In general, crisis seems to describe an event which is sudden in onset, requires rapid action, tends to establish a demarcation line, and is limited in time. A stress situation, on the other hand, usually develops gradually, demands less in terms of action, is difficult to isolate, and often continues for a prolonged period. Consequently, a crisis situation may be more easily identified and dealt with more readily by those in crisis as well as members of the health team. This places an added burden on members to remain alert for stress-producing situations because stress, when unrelieved, seems to have a greater potential for the development of neurotic behavior patterns.

Hill describes the course of adjustment to crisis graphically as the "truncated form of a roller-coaster."[4] The crisis, which may be dulling initially, is followed by a drop in organization as the individual or group realizes the implications of the event, the lowest point of disorganization. With the initiation of adjustment responses the recovery period begins, and a new level or reorganization is sought. The level of reorganization attained depends on the adequacy of the adjustment made for those involved.[5]

Both stress and crisis situations necessitate changes in a person's behavior if he is to resume the equivalent level of functioning he achieved prior to the disturbing event. Adaptation may include altering present behavior patterns, learning and using new behavior, or drastic reorganization of one's goals and life-style. Although certain events tend to produce stress or be viewed as a crisis almost universally, there is wide variation in response to situations both individually and culturally. An event which is stressful for one person or family unit may represent a crisis to a second and create only minor discomfort in a third. These situations represent the extremes; however, it is critical that the nurse and other members of the health team remain open intellectually and emotionally to the patient's and family's subjective views of potentially disturbing occurrences regardless of objective expectations.

GENERAL ASPECTS OF NURSING CARE

Through the nursing care provided, the nurse helps the patient and family unit cope with stress and crisis. Nursing care is composed of four major aspects, or elements. These are observation, interpretation, intervention, and evaluation.

Observation

Observation includes listening attentively, looking critically, and eliciting responses purposefully. What is the patient saying and with what inflection? How does the patient or family member appear? What is the degree of muscle tone? Is there much or little facial expression? Are questions answered or ignored? What is the response to encouragement of verbalization?

Interpretation

As the nurse gathers data, the process of interpretation is also begun. Comparison of the different kinds of information obtained is made for consistency. Does the patient's appearance correlate with his words? The nurse analyzes behaviors singly and as part of the whole picture. Lethargy may indicate depression or result from physical exhaustion. Cultural patterns and socioeconomic factors are reflected in the patient's behavior and responses. The Spanish-American woman who smiles cheerfully and agrees readily with all suggestions may be responding to what she believes are the dominant culture's expectations. Based on knowledge and observations, the nurse reaches some tentative conclusions about the situation.

Included as an integral part of nursing interpretation and intervention is validation of conclusions. Validation is accomplished in a number of ways. The nurse encourages the patient or family members to expand a statement by saying, "Tell me more about that." The nurse verbalizes an interpretation to the patient for confirmation or denial. It can be suggested that other people often feel a certain way under similar circumstances. These findings can then be compared with those of other caretakers. The nurse initiates action and contrasts patient or family reaction with nursing expectation.

Intervention

Observation and interpretation of the behavior of those for whom care is provided form a foundation for nursing intervention. However, observation, interpretation, and validation do not complete the process. These processes must be ongoing if nursing intervention (which includes nursing diagnosis), plan, and action are to be viable and productive. Whether in the hospital setting or outside, living is dynamic, and nursing care which is static and automatic does not promote growth in either the patient or the nurse. What then is nursing intervention? It is the purposeful use of self, of one's knowledge, of one's skills, and of prescribed approaches and treatments to help the patient (and family unit) regain his previous level of health and well-being, if possible, and to enhance his ability to cope with stress-producing or crisis-inducing experiences. It requires involvement with people and the ability to care for and about them. In practice, nursing intervention is making decisions about what the patient is experiencing, what his strengths and limitations are, and what needs the patient has—nursing diagnosis; determining means by which the patient's strengths can be used and limitations diminished, the patient's needs can be met, and the mutual goals of patient and nurse can be achieved—nursing care plans; and implementation of this plan—nursing action. Action is a stimulus which brings about a response or reaction, and this brings the nurse to the final aspect of nursing care—evaluation.

Evaluation

Evaluation is the process of deciding if and to what extent the nursing care given is effective. Are the patient's needs being met? Is progress being made toward the achievement of the goals? Are the patient and the family unit coping with the situation? Evaluation often results in a recycling of all or part of the process of nursing care. Continued observation may yield new information. Behavioral response may indicate a need for different interpretation. Failure of the patient to make satisfactory progress may require alterations in nursing diagnosis, care plan, and action and in the evaluation or reconsideration which follows. This process of nursing care continues for whatever period of time the nurse-patient relationship exists and regardless of whether there is frequent, prolonged contact, as in the hospital setting, or intermittent contact, as in the community health setting.

THE NURSE AND THE NURSING PROCESS

During the process of nursing care there is, in addition to the direct effect of planned intervention, a secondary and vitally important indirect effect. This effect is related to the person of the nurse. Culturally, socially, experientially, who the nurse is colors how the care is provided. Attitudes, values, and beliefs influence the nurse's behavior toward patients, often without the awareness of either patient or nurse. Much is written about why it is necessary for the nurse to understand and accept the patient, but not enough emphasis is placed on the importance of nurses understanding and accepting themselves. Nurses need to know who they are and where they are first. Achieving self-awareness and recognizing the impact of self on the patient-nurse interaction is difficult because it forces one to look honestly at oneself, and this may be painful. However, nurses cannot hope to understand and accept the recipient of nursing care until they are able to do it first for themselves, and respect how it modifies personal nursing ability as well as patient response.

Another essential consideration in regard to the nursing process is the fact that it is not only the patient and family unit who are acted upon and affected. Nursing care involves interaction between people, and through the experience the nurse can also grow, learn, and change. If the nurse refuses this opportunity or is unaware of the effect of nursing care rendered by others, the reward of sharing the experience will be lost, and the patient will not receive the level of care he might have had. Nursing care, then, involves interaction between a minimum of two people, and failure to recognize the implications this has for the outcome is very much like operating in a vacuum.

COMPLICATIONS OF CHILDBEARING

Complications of the childbearing process are a potential source of stress or crisis for the pregnant woman or new mother and her family unit. The nurse attempts to help those involved cope with and emerge from the experience at the highest health level possible. The term family unit as used in this chapter refers to the people who are closely tied to the patient emotionally whether or not they are related by blood or marriage. The definition of family and the individual's attachment to its different members will vary culturally. Currently in our society, the meaning of family is changing and is inconsistent across groups. The important consideration for the nurse is recognition and inclusion of significant others in the nursing process.

Complications of the childbearing process may occur in any phase of the cycle from conception until mother and infant have been assessed as healthy or normal. The particular kinds of stress or crisis and how the individual and the family unit cope with these complications as well as the therapeutic nursing intervention will vary and are influenced by several factors: the nature and severity of the complication, the phase of the cycle during which it occurs, the person(s) affected, the sociocultural background of the patient and family unit, the strengths and limitations of those involved, and their previous coping ability.

Complications of Early Pregnancy

Spontaneous abortion is one of the potential problems of the first trimester. During this early stage of pregnancy the woman has not yet experienced the feeling of movement and life within her body. Consequently she has not developed the same feeling of attachment to the embryo or fetus and the sense of the full reality of pregnancy which will evolve during the second trimester. Even though pregnancy has been confirmed and the woman has noted the early signs of pregnancy such as amenorrhea, fullness and tingling in her breasts, and unexpected episodes of nausea and vomiting, she does not have the feeling that "this is really happening to me."

Loss of the embryo or fetus through spontaneous abortion during the first trimester, therefore, involves different responses than does a stillbirth or newborn death. Particularly if this is a first pregnancy, the woman is likely to question her womanhood. Despite the current diminishing equation of womanhood and fulfillment with motherhood, many women are still emotionally and culturally tied to the older concept. Even if spontaneous abortion does not threaten her status as a woman, she may undergo a loss of self-esteem or a weakening of self-concept. She may well feel something is wrong with her. Why is her body incapable of completing this pregnancy? If the pregnancy was desired, the woman who aborts experiences frustration at not reaching her goal of motherhood. She will be concerned and more apprehensive about the outcome of future pregnancies. She may wonder whether or not she will become pregnant again. There are guilt feelings related to real or imagined failure to comply with restrictions and/or taboos imposed by pregnancy and the wish that she were not pregnant which every pregnant woman has at some time. Guilt feelings are further increased if the pregnancy was unwanted. In this instance, the feeling of relief at its termination provides another source of guilt. Spontaneous abortion may also cause the pregnant woman anxiety or fear for her own health or life. Particularly in the event of massive hemorrhage which may accompany incomplete abortion there is evidence to support her fears.

The woman's husband or partner also has feelings of his own to handle. His primary concern is likely to be for his partner's welfare and safety. "Is she going to be all right?" is his question, whether verbalized or not. Should death result from or be related to any phase of the pregnancy, he may experience guilt feelings as the person responsible for the pregnancy. If he was unhappy about the pregnancy, the husband may, like his partner, feel responsible for the loss of the embryo or fetus. The male's manhood is less vulnerable to the threat occasioned by spontaneous abortion than is his partner's sense of womanhood. Manhood is apparently related to sexual function and the ability to impregnate. However, production of an abnormal infant has singular implications for both partners. Another factor which may influence the attitude or response of the male whose partner aborts spontaneously is his disappointment over the loss and his need to blame someone. He may hold the physician responsible or he may blame his partner even though there is no reason to blame either. It is essential when dealing with psychological aspects to remember that feelings and emotions are not based on logic.

GUILT FEELINGS

Feelings of guilt are frequently associated with complications of the child-bearing process. When people are faced with unexpected, distressing events such as spontaneous abortion or the birth of an infant with a congenital anomaly, the frustration experienced seeks release through determination of cause. Responses and feelings dating back to their childhood years are also aroused. During the socialization process the child is taught cause and effect relationships very early. A great number of behaviors take on a right or wrong, good or bad connotation. If the child is right or good, he is rewarded. If he is wrong or bad, punishment follows. As his superego develops he becomes his own policeman. Even when the wrong or bad is not discovered by his parents, he feels guilty because he did something which is prohibited. He is blameworthy. Adults to a greater or lesser degree are subject to remnants of the early training process. At a time when anxiety is high and emotion affects intellectual processes, adults are particularly vulnerable to guilt feelings.

Guilt feelings are often expressed or alluded to verbally. "What did I do wrong?" or "I wonder if I took some medicine I shouldn't have," indicate feelings of responsibility for the abortion of the fetus or congenital defect of an infant. Sometimes these statements are related to a specific incident. In other instances they reflect a more general feeling that "there must be a reason for this to have happened." In order to help the person express these feelings and work through them the nurse can encourage the person to verbalize more about the concern. Appropriate responses to these kinds of questions or statements include, "I wonder why you feel you did something wrong," or, "You've asked why this happened several times. Is there something specific that concerns you?" Nursing intervention is designed to help the parents talk about and deal with their own feelings. It is rarely helpful for the nurse to speculate about possible causes.

There are instances when the nurse should not attempt to handle the problems that are uncovered. Help from other professionals with more background in psychological and psychiatric counseling should be obtained when defensive behavior such as withdrawal and hyperactivity are severe or prolonged. Additional help is also indicated when there is evidence that guilt is caused by attempted abortion or drug use during the pregnancy, or when the abortion or defective infant is perceived as deserved punishment for infractions unrelated to the pregnancy.

Guilt feelings may be particularly upsetting and difficult to handle when the complication occurs in an unwed pregnancy. Although pregnancy outside legal marriage is accepted more readily than in previous years, it remains a moral issue for many people. These attitudes tend to heighten the woman's and sometimes the man's guilt feelings. It, too, is a situation for potential perception of the complication as punishment by both the couple and others.

ECONOMIC FACTORS

At times complications of early pregnancy create economic problems for the couple. Added stress can be anticipated if they do not have health insurance, either private or through governmental agencies, to cover medical expenses and costs or if the wife's employment is a major source of income and she is unable to work for a period of time. Included among the former are a group of people in our society who have marginal incomes. They tend to manage as long as there are no major (for them) unexpected expenses. Unless they are employed by an organization which provides or requires health insurance, this item tends to be left out of the budget. Whether the problem is spontaneous abortion or total breakdown of the car needed for travel to work, the expense is too great for them to handle and is a source of stress. Many are faced with prolonged periods of payments to hospitals or loan companies which constantly threaten their frail financial balance. Others are unable to deal with this added stress and feel hopeless and helpless in their struggle for self-maintenance. The male's self-esteem is particularly vulnerable under these conditions, and his partner, as well as others, can further decrease his feelings of self-worth by her reaction and because of her own anxiety.

This kind of situation is especially difficult for a young couple early in marriage. It imposes an additional stress factor at a time when there are already many adjustments to be made and when their resources for dealing with stress and crisis as a couple are limited. The nurse cannot ignore this aspect of the lives of the people for whom care is given. The nurse will often have to involve other professionals and agencies in helping the family find and use resources, but the recognition of potential economic stress and the effect it has on the patient and family unit are well within the province of nursing care.

NURSING CARE

What then are the implications for nursing care in spontaneous abortion and other complications of early pregnancy which result in loss of the embryo or fetus and which may cause some concern for the pregnant woman's health or life? The nurse's initial contact with the woman is often in an emergency setting or an unplanned hospital admission. The primary responsibility of the health care team is to ensure the survival of the pregnant woman. However, during the period of emergency care, the nurse has an opportunity to observe the reactions of the patient and her husband or family. Appropriate reassurance of both is essential. The nurse who *makes* time to listen to the expressed fears of the patient and family can help them sort out the realistic fears from those which are not. This allows the nurse to give reassurance by briefly explaining what is being done and will be done to care for the patient. It also provides specific reassurance related to the source of fear and anxiety rather than stating such platitudes as, "Everything will be fine," which is generally not helpful. If verbal expression of fear is absent, the nurse can make use of behavioral cues such as facial expression or increased motor activity. The nurse might say, "You look worried. Tell me about it," or "You look upset. Let's talk about your concerns." If the father of the child or the family is separated from the patient for a period of time, it is important that they be given information about the condition of the patient at intervals. This gives those waiting accurate information with which to deal and lets them know that the health team cares about and understands what they are experiencing.

Following the initial emergency care for spontaneous abortion, the potential problems discussed earlier need to be considered to determine how the woman and family unit are coping with the event and its ramifications. In order to plan and carry out appropriate nursing care, the nurse needs to observe and make interpretations about the following: the relationship and communication of the couple or of the patient and significant other, patient and family source and use of support, expression of feelings by the couple related to self-concept, patient reaction to future pregnancy, patient and family response to loss, expression of guilt feelings by the couple, and socioeconomic and cultural data.

A nursing diagnosis based on the information obtained through observation and interpretation can then be made and appropriate nursing intervention planned. If the woman appears depressed and has talked little about what she has experienced, the plan might include provision for one nurse to give most of the patient's care, allowance for this nurse to spend extra time with the patient, and confrontation of the patient with feelings common to others in her situation. If the patient is able to share her feelings of decreased worth and the fear that a second pregnancy is too risky, the nurse has an opportunity to help the patient work out these feelings, deal with them realistically, and begin to direct her energies outward toward resumption of previous activities and development of new goals. However, if the patient does not show signs of coping, the nurse needs to involve other members of the health team, help initiate appropriate referrals, and aid the family in planning for continuing care. In too many instances hospital personnel think about the patients' care only in the hospital setting. This is a narrow and limiting outlook for both the patient and the nurse. Hospitalization is an extremely brief experience for most people and discharge rarely coincides with resolution of the patients' problems. The nurse, regardless of the employment setting, has a responsibility to help families plan for, and in some instances arrange for, continuing care.

Complications during the Second and Third Trimesters

Complications which arise during and after the fourth or fifth month of pregnancy pose different kinds of problems for the pregnant woman and family unit. Consequently, although the theoretical basis of nursing care is unchanged, the nurse will be dealing with different kinds of stress and crisis situations. Near the end of the fourth month, the pregnant woman experiences the first sensation of fetal movement. This is probably the single most significant and confirming sign of pregnancy for the woman. Other signs of pregnancy become more apparent than they were during the first trimester. These factors increase the sense of the reality of approaching motherhood and strengthen feelings of attachment for the fetus. Early feelings of disappointment or denial of pregnancy, unless deep-seated, have to an extent been resolved, and the pregnant couple begin to prepare physically and psychologically for the birth of the baby.

There is a second aspect of the later stages of pregnancy which also influences the consideration of complications. Potential threats to the woman's health and life increase as she nears term. Depending on one's viewpoint, the pregnancy itself may complicate a pre-existing condition, such as cardiac disease. Complications during the third trimester of pregnancy then have potential for causing ambivalent feelings in the pregnant woman and her family unit. Fear and anxiety about the health and life of the pregnant woman and her unborn child may arouse conflicting emotions. At times the family or some members of it are faced with making a choice which will provide a relative advantage for either the woman or fetus in terms of health and life. This is a difficult situation for everyone.

As with spontaneous abortion, guilt feelings are readily generated in the pregnant couple by any threat to the fetus. Because of the increased danger for his partner, the male is more likely to feel guilty, especially if the procreation of a child was of greater importance to him than to his partner. Failure to obtain early antenatal care and the response of health professionals to this omission also heighten the feelings of guilt.

Feelings of resentment toward the father may be engendered by complications of pregnancy. Again, the need to blame someone may be apparent. "You did this to me" or, "If it weren't for the pregnancy, I would be okay" are often nonverbalized but behaviorally expressed feelings of the pregnant woman whose health or life is threatened even temporarily by complications of pregnancy. These feelings pose a serious problem to communication and mutual support. If delivery is accomplished successfully for mother and baby, remnants of these feelings, if not coped with adequately, may negatively influence the development of a healthy mother-child relationship. They also may carry over to future pregnancies.

The woman's self-esteem may decrease as a result of her inability to carry out successfully a "normal" function of women. Both partners are likely to see themselves as less worthy if the potential danger to the fetus is great. There is often a feeling of "There must be something wrong with me," on the part of both. This phenomenon is particularly evident among individuals who have experienced limited or little success in life.

Economic factors are more often of greater concern with complications which occur in the later stages of pregnancy. Problems such as toxemia and cardiac disease usually require termination of employment. Increased medical care often associated with periods of hospitalization adds to the financial burden. The couple may have planned carefully with usual expenses in mind and the benefit of the woman's salary until very near term. This kind of budget may be destroyed by complications of the second and third trimesters. Insurance benefits may not cover the complications of pregnancy which affect either the mother or infant.

Fear for the survival or normality of the fetus is a very realistic concern with complications such as placenta previa or premature labor. The nurse and other members of the health team must be able to give the woman and family unit accurate information. Extreme optimism in the face of actual danger is unfair to the patient and insulting to her intelligence. Neither should the situation be presented as bleak when the outcome is questionable. Honest appraisal of the situation and communication with the woman and family unit establish a feeling of trust. Allowing or encouraging the patient to talk about her fears for the fetus often enables her to gain perspective, work through feelings, utilize support, and cope with the stress or crisis. If survival of the fetus is highly unlikely as with early premature labor or signs of severe fetal distress, anticipatory grief work may be initiated by the woman and/or her partner. Whether or not this improves coping ultimately depends on the extent to which it is accomplished and the eventual outcome of the pregnancy. Anticipatory grief work will be discussed in more detail later in this chapter.

Birth of an Ill or Deviant Infant

The birth of an ill, premature, or defective baby confronts the family unit with a realization of one of the most distressing fears during the pregnancy. If the pregnancy was desired and the infant's arrival eagerly anticipated, the parents are faced with concern for the infant's survival or reduced potential for normal development at a time when they expected to feel pleasure and fulfillment. If the pregnancy was unwanted, the crisis for the mother and father may be even greater because of guilt feelings and/or interpretation of the outcome as punishment.

Parents of infants who are seriously ill or who have a major defect at or shortly after birth invariably ask themselves one or more of the following questions: "Will the infant survive?" "What residual effects will there be?" "Will we be able to take care of the child?" "How will this complication change our plans and goals?" "Will we be able to afford the care this child needs, now and later?" "Why did this happen to me (us)?" "Did I (we) do something to cause the problem?" Other questions and concerns will also be formulated in the minds of the parents, but in general the above are the most common.

Although these concerns are generally felt by parents, they may not be expressed verbally. The failure of mothers and/or fathers to verbalize these questions and feelings is a warning signal to the nurse which indicates the need for further investigation.

DENIAL

Denial is one of the defense mechanisms employed by parents when told their infant has a congenital defect, particularly one in which most of the signs and symptoms are internal. Denial is an inability to acknowledge the reality situation because it is extremely painful or distressing. Instead, the opposite of the real facts is accepted as true. Denial serves a protective function initially. It allows parents time to gather their resources and find more constructive ways of dealing with an unpleasant reality. However, its continued use in the presence of evidence to the contrary is an unhealthy sign. Denial is difficult for nurses and other members of the health team to handle. It may result in hostile challenges of professional knowledge and ability. In addition, it is easy to reinforce the parents' denial by agreeing with him in regard to negative signs of defect. Generally, nursing intervention encourages parents to deal with the reality of the situation following the initial impact of the stress or crisis. Grief work over the loss of the expected normal child must be done, and feelings of frustration, guilt, and disappointment expressed. When parents have begun to deal honestly with their feelings, information regarding corrective procedures or habilitative measures provides them with knowledge which they can use in coping with the problem. When coping mechanisms are absent or seriously diminished, attempts to break down the defense mechanism of denial may leave the person unable to function. In this instance additional help is needed.

NURSING RESPONSIBILITIES

The nurse caring for the family of the infant with a problem such as respiratory distress syndrome or congenital heart disease must remain aware of and plan to meet the needs common to most new families as well as aid other team members in meeting these needs. Most mothers need to talk about their labor and delivery experience both to clear up any misconceptions they may have and to express their negative feelings about the experience. In this way the mother is able to finish the psychological work of labor and delivery and move away from the experience with a realistic picture of what took place and reassurance that she is a worthwhile person.

The mother who has delivered an ill or deformed baby has these same needs plus increased needs for care, attention, and help because of her anxiety about the infant's fate and her feeling of decreased self-esteem related to the production of an abnormal infant. However, if the concern of members of the health team as well as family and friends is focused mainly on the infant, the mother may be reluctant to discuss those experiences and feelings which center directly on her. The nurse must include the psychological work of normal labor and delivery in the patient care plan and demonstrate a genuine interest in and concern for the mother's well-being.

In addition the nurse needs to observe the father's behavior and his interaction with his partner carefully to determine whether or not he is able to provide the love and support he would normally give to her. He, too, may be overwhelmed with concern for the infant and his uncertain future and thus may be unaware of his partner's needs and be unable to meet them. If this is happening, the nurse and other members of the team must support and care for the father to help meet his needs and help him understand and meet his partner's needs.

There are, of course, many instances when a crisis of this nature brings marriage partners closer together and strengthens their ability to cope. However, this is far from universal and seems to be a function of the strength of the relationship and the success of the couple in coping with previous crises. It is imperative that the nurse make careful observations and interpretations of the behavior of the father and mother in relation to themselves and each other. In this way there is a basis for making a nursing diagnosis and planning appropriate nursing action.

The birth of an ill or defective infant often precipitates an economic crisis for the mother and father. Medical care of the seriously affected infant is extremely costly and may be prolonged for weeks, months, or even a lifetime. Not all health insurance policies cover unusual care for the newborn, and it is not impossible for families to incur debts under these circumstances which they are never able to pay. At times sufficient outside resources to help the family do not exist. However, there are many resources for financial aid such as handicapped children programs and tax-supported hospitals. Referral or making arrangements for help is part of the nursing responsibility. Depending on the setting, this may require nothing more of the nurse than referral to the Social Service department, or it may entail locating an appropriate resource and helping the family learn to use it. Unfortunately, nurses and physicians are frequently unaware of available resources or even of the extent of financial liability incurred by the family as a result of their care.

RELATIONSHIP FORMATION WITH PARENTS AND SIBLINGS

The birth of a deviant infant is almost always a crisis situation for the family unit, particularly if there is little hope of his approaching normal appearance, intellectual ability, or physical function. The response to the infant usually includes elements of rejection and overprotection. Either may be dominant, and both have serious implications for the satisfactory adjustment of the parents, child, and siblings. Inability to accept the abnormal infant as he is distorts the development of mother-child and father-child relationships. Parents may overtly neglect the infant or covertly punish him for the disorganization his birth caused. Necessary rearrangement of financial priorities and disruption of major goals may be blamed on the child. Guilt feelings caused by the birth of the deviant infant as well as their reaction to him may result in parents unnecessarily giving up important goals and providing less in time and material goods for other children in order to do everything possible for the deviant child. When this happens siblings feel loss and resentment; this distorts the sibling relationship with the abnormal child and may negatively affect their own growth and development.

Some families are unable to cope with a crisis of this nature and break up under the strain. Other families remain intact physically but at a tremendous emotional cost to all. Families faced with this kind of crisis need help and support from many sources. Health professionals, clergymen, extended family members, friends, and employers contribute to successful resolution. Nursing care which increases the family's coping ability utilizes individual and family strengths, allows for expression of feelings, supports and guides appropriately, and helps the family deal with the awful reality. Care for these families is initiated with the birth of the infant but does not end with discharge from the hospital. In varying ways and degrees it will be necessary for an indefinite period of time. The quality of early care, however, is extremely important and has tremendous implications for healthy adjustment and later care.

Mary, a Child with a Congenital Birth Defect

One situation in which the needs of the parents for care following the birth of a child with spina bifida were not met is described below.

When the nurse first met the child and her family, Mary was six years old, unable to walk, incontinent of urine and stool, mentally retarded, and exhibiting behavior characteristics of children who have never formed a warm, trusting relationship. Mary's parents were born and raised in another country and moved to the United States when Mary was three years old. There are three other children, one boy and two girls, all younger than Mary.

When the nurse first became acquainted with her, Mary was hospitalized for total evaluation and determination of rehabilitation potential. The parents had not sought evaluation earlier because they were afraid of psychological damage to Mary. She had been hospitalized three times for a total period of 10 months by the time she was fifteen months old. They were not allowed to hold her, and felt she did not respond normally when they finally brought her home to stay. This nurse first became interested in Mary because of her extreme seeking behavior toward anyone in sight. As the relationship developed, many further insights about Mary's behavior and needs were gained. Mary's mother did not visit, although the father came frequently. Mary's interaction with her father was superficial and falsely cheerful, and she displayed little affection when talking about her parents.

After evaluation Mary was discharged to be readmitted later for surgery to improve alignment of her feet and to stabilize her ankles. Because the nurse had only talked with the mother on the telephone and because of this nurse's concern that Mary be as well prepared as possible for another hospitalization and for surgery which Mary perceived as mutilating, a home visit was planned.

Midway through the visit, Mrs. H., Mary's mother, described Mary's relationship with the other children, stating that Mary consistently played with the next younger child until she was no longer able to compete.

Mrs. H. then said, "What happens when there's no more baby? I wonder if she would be happier if we gave her away."

Mr. H. asked, "Could you really give her away permanently?"

Mrs. H. answered, "She could be happier if she didn't have to try to keep up." Mr. H.'s reaction was one of complete surprise. Mr. and Mrs. H. continued talking with each other, often unaware of the nurse's presence. Then Mr. H. asked for information about the local residential facility for retarded children—he wanted to know what it was like and if they could visit. Later they related that some people had encouraged them to "give Mary away" at birth. Mr. H. said they would have had the same problems without her, but Mrs. H. did not agree. Mr. H. added that it might have been easier had Mary been born fourth rather than first. As this nurse listened and occasionally helped them clarify their thoughts or provided information, they communicated some of their feelings about this child to each other for the first time—6 years after her birth and following several years of experiencing the hardship and frustration with her care. They made no decision that evening, except to look into possible placement.

The nursing decisions made were to introduce a social worker into the situation (the parents accepted this idea), to maintain contact with the family until Mary was readmitted, to be present at the time of admission, and to work intensively with Mary, her parents, and the social worker during the hospitalization.

During the next 2 weeks the family worked on their problem of whether or not to give Mary away. They used the social worker and talked to personnel at the residential facility. By the time Mary was admitted for surgery, Mr. and Mrs. H. had made their decision—to keep Mary. They had reasons—"If we give her away, the other children might be afraid we will give them away too." Mr. H. expressed a real attachment for Mary, which this nurse had observed during his visits to the hospital. Mrs. H. expressed her feeling that Mary was their responsibility and that the child would be lonely and miss them if placed outside the home.

They had dealt with and resolved a serious problem, at least for the time being. They had grown in their ability to express and work through some of their negative feelings. They had been able to use resources outside the family. What would have been the situation, had appropriate nursing intervention been initiated 6 years earlier and followed through?

Complications Resulting in Death of the Infant

The death of a newborn is difficult for parents and professional health workers alike to accept. If the infant is seriously deformed or in danger of death at an early age, feelings are ambivalent and people try to rationalize the death. However, it is still a tragic event because of the sharp contrast between the occurrence and the expectation.

Material which has been covered earlier is applicable to this situation. Guilt feelings, loss of self-esteem, depression, withdrawal, inability to communicate effectively are common following the death of a newborn. Nursing care consists of the same basic elements. Support and appropriate intervention are essential. Although grief has been mentioned previously in this chapter, the grief reaction and grieving process have not yet been dealt with in depth.

GRIEF AND THE GRIEVING PROCESS

Grief is a normal physical and psychological reaction to loss. The loss may be of a loved person or an object for which the individual has developed strong attachments; it may be loss of a body part or function or a subjective loss of love or self-esteem. The loss itself, regardless of the object, apparently triggers a grief reaction. Although much research has been done on grief and grieving, Lindemann's classic study still forms the basis for identifying the characteristic symptoms and course of acute grief.[6] He lists the symptoms of the normal grief reaction as "(1) somatic distress, (2) preoccupation with the image of the deceased, (3) guilt, (4) hostile reactions, and (5) loss of patterns of conduct."[7] Recovery from an acute grief reaction and the amount of time required depend on the person's ability to do the grief work. Successful grief work requires that the person allow himself to feel the distress caused by the loss and to express these feelings. It involves "emancipation from the bondage to the deceased, readjustment to the environment in which the deceased is missing, and the formation of new relationships."[8] If the person is able to do the necessary grief work and the grief reaction is uncomplicated, the usual duration is 4 to 6 weeks.[9]

Even though Lindemann's work deals primarily with grief occasioned by the death of a loved person, his concepts and observations are applicable to grief resulting from other kinds of loss. The grieving process and grief work have many implications for those concerned with the psychological aspects of complications of the childbearing process. Grief reactions may follow death of the embryo, fetus, or infant; death of the mother; loss of self-esteem due to inability to carry the fetus to term or due to production of an abnormal infant; surgical removal of one or more of the female reproductive organs; and loss of the anticipated healthy infant with the birth of an ill or abnormal infant. In these instances a grief reaction in the woman and her husband should be anticipated by the nurse and other members of the health team. Nursing intervention should be geared to helping the family unit through the grieving process. Because the period of hospitalization is often brief, appropriate referral and follow-up in the community is essential. Initial emotional distress and expression of feelings should be present shortly after the stress or crisis situation. Absence of appropriate reaction should alert the hospital caretakers to the need for additional care.

If the woman and the family unit are experiencing and expressing the emotion associated with loss and grief, their potential for carrying out the necessary grief work is good. The person or persons deeply affected by the loss face the three major tasks outlined by Lindemann: (1) They must break the ties to the lost object or person. The parents of the newborn who dies must return home empty-handed and put away the clothing and furniture prepared for the baby. They have to deal with the fact that the pregnancy is over and the outcome was unsuccessful. (2) They must adapt to the altered environment. The parents of an infant born with an abnormality must grieve for the anticipated normal infant. In his place they must learn to accept and love an infant whose care may be complex and time-consuming, who may be in danger of death now or at some later time, and whose condition may require expensive care and equipment. (3) Finally they must develop new attachments. The woman who aborts spontaneously and feels her self-concept and her womanhood threatened by this event must recognize her other talents and abilities as a person and as a woman. She may plan to resume a successful career which previously brought many satisfactions or look forward to another pregnancy at a later time.

In addition to the grief reaction precipitated by actual loss there is another type of grief, anticipatory grief, which occurs with potential loss such as when a soldier leaves for war or during a critical illness in a loved person.[10] Anticipatory grief is a protective mechanism which allows the person to prepare for the crisis or loss in advance and plan for his adjustment to the loss. All of the symptoms of the acute grief reaction may be present. When the actual loss does occur, the normal grief reaction is diminished, and the loss is often accepted as inevitable and probably for the best. Statements such as, "At least he isn't suffering anymore," or, "She wouldn't have been normal," verbally indicate anticipatory grief work has been done. However, if the expected loss does not happen and anticipatory grief work has taken place, the person is faced with another stress or crisis. The emotional ties which have been broken must be rebuilt. Changed plans and altered goals must be rearranged to again include the surviving person.

Anticipatory grief can occur with some complications of the childbearing process. If the pregnancy has been difficult and there has been concern for the survival of the fetus, particularly in the later stages of pregnancy, anticipatory grief work may have been accomplished. To protect themselves from the impact of a fetal death near term or a stillbirth, the pregnant woman and her husband may have prepared for such an event and even started to plan individually or together for a future pregnancy or possible adoption. When this happens, the birth of a live infant will evoke a response which may be difficult to understand unless the nurse is aware of the phenomena of anticipatory grief. At a time when hospital personnel expect the new parents to be extremely delighted and happy, the nurse may encounter disbelief and a flat reaction instead. A mothering attitude may be slow to develop, and interest in and concern for the infant may be diminished. Guilt related to the parents' feelings of detachment from the infant may increase their distress.

Another occasion for anticipatory grief work is the birth of a baby whose condition is or becomes critical, such as in the case of a small premature infant or a baby with a serious cardiac defect. Parents are and should be aware of the fact that this infant may not live. They do not necessarily give up hope for their baby's survival, but they usually try to prepare themselves for the possible death of their infant. The amount and degree of anticipatory grief work done will vary with the duration of the critical period and their interpretation of the infant's chances for survival. Decreasing queries about the baby's condition and fewer visits to the nursery may indicate that anticipatory grief work is in progress. If the infant dies, the grief reaction will be less acute, but if he survives they will have to establish an attachment for him.

Nursing care must be planned to allow for gradual adjustment of the parents to the new circumstances. They may be baffled at their own reaction. Understanding acceptance of their feelings, provision of an environment in which they can discuss them freely, and information which will help them gain insight about what has taken place enable the parents to cope more effectively with this additional stress or crisis.

THE INFLUENCE OF CULTURAL FACTORS

The significance of cultural factors on the person's perception of stress or crisis, on his manner of dealing with complications, and on the effect on nurse-patient interaction has been alluded to previously. However, because the impact of culture is frequently ignored or responded to in terms of stereotyped expectations, it is important to emphasize culture specifically.

"Since culture defines *a way of life for a designated group of people*, the nurse must understand the particular way of life for a defined patient, family, or social group. . . ."[11]

The culture in which a person grows up influences attitudes, values, beliefs, and habit patterns substantially. Often this influence is unrecognized, and even when the person demonstrates intellectual awareness of these factors, emotional response may not be altered. The person's cultural background provides a basis for decisions regarding behavior under ordinary circumstances and when faced with new situations. Culture also influences his expectations of providers of care in terms of roles and functions and his perception of health and health practices. When a person enters a health care system or hospital dominated by people of another cultural group, misunderstanding and conflict often result.

The institution or agency itself is, in a way, a subculture with an in-group of employees and an outgroup of patients. In addition, the behavior, beliefs, and attitudes of individual members of the health care team are influenced by the particular cultural group to which each member belongs. In order to meet the needs of patients from different cultural settings, the nurse must develop cultural awareness as well as self-awareness.[12] Cultural awareness is gained by studying other cultural groups, contacting and interacting with people of differing cultural backgrounds, and by caring for patient members of diverse cultures.[13]

Aspects of life about which knowledge of cultural background is particularly relevant to the nurse include medical practices, religious beliefs, family relationships, and economic status. Some would not include economic status under cultural factors, but when poverty or wealth are of long duration, there is rationale for identifying the members of those groups as part of a particular culture or subculture. The cultural definition of pregnancy, belief or nonbelief in an afterlife, the role of grandparents, and whether the usual diet is high in starch with little protein or gourmet foods should influence nursing care. Listening to the patient, demonstrating behaviorally that the patient is a worthwhile person, and involving the patient in his own care plan enable the nurse to care for the patient culturally and individually.

CONCLUSION

Much of the material in this chapter has dealt with negative responses and distressing situations. This is done purposefully because of the nature of the subject and the importance of recognizing and caring for the various problems described. However, if application is made unthinkingly and without consideration of the people involved—nurse and patient—the goal of this chapter—to help people care for people—will be unmet. The nurse cannot and should not expect to have the capacity to meet every need presented by patients. The nurse will meet many of these needs well, and even under the distressing circumstances described there is satisfaction in providing care and observing growth.

REFERENCES

1 Blake, Florence G., F. Howell Wright, and Eugenia H. Waechter: *Nursing Care of Children*, 8th ed., Lippincott, Philadelphia, 1970, pp. 17–18.
2 Lazarus, Richard S.: *Psychological Stress and the Coping Process*, McGraw-Hill, New York, 1966, p. 10.
3 Parad, Howard J., and Gerald Caplan: "A Framework for Studying Families in Crisis," in H. J. Parad (ed.), *Crisis Intervention: Selected Readings*, Family Service Association of America, New York, 1965, p. 56.
4 Hill, Reuben: "General Features of Families under Stress," in H. J. Parad (ed.), *Crisis Intervention: Selected Readings*, Family Service Association of America, New York, 1965, p. 45.
5 Ibid., pp. 45–48.
6 Lindemann, Erich: "Symptomatology and Management of Acute Grief," *American Journal of Psychiatry*, 101:141–148, 1944.
7 Ibid., p. 142.
8 Ibid., p. 143.
9 Ibid., p. 144.
10 Knight, James A., and Frederic Herter: "Anticipatory Grief," in Austin Kutscher (ed.), *Death and Bereavement*, Charles C Thomas, Springfield, Ill., 1969, pp. 196–201.
11 Leininger, Madeline M.: *Nursing and Anthropology: Two Worlds to Blend*, Wiley, New York, 1970, p. 99.
12 Ibid., p. 98.
13 Ibid., pp. 97–99.

BIBLIOGRAPHY

Baldwin, Alfred L.: *Theories of Child Development*, Wiley, New York, 1967.
Blake, Florence G.: *The Child, His Parents, and the Nurse*, Lippincott, Philadelphia, 1954.
Erickson, Erik H.: *Childhood and Society*, 2d ed., Norton, New York, 1963.
———: *Identity: Youth and Crisis*, Norton, New York, 1968.
Hinshaw, Ada Sue: "Early Planning for Long-term Care of Children with Congenital Anomalies," in Betty Bergerson et al. (eds.), *Current Concepts in Clinical Nursing*, Mosby, St. Louis, 1967, pp. 284–291.
LeMasters, E. E.: *Parents in Modern America*, Dorsey, Homewood, Ill., 1970.

Leslie, Gerald R.: *The Family in Social Context*, Oxford, New York, 1967.

Murphy, Lois: *Personality in Young Children*, Basic Books, New York, 1956.

Redmann, Ruth E.: "Black Child—White Nurse: A Nursing Challenge and Privilege," in Margery Duffey (ed.), *Current Concepts in Clinical Nursing*, vol. 3, Mosby, St. Louis, 1971, pp. 106–114.

Rubin, Reva: "Cognitive Style in Pregnancy," *American Journal of Nursing*, 70:502–508, 1970.

Schoenberg, Bernard, et al. (eds.): *Loss and Grief: Psychological Management in Medical Practice*, Columbia, New York, 1970.

Scott, Diane: "Crisis Intervention," in Betty Bergerson et al. (eds.), *Current Concepts in Clinical Nursing*, Mosby, St. Louis, 1967, pp. 392–399.

Selye, Hans: *The Stress of Life*, McGraw-Hill, New York, 1956.

Wiedenbach, Ernestine: *Clinical Nursing: A Helping Art*, Springer, New York, 1964.

————: *Family-centered Maternity Nursing*, Putnam, New York, 1967.

31 | HIGH-RISK PREGNANCY

Joanne M. Juhasz and Rosemary Cannon Kilker

CONTRIBUTING FACTORS TO HIGH-RISK PREGNANCY

Toxemia of Pregnancy

Toxemia, a specific disease of pregnancy, is a very old and very common complication. In the United States today it occurs in approximately 5 to 7 percent of all pregnancies. Toxemia is a vascular disease manifested by sodium and water retention. However, the specific cause of the disease still remains unknown. Toxemia has a triad of symptoms—hypertension, edema, and proteinuria—which usually develop in the last trimester of pregnancy. Certain women, however, are more predisposed to toxemia, such as those who have diabetes, hypertension, vascular disease, a multiple pregnancy, or hydatidiform mole. These women will develop the disease the first or second trimester of pregnancy.

Toxemia occurs most frequently in the young primigravida (twenty years

The authors wish to acknowledge the assistance of Dr. Walter B. Cherney, Director of Postgraduate Education, Department of Obstetrics and Gynecology, Good Samaritan Hospital, Phoenix, Arizona, in the preparation of this chapter.

old and younger), and the primigravida over thirty years old who is impoverished or culturally disadvantaged. It occurs in multigravidas with similiar backgrounds who are thirty-five years of age or older or who have had five or more previous pregnancies. It is also a disease that occurs more frequently among nonwhites. Thus, it may be said that there are approximately six known factors that predispose to toxemia: (1) age, (2) parity, (3) race, (4) socioeconomic status, (5) multiple gestation, and (6) pre-existing diseases.

Toxemia is differentiated on the basis of its severity. It is divided into two categories—preeclampsia and eclampsia. Eclampsia is manifested by convulsions and coma; preeclampsia is further subdivided into mild and severe degrees. A blood pressure of 160 over 110 or above, marked proteinuria, oliguria, cerebral or visual disturbances, or massive edema is evidence of severe preeclampsia. Anything less is considered mild preeclampsia.

A pregnant woman with toxemia is a high-risk mother, and as such her baby will be a high-risk baby. The increased perinatal loss is about 5 percent. At birth both the baby and its placenta will weigh less than those of a nontoxemic mother of the same gestational age. The baby's difficulties may be further compounded by his being delivered before full term, as early delivery is often advisable. Termination of the pregnancy is the only cure for toxemia.

Toxemia in pregnancy is a disease which has existed for many ages. It was a problem in the days of Hippocrates as well as today. Various methods of treatment have been expounded; however, the basic mode of treatment in 1971 remains unchanged from the first part of this century with one exception: the nursing component.

The first member of the medical team the pregnant woman meets is the nurse. The member of the medical team she sees most often is the nurse. The member of the medical team she communicates with most frequently is the nurse. Therefore, the nurse must be most exact in making the initial antepartal assessment so that a baseline of health can be established. From this assessment, objectives are formulated to guide the patient through an uneventful pregnancy that will terminate with a healthy mother and baby. For the most part, toxemias can be prevented or, if not prevented, controlled. This prevention and control is begun at the first antepartal visit. Those characteristics which predispose to toxemia—age, parity, weight, diet, marital and socioeconomic status—are noted. The patient's knowledge and understanding of her own body functions and changes that will occur during pregnancy are determined. Socioeconomic information is obtained so that plans and changes that might be necessary to make, such as living arrangements and finances, may be completed early. All the tests and examinations of this particular clinic or office are explained to the patient in full detail to eliminate her stress and anxieties.

At each subsequent antepartum visit, the nurse makes a reassessment of the pregnant woman's health. This assessment is then compared to the last visit. The urine is tested for protein, the blood pressure and weight are recorded on the antepartum chart, and inquiries are made into any problems that she might have encountered since her last visit. The nurse explains the results of all tests and helps her to understand their meaning.

When the blood pressure first begins to slowly rise, the weight gain exceeds 1 to 1½ pounds per week, and protein appears in the urine, vigorous treatment must begin. The nurse must review with the woman her daily diet to determine the sodium and calorie intake so that proper adjustments can be made. Often the nurse finds that the problem in the diet is not the food itself but the preparation. For example, Mrs. T., an eighteen-year-old primigravida, 32 weeks pregnant, was beginning to gain weight too rapidly, and her hands and feet were edematous. Her diet seemed to be adequate; however, when asked about the preparation of foods, the nurse learned that she used bacon and pork fat for flavoring along with liberal amounts of chili sauce. Besides explaining the high sodium content of these foods to Mrs. T., the nurse also explained the necessity of reading the labels on all canned and frozen foods to eliminate those products that were preserved with large amounts of sodium.

The nurse must help the patient plan rest periods in the morning and afternoon and encourage her to sleep at least 8 hours each night. While talking with the woman, family problems are often discussed, and the nurse can perhaps help resolve some situations or refer the patient to other agencies. Medications the physician may prescribe, such as sedatives, tranquilizers, and diuretics, need to be explained again after the physician's conference. The nurse must reinforce the physician's orders and instruct the patient regarding the signs and symptoms she needs to report immediately, such as headaches, blurred vision, epigastric pain, increased edema, nausea, vomiting, and scanty urine. The nurse needs to reinforce the seriousness of the situation many times, and to restress the importance of the guidance given her by the doctor. Many times the patient will feel she is improving and will not keep her antepartum visit. This must be foreseen by the nurse and much emphasis must be placed on the importance of all antepartum visits. There are times when the woman's condition has not improved significantly but has not deteriorated enough for inhospital therapy. At this time the nurses should make a "phone visit" to inquire about the patient's condition and to let her know that there is concern for her.

There are times when the regimen of diet, rest, and medication is not effective in controlling the development of preeclampsia on an outpatient basis. For unknown reasons, the patient's condition may continue to deteriorate. When this occurs it is necessary to instigate more rigorous therapy with hospitalization.

On admission to the hospital, a rigid regimen is inaugurated. The physician's orders may include the following: complete bed rest; checking weight daily, fluid intake and output, vital signs, and fetal heart tones; use of a Foley catheter; low-sodium and low-calorie diet; blood studies; 24-hour urine proteins; fetal age determinations; restriction of visitors; and eclamptic precautions. Eclamptic precautions include a darkened quiet room which excludes as much external stimuli as possible. The medications would include sedatives, diuretics, antihypertensives, and anticonvulsive drugs.

The nursing assessment of this woman during the antepartum period should be available to those caring for her in the hospital. This will enable the nurses to have a complete picture of the patient's health and needs on an outpatient basis. However, an inhospital assessment is necessary as soon as possible in order to better evaluate her progress. The nursing assessment at this point will include an evaluation of the woman's general appearance; alertness; condition of skin; edema of face, hands, and feet; reflexes; attitude toward hospitalization; and family relationships as well as vital signs, fetal heart tones, weight, and blood pressure. Most of these assessments must be reevaluated every 2 to 4 hours to determine the patient's health progress and new health needs. The nurse must allay fears of the woman and her family as much as possible by explaining the reasons for the equipment present in the room and for all the procedures that must be done. Many patients would never request a private room because of financial reasons. However, in the case of preeclampsia, private rooms are necessary for the quiet that is required in the treatment. The rationale for this private room must be given to the patient, her husband, and other members of the family. In a crisis situation, such as in the situation with preeclamptic patients, they are admitted for vigorous treatment; therefore, only the husband or another member of the family is permitted to remain. This, too, must be explained to lessen anxiety. Eclamptic precautions involve (1) close, almost constant observation of the patient by the nurse or a nursing aide and (2) the availability of the toxemia tray at the bedside. The contents of the toxemia tray, which include medications, airways, syringes, needles, and tourniquets, should be explained completely to the relatives, though perhaps only in simple terms to the patient. In all high-risk and crisis situations, intravenous therapy is the rule. Before the therapy is started, the equipment and the purpose for it needs to be fully explained to both the patient and the family. The intravenous infusion must be checked every 30 to 60 minutes to control the infusion rate. Too rapid an infusion can overwhelm an already water-logged body. If the woman's condition does not improve after 4 to 8 hours, all oral intake may be restricted. Good oral hygiene is a must and is provided by the nurse and, after careful instruction, by the family member who is present. This is accomplished by cleansing the mouth and teeth and moistening the lips with a damp cloth. Cracking of the lips is prevented by use of a skin softener. When a catheter is inserted and connected to continuous drainage, instruction as to the value of the intake and output is given. With the heavy sedation that is necessary in the treatment of preeclampsia, the safety measure of side rails is a necessity. Side rails frequently irritate the patient and her family, and their value may have to be explained many times. Before injections are given to the patient, she must be prepared for the discomfort that they may cause, particularly for the burning sensation of magnesium sulfate when a local anesthetic agent is not used. If the nurse does not forewarn the patient about these injections, the pain could be enough of an irritant to trigger a convulsion. These injections also should be explained to the family.

Close nursing observation must be maintained around the clock for signs of eclampsia and labor. This close observation is continued until her condition is under control. Many times labor begins, and the patient is not aware of it because of her deep sedation. Therefore, the nurse must be alert to periodic intervals of restlessness. These women are most apt to have a rapid labor, ending with a precipitous delivery. This can and must be prevented by close nursing observation.

As with labor, the patient cannot tell you of an impending convulsion. However, by constant assessment of her condition, this can be predicted. The nurse should investigate all of the patient's complaints. Even though highly sedated, many women will foggily complain of a severe headache, a tightness of the chest, poor vision, or epigastric pains. These can be prodromal symptoms of a convulsion. An assessment of her condition is necessary immediately, even though an assessment may have been made only a few minutes previously.

All convulsions cause intense anxiety in nurses. However, the nurse must always remain "cool." The onset of the convulsion, the progress of the convulsion, the body involvement, and the length of the convulsion must be observed. While making these mental notes, the nurse must provide expert nursing care for this woman. The patient must be protected from hurting herself during the convulsions but never restrained. Aspiration of any vomitus must also be prevented. As the convulsions decrease in intensity and finally cease, the patient will go into a coma which will last several hours. The treatment which has been prescribed previously will not be intensified. Repeated convulsions will depend on the woman's response to this treatment. Until her condition improves, constant observation is necessary.

Fortunately, once preeclamptic treatment is initiated, convulsions rarely occur. However, when the pregnant woman's condition is under control, most physicians terminate the pregnancy as soon as the fetus has attained a gestational age compatible with extra-uterine life, providing the uninterrupted pregnancy is of no threat to the well-being of the woman. Induction is usually accomplished by intravenous oxytocin and amniotomy.

During induction a nurse must be in attendance at all times. Frequent nursing assessments every 15 to 30 minutes must be made of the pregnant woman and fetus. Regardless of the gestational period, the nurse must prepare for the delivery of a high-risk baby. Emergency equipment for the baby, such as resuscitation and blood sampling equipment, must be available in the delivery room and the nursery and the pediatrician notified of an impending high-risk delivery. A husband or some other close family member should be allowed to stay with the patient at all times. With proper instructions, these relatives do not interfere with the care and treatment of the loved one. The nursing staff should keep other relatives informed of her progress.

Following delivery the signs and symptoms of toxemia rapidly fade, but the danger of convulsions remains for 24 hours. It is therefore advisable and good nursing judgment to again place this mother in a private room until the danger period has passed. Immediately after delivery, the mother's first concern is for her baby. Regardless of the condition of the baby, mother must be kept informed of his health and well-being. If the baby is very much premature, the nurse must begin instructing the mother and the family in the care of a premature and help the parents prepare for the baby's probable extended hospital stay and future homecoming.

Family planning must also be discussed by the nurse with this patient. It is in the interest of the mother's health that the next pregnancy be delayed for several years. Within 10 to 14 days the blood pressure usually returns to normal. However, about one-third of these mothers continue to have hypertension or have a recurrence of it in subsequent pregnancies. For this reason, extended health evaluations must be encouraged by the entire nursing staff.

Multiple Births

Multiple births are not thought of as mysteries and dangers today as they were in the past. Twins are the most common multiple birth, occurring approximately once in every 54 births in the white race and once in every 39 births in the nonwhite race, and quintuplet births are the greatest exception. Heredity is the largest causative factor in multiple births followed by race and age. However, with the use of hormone therapy for infertility, multiple births are becoming more frequent.

Twins may be either identical or nonidentical. Identical twins develop from a single egg and are called single-ovum twins. Fertilization takes place in the usual way, but the ovum divides into two identical parts instead of developing as a single individual. Nonidentical or fraternal twins develop from the fertilization of two ova by two sperm and are known as double-ovum twins. The resemblance of these twins to each other is no greater than that of siblings. Single-ovum twins have one placenta and one chorion but usually have two amnions and umbilical cords. Each double-ovum twin has its own chorion and placenta. Sometimes in the double-ovum twins the placentas may be fused and thus will resemble one large placenta. The double-ovum twins are the most common of the two types.

The diagnosis of multiple birth is usually made during the last several months of pregnancy. It is made on the basis of constant assessment of the pregnant woman's uterine growth. Multiple birth is suspected when the uterine size is greater than it would be for that particular time in pregnancy. It is suspected if an excessive number of small parts are felt during palpation of the uterus, when two fetal heart tones of different frequency are heard, and when there is a history of twins in the family. To make a positive diagnosis, an x ray is necessary. Multiple births usually occur 2 weeks or more before the due date. Therefore, plans must be made for early delivery, the care of prematures, and increased baby supplies. When multiple pregnancy does go to term, the babies are usually smaller than single full-term infants.

The added psychological and physiological burden of a multiple pregnancy predisposes to multiple complications. The pregnant woman experiences more discomfort in the lower abdomen and back. Sleeping is difficult; activity is awkward and slow. Because of the crowding of the stomach, small feedings are better tolerated than the usual three large meals a day. The nurse must go over all these discomforts with the woman to decrease her fear that something "horrible" is wrong. Many suggestions can be given to help the pregnant woman through the last few trying weeks of pregnancy. A well-fitting maternity girdle may be suggested to relieve some of the discomforts of locomotion. The placement of pillows to support the uterus when lying down will promote better rest and sleep. Edema of the lower extremities is common and can be relieved by support stockings and frequent elevation.

Women with a multiple pregnancy are more susceptible to major complications such as prematurity, toxemia, and postpartum bleeding. Therefore, the nurse's role in assessing and providing guidance to a woman with a multiple pregnancy is more intense. More frequent visits to the physician are necessary, and she must be encouraged to keep these appointments. She must be prepared differently for her labor. Sedatives will be given sparingly, the fetal monitor may be used, and the anesthetic may not be the patient's choice. The nurse also needs to prepare both parents for the physical appearance of premature babies and the possibility of premature complications. It is sometimes difficult to convey to parents that because of their low birth weight the babies may not be able to go home with mother but will have to remain in the hospital for several days or weeks. In the assessment of each individual woman's situation, home visits may be necessary to help her and her family prepare for this multiple birth. At the time of delivery, the nurse must be prepared for premature care and for postpartum bleeding complications of the mother. At no time, however, should the nurse's behavior cause undue anxiety in the mother or family.

If a multiple birth is undiagnosed until delivery, this can cause a psychological shock to both parents. One child has been planned for, but two may cause a financial and emotional crisis. The thought of the care of two new babies at the same time may be overwhelming. Problems such as feeding, diapering, and loving must be worked through with the mother and father. Plans must be made to double all the equipment that has been provided at home. All of these problems can be resolved, but it takes much help and support from the nurse and physician for the parents to make the transition from the hospital to the home. Home visits may be needed to help the family through the adjustment period. Methods of choice for family planning are reviewed. Parents of diagnosed and undiagnosed multiple births need understanding and empathy to help them construct a new type of family living.

Hyperemesis Gravidarum

One of the most common and troublesome complaints of pregnancy is nausea and vomiting, or "morning sickness." This occurs during the first trimester of pregnancy and usually responds quite readily to therapy. Today it is rare for this complaint to develop into pernicious vomiting or hyperemesis gravidarum. Since all women with hyperemesis gravidarum start out with a simple case of nausea and vomiting, all such complaints need to be treated with proper understanding and therapy. When ambulatory therapy does not alleviate the symptoms and hyperemesis is evident, hospitalization is required. Few women need to be admitted to the hospital for the care of this complication of pregnancy, and today very few critical cases are seen. Those few who are admitted to the hospital for treatment usually show very rapid improvement.

The exact etiology of hyperemesis is unknown. Many theories have been proposed. There are certain normal changes that occur in pregnancy that are basic to all causes of vomiting, such as the endocrine and metabolic changes. In addition to the psychic impact of pregnancy with the impending responsibilities of motherhood, the decreased motility of the stomach and the high levels of chorionic gonadotropin are possible causes.

The psychic factor has long been considered a major component in hyperemesis gravidarum. This is quite understandable as there is no greater confrontation in a woman's life than facing a new pregnancy, wanted or unwanted. After the first menstrual period is missed, there are days and sometimes weeks of uncertainty before a positive pregnancy diagnosis is obtained. Following this, the expectant mother's life is inundated with adjustments and plans for the present and the future. A woman's reaction to pregnancy goes back to her childhood days and her relationship with her mother. It goes back to when she met her husband, her relationship with her husband, and the prospect of the next 20 years. However, we must not let the psychic factor overshadow the organic processes that are also at work. Both aspects of this disease—psychic and organic—must be treated.

"Morning sickness" is the beginning of all cases of hyperemesis. As the condition worsens, the woman cannot retain any liquid or solid foods, and symptoms of dehydration and starvation occur. Dehydration is manifested by diminished urinary output, highly concentrated urine, and dry skin. If the condition continues uncontrolled, jaundice may develop, the pulse rate becomes accelerated, and a low-grade fever may be present.

Starvation is always present. It is manifested by weight loss and the presence of acetone and diacetic acid in the urine. In extreme cases there is an increase in the nonprotein nitrogen, urea acid, and urea. There is a marked vitamin deficiency. If there is a particularly marked decrease in vitamin B, polyneuritis develops.

The only treatment for hyperemesis is hospitalization. This in itself is therapeutic. The woman is taken away from her duties and responsibilities. She has a change in environment, she is protected, and there is a profound interest displayed by the physician, nurse, and family. The three principles of treatment are (1) combat dehydration by intravenous fluids, (2) combat starvation by intravenous glucose and vitamins, and (3) combat psychological symptoms by counseling and perhaps psychotherapy and sedatives.

Usually the nurse in the clinic or physician's office will have one or two visits with the patient before hospitalization becomes necessary. There are usually more phone communications rather than personal encounters. In even the shortest communication, however, it is necessary that the nurse convey warmth and concern. The relationships this woman develops with her doctor and the nursing staff are of great therapeutic value on both an in- and out-patient basis. On an outpatient basis the nurse must discover the woman's daily living habits, food and rest-taking priority; her relationship with her husband; and her feelings about herself and about this pregnancy. The nurse must reinforce the doctor's guidance and medication regimen.

On admission to the hospital, the nurse's assessment includes the patient's physical condition, her emotional state regarding herself and this pregnancy, and her family relationships. The nurse must be friendly, warm, and concerned in caring for this mother. The first 24 hours of hospitalization are crucial, and this must be carefully explained. A private room is a necessity and all visitors are excluded. The husband and family must realize the need for such restrictions and must be encouraged to call any time to inquire about the patient's condition. It is excellent practice for the nurse to arrange a time when the family can be contacted and report the patient's progress. This relieves many of the family's anxieties and builds security concerning their loved one's care.

Oral intake is discontinued the first 24 hours. Glucose and saline solutions are administered intravenously. Vitamins, particularly the B complex, and minerals are added to the intravenous solutions. The regimen for the first 24 hours gives the gastrointestinal tract complete rest. Accurate recordings of fluid intake and output are kept. The nurse's assessment needs to be made hourly during the first 24 hours to determine whether the woman is progressing with the treatment or if changes need to be made in regard to fluids, sedatives, and other medications. Intravenous fluids must be monitored carefully so that they do not infuse too rapidly and overwhelm the system or infuse too slowly and fail to accomplish the intended purpose. After 24 hours or when the vomiting subsides, small portions of food are given every 2 to 3 hours. Liquids and solids are given at alternate hours in small amounts. Foods must be either hot or cold, palatable, and attractive.

The nurse must help this expectant mother sort out her feelings concerning this pregnancy and help her and her family resolve some of their problems. One example of family cooperation is the case of Mrs. R.

Mrs. R, a thirty-five-year-old para 2 was admitted to the hospital for severe nausea and vomiting. Her last pregnancy was 9 years ago. Mrs. R was worried about telling her other two children about this pregnancy and how this baby would work into the family structure. Mr. R told the children about the expected new member of the family. They were delighted. Five days later, Mrs. R visited with the children in the off-floor waiting room. When Mrs. R saw how accepted this baby was, her mental and physical health improved rapidly. She was discharged 3 days later.

On rare occasions the pregnant woman's condition does not improve after the first 24 hours. Drastic measures, such as tube feeding, may then have to be instituted. The tube is passed into the woman's stomach and a high-calorie, high-vitamin formula is given. In this situation the nurse needs to give much psychological support as well as expert physical care.

With patience and understanding the most severe cases of hyperemesis will respond to treatment. It is only in very rare instances that patients will continue to vomit, and the interruption of pregnancy becomes necessary. Before discharge the nurse should help the woman begin to plan her activities during this pregnancy and for labor and delivery. Consideration for future family planning is also appropriate at this time.

COMPLICATIONS ASSOCIATED WITH BLEEDING DURING PREGNANCY

Bleeding as a symptom is probably one of the most serious concerns in pregnancy. Bleeding is never normal. To most people blood is equated with life, and the loss of blood threatens life. The pregnant woman depends on her blood supply to give life to her unborn child. When there is loss of blood, she fears that this means loss of life to her baby. Indeed, she is correct in believing that adequate amounts of maternal blood are necessary to her unborn child's life. Not only is blood necessary, but adequate circulation to deliver the blood is also necessary. This section discusses those conditions which have vaginal bleeding as their main symptom. Only the most common conditions are discussed. There are numerous conditions which cause vaginal bleeding in pregnancy, some innocuous, some serious. It is not possible within the scope of this text to discuss them all. Those conditions most commonly encountered are discussed in detail. Those which are less common are mentioned as possible causes. Remember that bleeding is *never* normal.

Abortion

GENERAL CONSIDERATIONS

The most common cause of bleeding during the first trimester is abortion. Abortion is the medical term used to describe the termination of pregnancy whenever it occurs before the fetus has reached a stage of viability. The interpretation of "stage of viability" is varied. Usually the weeks of gestation, inaccurate as they are, are used to determine viability. A fetus expelled from the uterus before 20 weeks is considered an abortus. A fetus weighing less than 400 grams is also considered an abortus. However, 28 weeks gestation and less than 1,000 grams have been used as criteria. With the advent of premature intensive care centers, however, many fetuses formerly considered abortuses have survived.

ILLEGAL ABORTION

Abortion as a medical condition affecting mainly the first trimester of pregnancy may be subdivided into spontaneous and induced, or planned, abortion. (Induced abortion as a therapeutic measure has been discussed in Chapter 12.) Induced abortion may also be illegal. The definition of an illegal abortion has been, in the past, termination of pregnancy without medical or legal justification. It is more difficult to accurately determine what is legal or medical justification now, since many states have modified their abortion laws. The incidence of illegal abortion is not known, but it is estimated that the rate is between 15 and 20 percent of all abortions.

If women were informed of complications arising from illegal abortions, possibly they would be less likely to resort to such drastic means. Severe hemorrhage, sepsis, acute renal failure, or bacterial shock can result from spontaneous abortion also but are more often a result of illegal abortion. One fact frequently alluded to in support of liberalizing abortion laws is the maternal morbidity and mortality associated with illegal abortion.

The nurse may be in a position to assist the woman who has a severe complication due to an illegal abortion. While the main focus of the nurse's care may be directed toward meeting the woman's critical physical needs, the emotional response of the woman to her own life-threatening crisis will require appropriate response from the nurse. As she faces the possibilities of death, long illness, or sterility, the woman may want to express her feelings and concerns to the nurse providing for her needs. Support for the grieving or dying patient is a subject covered very well in other publications. Nursing intervention planned for the crisis of serious illness as the result of illegal abortion must take into consideration all facets of the problem. The age of the patient is important in determining the approach. The very young girl may not fully realize the impact that sterility as a result of the abortion may have. Future problems may arise in her relationships with men. These problems can be anticipated and appropriate guidance offered. The need for long-term professional help and guidance will need to be identified and planned. The financial burdens resting upon herself or her parents are part of the problems faced by such a patient. The older woman may be ridden with guilt feelings if the illegal abortion and its complications cause sterility. The loss of the reproductive function and its impact on the woman must be recognized and dealt with.

SPONTANEOUS ABORTION

Spontaneous abortion results from natural causes and may be classified as follows:

Threatened abortion: The fetus is jeopardized by unexplained bleeding.
Imminent abortion: Abortion is inevitable.
Complete abortion:The entire products of conception are expelled.
Incomplete abortion: Part of the products of conception are passed and part are retained.
Missed abortion: The fetus dies in utero and is retained for 2 or more months.
Recurrent abortion: Abortion occurs in a number of successive pregnancies.

The incidence of spontaneous abortion is usually given as about 10 percent of all pregnancies or 1 in every 5 interrupted pregnancies. It is difficult to be accurate concerning these statistics because some women may abort in early weeks when they did not realize a pregnancy existed.

Causes

The causes of spontaneous abortion are discussed in the order of most frequent occurrence.

Early in pregnancy spontaneous abortion is usually preceded by the death of the embryo or fetus. The problem then becomes one of finding the cause of fetal death. The most common cause of fetal death or death of the embryo in the early months is abnormal development. The abnormalities are incompatible with life, thus the fetus dies, and the products of conception are expelled.

Knowledge concerning abnormal development of fetuses is increasing rapidly. Certain drugs are known to cause specific developmental abnormalities. Specific diseases also contribute to the abnormal development of the fertilized ova. As precise knowledge grows, cause and treatment may follow and may prevent some spontaneous abortions due to abnormal fetal development.

Recent studies have found that among aborted fetuses 67 percent had structural abnormalities and 41 percent were grossly pathological.[1] There is a high incidence of abnormal development in early abortion.

Other causes are attributed to faulty implantation or unfavorable intrauterine environment. With the advances in the knowledge and science of genetics, it is possible to determine and identify some chromosomal aberrations that cause abnormal embryonic and fetal development and their relation to spontaneous abortion.

Abnormalities of the placenta after the 20th week may lead to abortion or, more often, to premature labor. These abnormalities include placental insufficiency due to endarteritic changes in blood vessels of the villi, large placental infarcts, and later placenta previa and premature separation of the placenta.

Maternal disease as a cause of spontaneous abortion must be considered. Severe acute infections such as pneumonia, pyelonephritis, and typhoid may occasionally lead to abortion. These acute infections release toxins from the mother, causing fetal morbidity or mortality and consequent abortion. Specific bacterial invasion may itself cause death or illness in the fetus and its subsequent expulsion.

Although chronic wasting diseases such as tuberculosis or carcinomatosis are rarely causes for abortion, they can often cause premature labor.

Endocrine imbalance may be the cause of abortion. A thorough study of the maternal endocrine system may be necessary if no other cause for abortion is found. The secretion of progesterone by the corpus luteum maintains the decidua from which the growing embryo obtains its sustenance. If progesterone secretion is reduced or absent, this condition would contribute to fetal loss. Supplemental progesterone therapy may be necessary to maintain the pregnancy and prevent abortion. In gathering clinical data to rule out any endocrine disorder, the nurse may anticipate that the physician will order diagnostic tests to determine endocrine function. Preparation of the patient for these tests will serve to relieve some of her anxiety.

Occasionally, laparotomy during pregnancy is necessary. If the site of the surgery is in close proximity to the pelvic organs, the possibility of abortion increases. The physician may prescribe daily administrations of progesterone for 7 to 10 days postoperatively to reduce the chances of postoperative abortion. Progesterone is a life-supporting hormone to the fetus.

Abnormalities of the reproductive organs are not often the cause of abortion but are more important causes of sterility. The most significant abnormality responsible for abortion is the congenitally short cervix or the surgically shortened or amputated cervix. Cervical tears that are poorly repaired or that heal poorly may cause late abortion.

The so-called "incompetent cervix" is an important cause in recurrent abortion and is discussed later in this chapter.

Man is an inquisitive being, always seeking answers to his questions. When a woman aborts, her family, her doctor, and the nurse want a simple, clearly understood reason for it. The role assigned to trauma, psychic or physical, in the causes for abortion is difficult to prove. Indeed, severe physical trauma may be the cause of abortion, and usually abortion quickly follows severe trauma. The mechanism for both physical and emotional trauma is probably not fetal death. It is due to interference with proper uterine blood flow, causing separation of the placenta and thus resulting in abortion. In this case the fetus and placenta would be normal and show no signs of death preceding the trauma.

Emotional shock as a cause of abortion is most difficult to document. There is no doubt that in rare instances emotional trauma causes abortion. Accurate history taking and thorough physical examination to rule out other causes must be done before the physician assigns emotional trauma as the cause of abortion.

There remains only one other cause for abortion to be discussed. Many infections have been suspected of causing abortion. Viral infections may cause abortion. Some of these directly infect the embryo, and others cause fetal death through the response of the woman to severe toxicity and fever. Some viral infections implicated in abortion are rubella, influenza, and poliomyelitis. Such rare infestations as toxoplasmosis, malaria, and amebiasis may also be causes of early or late abortion.

Pathological findings in spontaneous abortion usually demonstrate decidual hemorrhage—that is, hemorrhage occurs in the decidua basalis, causing consequent necrotic changes in surrounding tissue, subsequent inflammation, and detachment in whole or part of the ovum. Fetal death has always been thought of as secondary to decidual hemorrhage, but a few recent studies seem to put the sequence of events in a different order in some cases of abortion.

Regardless of the cause of spontaneous abortion the woman is concerned for the safety of the unborn child and herself. Vaginal bleeding is frightening to the pregnant woman. It threatens her life and that of her child. If she is unsure that she is pregnant or unsure she wants to be, the threat and the fear take on different dimensions. In describing the thought processes of the woman during the early weeks of pregnancy, Reva Rubin[2] suggests that she is not ready to accept the *actuality* of her pregnancy. She experiences both pleasure and displeasure related to the fact of conception. She feels ambivalent and wants to be sure of the fact of pregnancy. Vaginal bleeding that signals threatened abortion can upset this whole cognitive process. All at once the unsure presence is threatened by the loss of life-giving fluid—blood. Suddenly the fetus, heretofore thought of only as perhaps being present, is dictating the mother's behavior. The treatment for threatened abortion is usually bed rest. She must now protect with every precaution a life she was not quite sure was there and was not quite sure she was ready to accept.

A second threat is that although her precautions may save the unborn child's life, the child may be permanently damaged. Fear and anxiety related to delivery of a defective, damaged child are then to be dealt with.

Threatened Abortion

Threatened abortion is a condition in which the major symptom is moderate amounts of bright red vaginal bleeding accompanied by minimal amounts of back and abdominal pain. In this condition the mother experiences the threatened loss of the fetus. The physician usually will prescribe bed rest and sometimes sedatives and progesterone therapy. The nurse will need to make the necessary assessments of blood loss, pain, and needs for support and sedation. In the way of support the woman may need reassurance that she is not to blame for this condition. If she does not lose her baby, she may want reassurance that it will be normal when it is born.

Imminent Abortion

If threatened abortion continues, it becomes imminent abortion. With this condition there are usually uterine contractions which are easily identified and increase in intensity. The woman has a feeling or sensation for the need to bear down. Support required for this woman is directed toward preparing her for the reality of the abortion. After examination of the patient confirms that cervical dilatation is present, the condition becomes an inevitable abortion. The nurse may discover that the amniotic sac has ruptured and there is an escape of some amniotic fluid from the vagina. This can be confirmed by the use of nitrazine paper to determine the pH and to discover whether the leakage is urine or amniotic fluid. More often, however, the pelvic examination will confirm the rupture of the membranes.

Again the nursing assessments which are made and the nursing interventions which are planned are crucial to the woman's satisfactory recovery and resolution of crisis.

Incomplete Abortion

If the products of conception are not completely expelled at the time of abortion (incomplete abortion), a dilatation and curettage may be required to completely evacuate the uterus and control bleeding. As long as part of the products of conception are in the uterus, there is danger of hemorrhage. The nurse will need to prepare the woman for surgery. The necessary general pre-operative teaching will be needed as well as additional information to meet the woman's special needs. Her special needs will be related to her desire and the family's desire for pregnancy and their response to the loss of this particular pregnancy. She will need reassurance that she may be able in the future to have more children if she so desires. She may require assistance with the financial burden imposed by bed rest, restricted activity, and loss of income. She may also need reassurance and assistance with regard to the care of her family. A social worker could be of great assistance in helping resolve social and financial burdens.

In complete abortion the entire products of conception are expelled, and there is very minimal, controlled bleeding. Special attention should be given to the mother's religious affiliation. It will be most important to Roman Catholic parents that the fetus has been baptized. This is very simply done by immersion of the fetus in water or pouring water over the fetus and repeating the following words: "I baptize you in the name of the Father, and of the Son, and of the Holy Spirit." Most other Christian denominations do not believe in baptism of the fetus. The Judaic religion has other customs associated with death of the fetus. The nurse should inquire regarding practices of the parents as part of the spiritual care of the patient.

Missed Abortion

A missed abortion is rare but occurs when the embryo or fetus dies and is retained in utero for months. The uterus increases in size until the third or fourth month when signs of a threatened abortion are exhibited. These signs are of short duration, and it is thought that the pregnancy is progressing normally until subsequent examinations demonstrate no further uterine growth. Why the uterus does not expel the dead fetus is unknown, but the dead fetus can remain in utero for months or even years without producing the symptoms of a foreign body. If there are no symptoms, no course of action is taken in hopes that a spontaneous abortion will finally occur; this is usually safer than operative interference.

Recurrent Abortion

Recurrent abortion is a condition in which a woman has three or more consecutive abortions. The older term "habitual abortion" has gradually been eliminated in recent medical literature. In keeping with this current trend the term "recurrent abortion" is used throughout this chapter. Much research in the past has been directed toward predicting those women who were likely to abort. Other research has concentrated on specific causes for abortion and their correction. The treatment of recurrent abortion depends on the cause found by the physician. After thoroughly investigating all possible causes for the abortion, the physician will usually counsel the couple in regard to future childbearing possibilities. In anticipation of the possible lines of investigation the physician will use to establish the cause of recurrent abortion, the nurse may give some guidance to the woman to prepare her for the tests she may undergo. The woman will need empathy, guidance, and possibly clarification whether she is hospitalized or treated on an outpatient basis.

The pathology involved and the etiologic factors for recurrent abortion are manifold. However, there are two main categories which include all possible factors: defective spermatozoa and/or ova or an unfavorable maternal environment.

To establish defective germ cells as the cause of recurrent abortion, the physician will need to order studies of both sperm and ova. Pathological study of the aborted embryo will give information regarding abnormal development, but the conclusion that these abnormal embryos are the results of defective sperm and ova cannot be made. Most often the germ cells are not defective, and the greatest cause of recurrent abortion has to do with the maternal environment. Genetic counseling is available when the defective sperm or ova cannot produce normal embryos. The physician counsels the parents regarding the probability of the couple producing a normal embryo. The couple may decide to undergo a sterilization procedure and adopt children. Their decision may be to remain a childless family. If they already have a child (or children), they may decide that they will not adopt nor try to have more. Whatever the decision, the nurse lends her support and reassurance to the couple and refrains from value judgment.

The causes of an unfavorable maternal environment are many; therefore, only the most common will be discussed.

Pregnancy and its healthy continuance depends to a great extent on hormones. Hormonal problems account for a large number of failures in pregnancies. The thyroid gland and its functions are important in reproduction, and dysfunction of this gland has been implicated as a principal cause of recurrent abortion in many women. In determining the functioning of the thyroid gland in cases of recurrent abortion the tests included may be PBI (protein bound iodine), BEI (butanol extractable iodine), GBI (globulin bound iodine), thyroid scans, and iodine uptake studies. If a thyroid disorder is found, therapy usually is begun prior to the next pregnancy.

Other hormones, such as progesterone, secreted by the corpus luteum are important in pregnancy. The corpus luteum secretes both progesterone and some estrogens which are necessary to the maintenance of the decidua basalis, which provides nourishment for the conceptus. If there is a deficiency in these hormones, it is probable that this condition may cause death of the embryo. If levels are low, the physician usually will give the woman some supplemental progesterone.

Later in pregnancy the placenta assumes the function of the corpus luteum. Failure on the part of the placenta to assume its function may be the cause of recurrent abortion. If pregnanediol levels in the urine are not high enough, the woman is usually started on hormonal therapy.

The relationship between maternal diet and growth and development of the fetus has been studied by many. Hytten and Leitch[3] discuss at length the relationship between maternal weight gain and nutrients and fetal weight and development. Certain vitamins are essential, and their absence can cause poor nutritional status and perhaps abortion in early pregnancy. As a cause of recurrent abortion, however, the mother's nutritional status must be considered.

Defects in the anatomy of the uterus may also cause abortion. Uteri with double cavities have accounted for a few cases of recurrent abortion. However, more than 75 percent of women with a bicornuate uterus have no problems.[4]

The *incompetent cervix* is a term which is applied to a condition in pregnancy in which the cervix dilates, usually without pain or accompanying bloody discharge. This usually occurs during the second trimester of pregnancy and is followed by spontaneous rupture of the membranes. The fetus is born but is usually so immature that it expires before, during, or after delivery. In a woman who has a history of these events, an operation may prevent further loss. This operation, named after the surgeons who perfected it, is called the Shirodkar or MacDonald procedure. The purpose of both procedures is to reinforce the cervix by some type of suture. They are usually performed between the 14th and 18th weeks of pregnancy. These sutures are left in place until the 38th or 39th week of gestation. They are then removed, and the patient is delivered vaginally. At times, however, the sutures are left in place and a cesarean section is performed.

COMPLICATIONS OF ABORTION

Severe hemorrhage, sepsis, acute renal failure, and endotoxic shock (bacterial shock) are serious complications which may follow abortion. The treatment of these complications does not differ greatly from their treatment when abortion is not the cause. However, the obstetric treatment is discussed in the following pages. It must be remembered that whether the cause is induced or spontaneous abortion, the complication and treatment can be the same.

Although temperature elevation often accompanies abortion, it is usually not a serious complication. The patient may have a temperature elevation before or after expelling the products of conception. When fever does occur every precaution is taken to rule out more serious complications. Fever, of course, may indicate infection, which is one of the complications of abortion. It does not often occur in hospital abortion, but when abortion takes place at home or en route to the hospital, the possibility of infection is greater. The usual causative organisms are in the coli and aerogenes groups. Other organisms can be the cause, such as anaerobic or hemolytic streptococci, staphylococcus, and clostridia. Infection, most often endometritis, can be treated conservatively with broad-spectrum antibiotics, rest, and fluids. If the uterus has not been emptied, the physician usually does this immediately. When the infection is more widespread, as in parametritis, localized or general peritonitis, and generalized septicemia, more vigorous treatment will be required. Early signs and symptoms of progressive infection must be carefully observed by the nurse. Although fever is usually the first sign, others which include pain, local tenderness, rise in pulse rate, and drop in blood pressure should be carefully observed and reported by the nurse.

Occasionally infection may develop into a chronic pelvic abscess. This usually means a long hospitalization and recovery period for the patient. Surgical drainage of the abscess is undertaken if it can be done vaginally. Sometimes, however, the abscess will require abdominal surgery. Care for these women includes, in addition to physical aspects, a great deal of supportive encouragement. Chronic pelvic infection and abscess are debilitating and require lengthy hospitalization. The family should visit as often as they can and as often as the patient's condition allows. The nurse should be attuned to the patient's fatigue level.

Fatal hemorrhage due to spontaneous abortion is extremely rare. However, hemorrhage can and does occur, and the treatment includes transfusion and, when necessary, emptying of the uterus. In unusually severe hemorrhage it may be necessary to ligate the hypogastric arteries which supply the uterine vessels. On very rare occasions it may be necessary to remove the uterus when hemorrhage cannot be controlled. This sudden loss of the uterus can cause deep emotional disturbances in the woman. The nurse's skill in giving emotional support to the woman who is faced with such a loss is most important to the woman's difficult adjustment.

Bacterial endotoxic shock, usually caused by E. coli, is a rare complication associated with spontaneous abortion and can be fatal, depending on the degree of renal involvement. In such conditions the patient is given fluids parenterally with an antihypotensive drug and large doses of antibiotics. There is grave danger that before the patient responds to the drugs, water intoxication may occur. The nurse must closely monitor the fluid intake and output. The urine output must be at least 30 cc per hour or more to indicate maintenance of adequate circulation and kidney function. The care for such patients is not greatly different from any other patient who suffers from overwhelming infection.

Acute renal failure may be associated with endotoxic shock, but more often it is the result of shock and infection. Death from acute renal failure was at one time extremely common. With the present state of medical knowledge and skill, the physician has time to allow the kidney to recover while the patient is on artificial dialysis. It is most important to recognize early the signs and symptoms of acute renal failure. Urinary output should be carefully observed and recorded.

Accidental perforation of the uterus can occur during dilatation and curettage whether the surgeon uses a curette or the uterine suction apparatus. Very small holes will heal spontaneously. The patient will require close observation by the nurse to detect early signs and symptoms of complications; such as weak, thready, or increased pulse rate; drop in blood pressure; pallor; and diaphoresis. If the perforation is the result of illegal abortion, it can be a much more serious complication. Usually the hole in the uterus is large and may involve blood vessels, or even the bowel or bladder. The nurse must be observant for signs and symptoms of peritonitis, pelvic infection, and bleeding into the peritoneal cavity. In peritonitis or pelvic infection, the woman would be observed for elevation of temperature, abdominal pain, tenderness, rigidity, and referred pain to the shoulder.

The doctor will want to have a flat plate of the abdomen taken. Following this a laparotomy is done. The patient must be prepared for these procedures in a very short period of time. She will need a great deal of physical and emotional support during this acute physical crisis. Because of her intense pain, the patient requires total physical care in bathing, changing position, and monitoring fluid intake and output as well as monitoring vital signs. No one is in greater need of acceptance and empathy than this woman.

Another complication which may accompany abortion is transplacental hemorrhage. Although the actual amount of blood lost may not be significant in terms of causing maternal shock, fetal erythrocytes in the maternal circulation cause another problem. Isoimmunization can result from the presence of fetal blood in the maternal circulation following spontaneous abortion. As part of accurate history-taking in women who are Rh negative, determining previous abortion is crucial. Abortion may have caused Rh sensitization. The physician may prescribe immunoglobulin to prevent the development of antibodies.

Ectopic Pregnancy

The second greatest cause of bleeding during the first trimester is ectopic pregnancy. Ectopic pregnancy is a pregnancy which is implanted outside the uterine cavity. There are several locations where an ectopic pregnancy might occur, but the majority of these occur in the fallopian tubes. Other sites include ovaries, anatomically underdeveloped portions of the uterus, cervix, and areas of the abdomen.

The clinical signs and symptoms of ectopic pregnancy are not always clearly discernible. If a woman misses one or two menstrual periods, she assumes she is pregnant. The uterus itself undergoes changes as in a normal pregnancy. When the embryo dies, there is some vaginal bleeding usually associated with pain in one quadrant of the abdomen. Many times pain is referred to the opposite quadrant of the abdomen or some other area of the abdomen or even the thorax.

Recently, there is some evidence that intrauterine devices used for contraception may cause tubal implantation of the ova.[5] Since conception generally occurs in the outer third of the uterine tube, any condition which impedes the progress of the fertilized ovum on its way to the uterus could result in tubal pregnancy. Such conditions include chronic salpingitis, congenital abnormalities of tubal development, corrective surgery performed on the tubes, adhesions caused by previous infection, and pelvic tumors near the tube. One other cause of tubal pregnancy may be the presence of endometrial implants in the mucous membrane lining of the tubes.

An implantation may occur anywhere along the tube. Usually the patient is symptomless until the tubal area of implantation becomes severely distended with the products of conception. The tube may then rupture, forcing the products of conception through the fimbriated end into the peritoneal cavity. Bleeding will occur either into the lumen of the tube or into the peritoneal cavity. Signs of shock usually accompany the rupture and subsequent bleeding. In rare instances when the ova is extruded intact it may find a suitable site for growth and development and become an abdominal pregnancy.

The woman who has a tubal pregnancy usually feels no other symptoms than those of beginning pregnancy. Until the pregnancy grows to sufficient size to cause rupture, the woman will notice no particular symptoms. Pain usually followed by vaginal spotting and fainting or "lightheaded" feelings may be the first signs. On examination the physician will find that the woman has extreme vaginal tenderness and abdominal tenderness and rigidity. Blood pressure falls, and the pulse rate increases.

If the woman has a slowly progressing rupture, the signs and symptoms may be quite different. The rupture causes slow leakage of blood, and, therefore, the body adjusts to the slow loss of blood. If the blood forms a pelvic hematocele, this may rupture and cause signs of shock. The hematocele may eventually form an abscess.

After tubal pregnancy has been treated and the woman is recovering, attention must be given to her response to the situation. The nurse will establish an environment and a relationship which facilitates verbalization of feelings. The woman's concerns for future childbearing will need expression and clarification.

If the tubal pregnancy was due to pelvic inflammatory disease or a tubal anomaly, chances are that the condition is bilateral. Therefore, the woman may be subject to another tubal pregnancy. This fact may influence her decision to practice contraception. Support for her decisions from the nurse will give the woman reassurance.

Ovarian pregnancy in which the conceptus implants in the ovary is rare. It usually results in rupture or degeneration of the embryo at an early stage.

TABLE 31-1
ANALYSIS OF BLEEDING COMPLICATIONS WITH RECOMMENDED INTERVENTIONS

Type of bleeding	Onset	Associated symptoms	Possible causes	Medical and nursing care
Slight to moderate bright red vaginal bleeding	During 1st trimester; rarely 2d trimester	Minimal back pain; minimal abdominal pain	Threatened abortion	Bed rest; progesterone therapy and/or sedatives; observe amount and kind of vaginal bleeding
		No pain	Cervical polyps / Cancer of cervix / Blood dyscrasias	Observe vaginal discharge
		Expulsion of part of products of conception	Incomplete abortion	Continuous observation; may receive oxytocic drugs; D&C may be required
	Beginning about 12th week	Enlargement of uterus out of proportion to duration of pregnancy	Hydatidiform mole	
Copious bright red bleeding accompanied by clots	During 1st trimester usually	Identifiable uterine contractions of some intensity; "bearing down" sensation	Imminent abortion	Strict bed rest; sedatives; progesterone therapy; observe amount and kind of vaginal flow and discharge
		On pelvic exam cervical dilatation / Rupture of amniotic sac	Inevitable abortion	
Minimal to controlled vaginal bleeding	Usually 1st trimester; rarely 2d trimester	Usually accompanied by feeling of relief from abdominal pain and back pains, "bearing down" sensation, and passage of all products of conception	Complete abortion	Observe for amount and kind of bleeding; prevent shock; oxytocics may be ordered
"Spotting"; occasional minimal vaginal bleeding	1st or 2d trimester or any time	Pain, amenorrhea	Ectopic pregnancy	Laparotomy
		None: usually discovered on pelvic exam or microscopic study of cells	Cancer of cervix	Possible laparotomy; vaginal hysterectomy; radiation treatment
		Periodic abdominal pain	Endometriosis	Hormonal therapy, laparotomy

Abdominal pregnancy is a rare condition. There are cases on record, however, and discussion of case histories may be found in obstetric literature. Even more rare are pregnancies occurring in the area of the cervix. In either case, painless vaginal bleeding at the time of implantation occurs, and subsequent bleeding requires surgical termination of the pregnancy.

Isoimmunization may follow ectopic pregnancy just as it may follow abortion and normal pregnancy. A maternal history of any ectopic pregnancy must be carefully noted.

Hydatidiform Mole

The importance of observing the quantity and quality of vaginal bleeding and its associated symptoms cannot be overemphasized. Often the description of vaginal discharge will enable the physician to make a diagnosis that will save the patient's life. In cases of hydatidiform mole the discharge containing the grapelike vesicles is diagnostic. Hydatidiform mole represents a degeneration of the villi accompanied by proliferation of the epithelium of the chorion. The degenerating cells of the villi become swollen with fluid, resulting in clusters of fluid-filled vesicles. Other signs and symptoms include uterine growth in advance of length of gestation and absence of "lightening." Bleeding may be either scant and spotty, or there may be gross hemorrhage. Hyperemesis is usually more severe than in pregnancy and is a frequent additional symptom. There also may be concomitant uterine infection.

Treatment consists of emptying the uterus of the mole, preventing further blood loss, and in the presence of infection giving antibiotic therapy. The surgeon uses great care in curetting the uterus, as its lining and musculature become soft in response to the mole and it could be easily perforated.

The woman will need additional support in adapting to the fact that she is no longer pregnant. These patients are more often met on the gynecological service than the obstetric service.

A few of these women develop recurrent moles or choriocarcinoma. These conditions can be responsible for bleeding in pregnancy. Choriocarcinoma, though rare, is a highly malignant cancer and survival rates beyond 1 year are uncommon.

Other Causes of Bleeding during Pregnancy

Bleeding during pregnancy at any stage can also be caused by cervical or vaginal polyps, carcinoma of the cervix, blood dyscrasias (e.g., thrombocytopenic purpura, leukemia), and vaginal varicosities. Bleeding later in pregnancy may be related to complications of labor and delivery. Placenta previa and abruptio placentae are the most common causes of bleeding in the latter half of pregnancy. These conditions are discussed in Chapter 32. Table 31-1 summarizes types of bleeding and possible causes.

COINCIDENTAL COMPLICATIONS OF PREGNANCY

Cardiovascular Problems

HEART DISEASE

During pregnancy the heart is called upon to increase its output by 30 to 40 percent. The heart is able to handle an increased blood volume of about 30 percent.[6] Heart rate increases in the second and third trimesters. These changes result in changes in heart sounds and may be the cause of functional murmurs in pregnant women. Such murmurs make diagnosis of heart conditions in pregnancy difficult.

Heart disease in pregnancy and its management have changed considerably over the years. As medical knowledge regarding heart disease and its treatment has grown, more women with heart disease are able to carry pregnancies to term. Cardiac surgery for congenital defects and acquired problems has meant that more women with these problems can carry a pregnancy to term.

The woman with heart disease may require additional nursing care during all phases of pregnancy. She may be fearful for the lives of herself and her infant. Additional burdens of pregnancy may limit her activities so that she is concerned for the health and well-being of her husband and family. Regardless of the nature of the heart disease, care for women during this period is essentially the same, and the concerns the mother has for her life, her infant, and her family are also essentially the same. Because of this, rather than name and describe *specific* heart disorders and congenital heart defects, this chapter discusses the care of women with cardiac lesions by classification according to the severity of the disorder. The New York Heart Association[7] has used the following criteria for grouping patients into four functional classes:

Class I patients have no limitation of physical activity. Ordinary physical activity causes no discomfort; they do not have symptoms of cardiac insufficiency and do not have anginal pain.

Class II patients have slight limitation of physical activity. Ordinary physical activity causes excessive fatigue, palpitation, and dyspnea or anginal pain.

Class III patients have a moderate to marked limitation of physical activity. During less than ordinary activity they experience excessive fatigue, palpitation, dyspnea, or anginal pain.

Class IV patients are unable to carry on any physical activity without experiencing discomfort. Even at rest they will experience symptoms of cardiac insufficiency or anginal pain.

Usually mothers who are class I and II patients will experience a normal pregnancy and have few complications.

The principal goals in antepartum, intrapartum, and postpartum care are to provide adequate rest, prevent infection and physical stress, and prevent and treat fluid retention and venous congestion. These goals apply also to women in classes III and IV. However, women so severely affected need greater supervision to maintain health and prevent fatigue. At the first sign of heart failure they are immediately hospitalized and treated. Close observation of the woman as she is seen in the clinic, office, or at home will help to detect any signs and symptoms of problems early. The implications of such a course of action are great for the woman and her family. The fear of death for both the woman and the fetus prevails. Emotional support in the form of listening and providing a reassuring attitude will be needed. False hope and reassurance are not helpful, but realistic goals in terms of care and treatment will provide women with the necessary support.

Dietary control is planned for preventing excessive weight gain and fluid retention. Low-sodium and low-calorie intake will need to be explained. Provision of consultation with the dietitian will assist the patient in understanding her limitations.

These women will be placed on diuretics. The selection of the diuretic and route of administration will be medical decisions. The nurse's responsibility lies in making accurate observations of the patient's tolerance and responses to the diuretic therapy prescribed.

The use of digitalis may or may not be part of the treatment. When employed, the necessary care accompanying the use of digitalis is the same as it is for nonpregnant cardiac patients.

Despite the close supervision and care, some pregnant women develop congestive failure, pulmonary edema, infections, and/or anemias. Women who suffer from any of these require immediate attention. In addition to those steps taken when any cardiac patient suffers from complications, pregnant cardiac patients require consideration of the fetus and the pregnant state. The response of the woman and fetus to drugs and therapy must be closely observed and accurately reported. Women with reduced cardiac output are more prone to produce small-for-gestational-age infants.

VENOUS AND ARTERIAL COMPLICATIONS

The arterial side of the circulation does not respond to the state of pregnancy in the same way as the venous side. Whatever complications arise in the arterial system are the result of coincidence and not an effect of pregnancy. Since the occurrence of arterial complications is not frequent, the nurse may not come in contact with mothers who suffer from these conditions very often.

References in the bibliography at the end of this chapter may be used to pursue interest in any arterial complications.

VARICOSITIES

Varicosities occur quite commonly during pregnancy and most often affect the legs. As the pressure from uterine and fetal growth increases in the pelvis, additional stress is felt in the veins of the pelvis, vulva, and legs. Positional relief, though temporary, is usually advised for mothers who are afflicted with varicosities.

It is possible to treat varicosities during pregnancy by injection or surgical procedures, but there is disagreement concerning the advisability of these procedures.

Varicosities of the vulva and vagina occur and may be the cause of complications during labor and delivery. A ruptured vaginal varicosity will result in vaginal bleeding and this cause may be overlooked. The vagina is inspected for bleeding sites.

Renal Disease

According to Guyton,[8] the maternal urinary system undergoes specific functional changes during pregnancy, namely, increased reabsorption of sodium, chloride, and water; increased glomerular filtration rate; and ureteral dilatation. These changes normally cause no difficulty and are relieved at the termination of pregnancy, but they may be the cause of certain complications incidental to pregnancy.

INFECTIONS

The most frequently occurring urinary tract complication is acute pyelonephritis. It is most often the right kidney which is involved. The uterus rotates toward the right as it grows out of the pelvis during pregnancy, causing pressure on the right ureter as it passes over the pelvic brim. This increased pressure on the right side is often cited as the cause for the increase in right-sided pyelonephritis. The treatment for acute pyelonephritis is usually bed rest, increased fluid intake, and antibiotic therapy.

Careful attention is given to detecting other infections in the urinary tract during pregnancy. Bacteriuria in pregnancy is an important complication. Many women who have bacteria in the urine during pregnancy develop urinary tract infections requiring treatment. It is important that the urine of pregnant women be cultured for the presence of urinary bacteria because urinary tract infection is a predisposing factor to prematurity.

Infection in the form of bacteriuria, cystitis, and acute pyelonephritis occurs most frequently as the renal complications coincidental to pregnancy. There are, however, other conditions that need to be mentioned. There is not much information concerning the care and treatment of these rarely occurring conditions, but there are some readings available which are listed in the bibliography at the end of this chapter.

Renal tuberculosis rarely occurs now but may be seen occasionally in the pregnant woman. Congenital abnormalities such as polycystic disease of the kidney, pelvic ectopic kidney, renal artery aneurysms, and ureteropelvic obstruction may cause severe problems during pregnancy but, again, are of rare occurrence.

URINARY TRACT CALCULI; NEOPLASMS

Urinary tract calculi and neoplasms of the genitourinary system do occur, but not often, during pregnancy.

Endocrine Disorders

DIABETES MELLITUS

The history of pregnancy in diabetic women is ominous. Before the discovery of insulin, pregnancy rarely occurred in diabetic women. When a woman did conceive, it usually ended in spontaneous abortion or caused her to develop diabetic acidosis and coma. The rare diabetic woman who managed to carry a pregnancy to term usually produced a stillborn, an abnormal infant, or a neonatal death.

Now that medical knowledge concerning diabetes and its cause and treatment has grown to such a degree, pregnancy is no longer rare in the diabetic woman. Many women who exhibited signs of diabetes in childhood live to the childbearing age and do become pregnant. The outcome of the pregnancy will depend upon the severity of the disease and the management of pregnancy.

Even though most diabetic women live a normal life span and some do bear children, the fetal and neonatal death rates are still higher in comparison to that of normal women. The danger to the fetus even in well-controlled diabetes is still increased.

Complications, particularly the toxemias and polyhydramnios, are frequent and endanger the fetus. Women who already have nephropathy, neuropathy, and vascular involvement have the highest rate of fetal wastage and make up part of the group of high-risk mothers. Infants of these women who go to term are frequently small for gestational age.

For the purposes of describing diabetes in pregnancy, it is useful to view the classification of diabetes described by White in her classic article:[9]

Class A. Pregnant women whose glucose tolerance test is only slightly abnormal. Fetal survival is high. Dietary regulation is minimal, and no insulin is required.

Class B. Pregnant women whose diabetes is of less than 10 years' duration, whose disease began at age twenty or older, and who have no vascular involvement.

Class C. Pregnant women whose diabetes began between age ten and nineteen, whose disease has lasted from 10 to 19 years, and who have minimal vascular involvement.

Class D. Pregnant women whose diabetes has lasted 20 years or more, whose disease began before age ten, and who have greater vascular involvement.

Class E. Pregnant women in whom calcification of the pelvic arteries has been demonstrated on x ray.

Class F. Pregnant women whose diabetes has caused nephropathy.

Preclinical Diabetes

Pregnancy, acting as a stress factor, may cause the body to demand an increase in insulin output. If the woman is predisposed to diabetes, the increased demand may be too much for her to respond to and she develops some symptoms of pre-diabetes. These usually involve a history of having delivered progressively larger babies, of perinatal loss, a slightly abnormal glucose tolerance curve, and glycosuria.

These women should be carefully observed during the remainder of the pregnancy by more frequent antenatal visits. They are given careful dietary instructions, with emphasis on protein and carbohydrate intake. Laboratory tests at each visit may include examination of urine for glucose, acetone, and albumin. These patients are generally allowed to deliver at term. If the baby seems to be gaining an excessive amount of weight, the woman may be delivered early, but this is a controversial issue and seldom done.

Diabetes, Classes B through F

In women whose diabetes is known before conception, close management is required during the entire pregnancy. These women are seen frequently, usually every 2 weeks during the first and second trimesters and weekly during the third trimester. A careful watch is kept for complications and often the woman herself tests the urine daily for sugar and acetone. She will require guidance and encouragement to continue to be vigilant. Requirements of diet and insulin often are variable during pregnancy. Each individual woman must be closely managed with special attention to ensure a successful outcome. The obstetrician and internist collaborate closely on her care and progress.

Labor and delivery are added stresses so occasionally labor will be induced early under very careful scrutiny. Delivery of a high-risk mother should take place in a center where techniques and personnel are available for high-risk delivery. Monitoring of the fetus and of uterine contractions should be carried out. Intravenous glucose is usually administered with careful adjustment of insulin requirements.

Pregnancy should only be terminated early enough to prevent fetal loss from placental insufficiency or complications affecting fetal survival, but too early a termination resulting in prematurity is to be avoided.

THYROID DYSFUNCTION

General Considerations

According to Guyton, the normal response of the thyroid gland in pregnancy is to increase in size and production of thyroxine by about 50 percent.[10] This produces in the pregnant woman some symptoms which may imitate hyperthyroidism: increased metabolic rate, increased PBI values, increased I^{131} uptake. The thyroid gland and its increased activity return to normal following pregnancy. However, in a few instances the gland does not return to normal, and simple goiter results.

Hyperthyroidism

Pregnancy is not rare in women with hyperthyroidism. Although there is a fair amount of experience with pregnancy in hyperthyroidism, there is disagreement as to the effects of pregnancy on the hyperthyroid state. Some physicians have found that pregnancy does aggravate hyperthyroidism and some have found an improvement of the disease.

Most authors agree, however, that when the pregnant woman has thyrotoxicosis, the fetus is endangered. In this condition fetal loss is high. Uncontrolled hyperthyroidism leads to abortion and fetal or neonatal death.

When the disease is controlled fetal outcome is usually good. There are some physicians who advise mothers against breast-feeding the baby.

Methods of treating this disease have improved over the years since 1940. There are generally two ways to control this disease in pregnancy. The choice of method usually is agreed upon by the obstetrician and internist. The first method consists of antithyroid drugs and iodine administered from the onset of pregnancy until about the 25th or 26th week of gestation. Fetal outcome is generally good. The second method consists of the administration of antithyroid drugs throughout pregnancy with delivery at term.

The effects of thyroid disorders on the newborn include: congenital goiter (endemic and sporadic), cretinism, congenital myxedema, and congenital hyperthyroidism. These effects are all amenable to proper treatment.

Hypothyroidism

Hypothyroidism is easily enough controlled provided enough thyroid is given to allow a normal thyroid state to exist. Giving too much thyroid causing hyperthyroidism must be avoided. Fetal outcome depends upon early diagnosis and treatment and accurate control during pregnancy.

Myxedema

Myxedema is rarely seen as a complication of pregnancy. Usually women acquire this disease after the childbearing age. Also, myxedema usually causes sterility. There are cases reported in the literature of pregnancy after the disease has been controlled, but they are extremely rare.

OTHER ENDOCRINE DISORDERS

There are any number of other endocrine disorders that may be present in the pregnant woman and include adrenal dysfunction (including Addison's disease), Cushing's syndrome, pheochromocytoma, hyperparathyroidism, acromegaly, and diabetes insipidus. There are in the literature some case studies of pregnancy complicated by these diseases. Special interest in a woman with a specific problem should prompt the nurse to pursue literature related to the specific problem.

Hematologic Problems

Maternal Isoimmunization

Although maternal isoimmunization occurs unrelated to pregnancy, it becomes a complication of pregnancy when maternal antibodies cross the placental barrier and invade the fetal circulation. The resultant disease of the newborn, erythroblastosis fetalis or hemolytic disease of the newborn, varies in its severity from a mild anemia and/or hyperbilirubinemia to death from severe hydrops fetalis. The most frequently occurring antigen antibody formation is due to Rh_0 (D) antibodies.

There are many sources of information which clearly explain the genetics of blood types and groups.

THE ANEMIAS

"Iron deficiency is the most common cause of anemia in pregnancy."[11] Women in the childbearing age may have iron deficiency for a number of reasons. Some of the causes include unsupervised and unwise weight reduction diets, poor dietary and appetite habits, and excessive menstrual flow. A woman who begins pregnancy in an iron-deficient state further complicates matters because the fetus will need sufficient iron for growth and development. The woman may not be able to get enough dietary iron and may be sensitive to oral intake of iron.

The physician will usually order iron in some oral preparation to supplement the mother's intake. If the mother tolerates oral iron well, the hemoglobin level will respond accordingly. Iron in parenteral form is used only when oral therapy is not tolerated or severe iron-deficiency anemia is present.

Deficiencies in vitamin B_{12} and folic acid are serious causes of anemia in pregnancy. Many studies recently have pointed out the serious effects of folic acid deficiency on fetal development. The fetus needs large amounts of nucleoproteins for its growth and development. Deficiencies in vitamin B_{12} and folic acid result in disturbance of the production of nucleic acid and nucleoproteins. Without these building blocks in sufficient quantity the fetus cannot develop normally. Replacement therapy is the treatment when deficiencies are found in vitamin B_{12} and folic acid.

COAGULATION DISORDERS

Women in pregnancy are subject to any coagulation disorder found in the general population. To the pregnant woman these disorders pose a more serious threat. Bleeding during delivery and postpartum periods is usually well controlled, but in coagulation disorders bleeding may be uncontrolled and endanger the mother's life. Coagulation disorders may lead to the development of emboli and endanger maternal and fetal survival.

Infections

RUBELLA

Rubella contracted by the pregnant woman early in pregnancy frequently causes a variety of congenital malformations in the fetus. Depending on the gestational age when rubella is contracted, the virus attacks the developing embryo. Table 31-2 shows the probability of certain congenital defects occurring when pregnant women contract rubella in the first trimester. There is a congenital rubella syndrome which manifests itself in infants who were infected with rubella virus in utero. Some of the clinical manifestations are neonatal thrombocytopenic purpura, long bone defects, hepatosplenomegaly, hepatitis, hemolytic anemia, cardiac lesions, eye defects, and hearing loss.

The placenta is a barrier only in the sense that *some* molecules, viruses, bacteria, or toxic substances are too large to cross over to the fetus. But the placenta in some instances is unable to differentiate what is allowed to pass through its circulation to the developing child. Thus, the virus of rubella as well as other viral and parasitic organisms find their way into the fetal circulation to cause destruction.

TABLE 31-2
IMPLICATIONS OF RUBELLA DURING PREGNANCY

Gestational age at which rubella was contracted by mother	Percent risk of congenital problems [12]	Probable types of defects
1–4 weeks	30–50%	Cardiac lesions Eye lesions (congenital cataract) Glaucoma
4–8 weeks	25%	Hearing defects (particularly organ of Corti defects)
9–12 weeks	8%	Psychomotor retardation
13–16 weeks	71%	Principally hearing defects

The use of gamma globulin in trying to prevent rubella after exposure is of questionable effectiveness. Deliberate exposure of young girls to rubella to prevent their contracting it during pregnancy is not effective. The susceptibility of individuals differs, and the child so exposed may not contract the disease. Even if the young girl has had rubella, exposure to the virus during pregnancy, though it may not make her ill, may affect the fetus. Nonpregnant susceptible females (no HI antibody present) may be intentionally exposed or vaccinated provided it has been established that they are not pregnant and will not conceive for at least 5 months after inoculation.

OTHER VIRAL DISEASES

The effects of measles, chickenpox, smallpox, and mumps on pregnancy and the developing fetus are not easily evaluated on the basis of current information. Some facts are known about each of the diseases mentioned and may be found in reference readings.

Other viral infections and their effects such as poliomyelitis, cytomegalic inclusion disease, and influenza may also be found in reference reading.

One virus disease which is fairly common bears mention here. Herpes simplex causes a very mild illness in the adult. The virus may be present in the external genitalia, mouth, or gums of the mother. This virus causes an extremely serious and often fatal illness in the newborn. It is advised that newborn infants be isolated from mothers with herpes simplex until manifestations of maternal disease subside.

COMMON INFECTIONS

The common cold, although easily contracted by everyone, seems to occur with more frequency in the pregnant woman. The cure is the same: rest, fluids, and aspirin for fever. The pregnant woman should, however, always consult her obstetrician before she takes any medication, even aspirin.

Miscellaneous Disorders

CHRONIC LUNG DISEASE

Women who suffer from a chronic lung ailment, such as emphysema, pulmonary tuberculosis, and asthma, may also become pregnant. The effect of pregnancy on these diseases depends on the severity of the illness. Usually in mild disease sufficient rest and supportive therapy are all that is needed. In the case of pulmonary tuberculosis modern chemotherapeutic agents do not harm the fetus and can be used safely.

VENEREAL DISEASE

Syphilis and gonorrhea, the most common of the venereal diseases, are considered among the most serious public health problems today. Since both are preventable and easily treated, it becomes a problem of public health education to treat mothers during pregnancy. Congenital syphilis can be prevented if the mother is treated. Likewise gonorrheal infections can be prevented and treated. Broad-spectrum antibiotics are effective against both diseases.

COLLAGEN DISEASES

This general category of illnesses includes systemic lupus erythematosus, rheumatoid arthritis, scleroderma, and rheumatic fever. These occur rarely and are uncommonly associated with pregnancy. If pregnancy does occur it is likely to end in abortion or fetal death.

MYASTHENIA GRAVIS

Myasthenia gravis in a pregnant woman may cause problems for the mother and infant. Both improvement and exacerbation in women with this disease have been reported. These women are followed very closely during pregnancy to maintain control of the disease and to prevent fetal loss.

During labor and delivery it is often necessary to administer anticholinesterase drugs. Anesthetic agents which have curare-like effects are not given. Likewise scopolamine is contraindicated.

The baby may have a transient form of this disease at birth and will require close observation and treatment. The mother may or may not be advised to breast-feed.

NEUROSES AND PSYCHOSES

Pregnancy in association with neuroses and psychoses is not uncommon. Many normal fears and anxieties plague the pregnant woman. Programs designed to increase the pregnant woman's knowledge regarding pregnancy, labor, delivery, and child care are valuable in allaying fears and anxieties. When anxieties are out of hand and uncontrolled, professional assistance may be necessary.

The relationship between maternal mental states and their effect on pregnancy has been studied.[13]

For the truly psychotic woman, the psychiatrist may recommend termination of pregnancy. If the woman develops a psychosis during the postpartum period, this is not considered distinct from a psychosis developed at any other time. Professional care is required and is given usually in the mental health unit.

DRUG ADDICTION

Maternal drug addiction is a growing, serious problem in this decade. It is important for the health of mother and baby that every effort be made to withdraw drugs from the mother during pregnancy. If the mother is addicted at the time of delivery, the infant will also be drug dependent and experience withdrawal symptoms. This subject and related knowledge are discussed in much of the current literature. The nurse involved in serving pregnant women and newborns must be aware of current knowledge and treatment of drug addiction.

REFERENCES

1 Stratford, B. F.: "Abnormalities of Early Human Development," *American Journal of Obstetrics and Gynecology*, 107:1223–1232, 1970.

2 Rubin, Reva: "Cognitive Style in Pregnancy," *American Journal of Nursing*, 70:502–508, 1970.

3 Hytten, Frank E., and Isabella Leitch: *The Physiology of Human Reproduction*, Davis, Philadelphia, 1963.

4 Hellman, Louis, and J. Pritchard: *Williams Obstetrics*, 14th ed., Appleton-Century-Crofts, New York, 1971.

5 Breen, James L.: "A 21-year Survey of 654 Ectopic Pregnancies," *American Journal of Obstetrics and Gynecology*, 106:1019, 1970.

6 Guyton, Arthur C.: *Textbook of Medical Physiology*, 4th ed., Saunders, Philadelphia, 1971, p. 982.

7 Criteria Committee of the New York Heart Association, Inc.: *Nomenclature and Criteria for Diagnosis of Diseases of the Heart and Blood Vessels*, 5th ed., The New York Heart Association, New York, 1955.

8 Guyton: op. cit., p. 983.

9 White, P.: "Pregnancy Complicating Diabetes," *American Journal of Medicine*, 7:609, 1949.

10 Guyton: op. cit., p. 981.

11 Rovinsky, Joseph J., and Alan F. Guttmacher (eds.): *Medical, Surgical and*

Gynecologic Complications of Pregnancy, Williams & Wilkins, Baltimore, 1965, p. 536.

12 Ibid., p. 675.

13 Richardson, Stephen A., and Alan F. Guttmacher (eds.): *Childbearing— Its Social and Psychological Aspects*, Williams & Wilkins, Baltimore, 1967, pp. 53–73.

BIBLIOGRAPHY

Barnett, Henry L.: *Pediatrics*, Appleton-Century-Crofts, New York, 1968.

Blechner, Jack N., et al.: "Oxygenation of the Human Fetus and Newborn Infant during Maternal Metabolic Acidosis," *American Journal of Obstetrics and Gynecology*, 108:47–55, 1970.

Breen, James L.: "A 21-year Survey of 654 Ectopic Pregnancies," *American Journal of Obstetrics and Gynecology*, 106:1004–1019, 1970.

Caplan, Gerald: *Concepts of Mental Health and Consultation: Their Application in Public Health Social Work*, U.S. Department of Health, Education, and Welfare, Social Security Administration, Children's Bureau, Washington, D.C., 1959.

Carroll, R., et al.: "Bacteriuria in Pregnancy," *Obstetrics and Gynecology*, 32:525–527, 1968.

Charles, D.: "Infection and the Obstetric Patient," *Modern Treatment*, 7:789–817, 1970.

Coates, J. B.: "Obstetrics in the Very Young Adolescent," *American Journal of Obstetrics and Gynecology*, 108:68–72, 1970.

Coodley, E. L.: "Heart Disease in Pregnancy," *Postgraduate Medicine*, 47:195–199, 1970.

Cooper, L. Z.: "Rubella in Pregnancy," *Postgraduate Medicine*, 46:106–107, 1969.

Delaney, James J., and John Ptacek: "Three Decades of Experience with Diabetic Pregnancies," *American Journal of Obstetrics and Gynecology*, 106:550–556, 1970.

Dhodine, R. R., et al.: "Chromosomal Anomalies in Spontaneously Aborted Human Fetuses," *Lancet*, 2:20–21, 1970.

Donnelly, James F.: "Toxemia of Pregnancy," *American Journal of Nursing*, 61:98–101, April 1961.

Dudgeon, J. A.: "Intrauterine Infection, I," *Nursing Times*, 66:939–941, 1970.

———: "Intrauterine Infection, II," *Nursing Times*, 66:973–975, 1970.

———: "Intrauterine Infection, III," *Nursing Times*, 66:1007–1009, 1970.

Eastman, Nicholson, and Louis Hellman: *Williams Obstetrics*, Appleton-Century-Crofts, New York, 1966.

Fitzpatrick, Elise, N. Eastman, and S. Reeder: *Maternity Nursing*, 11th ed., Lippincott, Philadelphia, 1966, pp. 444–455.

Flowers, Charles E.: "Magnesium Sulfate in Obstetrics," *American Journal of Obstetrics and Gynecology*, pp. 763–776, March 15, 1965.

Freda, V. J., et al.: "The Threat of Rh Immunization from Abortion," *Lancet*, 2:147–148, 1970.

Garnet, James D.: "Pregnancy in Women with Diabetes," *American Journal of Nursing*, 69:1900–1902, 1969.

Gerber, A. H., et al.: "Active Management of Missed Abortion," *Obstetrics and Gynecology*, 32:312–315, 1968.

Goldman, J. A., et al.: "Transplacental Hemorrhage during Spontaneous and Therapeutic Abortion," *Obstetrics and Gynecology*, 35:903–908, 1970.

Grollman, Arthur: "Diuretics," *American Journal of Nursing*, 65:84–89, January 1965.

Gusdon, John P., Jr., et al.: "Amniotic Fluid Antibody Titers and Other Prognostic Parameters in Erythroblastosis," *American Journal of Obstetrics and Gynecology*, 108:85–90, 1970.

Guyton, Arthur C.: *Textbook of Medical Physiology*, 4th ed., Saunders, Philadelphia, 1971.

Harris, R. E., et al.: "Endocrine Complications of Pregnancy," *Postgraduate Medicine*, 46:123–129, 1969.

Hause, T. E., et al.: "Pregnancy Complicated by Urinary Tract Infections," *Obstetrics and Gynecology*, 34:670–674, 1969.

Haynes, D. M.: *Medical Complications during Pregnancy*, McGraw-Hill, New York, 1969.

Hellman, Louis, and J. Pritchard: *Williams Obstetrics*, 14th ed., Appleton-Century-Crofts, New York, 1971.

Highley, B.: "Antepartal Nursing Intervention," *Nursing Forum*, 2:62–80, 1963.

Hogue, Carol, and M. Couch: "Care of the Patient with Toxemia," *American Journal of Nursing*, 61:101–103, April 1961.

Hytten, Frank E., and Isabella Leitch: *The Physiology of Human Pregnancy*, Davis, Philadelphia, 1963.

Jorgansen, J.: "Rhesus-antibody Development after Abortion," *Lancet*, 2:1253–1254, 1969.

Laros, R. K., et al.: "Sickle Cell, Beta Thalassemia and Pregnancy," *Obstetrics and Gynecology*, 37:67–71, 1971.

Lerch, Constance: *Maternity Nursing*, Mosby, St. Louis, 1970.

Litwak, O., et al.: "Fetal Erythrocytes in Maternal Circulation after Spontaneous Abortion," *Journal of the American Medical Association*, 214:531–534, 1970.

MacLaverty, Michael, Robert Paulic, and Charles Smith: "Program for Toxemia Control," *American Journal of Obstetrics and Gynecology*, pp. 100–105, May 1, 1965.

Margolis, R. R., et al.: "Heparin for Septic Abortion and the Prevention of Endotoxic Shock," *Obstetrics and Gynecology*, 37:474–483, 1971.

Maternal Nutrition and the Course of Pregnancy: Summary Report, Committee on Maternal Nutrition/Food and Nutrition, National Academy of Science, Washington, D.C., 1970.

Montague, M. F. Ashley: *Prenatal Influences*, Charles C Thomas, Springfield, Ill., 1962.

Naib, Z. M., et al.: "Association of Genital Herpetic Infection with Spontaneous Abortion," *Obstetrics and Gynecology*, 35:260–263, 1970.

O'Neill, R. T., et al.: "Immunization in Spontaneous Abortion and Ectopic Pregnancy," *Obstetrics and Gynecology*, 36:264–267, 1970.

Pharoon, P. O., et al.: "Neurological Damage to the Fetus Resulting from Severe Iodine Deficiency during Pregnancy," *Lancet*, 1:308–310, 1971.

Phillips, C. A., et al.: "Intrauterine Rubella Vaccine," *Journal of the American Medical Association*, 213:624–625, 1970.

Potter, J. F., et al.: "Metastasis of Maternal Cancer to the Placenta and Fetus," *Cancer*, 25:380–388, 1970.

Pritchard, J. A., et al.: "Infants of Mothers with Megaloblastic Anemia Due to Folate Deficiency," *Journal of the American Medical Association*, 211:1982–1984, 1970.

Rashid, S., et al.: "Suction Evacuation for Incomplete Abortion," *Journal of Obstetrics and Gynaecology of the British Commonwealth*, 77:1047–1048, 1970.

Rovinsky, Joseph J., and Alan F. Guttmacher (eds.): *Medical, Surgical and Gynecologic Complications of Pregnancy*, 2d ed., Williams & Wilkins, Baltimore, 1965.

Rowan, D. F., et al.: "Virus Infections during Pregnancy," *Obstetrics and Gynecology*, 32:356–364, 1968.

Smith, J. W., et al.: "Bacteremia in Septic Abortion: Complications and Treatment," *Obstetrics and Gynecology*, 35:704–708, 1970.

Sparkes, R. S., et al.: "Inherited 13/14 Chromosomal Translocation as a Cause of Human Fetal Wastage," *Obstetrics and Gynecology*, 35:601–607, 1970.

Stone, M. L., et al.: "Narcotic Addiction in Pregnancy," *American Journal of Obstetrics and Gynecology*, 109:716–723, 1971.

Streissguth, A. P., et al.: "Mental Development of Children with Congenital Rubella Syndrome," *American Journal of Obstetrics and Gynecology*, 108:392–399, 1970.

Van der Werf, A. J., et al.: "Metastatic Choriocarcinoma as a Complication of Pregnancy," *Obstetrics and Gynecology*, 35:78–88, 1970.

Weekes, L. R., et al.: "Thromboembolic Disease in Pregnancy," *American Journal of Obstetrics and Gynecology*, 107:649–650, 1970.

Wilson, M. G., et al.: "Teratogenic Effects of Asian Influenza," *Journal of the American Medical Association*, 210:336–337, 1969.

Zuspan, F. P.: "Symposium on Toxemia of Pregnancy," *Clinical Obstetrics and Gynecology*, pp. 859–990, December 1966.

32 | COMPLICATIONS DURING LABOR AND DELIVERY

Karyn Smith Kaufman

Labor and delivery is the process whereby the mature products of conception are expelled by the action of rhythmic uterine contractions. When studying this process, it is often helpful to examine its three primary components:

1 The powers—uterine contractions
2 The passengers—fetus, cord, placenta, membranes, and amniotic fluid
3 The passage—maternal pelvis and reproductive organs

In order for a normal labor and delivery to occur each of these components must be normal. When abnormalities are present in one or more of them, a complicated labor and delivery exists to some degree.

The primary abnormalities of these three components will be discussed in this chapter. It is necessary, however, to emphasize the interrelatedness of the powers, the passengers, and the passage. An abnormality in one of them will frequently occasion abnormalities in the other two. However, by assessing each component individually, cause and effect relationships may be established.

POWERS

Premature Labor

When the rhythmic contractions of labor begin before the 37th week of gestation, premature labor exists. The incidence of this complication is 7 to 15 percent of all births. Because of the immediate care needed at delivery, this is considered a complication of the intrapartum period, even though the actual labor and delivery may be uncomplicated. The cause of many premature labors is unknown. Less than half of them are associated with maternal disease conditions such as toxemia, heart disease, or chronic hypertension.[1]

Nursing care of the woman in premature labor will be influenced by the presence of any of these disease conditions. In addition, the care will be influenced by knowledge that prematures have a lower margin of reserve for tolerating the stress of labor and can become hypoxic more quickly than the full-term infant. During labor, therefore, the pregnant woman will receive little or no systemic analgesia in order to prevent central nervous depression of the fetus. Careful monitoring of the fetal heart rate for patterns of distress is very important in view of the lowered tolerance of stress. The greater incidence of malpresentations may contribute to additional problems which will be considered later in this chapter.

The actual gestational age of the fetus is also taken into consideration in the nursing care of this patient. Preparation for delivery begins early in the labor and varies for the 28-week fetus as compared with the 37-week fetus. If multiple gestation is the precipitating factor in the premature labor, preparations for more than one infant have to be made. The following is suggested as a guide which can be adapted to individual situations.

1 Warming equipment in the delivery room turned on ahead of time. A servo thermal controlled unit is preferable for smaller prematures.
2 Resuscitation equipment in the delivery room with appropriate size masks, endotracheal tubes, and laryngoscope blade.
3 Equipment to monitor infant temperature, pulse, and respirations.
4 Personnel in attendance who are skilled in immediate newborn care.
5 Equipment available that provides warmth and oxygen for transporting the infant to a premature facility.
6 Informing nursery staff of expected premature infant, gestational age, significant maternal conditions, evidence of fetal distress in labor.
7 Discussing with parents the potential problems and preparations being made for their infant.

Uncertain estimated delivery date (EDC) or disease conditions of the mother or placenta that alter normal growth patterns of the fetus sometimes make it difficult to know what size infant to anticipate at delivery. Tests to establish fetal age and maturity are available and can be a useful adjunct in making specific preparations for delivery.[2, 3]

When the premature infant is delivered, it is important that trauma to the soft premature skull is minimal. Frequently an episiotomy is performed to reduce perineal resistance when the head is delivering. A spontaneous delivery is generally preferred. The nurse can assist the mother to push at appropriate times and to avoid long, forceful pushing.

The cord is clamped and cut quickly, and the baby placed in the heated crib for care. The nurse can participate in the immediate newborn care, keep the parents informed about the infant's condition, and alert the premature facility to the infant's birth and condition.

Dysfunctional Labor

Uterine contractions normally increase in frequency, duration, and intensity as labor progresses, but with full relaxation of the muscle between contractions. During this resting stage there is the minimum of intrauterine tension. This minimum tension, called tonus, is in the 8 to 12 mmHg range.[4] Normal labor contractions may reach an intrauterine pressure of 50 to 60 mmHg at the acme of the contraction. The contractions effect dilatation of the cervix and descent of the fetus over a period of time. Graphically, labor progress is seen to be an S-shaped curve (Figure 32-1).[5] These curves are based on mean values for duration of labor in primigravidas and multiparas. Limits of normal variation have been statistically derived, but clinically, when values outside those time limits are seen, the labor process is abnormal.[6]

PRECIPITOUS LABOR

Graphically, precipitous labor is an abnormally accelerated curve in which the total time for the labor and delivery process has been defined by some to be under 3 hours.[7, 8] The uterine contractions are increased in frequency, duration, and intensity. Intrauterine pressures are often above 50 mmHg with each contraction. The high level of uterine activity allows little rest time between contractions. Uterine blood flow may be sufficiently reduced to impair oxygen transfer across the placenta, culminating in fetal distress. The forceful contractions, particularly combined with minimally resistant maternal tissue, may propel the fetus rapidly through the maternal passage. The dangers of this are damage to the fetal head from rapid expulsion and/or an unattended delivery.

Whenever high levels of uterine activity are observed the nursing care must include close observation of fetal heart rate patterns and insurance that the patient is not left alone. If delivery is rapid and uncontrolled, the fetus should be carefully evaluated for injury. The circumstances of delivery should always be reported to the nursery staff to insure ongoing assessment. Intra-

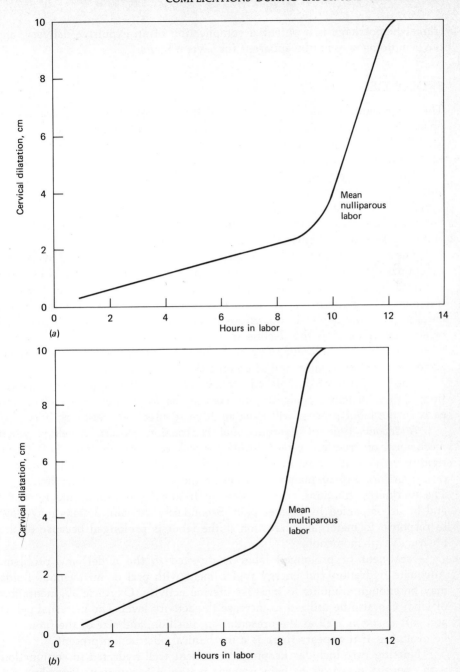

FIGURE 32-1
Labor progress curves (mean values).
(From Emanuel Friedman, "Synthetic Oxytocin," American Journal of Obstetrics and Gynecology, 74:1118–1124, 1957.)

cranial hemorrhage is a potential complication of an expulsive delivery, and the symptoms may not be apparent for several hours.

PROLONGED LABOR

The upper limits of normal duration of the various phases of labor (latent phase, active phase, deceleration phase, and second stage) have been defined.[9] Total length of labor is not as valuable an index of prolonged labor as assessment of progress of each phase of labor. Prolonged labor would therefore be an appropriate label for several different labor patterns, e.g., labor which begins slowly and progresses minimally for 12 to 15 hours, labor which progresses normally for a time and then fails to progress for several hours, or labor which progresses normally to near the end of the first stage and then is protracted beyond 1 to 2 hours[10] (Figure 32-2).

These dysfunctional labor progress curves will be associated with dysfunctional uterine contractions. One type of contraction pattern will be characterized by a decline in the frequency, duration, and intensity of the contractions. This pattern may occur in response to maternal exhaustion. When energy stores are depleted, the uterus cannot contract efficiently. If maternal exhaustion is causing the decline in uterine activity with resultant loss of labor progress, the accompanying symptoms will be dry mucous membranes, acetonuria, elevated pulse, and often an elevated temperature.

Another cause of diminished uterine activity is the influence of medication. Either systemic analgesics or continuous local anesthetics given too early in the labor process will have an adverse effect on uterine activity.

A second type of dysfunctional contraction pattern develops when mechanical obstruction is responsible for lack of labor progress. Soft tissue rigidity, inadequate emptying of the bladder or bowel, relative cephalopelvic disproportion, and/or malpresentation of the fetus occur in these instances. The uterine contractions may increase in frequency, duration, and intensity and be accompanied by greater pain. Secondarily the contractions may slow in response to maternal exhaustion if the labor is prolonged because of the obstructive phenomenon.

Treatment of prolonged labor is directed to the underlying problem. Adequate hydration and energy replacement with oral or intravenous fluids may be enough stimulus to increase uterine activity. Oxytocic augmentation of labor can also be utilized to increase the activity level. The maternal pelvis and soft tissue as well as the presentation, position, and size of the fetus will be evaluated if it appears there is a mechanical obstruction present.

Nursing care includes keeping the patient well hydrated in conjunction with comfort measures to help prevent maternal exhaustion. Providing for elimination needs will keep the bladder and bowel from impeding labor progress. When prolonged labor occurs, close attendance is desirable to encourage the patient who often feels fatigued and discouraged because of slow

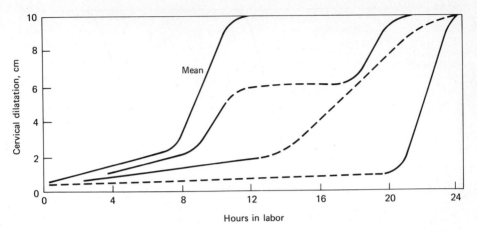

FIGURE 32-2
Major labor aberrations compared with the mean labor curve of nulliparas.
(*Adapted by Emanuel Friedman from J. P. Greenhill, Obstetrics, 13th ed., Saunders, Philadelphia, 1965.*)

labor progress. The fetus must also be evaluated for any symptoms of distress. Prolonged labor may tax the ability of the fetus to cope with the repetitive stress of contractions.

Induced Labor

A decision may be made to induce labor rather than await the spontaneous onset of uterine labor contractions. The decision can be *elective*, i.e., without medical indication, or *indicated* because of an unfavorable prognosis in awaiting spontaneous labor.

The method of induction may be rupturing the membranes artificially and then waiting for the onset of contractions. When the cervix is soft and partially dilated, contractions will often begin within a short time. Once labor begins, the progress is like that of a normal labor of spontaneous onset.

Administering oxytocics is a frequently used method of inducing labor contractions. These drugs may be given by buccal or parenteral routes. An intravenous drip of a diluted oxytocic is a common method. Amniotomy sometimes accompanies oxytocic administration. The resulting labor is accelerated when compared to the graph of normal labor.[11] (See Figure 32-3.) When the cervix is favorable, contractions usually begin within a short time of initiating the oxytocic. The frequency, duration, and intensity of contractions are monitored carefully, and increments in dose are based on the contraction pattern. The uterine tonus is often elevated when oxytocics are used.

Nursing observations include timing the contractions and noting whether relaxation of the uterine muscle occurs between contractions. Prolonged con-

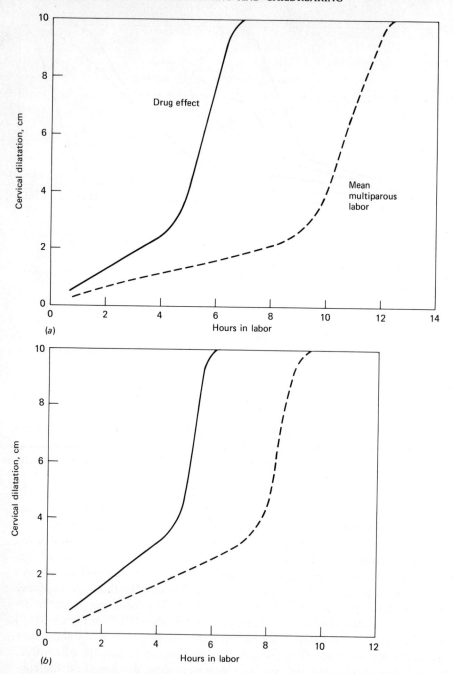

FIGURE 32-3
Comparison of labor curves when oxytocin is used.
(*From Emanuel Friedman, "Synthetic Oxytocin," American Journal of Obstetrics and Gynecology, 74:1118–1124, 1957.*)

tractions and/or inadequate uterine muscle relaxation may impair uterine blood flow and result in fetal hypoxia. The patient may need assistance to cope with the contractions of an induced labor because she may experience frequent, strong contractions from the onset, as opposed to spontaneous labor where the frequency, duration, and intensity of contractions increases gradually.

Third and Fourth Stage Complications

When delivery of the fetus is completed, the uterus must continue to contract to expel the placenta and membranes. Faulty contractions in the third stage may fail to accomplish placental separation, and the placenta will be manually removed.

In the fourth stage the uterus must contract around the exposed blood sinuses to prevent postpartum hemorrhage. When the uterus has contracted inefficiently during labor, it can be anticipated that there will be greater difficulty with uterine contraction in the fourth stage. If contractions were stimulated during labor with oxytocin, then this stimulation will usually be necessary after delivery. In practice most patients receive some amount of oxytocin during the third and fourth stages for prophylactic reasons.

PASSENGERS

Fetus

PHYSIOLOGICAL RESPONSE TO LABOR

With current knowledge we cannot predict exactly which fetus will not tolerate the stress of labor. Rather, a designation of high risk is applied to those instances in which the likelihood of fetal problems is high. A fetus of the diabetic, toxemic, Rh sensitized, hypertensive, or hypotensive mother is at risk. The premature fetus is at risk. However, since the ability to predict distress is so limited, every fetus must be continually assessed during labor.

Disturbances in fetal physiological functioning can be detected by evaluating the fetal heart rate pattern in relation to uterine contractions. Fetal monitoring equipment is the preferred method of obtaining fetal heart rate patterns. Three primary patterns are identified and described by Hon.[12] (See Figures 32-4, 32-5, and 32-6.)

The early deceleration pattern is apparently an innocuous fetal heart rate pattern. It develops in response to an increased pressure on the fetal head during uterine contractions.

The late deceleration pattern is an ominous pattern, particularly when persistent. Fetal hypoxia and acidosis result from this pattern, which is a reflection of placental insufficiency. Fetal-maternal gas exchange is markedly reduced.

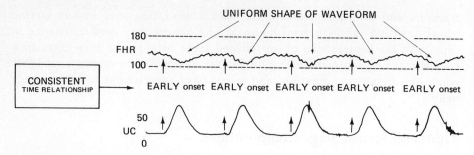

FIGURE 32-4
Early deceleration pattern. Head compression.
(From Edward H. Hon, An Introduction to Fetal Monitoring, Harty, New Haven, Conn., 1969.)

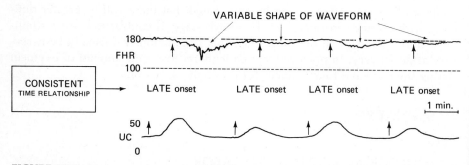

FIGURE 32-5
Late deceleration pattern. Uteroplacental insufficiency.
(From Edward H. Hon, An Introduction to Fetal Monitoring, Harty, New Haven, Conn., 1969.)

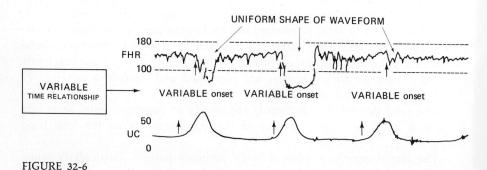

FIGURE 32-6
Variable deceleration pattern. Cord compression.
(From Edward H. Hon, An Introduction to Fetal Monitoring, Harty, New Haven, Conn., 1969.)

Variable deceleration patterns result from compression of the umbilical cord during uterine contractions. This pattern is seen in 85 to 90 percent of the clinically diagnosed cases of fetal distress. The pattern may be transient or may gradually become more severe. Metabolic acidosis less frequently accompanies this type of fetal distress.

The traditional criterion for defining fetal distress (heart rate above or below 120 to 160 beats per minute between contractions) has limited application. The late deceleration pattern may fall entirely within the acceptable range, yet the pattern is associated with marked fetal distress. Listening to the fetal heart rate between contractions with a conventional fetoscope makes identification of these patterns difficult, if not impossible. There may be some merit in listening through a contraction and on into the relaxation phase to detect heart rate response to the contraction and the speed with which it returns to the base-line rate. In practice this is difficult to do, and continuous monitoring in this fashion is uncomfortable for the pregnant woman and impractical for the nurse.

The base-line fetal heart rate is simply the rate seen most of the time. A base-line tachycardia (above 160 beats per minute) may accompany a late or variable deceleration pattern and is further suggestive of fetal distress. A base-line tachycardia without these deceleration patterns may be a symptom of early distress, but it is also associated with maternal fever and fetal immaturity.

A direct fetal electrocardiogram can be recorded from a fetal scalp electrode that is used with some monitoring systems. The ECG may provide information about changes in cardiac conduction that precede actual deceleration patterns. This would mean that fetal distress could be detected early in its occurrence, before the fetal reserve margin is exceeded.

It is also possible to assess acid-base status by sampling small amounts of fetal scalp blood. Correlation of blood pH values with heart rate patterns provides additional information about the type and degree of fetal distress.

The passage of meconium by the fetus in a cephalic presentation is assumed to be evidence of hypoxia. The presence of meconium is not a consistent finding with the heart rate patterns associated with fetal distress.[13]

Medications administered to the mother may also affect the fetus. For example, local anesthetic agents injected into the paracervical region for labor analgesia may produce a fetal bradycardia persisting for several minutes. The cause of this bradycardia is not well understood and is not well correlated with other symptoms of distress during labor or low Apgar scores at delivery.

Systemic narcotic analgesics given to the mother in labor will cross the placenta and can depress the fetal respiratory center. If delivery occurs while the drug is exerting its peak effect, the fetus may have difficulty initiating spontaneous respirations. The timing of administration of medications to the mother is as important as the dosage.

Whenever symptoms of fetal distress are observed, they should be brought to immediate medical attention. If the distress does not respond to treatment and becomes progressively more profound, operative delivery may be necessary if vaginal delivery is not imminent. Regardless of the mode of delivery, preparations for immediate infant resuscitation should be made ahead of time. Equipment such as described earlier in this chapter will be needed. The addition of equipment for umbilical catheterization is helpful. Medications can be administered via umbilical vessels to correct acidosis in severely depressed infants.

PRESENTATION, POSITION, AND SIZE

Abnormal presentation, position, and size of the fetus increase the incidence of complications because of the following:

1 If the presenting part is smaller than the vertex, which is normally the presenting part, the potential for a prolapsed cord increases. Example: A foot presenting in a breech presentation predisposes to a prolapsed cord (Figure 32-7). Five percent of breech presentations are complicated by a prolapsed cord.[14]

2 A smaller presenting part descending in the maternal pelvis is not as efficient a dilator of maternal tissue as the larger bony head in a normal presentation. Therefore, larger aftercoming fetal parts may not descend easily, resulting in a difficult delivery.
Example: In a breech presentation the feet and legs may deliver easily, but the shoulders and head may deliver with difficulty. Special forceps may need to be used (Figure 32-8).

3 A larger than normal diameter may cause a relative disproportion between the fetus and the maternal pelvis.
Example: A very large baby in normal position, a face or brow presentation with a larger presenting diameter of the head, or an anomalous head or abdomen may not be able to deliver through an average pelvis (Figure 32-9).

4 An abnormal fetal position will affect the mechanisms of labor necessary for delivery.
Example: A posterior position of the vertex may rotate to a direct occiput posterior position for delivery. Delivery of the head will then be accomplished primarily by flexion rather than by extension, as in occiput anterior positions (Figures 32-10 and 32-11).

The most common malpresentation is a breech presentation. It accounts for 3 to 4 percent of the 5 percent of all deliveries in other than the vertex presentation.[15]

There are some specific nursing care measures pertinent to the care of

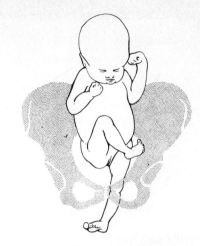

FIGURE 32-7
Footling breech.
(From Harry Oxorn and William Foote, Human Labor and Birth, Appleton-Century-Crofts, New York, 1964. By permission of the publisher.)

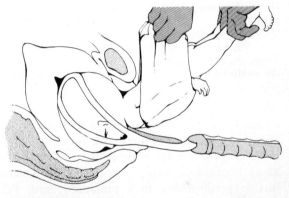

FIGURE 32-8
Forceps to the aftercoming head.
(From Harry Oxorn and William Foote, Human Labor and Birth, Appleton-Century-Crofts, New York, 1964. By permission of the publisher.)

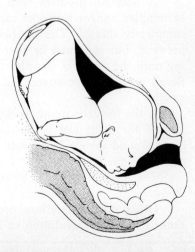

FIGURE 32-9
Lateral view of a face presentation.
(From Harry Oxorn and William Foote, Human Labor and Birth, Appleton-Century-Crofts, New York, 1964. By permission of the publisher.)

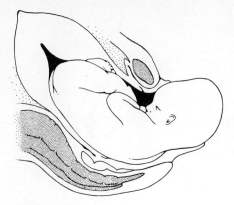 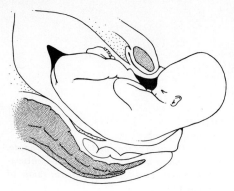

FIGURE 32-10

Flexion beginning in the occiput posterior position.

(From Harry Oxorn and William Foote, Human Labor and Birth, Appleton-Century-Crofts, New York, 1964. By permission of the publisher.)

FIGURE 32-11

Flexion completed in the occiput posterior position.

(From Harry Oxorn and William Foote, Human Labor and Birth, Appleton-Century-Crofts, New York, 1964. By permission of the publisher.)

a patient with the fetus in a breech presentation. Knowing that the possibility of a prolapsed cord is increased, the nurse should carefully observe the fetal heart rate pattern for symptoms of cord circulation interference (see Figure 32-6). Because of poor fetal-pelvic fit, the membranes tend to rupture early, further predisposing to a prolapsed cord. When membranes rupture, the perineum should be promptly observed for any obvious cord prolapse, and the fetal heart rate evaluated. The presence of meconium in a breech presentation is *not* a good indicator of fetal distress but is related to pressure on the fetal abdomen as descent occurs.

A frequent problem with breech presentations is that the small lower extremities and/or buttocks can reach the pelvic floor before the cervix has completely dilated. The mother develops an urge to push because of this pressure, but she must be coached in breathing techniques to prevent pushing until the cervix is completely dilated. Successful delivery of the head in a flexed position necessitates full dilatation of the cervix unless the fetus is small.

If the lower extremities deliver through the vaginal introitus before the rest of the fetus can be delivered, it is probably helpful to keep a warm cloth around them while awaiting completion of the delivery to help prevent cooling of the fetal body.

The mechanisms of a breech delivery are illustrated in Figures 32-12 to 32-20.

Other malpresentations occur less commonly than the breech presentation. If the malpresentation or large fetal size predisposes to a cephalopelvic

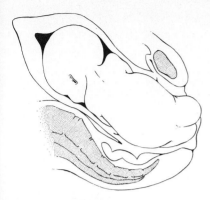

FIGURE 32-12
Breech crowning.
(From Harry Oxorn and William Foote, Human Labor and Birth, Appleton-Century-Crofts, New York, 1964. By permission of the publisher.)

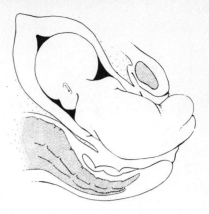

FIGURE 32-13
Birth of posterior buttock.
(From Harry Oxorn and William Foote, Human Labor and Birth, Appleton-Century-Crofts, New York, 1964. By permission of the publisher.)

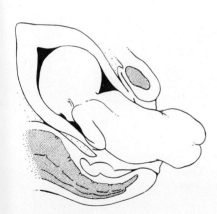

FIGURE 32-14
Birth of anterior buttock.
(From Harry Oxorn and William Foote, Human Labor and Birth, Appleton-Century-Crofts, New York, 1964. By permission of the publisher.)

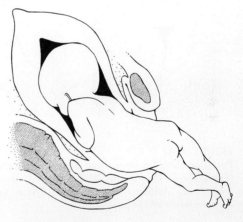

FIGURE 32-15
Feet born, shoulders engaging.
(From Harry Oxorn and William Foote, Human Labor and Birth, Appleton-Century-Crofts, New York, 1964. By permission of the publisher.)

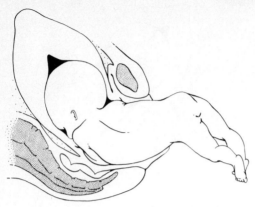

FIGURE 32-16
Descent and internal rotation of shoulders.
*(From Harry Oxorn and William Foote, Human
Labor and Birth, Appleton-Century-Crofts, New
York, 1964. By permission of the publisher.)*

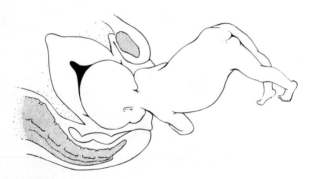

FIGURE 32-17
Posterior shoulder born, head has entered pelvis.
*(From Harry Oxorn and William Foote, Human Labor
and Birth, Appleton-Century-Crofts, New York, 1964.
By permission of the publisher.)*

disproportion, the dysfunctional labor curves of prolonged labor often appear.
Certain face presentations and brow presentations that spontaneously correct
themselves with good flexion of the fetal head may prolong labor until the
flexion occurs, but labor progress and delivery subsequent to flexion should
be normal. Large infants in normal position may cause difficulty at delivery
because of increased head and shoulder size. Whenever the labor is prolonged
and/or the delivery is difficult, the infant may be depressed at delivery. In
addition to adequate resuscitation, he should be examined for possible birth
injury. Cephalhematomas, brachial or facial nerve injury from pressure on

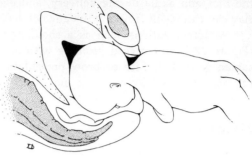

FIGURE 32-18
Anterior shoulder born, descent of head.
(From Harry Oxorn and William Foote, Human Labor and Birth, Appleton-Century-Crofts, New York, 1964. By permission of the publisher.)

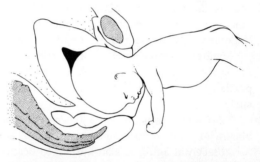

FIGURE 32-19
Internal rotation and beginning flexion of head.
(From Harry Oxorn and William Foote, Human Labor and Birth, Appleton-Century-Crofts, New York, 1964. By permission of the publisher.)

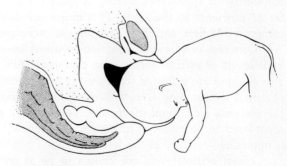

FIGURE 32-20
Flexion of the head is complete.
(From Harry Oxorn and William Foote, Human Labor and Birth, Appleton-Century-Crofts, New York, 1964. By permission of the publisher.)

the face and axilla during delivery, and even broken bones (most often the clavicle) can result from a traumatic delivery.

Malpresentations such as a shoulder presentation with a transverse lie (Figure 32-21) or a cord prolapse with any presentation will necessitate cesarean section. If face or brow presentations cannot deliver vaginally, then cesarean section delivery is also indicated.

Placenta

PLACENTAL FUNCTION

During labor the placenta must continue to provide the maternal-fetal gas exchange. Placental function is dependent on blood flow through the intervillous space where diffusion of gases takes place. Strong uterine contractions can effectively reduce uterine blood flow and therefore affect the gas exchange. Maternal toxemia or chronic hypertension can interfere with normal blood flow to the intervillous space because of vessel constriction. Maternal hypotension will also reduce the uterine blood supply.

Maternal-fetal gas exchange is also influenced by the amount of placental surface area available. A small placenta, an infarcted placenta, or a partially prematurely separated placenta will reduce the available exchange surface.

An edematous placenta (seen with diabetic mothers and with erythroblastosis) may compromise gas diffusion across the intervillous space.

Placental aging is also known to occur. Placental function may peak any time in the last weeks of pregnancy and then follow a downhill course. If the onset of labor occurs when placental functioning is less than optimal, gas exchange with the added stress of labor contractions may be compromised. This phenomenon is witnessed with postmature infants who often have a malnourished appearance. Placental aging is responsible for diminished transfer of nutrients to the fetus. This more complicated function is likely to be compromised first, and then later the gas exchange function.

One test of placental function in use is assay of maternal urine for 24-hour levels of estriol. Serial urine samples (daily, every other day, or 3 times a week, etc.) are collected from the pregnant woman when it is suspected that placental dysfunction is complicating her pregnancy. Estriol is produced by the placenta from fetal precursors. Levels of 12 mg or less per 24 hours are considered to be evidence of significant placental dysfunction. The treatment is immediate delivery of the fetus.

When estriol levels are known to be at critical levels, or when any of the previously described conditions that interfere with maternal-fetal gas exchange are present in labor, the fetal heart rate pattern is carefully evaluated for late deceleration curves. (See Figure 32-5.)

This characteristic deceleration of heart rate after the peak of the con-

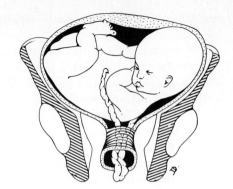

FIGURE 32-21
Transverse lie with a prolapsed cord.
*(From Harry Oxorn and William Foote,
Human Labor and Birth, Appleton-Century-
Crofts, New York, 1964. By permission of
the publisher.)*

traction with slow return to the base-line rate is symptomatic of diminished
gas exchange. In response to the low oxygen levels the fetus develops a relative bradycardia. Administering 6 to 7 liters of oxygen by mask to the woman
to raise the maternal blood concentration of oxygen and increase the gradient
at the placental exchange site may assist in correcting the pattern. If the contraction pattern is one of high activity, the uterus may need to be rested to
increase the uterine blood flow and promote better gas exchange. Placing the
patient in the lateral position may help reduce uterine activity. If oxytocin is
being administered the infusion rate may have to be reduced to lower uterine
activity. Because the placental insufficiency pattern is an ominous sign, corrective steps should be taken as soon as it is detected.

PLACENTA PREVIA AND ABRUPTIO PLACENTAE

The placenta is normally implanted on the upper wall of the uterus. When
abnormal implantation of the placenta occurs, complications result when the
placenta encroaches on the cervical opening. Blood vessels are exposed near
the cervix, and vaginal bleeding is the first symptom of placenta previa. This
bleeding is classically described as painless, bright red, and rarely of sufficient
amount with the initial episode to produce maternal fatality. The incidence of
this complication is about 1:200 deliveries. The cause of the abnormal implantation is unknown.[16]

The initial bleeding episode may occur in the latter part of pregnancy
without the presence of labor. When the fetus is quite immature and the
initial amount of blood is not great, the pregnant woman may be treated with
bed rest and close observation for any recurrence of bleeding. Continuing
hemorrhage, the presence of labor contractions, or a distressed fetus necessitate prompt delivery. As the cervix dilates in labor, a small or large portion
of placenta may be exposed, depending on its actual location. The cervical
dilatation is apt to tear through more blood vessels, resulting in further
bleeding. Unless there is only a margin of placenta near the dilating cervix

and labor is progressing quite rapidly, delivery is most often accomplished by cesarean section.

A normally implanted placenta that separates from the uterine wall before the fetus has delivered is called abruptio placentae. Varying degrees of abruption are apparently possible. Only a small marginal area may separate, or the entire placenta may detach from the uterine wall.

The symptoms of severe abruptio placentae are vaginal bleeding, a rigid tender uterus, pain, and fetal distress or death. In perhaps 20 percent of cases there is no apparent vaginal bleeding. These cases are described as concealed hemorrhage, i.e., blood from the exposed vessels remains retroplacental and is trapped between the placenta and the uterine wall. Uterine tenderness is very evident, and maternal vital signs may reflect the blood loss even though no external bleeding is evident.[17]

The greater number of cases involve a separation of only one or two cotyledons. This may produce some vaginal bleeding, but maternal vital signs are stable and fetal distress is not evident. In milder forms the most characteristic symptom may be failure of the uterus to relax between contractions. Again, the amount of maternal blood loss, status of labor, and/or the presence of fetal distress will influence the mode of delivery.

A secondary complication of abruptio placentae is hypofibrinogenemia. Whenever abruptio placentae is suspected, clotting times are checked to detect this problem.

The nurse must recognize that any vaginal bleeding developing during labor (as distinguished from normal bloody show) or present at labor onset is abnormal. The immediate cause of the bleeding may not be apparent, but placental bleeding is always suspected. It is important to estimate the amount of blood being lost. Pads, linen, etc., can be weighed and their amounts compared to comparable dry articles. Vital signs must be monitored every 10 to 15 minutes. Pulse rates generally change before blood pressure readings. The presence of other symptoms are also evaluated: pain, uterine tenderness, and uterine rigidity between contractions. Whenever placenta previa is suspected, the cardinal rule is *no* vaginal or rectal examination unless it is done under circumstances where an immediate cesarean section can be performed because massive hemorrhage can result if placental tissue is torn when an examination is attempted.

The fetus must be closely evaluated since placental bleeding obviously compromises placental function. Profound distress or death can occur swiftly in severe cases. In milder cases in which labor is progressing, the nurse should watch for late deceleration patterns as evidence of placental dysfunction.

Blood is drawn for clotting time and is typed and cross matched in the event blood replacement is needed. An intravenous infusion should be in place. Preparations for emergency delivery and infant resuscitation should be made when indicated.

Umbilical Cord

The vessels of the umbilical cord are responsible for transporting nutrients, oxygen, and waste products between the fetus and placenta. Interference of cord circulation predisposes the fetus to distress.

Mechanical interference occurs if the cord becomes compressed between the fetal presenting part and the maternal pelvis. When an overt prolapse occurs, this is treated as an emergency situation and immediate delivery is accomplished. When the cord is visible at the vaginal introitus, it is observed for pulsation. If pulsation is slowing, it is sometimes possible to place gloved fingers against the presenting part firmly enough to take pressure off the cord while preparations are made for delivery. Placing the pregnant woman in the Trendelenburg position may also aid in reducing pressure on the cord. The nurse can protect the protruding cord by packing it with wet, sterile normal saline packs. If this is done, precautions must be taken *not* to compress the cord. Emergency intervention is not indicated if cord pulsation is absent, since this is evidence of fetal death.

If the cord is positioned so that each contraction produces cord compression, a variable deceleration pattern will be seen on a fetal monitor tracing. (See Figure 32-6.) The immediate treatment is to change the pregnant woman's position, since this may also change the position of the cord. If the pattern continues, the woman's position is changed again (side to side, to Trendelenburg, to sitting, etc.) until the pattern is corrected. In most instances the pattern improves with this measure. If no response is evident and the pattern becomes progressively worse (longer, lower decelerations), operative delivery may be necessary. Prolonged cord compression can produce considerable fetal distress and is probably associated with sudden sinus arrest.[18]

Loops of cord around the fetal neck or abdomen, a knot in the cord, or an abnormally short cord represent other potential interferences with cord circulation. The observations and treatment of fetal distress are those described above.

Membranes and Amniotic Fluid

Rupture of membranes normally occurs at any time during the labor process. When membranes have been ruptured 24 hours prior to the onset of labor, this is termed premature rupture of membranes. Such a premature rupture predisposes the woman and fetus to infection. The pregnant woman may develop amnionitis, an intrauterine infection, and the fetus may develop pneumonia or septicemia. The classic signs of such infection will be maternal symptoms of increased pulse rate, elevated temperature, and presence of a foul-smelling vaginal discharge. During labor the fetal heart rate may show sustained tachycardia in response to maternal fever. At delivery the infant will often possess the same characteristic odor of the infected uterine contents. Respiratory distress may be evident. Both mother and infant will need close observation following delivery.

Rupture of membranes is also related to prolapse of the umbilical cord. Whenever there is a poor fetal-pelvic fit, the sudden release of fluid from the uterus when membranes rupture may "wash" the cord down along or past the presenting part. It is always important to evaluate fetal heart rate when membranes rupture, and particularly so when a malpresentation or a high presenting part occurs.

There is normally about a liter of amniotic fluid present by the end of gestation. The fluid is normally clear, although suspended particles such as vernix, lanugo, and epithelial cells are usually seen. Discolored fluid is not normal and reveals fetal difficulties. Green-tinged amniotic fluid is stained from meconium and is evidence of an episode of fetal hypoxia. Yellow fluid is seen with erythroblastotic infants; bilirubin in the amniotic fluid causes this discoloration. Bloody amniotic fluid is usually symptomatic of fetal blood loss into the amniotic sac.

Abnormally large amounts (polyhydramnios) or small amounts (oligohydramnios) of amniotic fluid have been associated with fetal anomalies. Fetal swallowing and urination play a role in amniotic fluid formation. Esophageal and central nervous system anomalies have been found with polyhydramnios, and urinary system anomalies have been found with oligohydramnios.

The close association between amniotic fluid status and fetal status have led to widespread testing of the amniotic fluid as a reflection of fetal problems. Amniocentesis is now a low-risk method of obtaining samples of fluid for study. The nurse needs to understand this close relationship and observe amniotic fluid for clues to the possible presence of fetal complications.

PASSAGE

Pelvis

The obstetric or true pelvis is a complete bony ring bounded laterally by the ischial bones, posteriorly by the sacrum, and anteriorly by the pubic bones. The various dimensions of the pelvis are the ultimate limits of the birth passageway. The fetal head must be able to negotiate these dimensions, or vaginal delivery will be impossible.

The primary planes of the obstetric pelvis are the inlet, the midplane (the plane of least dimension), and the outlet. (See Figure 32-22.) With reference to an average size, full-term fetus, there are identified average and minimum measurements for each of these planes.

The pelvic inlet is formed by the sacral promontory, the iliopectineal lines on the iliac bones, and the superior border of the symphysis pubis. The narrowest diameter of the inlet is usually the anteroposterior diameter. When this measurement is normal, then the inlet is assumed to be of adequate size.

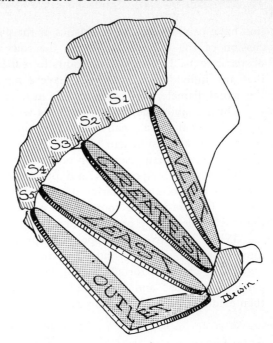

FIGURE 32-22
Planes of the pelvis.
(From Harry Oxorn and William Foote, Human Labor and Birth, Appleton-Century-Crofts, New York, 1964. By permission of the publisher.)

The minimum normal measurement for this anteroposterior diameter is 10 cm. This measurement would theoretically still allow the average term fetus with a biparietal head diameter of 9.5 cm to pass through the inlet.

The pelvic midplane passes through the ischial spines. The distance between the ischial spines forms the transverse diameter of the pelvic midplane and represents the smallest diameter of that plane. The minimum normal measurement of that diameter is 9.5 to 10 cm. A transverse diameter measuring less than that will not permit internal rotation of a normal size fetal head to the occiput anterior position.

The pelvic outlet is formed by the inferior border of the symphysis pubis, the ischial tuberosities, and the last sacral vertebra. The distance between the ischial tuberosities is the transverse diameter of the outlet. This distance and the angle of the subpubic arch influence the amount of space available at the outlet.

Architecturally the pelvis varies in shape and dimension. Four pelvic types have been described: the gynecoid, the android, the anthropoid, and the platypelloid. The characteristics of the ideal gynecoid pelvis make it most suitable to childbearing. Probably 40 percent or more of the female population have pelves with characteristics of the gynecoid pelvis.[19] A detailed discussion of the differences among the four types can be found in medical obstetric texts. The important points to realize are that classic pelves are rare, that any individual woman may have a mixture of characteristics, and that the actual diameters are relevant only in relation to fetal size.

During labor, therefore, the pelvis with "borderline" measurements may be no problem for a small fetus. A normal pelvis may be inadequate when contractions are insufficient to mold the fetal head and expel it from the passage or when a malpresentation occurs. The different pelvic shapes can contribute to fetal malpositions and presentations; e.g., the fetal vertex may rotate to the occiput posterior position for delivery rather than the occiput anterior if there is more room in the posterior portion of the lower pelvis, or the small breech may present when the pelvis is small and narrow.

When a relative cephalopelvic disproportion does occur in labor, symptoms of prolonged labor with cessation of progress will appear. X-ray pelvimetry is often performed during labor to obtain precise measurements of pelvic dimensions and fetal head size. A final diagnosis of disproportion is then made on the basis of the x ray.

Soft Tissue

The soft tissue of the maternal generative tract lies between the pelvic bones and the fetus. Abnormalities of the soft tissue can also reduce the size of the birth passage.

Tissue resistance can influence labor progress. A rigid cervix will dilate slowly and lead to prolonged labor. Stretched tissue and poor muscle tone can contribute to rapid precipitous labors. Tissue resistance is primarily responsible for the longer primigravid labor as compared to subsequent labors.

Space-occupying tumors, such as uterine fibroids, may contribute to malpresentations. Small fibroids located high in the fundus are compatible with normal labor and delivery, but fibroids in the lower segment or cervical area may prevent descent of the fetus.

Congenital anomalies of the uterus, cervix, or vagina may influence whether normal labor and delivery is possible. Severe anomalies that play a role in infertility or repeated spontaneous abortion obviously prevent normal labor and delivery. Slight anomalies may not even be discovered until the time of labor and delivery. A partial septum in the uterus may reduce the available space for fetal growth and predispose to premature delivery. A septum in the cervix will prevent normal cervical dilatation in labor. An incompetent cervix which dilates without the presence of labor contractions is associated with premature delivery.

Trauma to maternal tissues is a complication of vaginal delivery. The cervix or the vaginal mucosa may sustain lacerations in the delivery process. The perineum may also be torn. Perineal tears are classified according to the tissue involved in the laceration. First-degree tears involve the vaginal mucosa at the vaginal outlet, and/or the perineal skin and fourchette. Second-degree tears involve torn muscle in the perineal body. Third-degree tears involve the perineal body and the rectal sphincter. Fourth-degree tears extend through the rectal spincter and involve the rectal mucosa. Third- and fourth-degree lacerations can result from extensions of an episiotomy. Lacerations along the labia minora and around the urethra can also occur. It is important that lacerations are identified and repaired to effect hemostasis and to promote proper healing and perineal muscle support.

In the fourth stage of labor it is important for the nurse to detect any vaginal bleeding that is unrelated to uterine atony. A laceration of the cervix or vagina that may have been overlooked can produce a constant trickle of bright red blood in the immediate postpartum stage. Reexamination of the patient and suturing of the laceration may be necessary to prevent undue blood loss.

Hematomas can also form under the perineal skin. If they are small, they will be noticeable only by the skin discoloration and tenderness they cause. Large hematomas can form under the vaginal mucosa and may cause extreme pain and symptoms of shock if the blood loss is great. The nurse should be particularly concerned about complaints of rectal pressure during the fourth stage, since this may well be symptomatic of a hematoma.

FORCEPS DELIVERY

Forceps delivery is a means of assisting the pregnant woman to deliver the fetus through the normal passage. Forceps are applied by a skilled physician to the fetal head. During a uterine contraction, pull is exerted on the forceps while the woman pushes, if possible. The pull on the forceps always coincides with a contraction since this obtains maximum force. The sum of the pushing force plus the pulling force is needed for effective use of forceps.

Outlet (low) forceps are used when the fetal head has reached the perineal floor and the position of the head is occiput anterior. The outlet (low) forceps delivery assists the woman in the final expulsion of the fetus through the vaginal outlet.

In a midforceps delivery the forceps are applied after engagement of the fetal head in the pelvis. The station is at least 0 and it may be +1 or +2, and the cervix is completely dilated. This is a more difficult delivery and may involve a rotation of the fetal head to the occiput anterior position.

Many different kinds of obstetric forceps are available. Some forceps have special uses; e.g., Piper forceps are applied to the aftercoming head in a breech presentation. (See Figure 32-8.) Forceps are curved to fit the fetal head (cephalic curve) and also to fit the maternal pelvis (pelvic curve). A forceps application is illustrated in Figure 32-23. The choice of particular forceps for delivery rests with the physician.

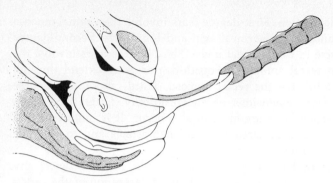

FIGURE 32-23
Correct forceps application.
(From Harry Oxorn and William Foote, Human Labor and Birth, Appleton-Century-Crofts, New York, 1964. By permission of the publisher.)

CESAREAN SECTION

Cesarean section is an operative procedure for delivery of the fetus. An incision is made into the abdominal wall and into the uterus itself. The infant, as well as the placenta and membranes, is delivered through the incision. The uterus and abdominal wall are then sutured. Generally the uterine incision is made in the thinner lower segment in a transverse direction. This incision is associated with less blood loss, and less tendency to rupture at the incision site in successive pregnancies. The alternative incision is the "classic," longitudinal midline uterine incision. This incision is now used less frequently than the low transverse incision. It may, however, be the choice when cesarean section is performed because of a low-lying placenta.

Cesarean section is now associated with low maternal mortality and morbidity figures. The availability of good anesthetics, skilled nurse anesthetists, anesthesiologists, and obstetric surgeons, blood banks, and antibiotics have reduced the risks to a minimum level. Care of the patient after cesarean section is similar to that of a patient undergoing abdominal surgery.

Fetal mortality and morbidity figures are higher for emergency cesarean section deliveries than for vaginal deliveries. Many cesarean sections are performed because of a jeopardized fetus, so these higher rates are expected. The incidence of respiratory distress is also higher in infants delivered by cesarean section, particularly in premature infants; this could be the result of a combination of factors. When the fetus passes through the *birth canal*, pressure on the chest helps rid the fetus of amniotic fluid accumulated in the lungs and bronchi. This, of course, is not the case with cesarean section delivery. An emergency cesarean section is not done unless the fetus and/or the mother is in difficulty.

IMPLICATIONS FOR THE NURSING PROCESS

Nursing the patient in labor demands continual assessment because of the dynamic nature of the labor process. Complications may occur at any point in the labor or may be present at its onset.

An initial assessment takes into consideration significant past and present history related to labor and delivery. The presence of maternal disease conditions that influence placental function is very important information. Obtaining information about the pattern of contractions prior to hospital admission, status of fetal membranes, history of any vaginal bleeding, length and description of past labors, and the gestational age of the current pregnancy helps the nurse plan the patient's care.

In addition to this history the current status is assessed. Observing hydration status, level of fatigue, and the amount and type of discomfort provides more information for the nursing care plan. Measuring the vital signs, the frequency, duration, and intensity of contractions, and the fetal heart rate contributes data about maternal and fetal response to this labor. By palpating the abdomen the nurse can obtain information about fetal position, presentation, and size. A nurse properly trained in vaginal or rectal examination procedure can obtain information about fetal position and station and status of membranes as well as cervical dilatation and effacement.

As labor continues, the nurse is particularly alert for signs of fetal distress, dysfunctional labor progress, and symptoms of altered maternal homeostasis, such as altered vital signs, dehydration, or abnormal bleeding.

The patient who exhibits some type of complicated labor and delivery needs the emotional support and comfort measures of any labor patient. In addition, the nurse will need to implement specific care for the complication that exists. Nursing care measures for specific problems have been mentioned throughout this chapter.

The nurse must also be aware of what the complication means to the patient and her family. When a family is faced with a complication of what is optimally a normal, happy situation, they are in a crisis. The skillful nurse will be able to help the family cope with the crisis, perhaps only by helping them acknowledge that a crisis does exist and that there is a reason for concern. Avoiding questions or providing false reassurance will not improve their coping abilities. Studies in crisis intervention have shown that the only way to successfully survive a crisis is to be aware that it exists. [20, 21]

When fetal outcome is threatened, as in cases of very premature labors, fetal distress, or erythroblastosis, the parents may want to know about preparations for the baby. They need the concern of others and want to know the possibilities for a successful outcome.

In an acute situation such as maternal hemorrhage or prolapsed cord the threat to life is very real. The professional personnel will also be coping with the crisis situation, but the crisis for the patient and family and their concern cannot be overlooked. Someone can and must talk to the patient about what is happening and what is being done. And someone must talk with the family as well. Again, allowing expression of grief and anxiety is beneficial to their ability to cope with the situation. Providing information as needed and acknowledging realistic concerns are also helpful.

The ability to work as a member of a team is important when caring for the patient with a complication of the labor and delivery process because many health professionals are likely to be involved in her management. Communicating pertinent information and taking initial corrective steps, as when fetal distress is first detected, may prevent a complication from becoming worse. In acute situations the nurse must know what has to be done to prepare for emergency intervention and should begin that preparation. The nurse must continue to communicate pertinent observations and be able to function when rapid decisions and actions are necessary. Interdisciplinary team work greatly increases the chance of successfully resolving a complication of the labor and delivery process.

REFERENCES

1 Eastman, Nicholson J., and Louis M. Hellman: *Williams Obstetrics*, 13th ed., Appleton-Century-Crofts, New York, 1966, pp. 535–537.
2 Hasselmeyer, Eileen G.: "Indices of Fetal Welfare," in B. Bergerson et al. (eds.), *Current Concepts in Clinical Nursing*, vol. 2, Mosby, St. Louis, 1969, pp. 298–318.
3 Gluck, Louis, et al.: "Diagnosis of the Respiratory Distress Syndrome by Amniocentesis," *American Journal of Obstetrics and Gynecology*, 109:440–445, 1971.
4 Oxorn, Harry, and William R. Foote: *Human Labor and Birth*, 2d ed., Appleton-Century-Crofts, New York, 1968, p. 361.
5 Friedman, Emanuel A.: *Labor, Clinical Evaluation and Management*, Appleton-Century-Crofts, New York, 1967, pp. 27–31.
6 Ibid., pp. 36–37.
7 Eastman and Hellman: op. cit., pp. 835–836.
8 Oxorn and Foote: op. cit., p. 366.
9 Friedman: op. cit., pp. 36–39.
10 Ibid., pp. 45–50.
11 Ibid., pp. 314–315.
12 Hon, Edward H.: *An Introduction to Fetal Monitoring*, Harty, New Haven, Conn., 1969, pp. 21–60.
13 Ibid., p. 46.
14 Oxorn and Foote: op. cit., p. 195.

15 Ibid.
16 Eastman and Hellman: op. cit., pp. 612–637.
17 Ibid., p. 626.
18 Hon: op. cit., p. 36.
19 Eastman and Hellman: op. cit., pp. 302–306.
20 Caplan, Gerald: *Principles of Preventive Psychiatry*, Basic Books, New York, 1964, pp. 288–296.
21 Parad, Howard J. (ed.): *Crisis Intervention: Selected Readings*, Family Service Association of America, New York, 1965.

COMPLICATIONS OF CHILDREARING

33 | POSTPARTUM CARE OF THE HIGH-RISK MOTHER

Virginia Gramzow Kinnick

Much of the literature about the high-risk mother and her infant is oriented to the mother's pregnancy, the hazards for her fetus, and to the condition and care of the baby following delivery. Although much has been written about the role of the nurse in working with parents who have produced a stillborn or a high-risk baby, little has been written about this care in relation to the mother when her condition continues as a high-risk puerperium.

During the first 48 hours after delivery the high-risk mother may have many more physical problems than one whose maternity cycle has been uncomplicated, whether a "perfect" baby has been produced or not. The chances of an abnormal baby, however, whether he is premature or has congenital defects, are much greater for her, too. She will be concerned about the welfare of the baby but, due to her physical condition, will have less energy to cope with what she may perceive. Her concern about her ability to care for this child may be magnified and distorted during this time.

The purpose of this chapter is to present some implications of what a continued high-risk condition of the mother in the puerperium means to her, to her family, and to her mothering role, when accompanied by either a normal baby or a high-risk condition of the baby. Certain basic nursing considerations will then be discussed in relation to the needs presented by the mother's condition and condition of the baby. Specific high-risk conditions that can continue into the puerperium will be presented, and implications for the physical care required for these specific complications will be discussed.

CONCERNS CREATED BY THE MOTHER'S CONDITION

The Taking-in Phase

There is now more awareness of the emotional changes that a woman goes through with a normal puerperium. Rubin has written fairly extensively on the readjustments a woman must make following delivery and the phases she goes through.[1] She describes the first phase, the taking-in phase, as being a passive and dependent phase for the mother. This usually lasts 2 or 3 days. She likes to be taken care of and have simple decisions about her care made for her. During this period, she seems more aware of her needs than her baby's. She is talkative about her labor and delivery, reliving it to some extent, and this helps her to regard her baby as a separate individual rather than the previous extension of herself.

In the woman who has complications in the early puerperium this early phase may be more obvious and will probably last for a longer period. The early puerperium has extensive physiological changes which may cause a crisis in many medical complications or overlapping complications of pregnancy. Until the mother's physical imbalance has been restored, she may not have fully become a part of the taking-in phase as described for the mother with a normal puerperium. If she has not delivered a healthy or normal baby, this phase will be extremely difficult. She will probably be more concerned about her baby during this phase than the mother of a healthy baby. She will also be besieged with a mixture of feelings of grief, anxiety, and guilt about her role in not producing the "perfect" baby.

It is also important for the high-risk mother to have an opportunity to relive her labor and delivery experience and resolve some of the fantasies she may have about them. The nurse should encourage the mother in her efforts to do this and should help her realistically appraise a difficult labor and delivery experience and/or her role and her partner's role in producing an abnormal baby if this has occurred. It is important to this couple that they have been "good parents" throughout the woman's maternity cycle. If the mother encounters these particular anxieties and resolves her fantasies of guilt, she will be more ready to enter the taking-hold phase of the puerperium and to develop a healthy self-concept of her maternal role.

THE FATHER'S CONCERNS

Initially, many demands will be made upon the father. Depending on the degree of complications in the mother's conditions, his greatest anxieties will be with her. However, he will probably have innumerable anxieties. Other predominant concerns could involve the baby's condition if a healthy baby was not produced, feelings of guilt about his role in the problems involved with his partner's condition, economic considerations, and concerns about other children. He needs the opportunity to express some of his feelings and resolve his anxieties so that he can be more supportive to his partner and family. He also needs to know what is being done for his partner, which frequently involves clarification of information presented to him by the doctor.

The parents' ability to cope with the problems that confront them will depend on multiple factors which include their own existing personalities, previous encounters with the maternity cycle, their relationship with each other, and the number of stressful situational factors occurring at the time of this crisis. Situational factors include the kind of nursing and medical attention they receive during the mother's hospitalization.

NURSING IMPLICATIONS

The intervention of nursing and medical personnel during the early puerperium can have strong influence in how this couple copes with the problems that confront them. Fear of criticism or disapproval of the feelings they express will create increased and unresolved anxieties within the parents, and in turn, they will begin to project blame on others or themselves. Other children or the spouse may become the scapegoat for these unexpressed anxieties.[2]

To help the couple ventilate some of their concerns, the nurse must help them to develop trust in the health team. It is important then that this couple be assigned the same nurse each day so that this person becomes a familiar figure to both parents. The concern and respect the health team shows for them, the truthfulness and objectivity of answers to the parent's questions, and the skill and thoughtfulness by which the nurse carries out physical care of the mother will all be factors in developing this trust. If the mother is not fully conscious during the first 48 hours after delivery, when a medical crisis may occur, the nurse will be directing intensive physical care to the mother and intensive emotional support toward the father.

During periods of stress, people do not accurately hear what is being said to them. The nurse must recognize that the father may need an opportunity to ventilate certain anxieties before he can understand some of the explanations the health team has for him of the mother's condition. During these times, the father may become quite sensitive to nonverbal communication. When nursing personnel retreat or seem to avoid communication with him, they may be reinforcing his fears that he is not being told everything. The patient, depending on her awareness, may react in the same way. She will be especially sensitive to nonverbal or verbal communication in relation to the condition of her baby. The anxieties of both parents will be increased if their questions are avoided.

The nurse needs to be aware of what the couple has been told about the mother's condition. Facts may need to be repeated and reinterpreted, and the feelings expressed by both should be accepted. The nurse may be available almost constantly until the physiological equilibrium has been restored and will become a familiar and important person to both parents. The nurse who becomes a symbol of trust to them will be of utmost assistance to the couple throughout the taking-hold phase for the mother. This relationship is of extreme importance in helping the mother to gain confidence in her mothering role and helping the couple to prepare for the adjustment from the hospital into the home setting.

CONCERNS OF THE NURSE

Nursing personnel may find it difficult at times to handle their own feelings and concerns for this family, especially if the mother does not go through the first 48 hours without superimposed complications. The nurses working with the couple should have the opportunity to express their feelings to someone available to them outside the immediate nursing situation. Conferences should be held daily by the health team to discuss some of the problems involved and to develop an ongoing care plan.

The concerns of this couple will also involve the baby they have produced. Those concerns and further implications for nursing care in relation to them will be discussed in the section on Concerns Created by the Infant's Condition.

The Taking-hold Phase

The second phase, taking-hold, usually lasts about 10 days and may be an extremely difficult period for the mother who has had complications in the early puerperium. This phase is involved in regaining control of body functions. The healthy mother is frequently afraid that more has been lost from her body than the baby. Her concern for her baby and her ability to care for him are greater at this time, but she is also ready to begin learning.[3]

A woman who has been ill in the early puerperium will have a greater sense of body loss. Her anxieties will not only be increased by her lack of control over her body, but her concerns will be increased for her baby, whom she may not have yet seen. Additional anxieties include her ability to cope as a mother in the presence of her physical incapacities, her concern of how this experience will permanently affect her body function and ability to function as a mother, and the effect of these multiple stresses on the family unit. She may feel overwhelmed by the problems that confront her.

Since the mother's illness may have prevented contact with her baby, it is important that contact be promoted as soon as her condition allows. Maternal feelings do not come automatically, and the mother needs to be aware that early and continuous contact with her baby will encourage the growth of her feeling for him.[4] Also of importance in helping this woman develop maternal feelings is support and encouragement of her ability to fulfill the mothering role in spite of medical problems or other physical problems that affected her in the early puerperium. A healthy woman usually has concerns about her ability as a mother, and the concerns of the high-risk mother in the puerperium must be even greater.

The area of feeding seems to be an important test to the woman in this period of questioning her ability to be a good mother.[5] Feeding time is an important time, and she should be assisted and supported throughout. It is important that the baby be brought to her for feeding when he is hungry, rather than on the nursery schedule when the baby may be sleeping. The nurse should stay with the mother throughout the early feeding periods to guide and support her as necessary. This period is when mothers have most of their questions about their babies and when progress can be made in their gaining confidence in the mothering role.

As this mother becomes acquainted with her baby, she will also be involved in the restoration of her body function. Rubin stresses the importance of the motivating factor that intolerance of inadequacies plays.[6] The woman who is intolerant of the inadequacies of her body must be taught how to cope with these inadequacies appropriately as well as to stabilize them so that she can regain control. For the patient with hyperthyroidism, it may be a rapid process involving the basic body functions of a normal puerperium plus taking medications for her condition. For the patient with cardiac disease, it may be a very slow and frustrating process that also involves a great amount of bed rest that seems incompatible with the mothering role in the weeks to follow. She may find it difficult to accept the help that she will need.

THE FATHER'S CONCERNS

During this period of time, the father's concerns will still involve economic needs of the family. A new concern may involve the future relationship he will have with his partner. The resolution of this anxiety will depend on many factors such as the previous stability of their marriage, their ability to communicate with each other, the resolution of guilt felt by both parents toward the mother's condition, and the handling of their feelings if the baby produced did not fulfill their expectations.

NURSING IMPLICATIONS

The nurse plays an important role in coordinating the rehabilitation activities of the new mother and her care of her newborn. The patient must be taken at the pace compatible with her emotional and physical health and the health of her baby. It is also important for the nurse to support the father and increase his awareness of the support his mate needs from him. Both parents must be involved in plans made for the care of the baby and mother in the home. The family unit can be strengthened through sensitive nursing care.

The couple must become fully aware of how the mother's health will be permanently affected by the complications in her pregnancy and puerperium as soon as the medical team know. If the physiological equilibrium has been reestablished during the first 48 hours following delivery, there is probably minimum change from her nonpregnant physical condition. The prognosis of specific conditions, however, does vary and will be discussed in a later section.

Communication between the couple can be encouraged by the health team by involving both parents in all reports and discussion of the mother's and baby's condition. The father needs the support of the health team but also needs to be made aware of what to expect of his partner's behavior and how he can be of help to her.

FAMILY REORGANIZATION

How both parents are assisted through the early puerperium has profound implications on the reorganization of the family. Both parents must be aware that when they return to the home, other children in the household cannot be expected to assume roles of an older age group. For example, toddlers cannot be expected to suddenly have little need for time and attention from their mother. Caplan feels that family equilibrium is determined by whether individual needs are "perceived, respected, and gratified."[7] He does not believe that the individual would suffer greatly if his needs were perceived and respected even though the family may not be able to fulfill them.

Mothers may feel overwhelmed by the demands made upon them with possible limited physical capacities and a new baby plus other children in the home. The father, too, may feel frustrated by the new demands that will be made on him initially. Each parent can be helped to become aware of what these demands mean to each other and to other children in the family and how to handle them. For example, they can be prepared to expect periods of regression from the toddler as being the norm; and just as importantly, they can learn to perceive and respect the needs for attention in this toddler in order to reestablish family equilibrium and to promote healthy, emotional development in their child.

If both parents have been allowed the opportunity to ventilate their anxieties and frustrations, they will be better able to make plans for return of mother and infant to the home. The nurse should encourage them to discuss needs of other children in the home and guide them in making plans for how the mother can divide her time among her family, including her husband, and still get the rest she needs. Home planning should be discussed with the mother and father as a team. Both parents should be made aware of community agencies which can be of assistance to them in their adjustment into the home.

IMPLICATIONS OF FAMILY PLANNING

The need for family planning is an important area for these couples. Not only is it important in respect to the mother's health and the health of future babies, but it is important in the relationship between the husband and wife.

The couple should be encouraged to discuss the subject of birth control together. The most effective family planning method is probably that method freely chosen by the couple after careful education to what is available and what is most appropriate for the mother's condition. With some medical conditions, the need for specific measures may be essential for the mother's health so that few, if any, alternatives are available. However, if the couple is not encouraged to privately discuss the subject and what it means to each of them after the crisis they have encountered with this pregnancy, their sexual relationship may suffer profoundly as a result of their mixed feeling and fears of a future pregnancy. They should be encouraged to seek early assistance from the physician.

When the primipara has a high-risk pregnancy and she produces a stillborn or a baby with anomalies, the couple may have many mixed emotions about family planning. They need the opportunity to ventilate some of these mixed feelings in an accepting atmosphere. Genetic counseling services may be of help in contributing to their knowledge of their risk in future childbearing.

In some situations, the physician may strongly advocate sterilization of the woman. Sterilization may be very difficult for any female to accept, depending on multiple factors which include number of living children, religious orientation, and marital relationship.

CONCERNS CREATED BY THE INFANT'S CONDITION

Women whose pregnancies are classified as high-risk pregnancies have an increased chance of not being able to produce a normal, healthy baby. A nurse who is caring for the high-risk mother in the puerperium may also be caring for the mother of a stillborn baby, premature baby, or a baby with a congenital defect. The chances of this are even greater if the mother's condition continues to require intensive physical observation and care after delivery. Parental response to the baby's condition and the nurse's role in the situation are significant aspects of postpartum care.

Parental Response to Stillborn or Neonatal Death

GRIEVING PROCESS

Parents who have lost a newborn are besieged with grief and anxiety. Several authors have written about the progressive and universal process of grief.[8, 9] Individuals may proceed through each phase at different rates, but each phase must be thoroughly resolved for a healthy outcome.

The parents' initial response to the announcement of the loss of a newborn baby may be disbelief and shock. The emotional impact of loss may not immediately be felt. The father may remain in this phase longer than the mother since there will be many extra demands made upon him in this period. As the individual becomes aware of the reality of loss, crying becomes a typical reaction. When the emotional impact is felt, crying seems to be an important factor to help bring about a healthy resolution. Our society makes it difficult for men to resolve their loss in this way, but they may be able to successfully fulfill this need by grieving inwardly.[10]

Anger may also be expressed at this time and may be directed at personnel who come in contact with the patient or even toward the partner. It may be an expression of the person's own feelings of guilt.[11] Feelings of guilt are even greater when the pregnancy was not wanted, for any of several reasons, including deterioration of the mother's health from the effect of pregnancy. If it was a woman's first baby, however, she may question her adequacy as a woman.

The last phase of grief is usually the longest. During this time, the mother begins to resolve her loss. The cultural rituals which accompany death and mourning, such as funerals, usually begin the preparation for this phase. Initially, the mother will be preoccupied with thoughts of her lost baby and an idealization of the baby and its role in their lives if it had lived. Gradually, she will begin to replace thoughts of her loss with other interests and relationships. This phase may last anywhere from 6 months to a year.

It is an extremely difficult time for the husband, doubly so if he is also concerned about his wife's high-risk condition. He may appear devoid of affect as he makes necessary decisions about the baby and checks on his wife. If this is the situation, it is important that he not be encouraged to express his feelings at this time or he may lose the protective mechanism that allows him to function at a time when he is needed by others of his family.[12] It may also make him feel guilty that he is not reacting as others would expect. However, if he is experiencing the emotional impact of his loss at this time, he must be encouraged to do so and should be supported appropriately.

CONCERNS OF THE NURSE

The nurse may also grieve for this family, making it difficult to function in a meaningful relationship with the parents. It is important that feelings of grief do not blind the nurse to the emotional response of the parents and an understanding and accepting of its meaning. This problem may easily arise when the parents' reaction does not meet the expectations of what the nurse thinks it should be. It is important that nurses working with these couples have someone to whom they can freely ventilate their feelings of grief and anxieties created by the situation. If not, it will be difficult for the nurse to work effectively with the patient and her partner in their grief.

NURSING IMPLICATIONS

It is necessary that the nurse caring for the patient in the puerperium know what the couple has been told about their baby, whether the baby was a stillborn or is in critical condition in the nursery. If the patient was not conscious during delivery, she may not know about her baby in the early puerperium. When she regains consciousness, the doctor may not be present. Since it is usually the doctor who informs the parents of a baby's death, he must be made aware of the urgency of his presence when the patient is alert enough to begin asking about her baby.

The nurse will find it very difficult to work with the parents if they have not been told the truth about their baby. In the situation with a stillborn, both parents are probably aware of the death unless the mother was unconscious at the time of birth. If the baby was born alive, but in critical condition, they may not have been made aware of the seriousness of the situation. It is important that personnel do not give the couple unrealistic hope. When the baby dies, the shock and grief are greater when the parents have not been prepared for it.

When the death does occur, it is better that the couple be told together. The nurse should be available to them when the announcement is made. Observations of the couple's reactions and behavior will help the nurse determine how to respond. The nurse must be able to accept the behavior and feelings they express, and provide the necessary privacy for the couple in their expression of grief. The parents may want to be alone, but it is reassuring for them to know that a nurse is available if needed. They may want the nurse to remain with them. If so, the couple does not want someone with them who tries to offer explanations or such platitudes as, "at least you have another child at home." They want someone with them who cares and understands their feelings of loss. The mother's crying should be accepted and encouraged. The nurse should not appear rushed. During this time the parents should be consulted as to whether they would like spiritual counseling from a minister or other person.

The nurse must encourage an environment of trust so that the mother has an opportunity to share her feelings. It is important that the mother can express her feelings in order to help resolve her guilt fantasies.[13] She needs reassurance that she did nothing to cause the death of her baby.

Suggestions of how a trust relationship can be established have been discussed in a previous section in this chapter. It should be emphasized that members of the health team should be able to accept and understand the anger that may be directed at them. The individual who reacts with hostility will increase the anxiety felt by the parents and will be unable to work effectively with them.

It is important in the days to follow that the couple's loneliness is not reinforced by the nursing personnel. The nurse caring for the patient should be available to them when needed and should not appear rushed when involved in the care of the mother. As the mother prepares for dismissal from the hospital, the nurse can encourage her to ventilate the anguish and anxiety she feels in returning home without a baby.

One author feels that it is important for the parents to see the baby, especially if he was abnormal.[14] Seeing the baby will be extremely painful for the parents. If they are shown the baby in the hospital, the nurse again should be available to them as they reexperience new grief. However, the couple may have made funeral arrangements at which time the mother will see the infant. Seeing the infant helps the mother to complete the maternity cycle rather than leaving something unfinished. It also helps to eliminate or diminish distorted fantasies about her baby.

Parental Response to Prematurity

Even though the mother has had complications throughout her pregnancy, premature labor is still a shock. Neither parent has had the opportunity to complete psychological preparation for the baby or sometimes not even preparation in the home. Many women who have experienced a premature delivery will describe it as having unreal qualities. However, following delivery, these parents tend to have increased anxieties about whether their baby is alive or if it will live. There is also great concern about the presence of deformities and mental retardation.[15]

Accompanying the concern about their baby may be feelings of guilt. Their guilt feelings usually involve anxieties that they did something to cause the premature labor.[16] They may experience some feelings of grief also. Their grief is usually for the perfect baby expected or of their own failure to produce such a baby. However, the mother who has lost babies previously will probably experience a sense of achievement if her baby lives.[17]

NURSING IMPLICATIONS

It is important that the mother see her baby as soon as she is ready in order to help her minimize some of the fantasies that she may have created. If the mother's condition prevents her from seeing the baby early, her husband can assist her by reporting his observations. A nurse should be with the parents to help them express the concerns about what they see and support them as necessary. The early visits may be upsetting to the parents when they see the small size and general appearance of their baby with accompanying intravenous tubings and incubator.

It is again important that there are not multiple relationships with the parents. As in the other conditions described in this chapter, a relationship of trust continues to be important. Some suggestions in establishing this relationship have already been discussed. The most difficult area with these parents will be in objectively and truthfully answering questions they ask about their baby's condition. There is a tendency to reassure them when reassurance is not appropriate. If a baby dies, the shock and grief are greater if the parents have not been told about a decline in their baby's condition. It is easier for the parents to cope when they are given the facts rather than not knowing anything.

Frequently, the premature nursery is not on the maternity floor where the mother is hospitalized. Open lines of communication between the nursery and parents will be important to help minimize their anxiety about their baby. Effective methods in establishing these lines of communication will need to be coordinated by the nurse caring for the parents and the nurse caring for the baby. Coordination is necessary, since opening these lines of communication should later include opportunities for the mother to touch and/or hold her baby when it is physically possible for both.

Minimizing separation between the newborn baby and mother is always important in the development of a healthy maternal role. The premature baby's condition, as well as the mother's, makes this goal difficult to achieve. The ingenuity of the nurse will be important in helping this baby become an individual to the mother. This process will involve reports which include the baby's behavioral characteristics and feeding pattern. When the mother is able, she should be wheeled to the nursery to see her baby and supported as necessary with her first glimpse of the baby, as discussed previously.

In her early visits to the nursery, she may feel increased concern about her capabilities in caring for the baby, especially as she observes the nurse's skill in doing so. It will be extremely difficult for the mother if the personnel do not help her to feel that this baby is hers, and if she does not have an opportunity to touch, hold, or feed her baby before she leaves the hospital. Her increased anxieties will probably interfere with her maternal feelings toward the baby and affect her behavior toward all members of the family. For example, this increased anxiety could cause her to become overprotective of the baby to the detriment of other members in the family and the baby himself.

Personnel must be patient and supportive with the mother in her mothering role. She will probably need much reassurance and guidance in the feeding experience which will probably be the basis of her attitude in the total care because it will be her first mothering task and thus, a very important one in which to be successful. The goal of the personnel at this time will be to help her gain confidence in her capabilities to care for her baby. She also needs to be aware that the development of maternal feelings is a gradual process, even with mothers of full-term babies, so that it is common for a greater emotional lag to occur with mothers of premature babies because of their separation and lack of contact.

It may be difficult for this mother to return home without a baby. She and her husband must be made aware of the importance of the mother being able to return to the nursery for feeding experiences. The nurse should also give the mother certain times during the day to call about her baby when the nurse will be available to give the mother information.

Both parents must be prepared for the baby's arrival in the home; they should understand how their baby's needs will vary from a normal baby in special areas, such as feeding patterns and growth and development, and also how this baby is "potentially normal."[18]

Upon return of both mother and baby in the home, appropriate community referrals should be made.

Parental Response to a Defective Infant

The reactions of parents to the birth of a child who has a deformity are based on several factors, the primary factor being the severity of the deformity. Other factors include when they are informed, their amount of energy at the time, and their past experience with the condition.[19]

It is important that parents be told about the presence of a deformity in their baby soon after delivery. A perfect baby is expected, and the longer they assume this perfect baby has arrived, the more they suffer when eventually informed otherwise. This delay also causes distrust of personnel and bitterness which could be directed toward the child as well as those working with the couple.

Initially, the parents will feel shock and shame. It will be especially difficult for the woman who has a high-risk puerperium and, thus, already a sense of inadequacy about her own body. Since the baby is still considered an extension of herself, her sense of inadequacy and failure as a woman will be heightened.[20]

Both parents will need to grieve for the loss of the idealized baby before they are able to accept the defective one in its place. They will pass through the grieving process as described in the section on the stillborn. In this situation, more anger and hostility may be expressed than with a stillborn. The behavior of these parents must be accepted and understood by the personnel in order for the parents to move through this process more rapidly and thoroughly. Neither parent, especially the mother, will be ready to accept their baby until they have had an opportunity to express their grief and release some of their feelings of disappointment and failure.[21, 22] If these feelings are not expressed to someone, the formation of the relationship of this mother with her child can be detrimentally affected. Sometimes personnel accuse these mothers of rejecting their babies during this period, since they are not yet ready to accept them. However, this process is important in the mother's formation of her relationship with her baby and should be understood rather than frowned upon. Both parents need to be aware of the normality of this behavior.[23]

NURSING IMPLICATIONS

A nurse should be available to parents when they are informed of the baby's abnormality. It is important that all personnel be aware that anger or hostility could be directed at them and understand its basis. The nurse must be able to accept this expression of their feelings and support them in their mourning.

The parents' perception of the attitudes and behavior of personnel toward them immediately after the birth of their baby has great influence on the family's attitude toward their baby and how they cope with the problems created. The nurse demonstrates caring and respect for the parents even though they have produced an imperfect baby. Our society places great emphasis on the physical and intellectual "wholeness" of its people. The health team will be the first contact these parents have with attitudes toward them and their baby. This contact is at a particularly sensitive time for them, and they will be intensely aware of nonverbal communication of the health team.

The acceptance they perceive at this time and throughout their hospitalization will strongly affect their acceptance of the baby. The parent's acceptance of their child will in turn affect each member of the family. For example, if the mother is not able to express her feelings of guilt, she may become oversolicitous toward the baby and neglect the needs of other members of the family.

Basic principles of emotional support of these parents include those involved in support given to parents of premature babies. Even greater emphasis must be placed on the acceptance the health team demonstrates toward the baby and his parents. The parents must be helped to get to know their baby as one that can be loved although he has one or more problems. Personnel can help to demonstrate this concept by showing as much love and warmth to this baby as to others in the nursery. If parents observe the personnel demonstrate feelings of horror and shock at the baby's appearance or condition, their feelings of failure and shame will be increased, thus delaying their ability to form a healthy relationship. The parents will be extremely sensitive to all nonverbal communication and behavior that they observe either through the nursery window or at the mother's bedside.

As the mother begins to cope with her feelings and is ready to begin the basic mothering task of feeding her infant, the nurse must continue to support and reassure her in her abilities and in the nurse's acceptance of her and her baby. The health team must begin to teach the parents about the anomaly and what it will mean to the child as well as discuss realistic plans for rehabilitation. Appropriate referrals will be essential for this family.

The parents must also be helped to prepare for the handling of reactions from other children. They must be aware that sibling rejection is normal with a healthy child and does not arise because they have not presented a perfect baby.[24]

Another great concern of parents who give birth to a defective child is their probability of producing another child with the same problems. This subject is discussed in Chapter 13 in the section on genetic counseling.

CONCERNS OF THE NURSE

Nursing care of parents and babies in the presence of an anomaly can be very difficult because of multiple feelings within the nurse. Feelings of shock, distaste, or pity toward the baby may be prominent negative feelings. If these feelings are present, it becomes difficult for the nurse to either develop or maintain a meaningful relationship with the parents in helping them through the process of developing their own healthy acceptance of their baby. It is again essential that nursing personnel be aware of their own feelings and can discuss and ventilate them with others so that these feelings are not resolved at the expense of the parents and their child.

The nurse must be aware of feelings aroused by the parents' reactions toward the baby, too. More discussion of how the individual nurse is personally affected when caring for these babies and their families can be found in Chapter 34.

SPECIFIC HIGH-RISK CONDITIONS

There are many conditions in a high-risk pregnancy that are not abruptly terminated with delivery of the baby. Obvious examples include women who have a coincidental medical complication such as diabetes or cardiovascular disease. Since many nursing textbooks are oriented to the normal maternity cycle, nurses are often at a loss in knowing how these conditions are affected in the puerperium. Furthermore, they are probably not accustomed to caring for maternity patients with medical complications unless they work in high-risk centers where these high-risk mothers may be referred for their care. The majority of maternity nurses in general hospitals may suddenly be called upon to use knowledge and skills not commonly needed. It is extremely important for the patient involved that these nurses be aware of the physical care involved or have immediate access to this information.

The nurse needs to be aware of how the puerperium affects the coincidental conditions and how, in turn, these conditions may affect the puerperium. The first 48 hours after delivery involve significant changes in the body which produce a crucial period for many complications. The nursing care in this period is of utmost importance for these patients.

The following sections will discuss how continuing complications of pregnancy are affected by the physiological adaptation of the puerperium and, in turn, how they affect the puerperium. Nursing implications of integrating physical care of the two conditions will be discussed. However, specific nursing care of a medical condition will not be covered, since this is done thoroughly in any medical nursing textbook which should be found on maternity wards. It should be the responsibility of the nursing staff to hold conferences for purposes of refreshing the knowledge of nurses who care for these patients and helping auxiliary personnel in observing and understanding symptoms that are presented by the patient's condition.

Coordination and continuity of nursing care will be of utmost importance in the care of these patients with the multiple problems presented with both their condition and that of their babies. These patients have a greater need for rest than others, but many more demands for tests and treatments will be made upon them. Rather than one doctor, they may be seeing the obstetrician, pediatrician, internist, and even interns or residents in hospitals where they are present. Dietitians, social workers, and laboratory personnel may also have contact with the patient. It will be the nurse who will have prime responsibility for coordinating the activities of all these people so that the needs of the patient will be best fulfilled.

Discussion of emotional support is found in the previous sections. The following sections will include basically the physical care of each complication discussed.

CARDIOVASCULAR CONDITIONS

Cardiac Disease

After delivery occurs, there is a 20 to 40 percent increase in blood volume.[25] The blood that previously supplied the uterus is emptied into the general circulation, increasing cardiac output. For the person who has cardiac disease, the danger of congestive heart failure is again present in the first 48 hours following delivery—the first hour is the most crucial.

A moderate amount of blood loss following delivery reduces the total blood volume and aids the heart in its work. However, too much blood loss is a problem because of the anemia that results. If the cardiac patient requires blood in the postpartum period, packed cells would probably be given rather than overloading the circulatory system with whole blood.

The physiological diuresis of the body during the second to fifth days postpartum will help establish physiological equilibrium. However, the nonpregnant cardiac output level is not usually reached until almost 2 weeks postpartum.[26]

Psychic stimuli following delivery play a less important role in increasing cardiac output than during labor. Much anxiety is relieved by the termination of pain during the delivery process.[27]

The patient who develops puerperal infections and mastitis is also in danger of developing bacterial endocarditis. Most cardiac patients are put on prophylactic antibiotics following delivery and are often discouraged from breast-feeding by some doctors for this reason. Slight infections can also trigger congestive heart failure in cardiac patients. It is important that the patient be protected from upper respiratory infections as well as puerperal infections and mastitis.

Cardiac patients usually deliver vaginally at term and produce healthy babies which may be smaller than average size. Some doctors may discourage the mother from breast-feeding because they want to reduce any potential hazards of infection. However, most believe that mothers who are in classes I and II of the New York Heart Association's functional classifications may be allowed to do so if they so desire. Mothers in classes III and IV are usually discouraged from breast-feeding because of the increased demands on the fluid and metabolic status.[28]

When the woman has cardiac disease, especially if she has had congestive heart failure at any time, family planning will be important. Most doctors believe these patients should be prepared for a method of contraception before they return home. However, postpartal sterilization is usually not indicated for the patient whose condition is well compensated, and patients who have recently suffered congestive heart failure are poor surgical risks.[28]

NURSING IMPLICATIONS

Regardless of etiology, the greatest danger to these patients in the first 48 hours following delivery is congestive heart failure. Factors in the postpartum period which increase this possibility include the increased cardiac output at this time, slight puerperal infections, anemia from excess blood loss, and undue physical strain. Nursing care of cardiac patients during the postpartum will be directed at prevention of the abovementioned factors and intensive observation for early symptoms of congestive heart failure.

Two early symptoms of congestive heart failure are edema and shortness of breath; thus, the mother should be observed closely for the presence of edema and changes in the apical pulse as well as the rate of respirations. If she is bedridden, the edema will be found first in the posterior regions of the thighs and sacrum. If she is not on bed rest, the edema will probably be located in the area of the ankles. The mother's weight will probably not be a reliable indicator of edema during the early puerperium.[29] The apical pulse should be checked closely for any arrhythmias or changes. Nursing care of patients with congestive heart failure is thoroughly discussed in medical nursing textbooks.

The normal physiology of increased cardiac output cannot be changed. However, prevention of increased circulatory overload will be important. If an intravenous infusion accompanies the patient from the delivery room, the rate of flow should be determined by the doctor and regulated with great care by the nurse. As the patient begins to eat, low-sodium diets will be important in prevention of fluid retention. The patient will probably be on diuretics at this time for the same purpose. The total fluid intake and output should be carefully recorded.

It will be important for the nurse to closely observe the patient's blood loss and condition of the fundus in the early hours postpartum so that anemia from blood loss is checked as closely as possible. Oxytocics will probably be given, although Ergotrate is usually avoided because of its effect on the circulatory system.[30] Frequent manual determination of the condition of the fundus is essential, since an increased flow from a boggy fundus could be detrimental. The amount of blood loss that could cause anemia will vary with each patient, depending on such factors as previous hemoglobin and blood loss at delivery.

Although the patient may decide not to breast-feed, especially patients in classes III and IV, estrogen is not usually given to these patients for suppression of lactation because of the fluid retention that results. They will need to be assisted in the relief of breast engorgement when it occurs and in accompanying comfort measures.

Prevention of infection is always important in the puerperium. However, it becomes even more essential with the cardiac patient, since any infection will add increased stress and/or the increased risk of endocarditis. As mentioned previously, the patient will probably be on prophylactic antibiotics, but this factor should not cause a relaxation in good perineal and breast care.

Undue physical stress is also a factor in causing congestive heart failure. The amount of physical activity tolerated by each patient will vary. However, during this period of increased cardiac output, it will be important that activity be limited for all cardiac patients.

It is important for these patients not to strain when passing a stool. As the patient strains she tenses the thorax and holds her breath, causing changes in cardiac output and pressure. These changes may cause tachycardia and lead to cardiac arrest. This activity not only occurs when straining with a stool, but can also occur when getting onto a bedpan or moving around in bed. The patient should be taught to exhale during these activities rather than hold her breath.[31] Appropriate stool softeners, ordered by the doctor, should be started early in the puerperium to alleviate straining during defecation. The sluggish peristalsis of the bowel that occurs during labor and delivery and lack of early ambulation in the puerperium add to the problem of bowel elimination for the cardiac patient.

If the pulse is taken after exertion, it can be a good measure of impending congestive heart failure. Only a few minutes should be needed for the mother's pulse to return to normal after an activity has ceased, such as getting out of bed. A great length of time for the pulse to return to normal may indicate congestive heart failure.

The prevention of thromboembolic complications is important for the cardiac patient. The patient who is on bed rest should be encouraged to move her legs frequently and may be required to wear elastic stockings. Ambulation, as soon as it is considered safe, is advisable. Other methods of prevention are discussed in the section on thrombophlebitis.

LONG-TERM PLANS

Patients with cardiac disease must continue on the regimen necessary in the nonpregnant state. If congestive heart failure has occurred at any time throughout the pregnancy, a stricter regimen will probably be needed. It is essential for all of these mothers to have a strict pattern of rest in the following weeks to again prevent the possibility of congestive heart failure from overactivity and lack of rest. Long-term planning will be essential in the nursing care of these patients. Many community agencies may be of value to this family, such as those involved in household services, since help in the home will be essential for these mothers. The American Heart Association also has pamphlets available to help mothers find easier ways of accomplishing household responsibilities. Family members need to be aware of this need for help so as not to place undue expectations on the new mother.

Thrombophlebitis

During pregnancy and in the puerperium, the circulatory system undergoes some specific changes which can increase the tendency for venous thrombosis if preventive measures are not taken. Chances of thrombophlebitis are greatly increased during the puerperium when stasis of blood in the legs occurs and with the increased clotting ability of the blood at this time. The tendency is even greater with patients who have had cesarean sections and those who have been on bed rest in the last week or more of pregnancy, as in some high-risk pregnancies.

Phlebothrombosis is a venous thrombosis without the presence of an infectious process. The symptoms are usually masked. It is rarely encountered in the average, healthy, postpartum patient because it is formed more frequently in women over forty years old. There is a greater risk with emboli in this form of venous thrombosis than with thrombophlebitis.

The presence of a slight puerperal infection and direct injuries to a vein predispose to thrombophlebitis, which is a clot formed as a result of an inflammation of the walls of the vein. Thrombophlebitis can be present in the ovarian and uterine veins, and veins of the broad ligament, which would be referred to as pelvic thrombophlebitis; or it can be present in the veins of the leg, which is referred to as femoral thrombophlebitis.

PELVIC THROMBOPHLEBITIS

Symptoms indicating the presence of this condition begin with chills and a high fever. The causative organism is usually anaerobic streptococcus which can be cultured from the bloodstream only during a chill. Otherwise, its presence is difficult to detect. This condition does not usually appear until the second week postpartum. During the time of the chill and peak in her fever, the mother seems extremely ill. At other times she may appear and feel well.

The inflammation can rise higher and higher, or the thrombosis may limit it. As the inflammation extends, the thrombus can also be broken into a mass of pus with small emboli eventually breaking away. The result can be lung abscesses or even pleurisy or pneumonia. The metastatic infection can also occur in the kidneys.

The use of anticoagulants is important to prevent more clots from being formed and to decrease the possibility of pulmonary embolism. Penicillin will probably be the antibiotic used to combat the organism present in the bloodstream, since it is specifically for anaerobic streptococcus.

FEMORAL THROMBOPHLEBITIS

Symptoms indicating the presence of this condition usually do not occur until the tenth day postpartum. They begin with pain in the affected leg accompanied by a temperature elevation. As in most cases of phlebitis, the temperature fluctuates between high elevations and normal. However, the pulse remains elevated and ordinarily is elevated out of proportion to the temperature. The affected area will be hotter to touch than the rest of the leg or the other leg. Edema will be present; the degree of edema depends on the amount of obstruction in the vein.

Thrombophlebitis is often referred to as phlegmasia alba dolens, and also as "milk leg," especially when extensive edema is present. The latter phrase was used initially when it was believed that the edema was actually milk present in the leg. Perhaps this was because the skin over the area of swelling becomes tense and white, and lactation may cease when an acute febrile process is present.[32] It may take several weeks for the inflammatory process to heal, and recurring edema may continue to be a problem for years.

If thrombophlebitis is suspected, the patient is immediately put to bed and kept on strict bed rest with elevation of the edematous leg. Anticoagulants, pain medication as necessary, and antibiotics are usually given. The antibiotic most frequently used is penicillin.

NURSING IMPLICATIONS

The most important aspect of care is prevention. In the postpartum period, this would include early ambulation to prevent stasis of blood in the leg and the prevention of puerperal infection. Changing the position of patients who have had cesarean sections should be done frequently, and they should be encouraged to move their legs while in bed. If there is no contraindication for other conditions, elevation of the foot of the bed can be beneficial in assisting venous drainage for those requiring bed rest. The knee gatch should not be elevated and the patient should not lie in bed with legs or ankles crossed, since this would put added resistance to venous return.

When the patient is allowed to get up, she should be assisted in walking rather than allowed to sit. Sitting on the edge of the bed or sitting in a chair will only increase pressure on the veins in the legs, which are an additional source for clots. Elastic stockings may be ordered on those patients whose condition predisposes to the formation of clots, such as the cardiac patient who may be on bed rest.

With thrombophlebitis, a cradle is used to keep the bed clothes off the affected leg. The affected leg should never be rubbed or massaged and should also be handled very carefully so that an embolus is not dislodged. Sometimes heat is used to relieve the discomfort.

Pulmonary Embolism

Pulmonary embolism usually results from the development of phlebothrombosis rather than thrombophlebitis, making it difficult to detect warning signs before the actual damage occurs. However, knowledge of the conditions which predispose to phlebothrombosis will help preventive measures to be implemented. Predisposing conditions include congestive heart failure and hypothyroidism as well as the combining factors discussed in the section on venous thrombosis.

The seriousness of a pulmonary embolism will depend on the size of the embolus. A large embolus will cause sudden death within a few minutes or hours in a patient who previously appeared healthy. A smaller embolus will not be fatal, but there is a great possibility that other emboli, and larger ones, will be released into the bloodstream and that repeated episodes will occur which could be fatal.

Symptoms of pulmonary embolism include sudden and intense chest pain, severe shortness of breath, and cyanosis. The pulse is feeble and irregular. If the patient does not die soon after the attack, a high concentration of oxygen is given and anticoagulant therapy is started. The anticoagulant therapy does not affect clots that are already formed but does prevent formation of more. Medication, such as morphine, is usually given to help relieve apprehension.

NURSING IMPLICATIONS

The most important aspect of care is prevention of any form of venous thrombosis. In the postpartum period this would include early ambulation or some other measure to prevent stasis of blood in the legs and prevention of puerperal infection.

When the patient survives the first pulmonary embolism, she must be on strict bed rest and very quiet. Any movement may cause a fatal attack. Oxygen will be started immediately, and since anticoagulant therapy will also be ordered by the physician, the patient must be observed closely for unusual bleeding. Any apprehension must be relieved if possible. Most patients who are still alive after 9 hours will probably recover completely.[33]

ENDOCRINE DYSFUNCTIONS

Diabetes

Insulin needs of patients during the third trimester of pregnancy usually increase. During the immediate postpartum period there is an abrupt drop in the need for insulin, and if the dosage is not reduced prior to delivery or immediately following, insulin shock could occur. Other metabolic changes that normally occur as the body so rapidly returns to its nonpregnant state sometimes makes diabetes difficult to control in the immediate puerperium. The mother's diabetic condition should be fully stabilized within 72 hours postpartum.[34]

In the last weeks of pregnancy and during lactation, lactose is produced in the breast. If lactation is inhibited, lactose spills over into the bloodstream and is excreted into the urine. Lactosuria is sometimes misleading at this time, so blood sugar determinations are frequently done for a more accurate regulation of the insulin requirement. Lactosuria will still be found during lactation but is usually of insignificance clinically. The patient should check her urine during lactation following the early puerperium. Lactose demonstrates a negative test for glucose with the Clinistix although Benedict's solution tests positive for sugar.[35]

Diabetic women are more likely to develop toxemia and polyhydramnios in their pregnancy than other women. If eclampsia develops, the nurse will also be involved in the care of this condition as described in the section on postpartum eclampsia. Polyhydramnios will increase the mother's tendency to hemorrhage in the postpartum period. Thus, a diabetic patient may present multiple conditions which require intensive nursing care. However, with a

well-controlled diabetic condition throughout her pregnancy and close supervision of the pregnancy, toxemia may be prevented and her diabetic condition unchanged from her nonpregnant condition.

In women with diabetes, labor is sometimes induced approximately 2
weeks prior to term, since fetal death in utero seems to occur much more
frequently with these women when they are allowed to deliver at term. As a
result, prematurity is not uncommon, although the babies may appear large.
Increased incidence of abnormalities is also found in babies of diabetic
mothers.

Since diabetics are prone to infection, those mothers with a longer duration
of the disease are frequently discouraged from breast-feeding their babies.
Cracked nipples may be extremely difficult to heal and even develop into serious infections. Breast-feeding may also decrease the stability of their diabetic
condition, especially when weaning the baby, since their intake and lactation
needs will be varied. The decision to breast-feed will probably depend on the
seriousness of the patient's diabetic condition, her baby's condition, and her
doctor.

If the diabetes is well controlled throughout pregnancy, the mother's
diabetic condition in the postpartum period should gradually return to her
nonpregnant status. Women with gestational diabetes may find their condition returns to latent diabetes, but with each pregnancy and with age, clinical diabetes will eventually become permanent.[36]

Women who produce large babies, especially if the baby is a stillborn at
term, frequently are suspected of latent diabetes. Sometimes 2-hour post-
prandial blood sugars are done on them in the early puerperium. If unusually
high blood sugar is determined, a glucose tolerance test will be done. If latent
diabetes is detected, these patients will be warned of the role of weight gain
and counseled in the role that pregnancy and age plays in manifestation of
the clinical condition. Their future pregnancies will be closely supervised to
prevent intrauterine death at term.

NURSING IMPLICATIONS

Nursing care in the early puerperium of diabetic mothers will be directed at
factors which help to stabilize their diabetic condition and a healthy obstetric
condition. The mode of delivery, which is preferably vaginal, will also orient
nursing care. Cesarean sections are not done unless indicated by the obstetric condition. For example, a woman with a severe diabetic condition
whose cervix is unfavorable for induction will probably have a cesarean
section.

Fluctuation of the diabetic condition in the early puerperium will require
blood sugar determinations as well as the usual urine checks as ordered by
the doctor. In a mild form of diabetes, only frequent urine checks might be
done. Insulin dosage will be regulated accordingly. A short-acting insulin

may be used until stabilization occurs. The nurse must observe the patient for signs of hypoglycemia and impending insulin shock, which is most common during this period, and also must be alert for signs of diabetic coma.

The patient's diabetic condition begins to fluctuate in the presence of an infectious process, so good perineal care and breast care is again emphasized. The patient must understand the importance of good hygiene in relation to her postpartum care while she is in the hospital and in the home setting. Slight puerperal infections can make the management of the diabetic condition difficult, so infections should be reported immediately.

If polyhydramnios was present in pregnancy, the tendency toward hemorrhage is increased. These patients must be checked closely in the early puerperium for bleeding complications.

Thyroid Dysfunctions

HYPERTHYROIDISM

Physiology of the puerperium seems to have minimum effect on hyperthyroidism. The basal metabolic rate is increased during the last trimester of pregnancy but returns to normal within a week after delivery.

These patients have usually been on antithyroid medications during pregnancy to help produce a euthyroid state. The dosage of the antithyroid medication will probably be reduced in the first week of the puerperium. Since these drugs are excreted into the breast milk, these mothers are not allowed to breast-feed.[37]

If these patients are overtreated with antithyroid medications, their pregnancies will frequently result in abortions, fetal anomalies, and an overly suppressed fetal thyroid. Toxemia and postpartum hemorrhage could also occur with poor management of the hyperthyroid condition superimposed on pregnancy.[38]

NURSING IMPLICATIONS

Much of the nursing care in the puerperium of the patient will depend on the medical control of her thyroid condition. The nurse should be alert for increasing apprehension and tachycardia, suggesting an impending thyroid storm or crisis. Laboratory tests to determine thyroid status will probably be done until the thyroid condition is again stabilized to determine medication dosages.

Prevention of postpartum hemorrhage may be an important factor, depending on the status of the thyroid at the time of delivery. Toxemia may also be present. Otherwise, nursing care will basically involve a normal puerperium.

HYPOTHYROIDISM

There is little discussion in the literature on the postpartum care of the patient with hypothyroidism. The severe form of this condition is associated with sterility. When milder forms of the condition are present and untreated, the problems that occur are usually related to the ability to become pregnant and the maintenance of the pregnancy. Premature delivery and congenital anomalies are frequently present when the pregnancy is maintained.[39]

COMPLICATIONS SPECIFIC TO PREGNANCY

Postpartum Eclampsia

Convulsions in patients with eclampsia can continue to occur within the first 48 hours of the puerperium. Close observation of these patients is as essential during this time as it is prior to delivery. Obviously, the dangers are the same, with the potential threat of convulsions occurring during sleep. The blood pressure tends to be somewhat labile but usually high. Nursing personnel must not relax in their observation and care of these patients because delivery has occurred. Spontaneous recovery usually does not occur for 48 hours after delivery, so continued vigilance is important during this time.

Owing to sedation during this time, the mother may be unable to breastfeed until even the fourth or fifth day postpartum. Haynes states that with cases of posteclamptic patients reported that approximately half have developed postpartum psychosis.[40] These patients should be observed closely for signs of this condition.

NURSING IMPLICATIONS

Principles of nursing care of the eclamptic patient in the postpartum period are essentially the same as in the prenatal period. Basic differences, obviously, relate to the empty uterus. The nurse must use great care and gentleness in determining blood loss and checking the fundus so that convulsions are not triggered. Judgment as to fluctuations in blood pressure must be accurate in relation to blood loss and the eclamptic condition.

Since the level of hypertension may not return to normal for several weeks, these mothers should be put on low-sodium diets and maintained on these until there is a decrease in their blood pressure. It is difficult to determine immediately if permanent hypertension will result following postpartum eclampsia. However, it is more likely to persist in older women. Essential hypertension seems more likely to result when the patient is already predisposed to it.

Since the symptoms of postpartum psychosis may not appear until after the patient's dismissal, the family should be alerted to the possibility of changes in the behavior of the new mother. They should be aware of the need to seek help from their physician if unusual changes are observed.

Multiple Pregnancy

A woman with a multiple pregnancy is susceptible to multiple complications in the puerperium. Her chances of having toxemia, including eclamptogenic toxemia, are greatly increased compared to the woman with a single fetus. The danger of postpartum hemorrage is also heightened as a result of the overdistention of the uterus, which results in uterine atony after delivery. These patients should not only be checked closely for prevention of excessive blood loss, but preparations should be made to replace blood loss if necessary.

Premature labor is quite common with a woman who has a multiple pregnancy. Thus, prematurity as well as congenital abnormalities, fetal death, and fetal trauma at birth are more common problems with the multiple pregnancy than with a single fetus.

NURSING IMPLICATIONS

Immediate physical care of a woman with a multiple birth in the puerperium is basically directed at prevention of postpartum hemorrhage and appropriate nursing care in the presence of toxemia.

A combination of difficult emotional situations could be present, depending on the condition of the babies and whether a multiple pregnancy was expected or not. The nurse must be aware of a mother's need to grieve for a stillborn baby even though she has a second baby who is healthy and normal. If a second baby was not expected, it may not be as difficult for the mother because she would not have been prepared psychologically or made preparations in the home.

REFERENCES

1 Rubin, Reva: "Puerperal Change," *Nursing Outlook*, 9:753–755, December 1961.
2 Owens, Charlotte: "Parents Response to Premature Birth," *American Journal of Nursing*, 60:1118, August 1960.
3 Rubin: op. cit., pp. 754–755.
4 Caplan, Gerald: *Concepts of Mental Health and Consultation*, United States Department of Health, Education, and Welfare, Children's Bureau, Washington, D.C., 1959, pp. 62–63.
5 Henning, E., et al.: "A Dynamic Appraisal of the Puerperium," in Nancy Lytle (ed.), *Maternal Health Nursing*, Wm. C. Brown Co., Dubuque, Iowa, 1967, pp. 154–158.

6 Rubin, Reva: "Body Image and Self Esteem," *Nursing Outlook*, 68:20–21, June 1968.

7 Caplan: op. cit., pp. 42–43.

8 Thaler, O. F.: "Grief and Depression," *Nursing Forum*, 5(2):8–22, 1966.

9 Engel, G. L.: "Grief and Grieving," *American Journal of Nursing*, 64:93–98, September 1964.

10 Ibid., p. 95.

11 Ibid., p. 97.

12 Ujhely, G. B.: "Grief and Depression—Implications for Preventive and Therapeutic Nursing Care," *Nursing Forum*, 5(2):23–35, 1966.

13 Bruce, S.: "Reactions of Nurses and Mothers to Stillbirths," *Nursing Outlook*, 10:88–91, February 1962.

14 Owens, C.: "Parents' Reactions to Defective Babies," *American Journal of Nursing*, 64:86, November 1964.

15 Kaplan, D. M., and E. A. Mason: "Maternal Reactions to Premature Births Viewed as an Acute Emotional Disorder," *American Journal of Orthopsychiatry*, 30:541, July 1960.

16 Prugh, Dane G.: "Emotional Problems of the Premature Infant's Parents," *Nursing Outlook*, 1:461, August 1953.

17 Kaplan and Mason: op. cit., p. 542.

18 Ibid., pp. 544–545.

19 Kaullas, J.: "The Child with Cleft Lip and Palate—The Mother in the Maternity Unit," *American Journal of Nursing*, 65:121, April 1965.

20 Waechter, Eugenia: "The Birth of an Exceptional Child," *Nursing Forum*, 9:204, 1970.

21 Ibid., pp. 204–212.

22 Kaullas: op. cit., p. 122.

23 Waechter: op. cit., p. 209.

24 Ibid., p. 215.

25 Lerch, Constance: *Maternity Nursing*, Mosby, St. Louis, 1970, p. 109.

26 Haynes, D. M.: *Medical Complications during Pregnancy*, McGraw-Hill, New York, 1969, p. 69.

27 Ibid., p. 72.

28 Ibid., p. 99.

29 Shafer, K., J. Sawyer, A. McCluskey, E. Beck, and W. Phipps: *Medical-Surgical Nursing*, 5th ed., Mosby, St. Louis, 1971, pp. 314–315.

30 Mendelson, C. L.: *Cardiac Disease in Pregnancy*, Davis, Philadelphia, 1960, p. 77.

31 Johnson, B. J.: "Effects on Cardiovascular Function," *American Journal of Nursing*, 67:782, April 1967.

32 Fitzpatrick, E., S. Reeder, and L. Mastroianni: *Maternity Nursing*, 12th ed., Lippincott, Philadelphia, 1971, p. 498.

33 Barnes, Cyril: *Medical Disorders in Obstetric Practice*, Blackwell, Oxford, 1970, p. 236.

34 Babson, S. G., and R. C. Benson: *Management of High-risk Pregnancy and Intensive Care of the Neonate*, 2d ed., Mosby, St. Louis, 1971, pp. 74–78.

35 Barnes: op. cit., p. 276.

36 Ibid., p. 277.

37 Gerbie, Albert: "Endocrine Diseases Complicated by Pregnancy," in D. M. Haynes, *Medical Complications during Pregnancy*, McGraw-Hill, New York, 1969, p. 354.

38 Babson and Benson: op. cit., pp. 51–52.

39 Eastman, N. J., and L. M. Hellman: *Williams Obstetrics*, 13th ed., Appleton-Century-Crofts, New York, 1966, p. 786.

40 Haynes: op. cit., p. 54.

BIBLIOGRAPHY

Babson, S. G., and R. C. Benson: *Management of High-risk Pregnancy and Intensive Care of the Neonate*, 2d ed., Mosby, St. Louis, 1971.

Barnes, Cyril G.: *Medical Disorders in Obstetric Practice*, Blackwell, Oxford, 1970.

Bruce, S.: "Reactions of Nurses and Mothers to Stillbirth," *Nursing Outlook*, 10:88–91, February 1962.

Caplan, Gerald: *Concepts of Mental Health and Consultation*, United States Department of Health, Education, and Welfare, Children's Bureau, Washington, D.C., 1959.

———: "The Mental Hygiene Role of the Nurse in Maternal and Child Care," *Nursing Outlook*, 2:14–19, January 1954.

Eastman, N. J., and L. M. Hellman: *Williams Obstetrics*, 13th ed., Appleton-Century-Crofts, New York, 1966.

Engel, G. L.: "Grief and Grieving," *American Journal of Nursing*, 64:93–98, September 1964.

Fitzpatrick, Elise, S. Reeder, and L. Mastroianni: *Maternity Nursing*, 12th ed., Lippincott, Philadelphia, 1971.

Haynes, D. M.: *Medical Complications during Pregnancy*, McGraw-Hill, New York, 1969.

Johnson, B. J.: "Effects on Cardiovascular Function," *American Journal of Nursing*, 67:781–782, April 1967.

Kaplan, D. M., and E. A. Mason: "Maternal Reactions to Premature Births Viewed as an Acute Emotional Disorder," *American Journal of Orthopsychiatry*, 30:539–552, July 1960.

Kaullas, J.: "The Child with Cleft Lip and Palate—The Mother in the Maternity Ward," *American Journal of Nursing*, 65:120–123, April 1965.

Lerch, Constance: *Maternity Nursing*, Mosby, St. Louis, 1970.

Lytle, Nancy: *Maternal Health Nursing*, Wm. C. Brown, Dubuque, Iowa, 1967.

Makinson, D. H.: "Medical Disorders of Pregnancy," *Nursing Mirror*, 128:15–17, January 10, 1969.

———: "Medical Disorders of Pregnancy, Part II," *Nursing Mirror*, 128:42–45, January 17, 1969.

McLenahan, Irene G.: "No Baby to Take Home," *American Journal of Nursing*, 62:70–71, April 1962.

Mendelson, C. L.: *Cardiac Disease in Pregnancy*, Davis, Philadelphia, 1960.

Owens, C.: "Parents' Reactions to Defective Babies," *American Journal of Nursing*, 64:83–86, November 1964.

———: "Parents' Response to Premature Birth," *American Journal of Nursing*, 60:1113–1118, August 1960.

Prugh, Dane G.: "Emotional Problems of the Premature Infant's Parents," *Nursing Outlook*, 1:461–464, August 1953.

Rose, Patricia Ann: "The High Risk Mother-Infant Dyad—A Challenge for Nursing?" *Nursing Forum*, 6:94–102, 1967.

Rubin, Reva: "Body Image and Self-esteem," *Nursing Outlook*, 16:20–23, June 1968.

———: "Puerperal Change," *Nursing Outlook*, 9:753–755, December 1961.

Shafer, K., J. Sawyer, A. McCluskey, E. Beck, and W. Phipps: *Medical-Surgical Nursing*, 5th ed., Mosby, St. Louis, 1971.

Stevens, Bette A.: "Postpartum Eclampsia," *Nursing Mirror*, 123:331–332, January 13, 1967.

Thaler, O. F.: "Grief and Depression," *Nursing Forum*, 5(2):8–22, 1966.

Ujhely, G. B.: "Grief and Depression—Implications for Preventive and Therapeutic Nursing Care," *Nursing Forum*, 5(2):23–35, 1966.

Waechter, Eugenia: "The Birth of an Exceptional Child," *Nursing Forum*, 9:202–216, 1970.

Wiedenbach, Ernestine: *Family-centered Maternity Nursing*, Putnam, New York, 1967.

34 | CARE OF THE HIGH-RISK INFANT AND HIS FAMILY

Jane M. Brightman and Stephanie Clatworthy

The process of labor and delivery and the need for immediate adjustment to the external world create stress and crisis for all newborns. The majority of infants adapt well with little or no difficulty. Some, however—infants at risk —cannot or do not adapt with the same degree of ease. Predisposing the infant to difficulties during the adjustment phase of his life are certain maternal and environmental conditions. Also implicated are conditions which exist within the infant at birth or which appear soon thereafter. Table 34-1 lists the factors which commonly contribute to the vulnerability of the neonate. With or without any of the other factors noted in this table the majority of high-risk infants are premature or of low birth weight.

In an attempt to improve care and to decrease neonatal morbidity and mortality, those infants who are at risk during the first few days and weeks of life have been singled out for special attention. According to Nelson, the term "high-risk" infant has been coined to designate infants who should be under close observation by the most interested and experienced nurses available and visited frequently by a physician until complications arising from the circumstances leading to the increased risk may no longer reasonably be expected.[1]

The aim of special care for high-risk infants is not only to save lives but

TABLE 34-1
FACTORS WHICH COMMONLY CONTRIBUTE TO THE VULNERABILITY
OF THE NEONATE

Maternal high-risk factors

1. Age
   Under sixteen or over forty
   Current first pregnancy in a mother aged thirty-five or older
2. Prior pregnancy history
   Complications in previous pregnancies
   History of infertility (involuntary sterility)
   Rh sensitization
   Previous multiple pregnancies
   Previous premature births
   Previous births with malformations
   Previous births of infants 9 or more lbs. (even if previous studies for diabetes mellitus
   were negative)
3. Multiple pregnancy
4. User of drugs
5. Rh negative or maternal antibody sensitization
6. Bleeding after 20 weeks of gestation
7. Maternal medical problem
   Toxemia, hypertension, chronic renal disease, etc.
   Cardiac disease
   Persistent albuminuria
   Diabetes mellitus
   Obesity
   Chronic urinary tract infection
   Infectious disease (tuberculosis, syphilis, etc.)
   Viral (and protozoan) diseases: rubella, herpes simplex (especially cervicitis), cyto-
   megalovirus, toxoplasmosis
   Anemia
   Surgery during pregnancy
   Metabolic disease (e.g., hyperthyroidism)
   Drugs prescribed by physicians (e.g., iodides, propylthiouracil, rauwolfia, sulfas, etc.)
   Premature labor or threatened labor
   Postmature labor (2 or more weeks beyond expected date of confinement)

High-risk factors associated with labor or infant

1. Duration of active labor
   Primigravida: longer than 24 hours
   Multigravida: longer than 12 hours
   Second stage: longer than 2 hours
2. Ruptured membranes at 24 or more hours
3. Infant too large or too small for period of gestation
4. Maternal fever or infection
5. Placenta praevia or abruptio placentae
6. Any difficult delivery or Apgar score of 5 or less at 1 minute of life
7. High or midforceps delivery
8. Cesarean section (at least for brief observation)
9. Breech delivery (at least for brief observation)
10. Birth weight under 5½ lb (2.5 kg) or over 9 lb (over 4 kg)
11. Meconium-stained amniotic fluid

TABLE 34-1
FACTORS WHICH COMMONLY CONTRIBUTE TO THE VULNERABILITY OF THE
NEONATE (Continued)

High-risk factors associated with labor or infant

12. Multiple pregnancies
13. Any infant requiring resuscitation
14. Fetal distress by fetal ECG or by scalp blood sampling
15. Abnormalities in tests of fetal well-being and fetal age (e.g., estriol excretion, alkaline phosphatase, diamine oxidase, etc.)
16. Prolapsed cord
17. Respiratory distress syndrome or other respiratory distress
18. Malformation or other significant abnormality in newborn infant
19. Evidence of birth injury
20. Drug or other depression at birth
21. Evidence of infection in infant
22. Candidates for surgery, preoperatively and postoperatively

SOURCE: Louis Gluck, "Design of a Perinatal Center," *Pediatric Clinics of North America*, 17:778, November 1970.

also to afford this child the potential to attain maximum fulfillment. Inherent in this is the need to support family development in the crisis created by the birth of a high-risk infant.

For purposes of our discussion we will not include intrauterine growth defects, since they will be discussed in Chapter 35. We will limit our discussion to the problems most commonly associated with the infant at risk.

Depending upon the situation, certain needs have been identified as being common to all infants and families in this risk situation. The relative importance of specific needs may vary in each situation. For example, measures aimed at maintenance of respirations are of high priority for infants with respiratory distress syndrome.

THE NEEDS OF THE FAMILY

The birth of a child is considered to be a normal maturational crisis within any family unit. The response of the parents to their new child is individual and will be influenced by what the birth of a new baby means to them. Does the mother see this child as her gift to her husband—or perhaps to her mother? Does this family view this birth as an achievement in keeping with social status? What is their perception of their ability and desire to be parents of this child? At any rate, the parents' expectations invariably include that their child will surpass or at least attain their level of sociocultural accomplishment.

In most instances, the birth of a baby is a time of much joy accompanied by congratulations and wishes of well-being from family and friends. This is not the case when the infant is in a vulnerable situation. The atmosphere becomes one of watchful waiting, and responses are guarded. When a family first learns their baby is considered to be in a life-threatening situation, their initial response, a manifestation of their grief, is that of disbelief and denial: "No, it can't be, not my baby!" The parents are now beginning to mourn the loss of the perfect baby of their fantasies. As they begin to accept the reality of this situation, their greatest fear is that their baby will die.

The Nurse's Role

This is a very painful time for the parents. It is the responsibility of the nurse to help them to tolerate what they see, hear, and feel. Often, at this time, we impose separation upon the parents from their child—especially upon the mother—in an attempt to "spare them the pain." The baby is whisked off to a special nursery or even to another hospital; the mother is placed in a private room, usually at the end of the hall; and all our activities are supposedly geared to letting her rest. This careful neglect will not change the situation but will simply postpone dealing with reality. Rather than being helped to deal with the pain by caring professionals, the parents may be left to suffer alone. A nurse with insight will not be the instrument of such neglect. Fortunately, there is a growing awareness on the part of nursing and medical personnel of the needs of these families. Each of us needs help with a difficult situation at some time. It is not particularly easy to help parents to express and to deal with their sorrow. The nurse who is helping the family in crisis may also be in need of support.

Separation of mother and infant should be kept to a minimum. The early postpartum period is important in the development of effective mothering patterns. Studies have shown not only the immediate effects upon mother and infant, but also the enduring effects which separation has upon child-rearing practices. It is important to help parents to maintain the responsibilities of their roles. Mothers and fathers demonstrate that they have only delegated and not relinquished parental responsibilities by active involvement with the child. This may include actually caring for him or, as in the case of a very sick infant, watching and asking questions when they don't understand a particular treatment.

Development of Support

The nurse is a vital member of the health team to the family with a high-risk infant. Through this unique position, support and guidance can be provided to the family during times of stress. Assisting the family in coping with their grief as well as assuming the parenting roles is essential. The literature puts much emphasis on mothering patterns, but helping the father assume his role is just as important. It is our feeling that the man involved must be helped to assume his role and not be pushed into the role of "co-conspirator with the medical team" in an attempt to "spare the mother." The couple who are helped to deal openly with their feelings are in a better position to support each other.

Cognizance and insight into the nurse's own feelings and values are needed before support can be given. For example, if the nurse does not believe the family should grieve, an unawareness of the family's attempts to handle their grief may hinder or obstruct the family's coping mechanisms.

Being supportive may mean different things to each of us. Generally, we feel that it involves conveying a feeling of caring to the family. It means letting them know that we will be with them as they experience the pain of their crisis. It also means providing an environment in which the couple feels they can safely express feelings as they experience them. Initially the nurse must identify the strengths within a family and help sustain these strengths. This process may involve modifying established routines. For example, a couple may be adapting to the situation when they are together, but when forced to separate they are no longer able to cope. This is the family that needs extended visiting privileges with privacy provided as appropriate. Any routine not essential to the well-being of mother or infant should be questioned.

To be supportive, the nurse must deal with the situation openly and honestly. This is a time when the nurse and physician must confer in planning for this family and should discuss how questions will be answered. The parents at this time are searching for information and tend to ask similar questions of different people. Our answers need to reinforce each other if we are to help parents to understand what is happening and to foster a trusting relationship. Understanding of the situation and ability to adjust are further strengthened when the mother is allowed to remain on the maternity unit and is not forced into isolation within the unit.

With the average newborn, it is the father who is more likely to be excluded or separated from his child secondary to hospital policies and practice. However, when a child is transferred to a pediatric setting for more intensive care, the father is more likely to have closer contact with his child. The father may then become a major person to help the mother understand and deal with the reality of their problem. The father may be of similar help when the mother is unable to visit the nursery to see her child because of maternal complications, such as hemorrhage, or cesarean section.

The nurse is the key person to help the family become involved with their infant. The ability of the nurse to recognize the readiness of the family to proceed and develop their involvement with their infant will be of prime importance. As in any guidance situation, the nurse must proceed at the family's own pace.

Development of Trust

In dealing with the parents, the nurse may begin to identify clues that relate to the parents' feeling of guilt. Some degree of searching to place blame—on self, others, events, or fate—is not unusual. The mother may begin to recall events in the pregnancy which to her seem related. For example, "I shouldn't have gone on vacation"; "I fell during the fifth month"; "I took aspirin before I knew I was pregnant." Inherent in this are feelings of failure at not being able to produce a healthy child. The nurse should listen very carefully to notice whether guilt feeling persists or whether the mother's ideas begin to focus on the care of her child. Because guilt will be compounded when the parents cannot care for their child as they expected, the nurse should encourage the involvement of the parents with their child as soon as possible. When the mother's condition or the child's condition limits the contact, parents may vicariously share in the experiences through a trusted nurse. The nurse's approach to parents and the baby must convey respect for the responsibility with which the nurse is entrusted. It must never be forgotten whom this baby belongs to; otherwise the nurse may be viewed by the mother as a competitor. This will further any feelings of failure the mother may have.

Trust becomes even more important when the mother is discharged, but the child must stay for further care. Plans for discharge become of greater import for this family. Parents must return home, and the mother must become reacquainted with her other children and they with her. The children will need support for they have expected mother to return with a new baby. Plans will be needed to foster the continuance of the parents' involvement with their infant (see Figure 34-1). An infant who requires special care or extended hospitalization may present a financial burden to the family. The nurse must be cognizant of these factors and make appropriate referrals. During the period of hospitalization, the nurse has the opportunity to evaluate the family needs. Many families with high-risk infants will require additional nursing care over a period of time. When this is indicated the nurse should initiate plans for continuance of nursing care. The aid of a maternal–child health clinical specialist found within the community or the hospital may be enlisted. Referral to the pediatrician's nurse or the public health department may be appropriate. The nurse must be aware of the resources available within the community to facilitate appropriate aid for each individual family.

THE NEEDS OF A HIGH-RISK INFANT

Conservation of Energy

It is to be remembered that all newborn infants may have difficulty conserving their energy at birth, and with the high-risk infant this becomes

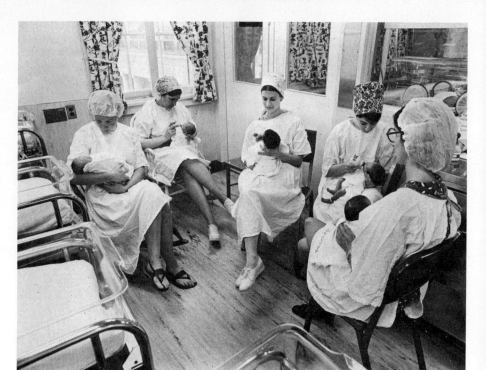

FIGURE 34-1
These two mothers (left and right), discharged without their infants, welcome the opportunity to return to the hospital to participate in the care of their babies. These nurses use this opportunity to encourage mothers to share their concerns for their infants and families.
(Courtesy of Boston Hospital for Women, Boston, Mass.)

imperative if life is to be preserved. Conservation of energy can be studied from a variety of approaches. For our purpose we will consider conservation of energy in each of several component parts: preservation and support of body temperature, support and maintenance of respirations, provision of adequate food and fluids intake, and prevention of infection.

Control of Body Temperature

The infant must be maintained in an environment that is neither too warm nor too cold. Either condition will stress his metabolic process as he attempts to adjust to this environment, creating a loss of energy and increasing his oxygen and calorie requirement. Immaturity of the central nervous system, lack of subcutaneous fat, and a high proportion of body surface to weight will contribute to loss of body heat. This process is accentuated to an even greater extent in the premature infant. In high-risk situations, maintenance of body heat reduces one demand on energy stores, allowing the infant to have more energy to expend in coping with the stresses of his situation.

The axillary area is the preferred site for measuring the infant's body temperature. Illness is reflected in changes of skin temperature before that of core or rectal temperature. Taking rectal temperatures may create additional stimulus and increase stooling. Excess stooling not only requires energy but also may cause loss of body fluids and electrolytes. Perforation of the rectum by the thermometer has been reported. The infant's temperature should be maintained at 36.5°C or 97.8°F by axillary measurement. His temperature will respond directly to the temperature of his environment; therefore, incubators are utilized to provide a more reliable means of stabilization of his environmental temperature. (See Figure 34-2.) Both the infant's body temperature and the temperature of the incubator should be recorded frequently.

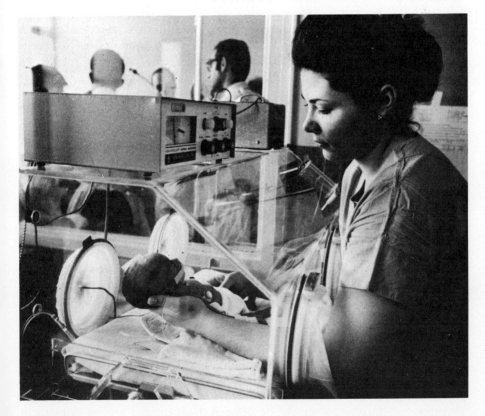

FIGURE 34-2
This infant's body temperature is being maintained through the use of an incubator. Note the apnea monitor and oxygen analyzer on top of the incubator. The tape on the infant's face is securing his feeding tube.
(*Courtesy of the Isolette Division of Air Shields, Inc.*)

While raising the infant's body temperature, the incubator should be 2 degrees higher than his body temperature. When the infant's temperature reaches 36.5°C (97.8°F) the nurse should adjust the incubator temperature in accordance with his needs. If the temperature of the incubator is 3.5° to 5.4°F lower than the infant's body temperature, it is likely that the infant is utilizing much of his energy reserve to maintain his temperature level. The temperature of the incubator may be influenced by direct sunlight, proximity to air-conditioners, outside temperature, or opening of portholes; thus infant temperature and incubator temperature should be checked and recorded at frequent intervals. Portholes on all incubators should be closed at all times, for a small active premature infant could fall through a porthole if the mattress is level with the openings. Air ventilation is provided by a motor which pulls in room air through a filter that removes very minute dust particles. There are a variety of mechanical devices available to assist the nurse in monitoring the infant's and incubator temperature which help reduce unnecessary handling of the infant; however, these devices must be checked frequently for accuracy by the nurse. For immediate awareness of temperature change, the infant and the incubator should be independently monitored for as long as the infant has difficulty in stabilizing his temperature.

Infants placed in incubators for temperature control must be left undressed and uncovered so the flow of warm air will have contact with the body surface. In addition, the infant who is uncovered is more easily observed by the nurse. When it is necessary to care for or handle the infant in an incubator, his temperature should be recorded before and after to determine the degree of heat loss and his ability to maintain his own body temperature. When he is taken out of the incubator, he should be wrapped in warmed blankets.

Care of Incubators

All incubators have various reservoirs for distilled water which are used to provide humidity. This, by the way, is a controversial issue, and humidity concentration is frequently determined by atmospheric conditions. Warmed humidity is definitely indicated when oxygen is administered. It is important that water be in these reservoirs when the heating mechanism is in use. This is necessary to prevent additional loss of fluids and dehydration. The humidity will assist in the dilution of the infant's secretions, enabling him to eliminate these with greater ease. The distilled water in its dark, warm reservoir provides a good medium for bacterial growth, particularly the *Pseudomonas*. Therefore, all incubators should be drained, cleaned, and refilled with fresh water every 24 hours. Another means of helping reduce the growth of *Pseudomonas* is that of using a weak silver nitrate solution (150 PPB or 0.84 ml of 0.5 percent silver nitrate per 5 gallons of distilled water).

If the incubator is no longer necessary for the care of the infant and his temperature has been stabilized, weaning from the incubator may be started. This is done by gradually decreasing the temperature of the incubator and frequently monitoring the infant's body temperature. As the temperature is lowered in the incubator, the infant may be dressed in a shirt, diaper, and receiving blanket. Once the incubator is at room temperature and the infant's temperature is maintained at 36.5°C or 97.8°F (axillary), he can be placed in a bassinet.

Maintenance of Respirations

Any infant having respiratory difficulties will be considered at risk. The degree of potential danger is directly related to the infant's energy stores and maturation and cause of his distress. The nursing care of such an infant is based upon his needs as well as the severity of his distress.

It must be remembered that breathing is a new experience for the infant. Respiration requires much energy, and priorities for maintenance of respiration must be second only to massive hemorrhage.

The Infant in Respiratory Distress

APPEARANCE

The appearance of the infant in respiratory difficulty follows a sequential pattern as the severity increases and is dependent to some degree upon the cause. The initial sign may only be increase in respirations that tend to be more rhythmic in nature. The apical pulse will become more rapid. Retractions will begin; usually the first to appear are subcostal, spreading to the substernal, intracostal, suprasternal, and clavicular areas. (See Figure 34-3.)

Initially the infant's color will be pink, but as his compensatory mechanisms become less effective, he will develop circumnasal-oral pallor and then cyanosis. At this time, nasal flaring on inspiration will occur. Depending upon etiology and energy stores, inspiratory stridor or expiratory grunt will appear. The infant's respirations will become abdominal, and see-saw breathing patterns will be evident. Since he is now utilizing a great deal of energy to breathe, his temperature may begin to drop and needs close surveillance. Too rapid cooling or warming tends to increase apnea. The cardiac system, in its attempts to compensate, may begin to evidence signs of failure, such as palpable liver and spleen and increased edema. Failure and death are impending when the heart rate begins to fall and respirations, although rapid, are frequented with increasing apneic spells. This resembles the Cheyne-Stokes breathing pattern.

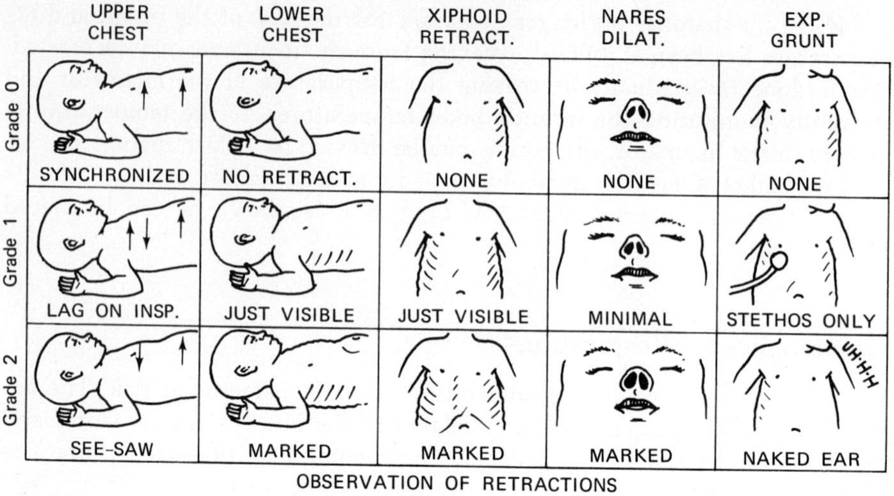

	UPPER CHEST	LOWER CHEST	XIPHOID RETRACT.	NARES DILAT.	EXP. GRUNT
Grade 0	SYNCHRONIZED	NO RETRACT.	NONE	NONE	NONE
Grade 1	LAG ON INSP.	JUST VISIBLE	JUST VISIBLE	MINIMAL	STETHOS ONLY
Grade 2	SEE-SAW	MARKED	MARKED	MARKED	NAKED EAR

OBSERVATION OF RETRACTIONS

FIGURE 34-3

Pictorial representation of retractions. This chart is used as an index of respiratory distress by grading each of five arbitrary criteria from 0 to 2: grade 0 indicates no difficulty; grade 1, moderate difficulty; and grade 2, maximum difficulty. The "retraction score" is the sum of these values; a total score of 0 indicates no dyspnea, and a score of 10 denotes maximum respiratory distress.

(Courtesy of Mead Johnson & Company, Evansville, Ind.)

POSITIONING

Positioning becomes of prime importance for the infant who is having respiratory difficulties and should be individualized. In some cases, elevation of the head of the mattress will allow less pressure on the diaphragm from the abdominal contents. Care should be taken to prevent the infant's arms from lying on his chest. This will only serve to increase the energy needed to lift the chest for inspirations. Flexion and abduction of the infant's arms will permit greater expansion of the thoracic area. It must be remembered that an infant in respiratory difficulty will utilize his abdominal muscles to a greater extent; therefore, diapers, if used, should be applied loosely around the abdomen.

To further enhance his respirations, it may be necessary to extend his neck slightly to prevent or lessen tracheal obstruction. This is easily done by placing a diaper roll under the infant's shoulders. Caution must be taken not to extend the neck too greatly, making it difficult for the infant to swallow his secretions. In addition, the nurse must watch that the diaper roll does not become displaced. An active infant can cause the roll to slide under his head, causing flexion of his neck with narrowing of the trachea, thus increasing his respiratory distress.

To facilitate drainage of fluids within the chest, the infant should be turned from side to back to side every 1 to 2 hours. This infant should not be placed in a prone position, for he then will be supporting his total body weight on his chest and abdomen.

FEEDING

Feeding the infant with respiratory difficulties may create medical and nursing problems. The infant who cannot breathe with ease will have difficulty in sucking and swallowing. The infant who is having mild respiratory distress and has no other contraindications, in rare instances, may be able to bottle-feed or breast-feed. Special attention should be given to clearing his airway prior to feeding. The clearer the airway, the easier he can nurse and the greater the amount of energy retained. Milk products tend to increase the amounts of mucus; in addition, milk that is aspirated will create more problems than clear fluids. For these reasons, the infant may be placed on clear fluids for a period of time. It must be remembered that sucking is a basic need of all newborns; therefore, whenever possible, bottle- or breast-feeding is preferable, providing it does not overtax his energy. Conservation of energy for recovery and growth is imperative. If the infant cannot tolerate the stress of sucking, then tube feeding will be necessary. Some infants do very well alternating bottle- or breast-feeding and tube feeding.

Evaluation of which schedule is best for the individual infant can be done as the nurse cares for the child. Many physicians allow the nurse to make this decision and will write appropriate orders providing the nurse some latitude of decision making based on observations and knowledge of the infant. When the physician does not share decision making with the nurse, it then becomes necessary to bring the needs and desires of the infant to the physician's attention.

Regardless of the method of feeding, there are two main considerations in feeding that infant in respiratory difficulty: (1) His stomach must not be distended. Overdistention will restrict the thoracic area and also increases the chance of regurgitation and vomiting and potential aspiration. (2) Energy reserves must be maintained. The infant may be able to feed well for 10 to 15 minutes for a total of 1 to 2 ounces and then be too fatigued to finish the feeding. For these two prime reasons, infants with respiratory difficulties do better with more frequent feedings of smaller amounts. For the infant who cannot tolerate oral or tube feedings, the parenteral route will be his only source of fluids and calories.

OXYGEN AND HUMIDITY NEEDS

The infant who has lowered blood PO_2 and increased blood PCO_2 levels or the infant who demonstrates clinical cyanosis or duskiness will require additional oxygen. Oxygen may be administered to an infant through an incubator, mask, or plastic hood.

Again, the temperature of the incubator should be regulated to conserve the energies of the infant. He should be undressed, not only for temperature control, but also for observations of his respiratory patterns. Humidity may need to be increased according to the severity and cause of the respiratory distress. There are a variety of humidifiers available: ultrasonic sound, fine misters, moist air, and warmed or cooled mist. The nurse must be knowledgeable as to the type of humidifier used on a specific infant. Nursing care of the infant receiving additional humidity will create several additions to the nursing plan of care. When warmed or cooled mist is utilized, the temperature of the incubator must be adjusted accordingly. The concentration of humidity should never interfere with observation of the infant.

For the past 30 years, optimal oxygen concentration and therapy for high-risk newborns has received and is receiving intensive study. Too little oxygen or too much oxygen may produce serious complications. Oxygen must be given at the direction of the physician; however, the nurse is the primary person who will be available to provide constant observation of the infant and who also will be the first one to recognize the need for oxygen. Through the nurse's constant attendance and knowledge, recognition of subtle changes in behavior and color can be made. The physician who visits once or twice daily may be less able to detect change. The nurse must be aware of the conditions of lighting (day, night, natural, or artificial light), since this may influence the infant's color. Changes in activity must be considered in relation to such things as feeding times and treatments.

The nurse will be able to observe for signs of hypoxia, but there is no clinical picture for oxygen toxicity. Blood PO_2 levels are the only guide.

Complications of Oxygen Therapy

Increased concentration of oxygen may have to be breathed by the infant to maintain a circulating PO_2 level sufficient to meet the cellular demands of the body. However, when increased oxygen is supplied, the risk of pulmonary oxygen toxicity is present. Increased amounts of oxygen create an increased inability of the lungs to assimilate the oxygen, thus increasing the need for more oxygen. High concentrations of oxygen (70 to 80 percent) given for even short intervals or slightly increased oxygen levels for a long period of time result in a loss of pliancy and a thickening of the alveolar and vascular structures, interfering with the gas exchange. This will lead to atelectasis and increased cellularity of the lung. The cilia become paralyzed, thus making the removal of secretions more difficult. Therefore, the infant may become dependent on the oxygen.

Hyperoxemia must exist before damage of tissue other than the lung develops. Of primary concern is that of retrolental fibroplasia. Hemorrhage and scar formation are identified with an ophthalmoscope. If scarring is found in the macular area, blindness will occur. The incidence of this condition is directly related to the maturity of the infant. Some feel that the infant less than 27 to 28 weeks of gestation is so susceptible that retrolental fibroplasia will occur if oxygen is supplied in the amount necessary to prevent brain damage. The only way of identifying toxic levels of oxygen is through measurement of oxygen tension of blood. It cannot be evaluated through observation nor through predictable regulated oxygen concentration. Frequent samplings of arterial blood for oxygen tension are vital.

The maintenance of a prescribed amount of oxygen is dependent on the concentration of oxygen within the incubator. The concentration will depend on the flow of oxygen (liters/minute) and the loss of oxygen through use of portholes, etc. It was believed that the concentration of 40 percent oxygen in the incubator was a safe maximum level in preventing retrolental fibroplasia. We now realize this figure is not an absolute, as the primary concern is the maintenance of adequate arterial oxygen tension. Each time the amount of oxygen is increased, the flow rate and oxygen concentration levels should be recorded to assist in the evaluation of the infant. If PO_2 levels are too high, oxygen should be decreased slowly, with careful monitoring of vital signs, oxygen concentration, and blood PO_2.

The nurse must be aware that the use of intravenous therapy to control acidosis may cause an abrupt rise in arterial PO_2. Arterial oxygen tension should be determined before and after any changes in oxygen or parenteral therapy and the infant should be closely observed.

It is imperative that the nurse working with infants requiring oxygen therapy be aware that oxygen supports combustion. The hazards of oxygen are increased with the use of electrical equipment. All electrical equipment should be grounded.

Suctioning

The infant with respiratory difficulties or any newborn during the first 24 hours of life may have difficulties handling his secretions. It is imperative that suction equipment be close at hand and that the nurse be skillful in its use.

Depending upon the size of the infant, a number 8 or 10 French catheter will be sufficient. A small container of water with a suction machine will be the only other equipment necessary. For the infant who is not apneic, it may be helpful to restrain his arms before beginning. The catheter may be lubricated with water. The infant's head should be held securely and the machine turned on. Gently insert the tube through the nostril. When obstruction is met, lift the tube straight up to make the natural turn of the nasal passage. The tube should then be passed until the infant gags (esophagus) or begins to cough (trachea). Once the tube is properly placed in the trachea, suction should be applied as the tube is slowly rotated and withdrawn. Care should be taken that suctioning be brief because air as well as secretions are being aspirated from the lung. This should be repeated in the opposite nostril. Each time the suction catheter is inserted, irritation of the mucosa occurs, creating an increase in the production of mucus. In addition, passage of a suction catheter or feeding tube may stimulate the vagus nerve, creating bradycardia. For these reasons, suctioning should be done only as necessary. Because of the strong potential of triggering the gag reflex, suctioning should be done prior to feedings.

Once the procedure is completed, all equipment should be discarded, and a new suction catheter and container of water are placed with the machine at the side of the incubator. Because of the potential traumatic effect of electrical suction, the de Lee mucus trap is preferred by many clinicians. Suctioning can be accomplished through the nose or mouth.

Resuscitation

Every nurse working with infants should be highly skilled in infant resuscitation. The need for this skill is extremely apparent when caring for infants with respiratory difficulties.

The infant demonstrating apnea may only require gentle stimulation to resume respiration on his own. A piece of gauze placed under the infant's axillary area or foot and tied to the top of the incubator for gentle tugging without having to open portholes will provide adequate stimulation for most infants. If this fails, rubbing the feet and legs or *gentle* squeezing of the chest will produce respirations. If these measures fail to produce respiration within 20 seconds, more vigorous resuscitation will be necessary.

Before resuscitation is begun, the airway must be cleared and the infant's neck slightly extended. This can be done easily with a diaper roll. Effective resuscitation of the infant, like the adult, is only done when he is lying on a hard surface. The new models of incubators have a firm enough mattress so that resuscitation can be instituted there; however, if the infant is in a bassinet or on a soft mattress, he should be placed immediately on a table or some other firm surface.

Once positioned, the first two fingertips (one finger on a premature infant) should be placed on the midsternum. Gentle, but firm, pressure should be applied to the sternum at 40 to 60 beats per minute. Every 10 beats should have two quick respirations. The respirations may be mouth to mouth, but most institutions now have a bag ventilator with a mask to fit snugly over the infant's nose and mouth. Insufflation should be strong enough to raise the chest but not so strong that a lung is ruptured. A bag ventilator should have an escape valve which prevents excessive air pressure. Sometimes air will be pumped into the stomach as well as the lungs. When abdominal distention occurs, a gastric tube should be passed to relieve the air pressure and thus increase the chest capacity.

Resuscitations of this nature must be started immediately to prevent brain damage and death. The physician should be notified immediately, but the nurse should not wait for his arrival to begin resuscitation.

When maintenance of respirations becomes a critical problem the infant may be intubated, and continuous respiratory assistance is provided with positive pressure. (See Figure 34-4.) Great nursing skill is now required, and the infant should not be left alone. If additional equipment or supplies are needed, the nurse caring for the infant must ask for someone else to bring them.

Food and Fluid Requirements

The required water, calorie, and electrolyte intake of the newborn baby is dependent upon his rate of expenditure and his body stores of these substances. When caring for an infant at risk, the need for additional calories, fluids, or electrolytes must be evaluated frequently in accordance to the needs of the individual infant. The nurse must have a sound base of knowledge of fluid and electrolyte balance and highly developed observational skills when collaborating with the physician in planning for the nutritional needs of a high-risk infant. It is not the purpose of this chapter to discuss in depth the physiological responses inherent in nutritional needs with pathological disorders but to center on nursing knowledge and skills necessary to help the infant maintain good calorie, fluid, and electrolyte balance.

ORAL FEEDING

The infant has strong oral needs at birth. Through his mouth, he will learn pleasure and fulfillment from hunger. By having his oral and hunger needs met promptly with a bottle to suck on and warm arms to snuggle in, he learns trust.

The infant is born with a sucking ability and a swallow reflex. However, the infant must learn to coordinate his sucking with his swallowing before bottle- or breast-feeding can bring pleasure and nutrition. Infants who cannot suck, swallow, or coordinate these activities are at risk. The inability to suck may be secondary to mouth or palate deformities, central nervous system depression, immaturity, or limited energy stores.

An infant who is considered at risk should be bottle- or breast-fed whenever possible to meet his oral needs and develop trust in a caring person. However, when the infant cannot be fed by bottle or breast, modifications of feeding must be instituted.

For the infant who has a weakened suck or who needs to conserve his energy while sucking, a variety of nipple and feeding tools are available. Most of these nipples are made of soft rubber. Some are longer or broader in length and diameter to assist the infant. Some nurses, in their attempt to get

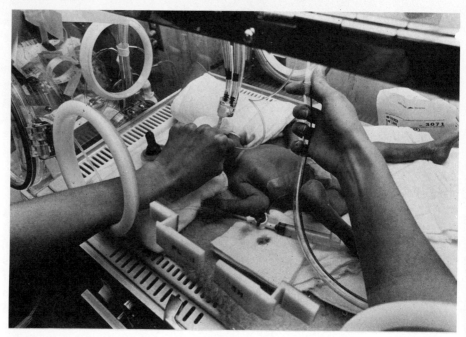

FIGURE 34-4
This infant's respirations are being assisted by means of a respirator. Also note the umbilical catheter in place and the syringe with stopcock for availability of blood for gas studies.
(*Courtesy of Boston Hospital for Women, Boston, Mass.*)

infants to eat, will enlarge nipple holes or pump the nipple so that the formula drips into the infant's mouth. This method of feeding is extremely dangerous because the infant will get too much formula and may aspirate or vomit. To have his mouth suddenly filled with fluid to a choking degree does not help him to develop trust or pleasure from his feeding.

BREAST-FEEDING

If the high-risk infant can tolerate it, he should be allowed the comfort and satisfaction of being breast-fed, when this is the method chosen by his parents. Although the basic principles of breast-feeding are applicable, some adaptation of the procedure may be necessary. For the infant with certain sucking disorders, a breast shield may be of help. The infant who needs to conserve his energy may need to be fed every 2 hours. Although it is generally considered unwise to give a breast-feeding infant a bottle, as this may interfere with his adaptation to the breast, the infant who needs to have his energy reserves maintained while meeting his nutritional needs may require supplemental bottle feedings. Nursing judgment is required to determine which pattern is most appropriate for a given infant and his mother. Some infants and mothers do very well if breast-feeding is supplemented by bottle-feeding. Other infants, with less energy, may have to alternate breast- with bottle-feeding. When the infant cannot tolerate full breast-feeding, or in some instances any breast-feeding, the mother must be strongly supported. Mother and nurse should plan together for the best means of maintaining a milk supply. This may be through manual expression and/or the use of breast pumps. The mother who wishes to breast-feed but cannot will need much encouragement. This is best done by praising her for those things she can do and by keeping her well informed of her infant's condition. This will assist in the reinforcement of reality. In addition, the mother who must keep pumping her breasts must be given reason and encouragement. This direct guidance can be very therapeutic to the mother in a crisis situation. It may also help her to accept her mothering role, for she can then feel that she is doing something for her baby and can see the results of her actions.

ARTIFICIAL FEEDING

For a baby who cannot tolerate sucking at all, such as those with cleft palates or cardiac conditions, other devices have been developed to assist the feeding. The eye dropper has been used successfully for many years, but it is a tedious method at best. Of greater assistance is the use of a 5 to 10 cc syringe with a rubber tube of about 1½ to 2 inches in length attached. The rubber tubing allows the formula to be placed further back in the infant's mouth. Neither of these methods of dripping formula into the infant provide him with the pleasurable feel of a nipple. The feel of a nipple is very important, and becomes of even greater importance to the infant who will not be able to feed with a bottle for a prolonged period, such as the cleft palate child. At times calorie requirement takes precedence over sucking needs, and the infant may be fed from a small cup.

Extreme caution must be taken whenever the drip method of feeding is utilized with the eye dropper or syringe, for the danger of aspiration is increased greatly. The infant should be held and area provided for him to lie down, if necessary. Suction equipment should be available. This type of feeding can be very fatiguing for the infant; thus, about 30 to 45 minutes should be allowed to provide for rest periods. Frequent bubbling will be necessary since the infant is more likely to swallow air. Again, the feeding should be as pleasurable as possible; both nurse and baby will enjoy the rest periods spent holding and cuddling. Once the stability of the infant is ascertained, the mother can be taught to use these devices when she demonstrates a willingness to do this.

TUBE FEEDING

The immature infant or the infant in respiratory distress may not be able to tolerate the stress of swallowing. Other infants who may have difficulty in swallowing are those with central nervous system disorders. For these, the primary method of feeding is by gavage.

Disposable gavage sets are available with a variety of sizes and length of tubes. The tube should be selected in accordance to the size of the infant. The infant's head should be elevated and his abdomen and chest exposed. His arms should be restrained to prevent accidental displacement of the tube. The tube should be measured from the bridge of his nose to the xiphoid cartilage.

The tube may be inserted into a nostril or the mouth. The nostril would be the choice selection if the tube were to be left in place. Some feel the nose is contraindicated, as it will cause irritation to the mucosa and create an increase in mucus secretions. The newborn breathes only through his nose and the foreign body will markedly decrease his breathing capacity. Some feel a tube should not be left in place as this will create a constant production of mucus. The newborn's eustachian tubes are broad and short; therefore, a nasogastric tube left in place provides a source for developing otitis media. Others feel that leaving the tube in place will be less traumatizing and less stressful, since it will not have to be passed every 2 to 3 hours. It is usually the practice to pass the tube through the mouth when it is not to be left in place. This eliminates irritation to the nasal mucosa, and the tube provides some oral stimulation simultaneously with the filling of the stomach, which is more normal and causes very little expenditure of energy for the infant when skillfully done.

Once the infant is elevated, chest and abdomen exposed, and his hands are secure, the nurse should hold his head in her hand, lubricate the tube with water, and insert the tube to the back of the throat. This may stimulate swallowing, which opens the glottis, allowing the tube to be passed with greater ease. Each time the infant swallows, the tube should be inserted another 1 to 2 inches. There is no reason to rush this procedure, as speed is not required. The tube should be inserted until the mark is reached which should place the tip of the tube within the stomach. If obstruction is met, stop. The procedure should be started over again, but the tube must not be forced.

There are three ways to ascertain whether the tube is in place:

1 Place the end of the tube in water; if bubbles appear and correspond to the infant's respirations, the tube is in the trachea. The infant will probably cough and choke. Some bubbles may appear if there was air trapped in the stomach, but these will cease and are not related to respirations.
2 Aspirate gently. The appearance of gastric contents will be proof that the tube is in the stomach.

3 Gently insert a small amount of air with a syringe into the stomach and listen with a stethoscope over the stomach for a bubbling sound. If any of these tests leave any doubt that the tube is placed in the stomach, withdraw the tube and begin again.

Once the tube is in place, it should be taped to the infant's cheek. With some infants it is necessary to aspirate the gastric contents to measure the amount of absorption of the previous feeding. The contents must be replaced in the stomach or the infant may lose vital electrolytes and enzymes necessary to absorb and utilize the next feeding. The amount returned should be considered when planning the amount to be administered at the current feeding.

The barrel of a syringe or a special cylinder is then attached to the feeding tube. Generally these are small to prevent the pressure of the flowing fluid from becoming too great. A 5 to 10 cc syringe can be used quite efficiently. It is wise to begin the feeding with 1 cc of clear fluid. Should the tube be misplaced, the infant would demonstrate immediate respiratory changes, indicating the tube to be in the trachea. Should this occur, clear water will create far less hazards than formula.

Observing the Infant during Tube Feeding

Once the feeding has begun, the infant's response should be carefully observed. The amount of solution may be ordered by the physician, but many times it is determined by the nurse from observations of the infant's tolerance to the feeding. The rate of flow should be slow; approximately 20 minutes will be needed for the average feeding.

To determine the infant's tolerance to the feeding, several factors should be considered. Distention of the abdomen will occur; however, caution should be taken to avoid overdistention, as this could lead to vomiting and aspiration and/or further embarrassment of respirations. The flow rate should be steady; however, if the infant shows distress, do not hesitate to stop the feeding and allow him to rest prior to its completion. When the fluid will no longer flow with gravity, maximum capacity has usually been attained. At *no* time should formula be pushed into the infant. If he does not tolerate the amount of feeding ordered, merely discontinue the feeding and report the results to the physician.

When discontinuing the feeding, clamp the tube securely and gently remove it. The infant should then be positioned comfortably and in a manner that will prevent aspiration if vomiting should occur.

The infant who can tolerate it should be held and cuddled following tube feeding, as he has been denied this aspect of feeding. Some infants prefer to be held and cuddled prior to the feeding. The nurse who communicates with the infant will learn his preference.

As the infant's needs for tube feeding decrease, he will begin to develop sucking motions while being fed. This should be supported with the use of pacifiers initially, and as his tolerance increases, he may be bottle-fed for one or two feedings each day. As he progresses, the number of bottle-feedings will gradually increase. Some infants, usually those who are more immature, may develop "lazy" tendencies and prefer the tube feeding to bottle, since hunger is relieved with little effort on his part. This phenomenon may also be increased with the infant who has not been taught that pleasure can be found in a nipple and that he can further benefit from being held. By introducing nipple feedings very gradually, this behavior can often be avoided.

INTRAVENOUS THERAPY

The infant who cannot have his fluid and calorie needs met by the above feeding methods will need parenteral therapy. It is recognized that parenteral therapy may be necessary for other reasons, such as administration of medication; however, regardless of the purpose, an intravenous administration of fluid and calories will influence his feeding needs. The preferable site for an intravenous infusion is felt to be in a peripheral vein. In some situations, the umbilical artery is utilized. An umbilical catheter with radiopaque markings is used, and its position after insertion is checked by x ray. The infant receiving parenteral fluids needs careful and astute observations. His fluid needs are greater than an adult's in proportion to his body surface and weight, and he can easily be placed in an unbalanced situation.

It is felt that an intravenous feeding is best administered with the use of an infusion pump which provides a more accurate and constant flow rate. This does not excuse the nurse from the responsibility of closely observing the infant. Some pumps will continue functioning after the drip chamber has emptied, exposing the infant to the danger of air embolism. A new model automatically sounds an alarm and stops pumping when the chamber is empty. Any of these pumps, however, will continue operating when fluid is going into the tissues, so that the infant must be watched closely for signs of infiltration. (See Figure 34-5.)

Several means can be utilized to assist the physician in the evaluation of the infant's needs for intravenous fluids. First, all infants receiving parenteral fluids should have their urine output measured so that an accurate record of total intake and output is obtained. Each time the infant voids, specific gravity should be measured as an indicator of the urine concentration. The urine should also be checked for glucose.

The weight of the infant is an indication of his adaptation to parenteral fluids. Some infants receiving parenteral fluids may be weighed as often as every 12 hours; others may be weighed every 24 hours. Initial base-line weights should include all equipment in use so that monitors do not have to be disconnected to weigh the infant. Generally, a weight gain or loss of 4

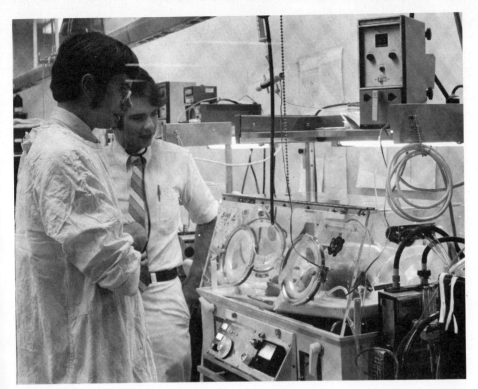

FIGURE 34-5
This infant's infusion is being monitored by an Ivac Corporation Model 500 Infusion
Pump. Should the burette of fluid become empty, this pump will automatically stop the
flow of solution and signal an alert. Every opportunity should be used to explain the
purpose of the multiple pieces of equipment to parents to help them understand how it
relates to the care of their child.
(Courtesy of Ivac Corporation.)

ounces or 100 grams over a 24-hour period is considered to be sufficiently
significant to alter the rate of flow.

CALORIE NEEDS

The fluid and calorie needs of the high-risk infant are basically the same as
for the full-term or "normal" infant. The difference must be based on the
specific needs demonstrated by the individual infant. The infant who is not
tolerating oral fluids well will obviously require additional fluids. The infant who is depleting his energy stores rapidly, such as in the case of an
infant with respiratory distress syndrome, will require additional calories.
The more immature the infant, the greater are his needs for carbohydrates, as
he will be expending a great deal of energy to adapt to the extrauterine en-

vironment. This is further complicated by his inability to store carbohydrates because of the immaturity of his body systems. For this reason the premature infant is often given formula containing 24 calories per fluid ounce. Carbohydrates should be maintained in proper amount. Too little carbohydrate can lead to hypoglycemia, a condition that attributes to central nervous system disturbances and mental retardation. This condition is found very frequently in the premature infant, infants of diabetic or prediabetic mothers, and the small-for-gestational-age infant. Hypoglycemia also becomes of great concern for the infant in stress situations, such as during cooling, respiratory distress syndrome, sepsis, or cardiac difficulties. It appears that whenever an infant is placed in a crisis situation, whether metabolic or environmental, that he is likely to deplete his carbohydrate levels rapidly.

Hypoglycemia has also been found with the infant who suddenly has parenteral fluids discontinued. It is felt that this is due to the fact that with the increase of circulating glucose from the fluids, the infant produces additional insulin. When the glucose is suddenly discontinued, the overproduction of insulin rapidly depletes the available gluscose levels; thus, hypoglycemia develops. If not severe, the infant will be able to compensate in time.

The infant who is hypoglycemic may not demonstrate any behavior indicative of the disorder. However, the hypoglycemic infant is likely to appear hyperirritable, jittery, restless, or lethargic. These symptoms are likely to occur with electrolyte imbalance, particularly of calcium and potassium imbalances; it becomes essential that blood be drawn immediately so that a laboratory diagnosis can be made.

Prevention of Sepsis

Prevention of infection is of prime importance in any newborn nursery. The import of these precautions becomes magnified when caring for the infant at risk. The infant whose energy reserves are being utilized to support life will have a decreased resistance to infection and thus will be more susceptible and vulnerable when exposed to infection. The additional stress of an infection may be all that is necessary for a complete collapse of the infant.

In addition to his increased susceptibility, the infant at risk is subjected to many procedures and treatments which may compromise his first line of defense, i.e., injections, suctioning, intravenous infusion, additional personnel, and prolonged hospitalization. It becomes obvious, then, that scrupulous adherence to aseptic technique be observed.

People are the primary source of infection in a hospital setting. For this reason, the number of people admitted to a nursery caring for high-risk infants should be limited to only those necessary to the care of these infants. Whenever possible, nursing staff should be permanently assigned to the special care nursery and should not be asked to "float" to other areas. Delivery of supplies should be made outside the nursery. Personnel coming from other departments should be limited so that whenever possible the same person comes from the x-ray area or from a particular laboratory.

It must be stressed, however, that parents *are* necessary to provide care for the infant and must be allowed to participate in the care of their child whenever possible. If one takes time to explain precautions necessary to safeguard their child, parents are usually quite willing and able to adhere to them. In fact, some become quite observant and may raise questions concerning others' observance of techniques.

Should an infant develop any symptoms indicative of an infectious process, he should be removed from the nursery at once. There is no way to effectively isolate an infant other than by room isolation. It is true that while an infant is in an incubator, he is isolated from other infants. However, whenever portholes are opened, transmission of airborne organisms becomes possible.

Effect of Drugs

NARCOSIS

An infant may require special attention in the first few hours of life if he is demonstrating the effect of analgesics or anesthetic drugs which his mother received during labor or delivery. He may be sleepy and have sluggish respirations. This baby needs to be observed closely so that supportive measures may be instituted, if necessary. This narcosis is usually transitory, and these babies tend to do well subsequently.

EFFECTS OF DRUG ADDICTION

Infants born to mothers addicted to habituating drugs such as heroin are being recognized and treated in increasing numbers. About 83 to 90 percent of infants born to actively addicted mothers will manifest withdrawal symptoms, and most of these infants will begin to show evidence of withdrawal within the first 24 hours of life. Supportive measures are generally used to control discomfort, irritability, and purposeless movements. The signs and symptoms which have generally been observed include tremors, irritability, hyperactivity, vomiting, poor food intake, high-pitched shrill cry, diarrhea, and fever. Dehydration and malnutrition occur secondary to the vomiting, diarrhea, constant activity, and wakefulness manifested by these infants. Among the first signs to appear and the last to disappear are hyperactivity and flushing.

Phenobarbital, diazepam (Valium), methadone, and chlorpromazine (Thorazine) are some of the drugs used in treating infants suffering from narcotic withdrawal syndrome.

Rather than dealing with affected infants, a better aim would be to treat women early in pregnancy. They prove, however, to be unreliable informants concerning their drug habits. There is evidence that later in pregnancy the fetus responds to the mother's withdrawal with hyperactivity so that it may be necessary to wait until after delivery and support mother and infant separately during the withdrawal process.

CONDITIONS COMMONLY AFFECTING THE HIGH-RISK INFANT

Thus far, the general principles of nursing care for any high-risk infant have been discussed in accordance with the general behavior or needs demonstrated. This will provide the reader with the basis for care of all infants in risk situations. The factors responsible for placing an infant in a risk situation have been included in the discussion. Since jaundice, respiratory distress syndrome, and prematurity are encountered so frequently, discussion of these conditions merits inclusion in this chapter in order to provide the nurse with the sound body of knowledge needed in caring for these infants.

Neonatal Jaundice

During the first few days of a baby's life, nurses make frequent, systematic observations of his skin to note the appearance of jaundice. The rise in serum bilirubin responsible for this yellow hue may have several causes. One of these, the phenomenon of physiological jaundice, was discussed in an earlier chapter. Other predisposing factors include high doses of vitamin K, drugs such as sulfisoxazole given to the mother during pregnancy, infections such as rubella, and maternal diabetes. The most common cause, however, is hemolytic disease of the newborn due to blood group incompatibility. Bilirubinemia beyond physiological bounds, or hyperbilirubinemia, exists when serum bilirubin levels approach 18 to 20 mg percent. The term hyperbilirubinemia of the newborn is usually reserved for infants whose primary problem is a deficiency of inactivity or bilirubin transference rather than an excessive load of bilirubin for excretion.

The liver of the newborn produces little or no glucuronyl transferase, the enzyme necessary for the excretion of bilirubin. In each of the aforementioned instances, the concern with rising bilirubin levels rests with the possibility of its being deposited in the basal nuclei of the brain. This results in a condition known as kernicterus which leads to cerebral damage or death. The critical level of serum bilirubin is approximately 20 mg percent, although lower levels may be significant in the premature. The bilirubin unconjugated by the liver is also referred to as indirect bilirubin after the laboratory procedure used in its determination. This circulating bilirubin is bound to albumin and, hence, is unavailable for deposition in tissues. The amount of free bilirubin in the tissues cannot be measured; however, it is felt that determining the degree of saturation of serum albumin can provide a clue to this.

Phototherapy

In order to help the body to excrete excess bilirubin, a therapeutic intervention whereby the infant is exposed to an artificial light source has been developed. Phototherapy breaks down tissue bilirubin into products which thus far seem to be nontoxic and easily excreted. The infant should be completely undressed when placed under the lights and should have his position changed about every 2 hours. The baby's body temperature should also be monitored closely and will be affected by such factors as (1) light source, whether cool blue light or a heat-producing source; (2) use of an incubator or an open crib; and (3) temperature of the room. The light source needs to be checked regularly, since the energy output of any bulb decreases markedly after 200 hours of use, resulting in a decrease in the rate of decline of serum bilirubin. Some record of the number of hours a bulb has been in use should be kept attached to the equipment. (See Figure 34-6.)

The full effects of exposure to light on the infant's biological rhythms is not yet known, which leads one to believe it should be used with caution. Careful observation of the infant's eating and sleeping patterns is important, since changes may indicate a need to reevaluate the therapy. Studies with experimental animals have demonstrated retinal damage. For this reason, it is imperative that the baby's eyes be protected. When applying eye patches, the nurse must be certain that the baby's eyes are closed to prevent corneal abrasion. A common side effect of phototherapy is loose stools which may appear greenish because of the increased excretion of bilirubin. The infant will need additional water to compensate for this fluid loss. The nurse caring for this infant must remember that he is not to be left suspended in this "limbo" indefinitely. Feeding time provides a good opportunity to take him away from the lights, remove the eye covering, and hold him. This infant still has need for visual and tactile stimulation as well as comfort.

Hemolytic Disease of the Newborn

The main characteristics of hemolytic disease of the newborn are hyperbilirubinemia and anemia. Although this condition can result from any blood group incompatibility, the difficulties usually arise when an Rh negative woman is carrying an Rh positive fetus. The Rh factor, a dominant trait, is an antigen present on the red blood cells of 85 percent of the white and 93 percent of the black population. Unlike the ABO system, there are no naturally occurring anti-Rh antibodies. An Rh negative person will produce anti-Rh antibodies upon exposure to Rh positive red blood cells, such as during a blood transfusion or an Rh incompatible pregnancy.

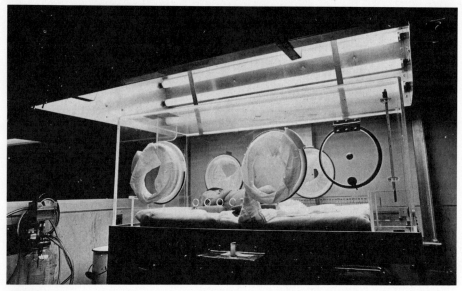

FIGURE 34-6
This infant is receiving phototherapy. In this instance it was necessary to open the port-holes for appropriate temperature control. To provide for safety, the mattress was lowered below the level of the open portholes.
(*Courtesy of Boston Hospital for Women, Boston, Mass.*)

It is important to remember that fetal and maternal circulations are sep-arate entities and that there is no mixing of blood. Late in pregnancy, and especially during the intrapartal period, there is appreciable placental transfer of fetal red blood cells to the pregnant woman. She responds by producing antibodies against the Rh factor which, on first exposure, begin to show up in her serum a few days after delivery. Since the production of antibodies takes time, the first Rh incompatible fetus usually escapes disease unless his mother has been sensitized by an Rh incompatible blood transfusion prior to this.

In subsequent Rh incompatible pregnancies, the woman will produce Rh antibodies earlier and in increasing numbers. These antibodies then cross the placenta and begin destroying the fetal Rh positive red blood cells. The fetus compensates by increasing red blood cell production, and hence, there appear increased numbers of erythroblasts in his circulation. In fact, the presence of these immature cells was the source of the older name for this disease— erythroblastosis fetalis. The problem usually increases in severity with each successive Rh incompatible pregnancy.

The affected infant will appear pale as a result of the anemia and will become jaundiced, usually within the first day of life. The immature liver is unable to conjugate for excretion the increased amount of bilirubin resulting from the destruction of erythrocytes. Thus, this infant may be in danger of developing kernicterus.

TREATMENT OF HYPERBILIRUBINEMIA

The goals of any treatment will be to reduce bilirubin levels and to correct the anemia. Keep in mind there are still circulating antibodies within the infant's system, causing hemolysis.

In severe cases, such as when the indirect bilirubin is approaching 20 mg percent (or cord bilirubin is greater than 5 mg percent) or the degree of anemia is severe, an exchange transfusion is performed. In this procedure, Rh negative blood is transfused usually via the umbilical vein. Using a three-way stopcock attached to a catheter, a small amount of the infant's blood is withdrawn (usually about 10 cc), and then a similar amount of the Rh negative blood is injected. This continues until the transfusion is complete. Using 500 cc of whole blood, it has been estimated that 85 to 90 percent of the infant's blood will be replaced. The amount of blood used depends upon the size and condition of the infant. The aims of an exchange transfusion are (1) to increase the hemoglobin level sufficiently to suppress production of Rh positive cells, (2) to keep serum bilirubin below dangerous levels, and (3) to remove both free antibodies and antibody-coated cells. Rh negative blood is used to prevent further hemolysis by remaining antibodies.

This is a stressful procedure for the infant. His body heat must be maintained and his vital signs must be frequently and carefully noted. Some nurseries have equipment which permits constant monitoring. The infant's extremities will be restrained. Restraints must be applied so that they are effective but not constricting. Resuscitative equipment must be at hand. The nurse usually has the added responsibility of recording the amounts of blood withdrawn and transfused along with the baby's reaction to the procedure.

Phototherapy is used by some physicians in conjunction with exchange transfusions to help reduce the number of transfusions necessary for any one infant. Phototherapy alone, except in mild cases, is not a treatment for hemolytic disease of the newborn, since it does not correct anemia, nor does it remove circulating antibodies.

In very severe cases, the anemia is accompanied by edema, fluid in serous cavities (hydrops fetalis), and heart failure. In an attempt to save those infants who previously died in utero, intrauterine transfusions have met with some success. Intrauterine deaths were usually the result of severe anemia. Rh negative cells are injected into the peritoneal cavity of the fetus where they are absorbed into the circulation. The need for this procedure can be determined by amniocentesis. This is performed when indicated by the pregnant woman's rising antibody titer. Spectrophotometric analysis of amniotic fluid bilirubin provides a guide in assessing the severity of the hemolytic process in the fetus.

PREVENTION OF HEMOLYTIC DISEASE DUE TO RH INCOMPATIBILITY

Since maternal antibodies are usually not present until a few days after the first delivery, and it is usually succeeding infants who are affected, prevention is aimed at suppression of maternal antibody production. A form of passive immunization has been used successfully for this. RhoGAM (Rho [D] immunoglobulin [human]) can be administered to the mother within 72 hours after delivery or abortion if she shows no evidence of antibody production. The mechanism of action is demonstrated in Figure 34-7. RhoGAM must be administered after every abortion and every Rh incompatible birth to prevent Rh sensitization.

ABO Incompatibility

Incompatibility of the ABO groups occurs more frequently than that caused by the Rh factor. It usually occurs when the woman is type O and the fetus is A or B. Hemolytic disease due to ABO incompatibility is usually less severe than that due to Rh incompatibility, although it can produce every gradation of disease seen with Rh. The main difference is that prior sensitization is not required, since A and B antibodies are already present in the mother's blood and thus the first-born can be affected.

Respiratory Distress Syndrome

Respiratory distress syndrome (RDS), formerly called hyaline membrane disease, is the chief reason for high perinatal death rates. It has been responsible for 30,000 deaths of newborns each year in the United States. The etiology of respiratory distress syndrome is still uncertain. The incidence, however, appears to be limited primarily to the premature infant usually less than 38 weeks of gestation who is apparently grown for gestational age. The disease has been found in 59 percent of infants less than 28 weeks of gestation but only in about 0.1 percent for full-term infants. Hyaline membrane disease has a tendency to be familial. It was previously thought that infants of diabetic mothers were more susceptible to the disease; however, recent studies indicate that diabetes is a predisposing factor only in that prematurity may be increased. Until recently, it was believed that cesarean section infants were more prone to develop the disease; however, it is now thought that only the reason for the cesarean section may influence its development. Racial factors do not seem to apply. Although asphyxia in the perinatal period is common, it is not a prerequisite. Third, hyaline membrane disease is found primarily in the immature infant, following a period of air breathing, usually in the first few hours of life.

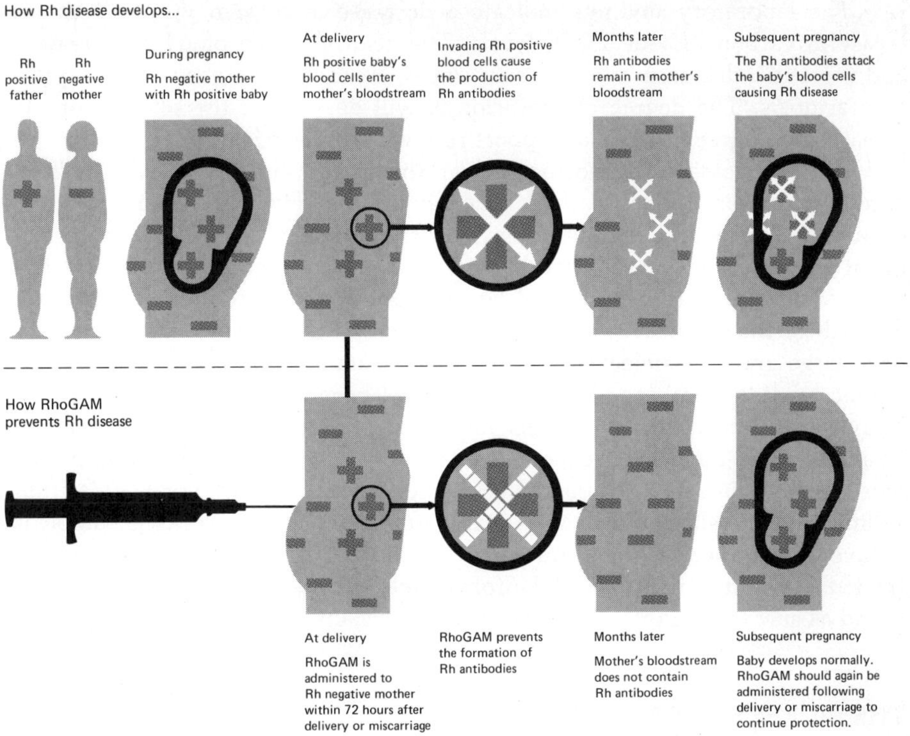

How Rh disease develops...

		During pregnancy	At delivery	Invading Rh positive blood cells cause the production of Rh antibodies	Months later	Subsequent pregnancy
Rh positive father	Rh negative mother	Rh negative mother with Rh positive baby	Rh positive baby's blood cells enter mother's bloodstream		Rh antibodies remain in mother's bloodstream	The Rh antibodies attack the baby's blood cells causing Rh disease

How RhoGAM prevents Rh disease

At delivery

RhoGAM is administered to Rh negative mother within 72 hours after delivery or miscarriage

RhoGAM prevents the formation of Rh antibodies

Months later

Mother's bloodstream does not contain Rh antibodies

Subsequent pregnancy

Baby develops normally. RhoGAM should again be administered following delivery or miscarriage to continue protection.

FIGURE 34-7
Mechanism of Rh disease production and the utilization of RhoGAM as a preventive measure.
(Courtesy of Ortho Diagnostics.)

CLINICAL MANIFESTATIONS

Clinical manifestations of the disease usually begin shortly after birth. Initially, the infant develops increased respirations and slight subcostal retractions. As the disease progresses, the respirations become more rapid and labored. Retractions on inspiration spread to include supra- and substernal and clavicular areas. Abdominal or see-saw respirations may develop. A grunt develops on expiration. The infant becomes cyanotic in room air, but his color will improve with oxygen. Nasal flaring develops, and tachypnea is evident. He tends to lie in a frog-like position with knees flexed, hips rotated out, and arms flaccid and slightly extended to his side. He may begin to develop edema in his extremities. Periods of apnea may develop; however, gentle tactile stimulation will usually restore respirations.

The laboratory findings indicate a decrease in oxygen PO_2 and an increase in carbon dioxide PCO_2 levels. The acidity of the blood is increased, and there is a decrease in buffer substances, creating a metabolic and respiratory acidosis. The degree of the acidosis will depend on the severity of the disease and degree of medical support received by the infant.

If the disease is not controlled at this point, the infant will develop severe retractions and greatly labored breathing. He will remain cyanotic even with increased amounts of oxygen. His apneic spells will be more frequent and resuscitation with mechanical assistance will become necessary. His pulse rate will begin to drop, and he will appear to be flaccid and exhausted. If he dies, the postmortem will reveal his lungs to be relatively airless and have large areas of atelectasis. Microscopic examination will reveal an eosinophilic hyaline membrane lining the terminal bronchioles and alveolar ducts. The reason for formation of this membrane remains in great controversy. Many theories have been expounded by authorities in the field, one of the most recent being that of Louis Gluck, who states that a ratio of 1:80 lecithin sphingomyelin (surface-tension-reducing substance) at 35 weeks gestation is a favorable indicator for extrauterine survival. This substance can be extracted from the amniotic fluid. Unfortunately, Dr. Gluck's work has not been found as successful in the hands of other physicians.

THE NURSE'S ROLE

Nursing care is of prime importance in the survival of these infants. The nurse is the one person who will be in constant attendance. The infant with respiratory distress syndrome is in an acute crisis and will require the attention of a single nurse in a one-to-one assignment. The observational skills of the nurse must be astute. Knowledge of the infant and of this disease process must be excellent to enhance observations. Too rapid a rise in the infant's temperature may produce further apnea, while inaccurate temperatures in the incubator may lead to loss of energy. High humidity may be necessary to dilute the secretions and make it easier for the infant to handle them; the increased amount of secretions are removed with suctioning. These infants will usually receive no oral food or fluid, and they cannot tolerate the stress of passing a feeding tube nor can their respirations tolerate a distended stomach following a feeding. Parenteral therapy is instituted; usually a 10 percent glucose solution is used to provide calories for energy. If parenteral therapy is not instituted soon enough, the infant may demonstrate symptoms of hypoglycemia as he uses up his energy stores. The immaturity of the renal system combined with the increase in glucose may create glycosuria. For this reason, the infant's urine must be collected and tested for sugar each time he voids. Specific gravity of urine will assist in evaluating the total amount of fluid needed for infusion. Glucose spilled in the urine will act as an osmotic diuretic, creating increased loss of electrolytes and fluids, thus defeating one of the purposes of parenteral therapy. Sodium bicarbonate may be added to the solution to increase the buffers. As the pH changes rapidly within the infant, blood analysis must be done frequently to evaluate the need for specific changes within the parenteral solution. In some acute care centers, the nurse does the blood analysis and alters the infusion.

The need for potential resuscitation and respiratory assistance is obvious. The nurse must be prepared to utilize special equipment in the care of this infant and must be knowledgeable, not only in the workings of specific equipment, but also in the behavior of the infant which indicates the need for such assistance. The nurse must also have the confidence to make a diagnosis when intervention is required and to activate appropriate measures. If immediate action is not taken, the infant may suffer the consequences. Action should be taken and the physician notified immediately. When the physician arrives, he may take over the resuscitative measures or have the nurse continue while he obtains additional data to alter the therapeutic regimen.

COMPLICATIONS

The infant with respiratory distress syndrome is a candidate for several complications. The development of these complications is greatly dependent upon the maturity of the infant and severity of the disorder. In addition to the apnea that has been previously mentioned, pneumothorax, pneumomediastinum, cardiac failure, sepsis, intravascular coagulation, intercranial hemorrhage, and hyperbilirubinemia may appear. These will need appropriate treatment if they occur. Again, it cannot be emphasized too strongly that it will be the nurse who will have the closest contact with these infants and that knowledge and observations may be the initial diagnostic tool.

The nurse caring for these infants will become very much involved and should be cautioned that there is an equally great need for communicating with and supporting the family. Because of the closeness of the nurse to the infant, giving the parents information and support becomes vital. If the parents cannot visit the nursery, the nurse should plan to spend some time each day with them. Whenever the parents are willing and able to enter the nursery, they should be encouraged to come in for a close look at their child and to touch him, even through the incubator.

When the infant begins to recover, the nurse should gradually transfer as much of the caretaking as possible to the mother. This may mean teaching the mother how to hold her baby while an intravenous infusion is in place or how to instill a gavage feeding. Mothers can be taught to do these things if there is someone who is willing to share the information.

The Premature Infant

The premature infant has the same needs for adjustment to his new environment as does the full-term infant. The difference with the premature infant is that he is more dependent on assistance from the health team, as he has been deprived of the warmth and security of his mother's womb. The closer his gestational age is to term, the more he will resemble the full-term infant in appearance and behavior. The degree of his immaturity will be relative to his gestational age. The younger, more immature infant has more difficulty adjusting to the external environment. (See Figure 34-8.)

An infant born prior to 37 weeks gestation is considered to be premature. Traditionally, emphasis has been placed on weight and a premature was described as an infant weighing 2,500 Gm or less at birth. Weight as a sole criterion is felt to be inadequate, since it fails to take into account the following: (1) one-half the infants who are premature by weight have a gestational age of 37 weeks or greater, (2) the infant whose low birth weight is due to genetic or racial factors and who exhibits no other sign of immaturity, and (3) those infants whose birth weight is greater than 2,500 Gm but who have a gestational age less than 37 weeks. The mortality rate of the third group of infants is 3 to 4 times greater than the term infant of equal weight.

Because of these factors, the premature or immature infant should be identified by evaluation of his weight and gestational age. When the nurse evaluates the gestational age of an infant, the history of the mother's last menstrual period is of great importance; however, this information is not always known or accurate. Therefore, there are other guidelines for determining the maturity of the infant. Table 34-2 lists some of the differing appearances of newborns with various gestational ages.

INCIDENCE

In 1961 the expert committee on Maternal-Child Health recommended that the term premature be replaced by the more appropriate term low birth weight and that the term premature be used only for infants born less than 37 weeks after the beginning of the mother's last menstrual period. Since the majority of statistical data available in the last 30 years included both premature and low-birth-weight infants, some concepts related to the premature may need alteration when new data, specific for the premature, have been acquired. Since the statistical emphasis on gestational age, as well as birth weight, is relatively recent, the real incidence of prematurity has not been adequately determined. In the United States, in 1965, the incidence of live infants born weighing 2,500 Gm or less was 12 percent for white infants and 13.8 percent for nonwhites.

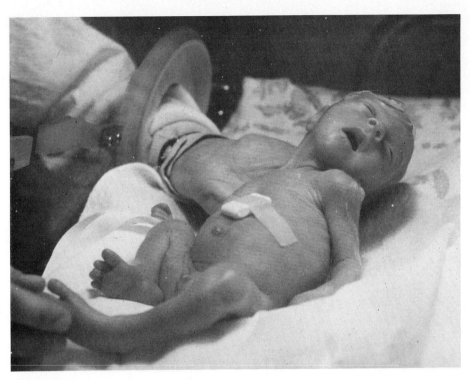

FIGURE 34-8
(a) A premature infant who is young and in a risk situation.
(Courtesy of New England Medical Center—Boston Floating Division. Photographed by Boston University School of Nursing, Media Services Department.)

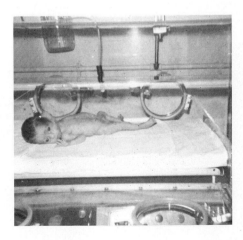

(b) A premature who is more mature and thriving. This newborn demonstrates the typical appearance of the premature infant. Note the lack of subcutaneous fat and the decrease of muscle tone. The infant's abdomen is distended following her tube feeding.
(Courtesy of St. Luke's Hospital, New Bedford, Mass.)

TABLE 34-2
INFANTS CLASSIFIED BY WEIGHT AND GESTATIONAL AGE

	Less than 3 lb 5 oz Group I	5 lb 8 oz (2,500 Less than 37 weeks 3 lb 5 oz to 5 lb 8 oz Group II
Percent of all deliveries	1	2
Neonatal mortality (%)	65	10
Appellations	Immature premature	Premature
Characteristics	Weight loss, 20% ± 10% Translucent and edematous skin Decreased tone Erratic extremity movement Periodic breathing Moderate jaundice Physiologic immaturity in enzymatic and functional development	Weight loss, 10% ± 5%
Complications	Respiratory distress syndrome common Susceptible to infection Asphyxial injury to capillaries, with hemorrhage	
Special requirements	Incubator care	
Exceptions	Some immature infants who are also malnourished and under-sized for their gestation, with some of the characteristics and nutritional requirements of Group III	

SOURCE: Modified from J. Yerushalmy, Bea J. van den Berg, C. L. Erhardt, and H. Jacobziner, "Birth Weight and Gestation as Indices of 'Immaturity,'" *American Journal of Diseases in Childhood*, 109:43, 1965.

TABLE 34-2
INFANTS CLASSIFIED BY WEIGHT AND GESTATIONAL AGE (*Continued*)

Gm) or less	*Over 5 lb 8 oz (2,500 Gm)*	
37 weeks and over	*Less than 37 weeks*	*37 weeks and over*
Group III	*Group IV*	*Group V*
2 to 4	2 to 4	90 ± 3
3 to 4	2	Less than 0.5
"Small for dates" Dysmature Postmature Pseudopremature Fetal malnutrition Intrauterine growth retardation Chronic fetal distress	"Pseudoterm"	
Minimal weight loss, less than 5% Malnutrition Dry and scaly skin Increased tone Restricted Moro reflex Increased oxygen consumption Minimal jaundice Cries for and has increased capacity for food Anxious, open-eyed appearance	Same as for Group II but less marked	Normal newborn infants
Respiratory distress syndrome rare Hypoglycemia common Reduced skeletal growth Increase in congenital anomalies May have had chronic intrauterine asphyxia	Respiratory distress syndrome occasionally Often neglected because of the false reassurance of their size	
Early water, glucose, calories, and vitamins	Same as for Groups I and II	
Infants who are biologically small due to race, family pattern, or early growth arrest; usually not malnourished		Up to 10% of normal infants, who have had some degree of fetal malnutrition as in Group III, particularly when of postdate delivery

RELATED FACTORS

Using the definitions of premature and low birth weight for gestational age, it is difficult to separate the causal factors associated with each. Thus far, certain factors have been identified as being associated with premature or low weight for gestational age infants. Nelson and Babson and Benson have attributed some of the maternal factors to include obstetric problems such as toxemia, premature separation of the placenta, placental insufficiency, intercurrent maternal disease, and incidental surgery. Also having some relationship to premature and low birth weight, although not necessarily causal, are the age and parity of the mother (primipara under twenty or over forty years old), her marital status, height, overwork, cigarette smoking, history of previous difficult pregnancy, fertility difficulties, race and low socioeconomic level, and poor nutritional status. Although largely theoretical, the paternal role is being investigated. The factors thus far implicated include older age of father, chronic alcoholism, diabetes mellitus, and the presence of Rh positive genes when the mother is Rh negative. Fetal factors associated with prematurity include multiple births, hydramnios, and abnormalities of the cord. The incidence of prematurity drops to a relative low of 5.6 percent in areas where there is a higher socioeconomic status. There are a number of reasons attributed to this discrepancy, although it is unclear which predominate. These include maternal education, nutrition, housing conditions, hygiene, interest in pregnancy, and antenatal care.

PROGNOSIS

The mortality and morbidity rates of premature infants and low-birth-weight infants are considerably higher than those of the full-term infant. Following discharge from the hospital, the mortality rate of low-birth-weight infants is three times that of full-term infants during the first 2 years of life. Since many of these deaths are attributable to infection, they seem at least theoretically preventable. Premature infants, barring any other physical difficulties, generally lag behind in growth and development, as compared to the full-term infant for the first 2 years of life. The larger the premature at birth, the more closely he will resemble the full-term infant in achievement of developmental tasks. The smaller the infant at birth, the greater the incidence of mental retardation, cerebral palsy, and neurological defects. This fact could be attributed to the higher incidence of cerebral anoxia and hemorrhage in the premature infant.

NURSING CARE

The nursery admission of a premature infant is often an emergency situation, as with any infant at risk. An initial evaluation is done to rapidly ascertain the need for immediate lifesaving measures. Because of the immaturity of his central nervous system and lack of subcutaneous fat, he will need support of his body temperature and incubator care. Depending on his color and respirations, oxygen may need to be administered. Parenteral therapy may be started immediately on infants who appear to be in respiratory difficulty or whose electrolytes are unbalanced. In most instances, these infants will have blood drawn to determine the status of electrolytes and blood gases. If sepsis is of concern, parenteral fluids may be started to facilitate antibiotic therapy. The maintenance of body temperature is imperative and must not be overlooked during the emergency admission procedure; therefore, the use of an infant warmer is of great benefit.

Once the emergency treatments have been completed, the infant will be placed in the incubator. Nursing care now becomes of primary importance for the survival of the infant. Frequent recordings of the infant's vital signs will be required. The temperature may be more liable in the premature than in the full-term infant. The premature should have his axillary temperature maintained at 36.5°C, or 97.8°F. Apical pulse rate will be weak, irregular, and rapid. Respirations are irregular. It is hard to establish norms for respiratory rates in the premature. According to Fitzpatrick et al., two patterns have been associated with a low mortality rate and have thus been described as "normal." In the first pattern, about 40 respirations per minute occur from birth onward without any significant fluctuations; in the second pattern, rates over 60 respirations per minute occur in the first hour with no significant increase and a subsequent decline. A significant increase would be a rise of 15 or more above that recorded for the first hour of life.[2] The earlier the gestational age, the more prone the infant is to periods of apnea. Gentle stimulation by rubbing the chest or gently compressing the thorax will usually be adequate to start respirations. It appears he sometimes just forgets to breathe. Because his pulse and respiration rates are irregular, they must be counted for a full minute. In addition to this, the nurse must observe for expiratory grunt and retractions which are indicative of respiratory distress. With the variety of electrical equipment available to assist the nurse in monitoring the vital signs of infants, it is imperative that the nurse be familiar with the equipment in use and cognizant of the potential electrical hazards. These may be compounded with the use of compressed gases and oxygen. The leads for these monitors are usually attached with adhesives or jellies, which can irritate the skin. It is therefore necessary, to maintain the integrity of the skin, that these leads be removed and then reapplied after the skin has been cleaned.

After the initial lifesaving measures have been instituted and the condition of the infant evaluated, the team must decide if this infant can be maintained in their nursery or if transfer to a regional neonatal referral center is necessary. This decision must be based not only on the condition of the infant, but on the availability of skilled nurses and physicians on a 24-hour basis. If transfer is determined necessary, a portable incubator with oxygen equipment attached should be used, and a registered nurse who is skilled in

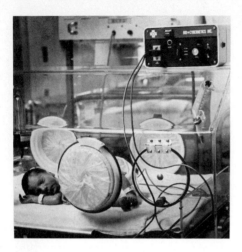

FIGURE 34-9
This premature infant's respirations are being monitored by a device which is connected to his mattress. Should his respirations cease, this apnea monitor will sound an alarm to alert the nurse to his needs. *(Courtesy of Bio-Cybernetics, Inc., Boston, Mass.)*

infant resuscitation should accompany the infant. Whenever possible, provision should be made for the mother to see her infant prior to transfer. The mother will need to be prepared by the nurse for the experience of seeing her infant in an incubator and perhaps surrounded by strange equipment. She may even be helped to hold or to touch her baby. This is a difficult period for the parents and for the nurse, since the possibility exists that this is the last time they will see the infant. The mother who has seen her infant is more ready to deal with the reality of his birth and the tasks of grieving.

There are many components to the care of the premature infant. One of the major concerns is the conservation of his energy and support of his immature systems. Maintenance of body temperature through use of the incubator is common practice. Because of the immaturity of his nervous systems, his sucking ability may be too weak to permit nursing a bottle, therefore tube feedings may be necessary. Vomiting is common because of an immature cardiac sphincter; therefore, small frequent feedings will be necessary. Prevention of aspiration and vomiting can be assisted by slightly elevating the head of the mattress. The elevated head may also assist the respirations.

POSITIONING

Positioning of the premature is of prime importance. His muscles are very weak and underdeveloped. The immaturity of his skeletal system permits molding of bones in relation to positioning. This is readily visible in his skull bones. He has little or no subcutaneous fat, allowing for pressure areas to be prevalent. His skin is thin and easily broken down. Therefore, sheepskin and bubble pads can be used to prevent breakdown of skin over bony prominences.

The premature infant should have his position changed every 2 hours.

This will enhance ventilation and expansion of his lungs and stimulate his circulation. Care must be taken, however, not to position the infant so there is constriction to his thoracic or abdominal area, as this may interfere with his respirations.

Care must be taken when applying diapers to a premature infant. If the diaper is too large, the hips may be hyperextended and externally rotated. If the hips are immobilized in this position for a period of time, deformities to the hips may occur. Therefore, if small diapers are not available, regular disposable diapers can be cut in half.

COMPLICATIONS

The premature infant has a tendency to bleed secondary to the fragility of the capillaries and low plasma prothrombin levels. This may be manifested as petechial or ecchymotic areas. Careful observation of the infant is required with special attention to the cord as it may be prone to secondary bleeding. Intercranial capillaries are particularly susceptible; therefore, observation should include watching for signs of increased intercranial pressure or bleeding.

Both the full-term and premature infant have a high hemoglobin concentration at birth. The cord blood on both a 1,200 Gm premature and full-term baby is approximately 17 Gm per 100 ml. In a premature infant below 1,200 Gm the hemoglobin is approximately 15.6 Gm per 100 ml. In both the premature and full-term infant there is a normal decline in hemoglobin concentration due to the interaction of several factors. The first is a relative decrease in the bone marrow erythropoietic activity. There is also a relative increase in the rate of hemolysis as well as a hemodilution due to the rapid expansion of the blood volume. The above factors are more extreme in the low-birth-weight infant and result in a more severe anemia at an earlier age. In the premature, the hemoglobin may drop to a level of 6 to 7 Gm per 100 ml at the third to seventh week. This guideline is helpful in evaluating whether or not an existing anemia is the result of a pathological process. In addition, a number of pathological processes and/or indiscriminate drawing of blood specimens may be superimposed upon this "physiological" anemia, creating a more severe anemia.

The majority of premature infants tend to become jaundiced on the second to fourth day of life. The level of serum bilirubin tends to be related to the gestational age of the infant. The immature liver is unable to conjugate the bilirubin created by the breakdown of red blood cells.

The premature infant has an increased susceptibility to infection and is less able to handle infection than the full-term infant. Also, his skin and mucous membranes are less protective. Treatments such as intravenous infusions may further break down this first line of defense and create new portals of entry. He has a lowered white blood cell count which does not respond with the expected elevation to infection. His ability to form antibodies is poor, and he is lacking in immune bodies transmitted via the placenta.

Particular care must be taken to assure that proper aseptic technique be carried out at all times. This may require repeated instructions to parents and hospital staff who visit and care for the premature infant. It has been our experience that parents can learn the necessary precautions quite readily and are usually quite eager to do what is best for their baby.

NUTRITIONAL NEEDS

Feeding practices for premature and low-birth-weight infants have undergone evaluation and change over the years and still vary. In general, it is felt that early feeding will contribute to a lower morbidity and mortality by preventing depletion of nutrients and maintaining biochemical homeostasis. Hypoglycemia and hyperbilirubinemia will be lessened. The premature infant in good condition with active peristalsis should be given 5 to 10 percent glucose water orally by 6 to 12 hours of age. Infants in poor condition, such as respiratory distress, should not receive oral feedings, but should receive parenteral fluids. According to the infant's tolerance, the water feedings will gradually be replaced by milk feedings until fluid and calorie needs are being met.

The premature infant will have to be fed more frequently than the full-term infant. Generally speaking, infants weighing less than 3 pounds will have to be fed every 2 to 3 hours. As the infant approaches 3½ to 4 pounds, his feeding schedule will approach 3 to 4 hours. The premature who is being bottle-fed initially needs to learn to coordinate his sucking and swallowing. The nurse must remember the importance of conservation of energy and not allow the baby to become chilled or fatigued during his feeding. Any feeding which takes longer than 20 minutes will probably be tiring to the premature. The smaller the premature infant, the less likely he is to demonstrate hunger; therefore, he may have to be awakened for feeding. The premature weighing less than 3 pounds may not have an adequate suck, swallow, or gag reflex and therefore may require tube feeding with a nasogastric tube or, in the case of an infant in severe respiratory distress, a gastrostomy tube. However, the insertion of a gastrostomy tube requires a surgical procedure and usually is not the first choice. An example of a feeding guide is demonstrated in Table 34-3.

EMOTIONAL NEEDS

It is difficult to distinguish specific emotional needs of the premature infant because similar needs have been demonstrated by other infants who have required prolonged care in incubators and separation from family. In general, the primary concern is the absence of opportunity for the infant to meet his developmental tasks at the same time or in the same manner as does the "normal" infant.

First, let us consider a few of the basic tasks that all infants must complete. If one considers Erikson's first stage of man, trust versus mistrust, or Freud's pleasure produces learning, and applies this to the premature or high-risk infant, one can immediately see inherent danger. The premature can have little trust when he has literally been pushed into supporting his own life far in advance of the full-term infant. The premature or any high-risk infant will have little development of pleasure if he is being stuck and poked frequently in pain or discomfort because of his medical disorder. He will hardly learn trust or pleasure if his primary contact with other people usually creates additional discomforts because of necessary treatments and procedures. In addition, the high-risk and definitely premature infants are frequently denied satisfaction of basic needs. The infant who is denied oral intake cannot suck unless a pacifier has been provided. The infant in an incubator has his vision blurred and distorted when looking through the plastic sides; should he require phototherapy, he is completely without vision. Also, the infant in an incubator has his hearing distorted. Within the incubator, he has the constant noise of the motor. It is possible that other noise may enter the incubator from people banging the incubator or talking in the near vicinity. It is also possible that such sound that enters the incubator may reverberate on all six surface areas, creating unpleasant sounds and perhaps painful stimuli.

Infants treated for risk conditions who have been denied pleasurable comforting contacts with a specific person have been observed to demonstrate behavior strongly suggestive of emotional disorder. Behaviors indicative of emotional disorder more frequently encountered are (1) lack or slowness of weight gain; (2) preference to look at ceiling lights rather than persons caring for them, as if afraid of the person or out of lack of trust; and (3) little crying, as if there were no reason to cry since it would bring no change—hopelessness. In essence, demonstration of the first developmental task of trust or pleasure is missing in these infants.

Longitudinal studies on premature infants have demonstrated the developmental lags for the first few years of life. One might hypothesize that these lags are related to early impedance in the development of the first tasks of trust and pleasure.

NURSING APPROACH

It becomes apparent that nursing care must be geared to assist the infant in meeting his first developmental tasks as well as his physiological needs.

The first nursing approach might well be the assignment of one nurse to be his prime caretaker for his entire stay in the nursery. This would provide the infant the opportunity to become familiar with her touch, smell, and sound of voice. Is this not what the "normal" infant experiences with his mother? The nurse would also become more cognizant of his communication patterns and means of satisfying his needs. Whenever care is to be provided,

TABLE 34-3
FEEDING GUIDE FOR PREMATURE INFANTS UNDER 2,000 GM (4 LB 8 OZ)

Formula	Age (in days)	Volume ranges ml/kg/day		ml/lb/day	
		Immature*	Undergrown*	Immature	Undergrown
10% glucose	0	20	30	9	14
Half, 10% glu-	1	30	45	14	20
cose and half,	2	40	60	18	26
full-strength	3	50	75	22	32
	4	60	90	26	40
	5	70	105	30	48
Full-strength	6	80	120	35	55
formula	7	90	135	40	60
(24 cal. per	8	100	150	45	70
30 ml)	9				
	10	110	160	50	75
	12	120	160	55	75
	15	130	160	60	75
	20	140	160	65	75

* *Immature* refers to the very small, weak, and hypotonic premature infant. *Undergrown* infants are those who are small for their gestational age and who have a greater need for calories.

1. The volume ranges allow a choice of feeding amounts. Most premature infants are more safely fed in the lower ranges. *Supplemental parenteral fluids will be necessary if dehydration, lethargy, or excessive weight loss occurs.*

2. Multiply infant's weight (kg or lb) by volume to be given for that day and divide by twelve (number of feedings) for amount to be fed at 2-hour intervals.

3. Infants on reaching 1.5 kg (3 lb 5 oz) should be placed gradually on a 3-hour feeding schedule (total volume given, divided by eight feedings).

4. Infants on the bottle and on reaching 1.8 to 2 kg (4 to 4½ lb) may be fed on a modified demand basis and at increased feeding intervals.
   Volume taken may range *above* 200 ml per kg (90 ml per lb).

Exceptions:

1. Infants in poor condition *for any reason* require a delay in oral feedings and the institution of parenteral fluids *from the first few hours of life.*

2. Any baby with distention, cyanotic or apneic attacks, or vomiting should have his feedings stopped and condition evaluated.

3. A stomach residual (at the time of the next gavage feeding) of over 1 ml indicates a delay in emptying time. Feedings should be reduced and the event reported to physician for evaluation.

4. Malnourished infants require glucose and water soon after birth to support brain metabolism, due to deficient glycogen stores in liver.

SOURCE: S. Gorham Babson and Ralph C. Benson, *Primer on Prematurity and High-risk Pregnancy,* Mosby, St. Louis, 1966, p. 107.

the nurse should talk to him and fondle him, even if this must be done through portholes. Holding his arm or stroking his head will provide contact with another person and will not endanger him in any way. As soon as possible, he should be held and cuddled.

Visual stimulation should be provided. This can easily be done with bright decals or small mobiles hung in the incubator. These should be placed where the infant can readily see them and yet not hinder the physical care necessary. Auditory stimulation is most effectively accomplished through the human voice. Caution must be taken in placing musical toys or radios inside the incubator. Further study is needed to determine the decibel increase and reverberation patterns of noise and its effects upon the infant's hearing.

The nurse who provides the infant with an opportunity to develop a sense of trust and pleasure in people and his world obviously provides him with a greater chance of emotional security.

FAMILY ADJUSTMENT TO THE HIGH-RISK INFANT

It should be obvious to the reader that the nurse caring for a high-risk infant must be acutely observant as well as informed. An infant in a risk situation poses a special threat to his parents. Their greatest fear—death of their child—is close to being realized. Parents seek to protect themselves from the pain of this threat by withdrawing from their association with the baby. They begin to grieve in anticipation of his death. Although this anticipatory grief begins as a protective mechanism, if the parents do not receive any assistance in dealing with their feelings, it is possible that they will grieve this baby out of their lives. This has tremendous implications for childrearing practices should this baby survive. If the parents have emotionally separated from this child, they will find it difficult to establish effective parenting patterns. They may tend to continue to consider this child vulnerable to serious illness or accident and even destined to die during childhood. To them, the child is only on tenuous loan and not really theirs.

The children involved in this process have been known to demonstrate a variety of problems. They may have difficulty with separation. These parents will rarely use baby-sitters but may leave the child with grandparents on occasion. Sleep problems may be manifest, and when the time comes these children may develop a school phobia. These parents may become overprotective and overindulgent, but since they tend not to set limits, the child may be overly dependent, disobedient, and uncooperative. Although the mother cannot seem to control this behavior, she may be quite restrictive of the child's activity, keeping him in the playpen excessively or forbidding such activities as bicycling. The mother, and later her child, may become overly concerned with body function, leading to hypochondriasis.

This is just an overview of some of the disordered childrearing practices that may result from a grief reaction which did not cease when the threat to the infant's life was over. Kaplan and Mason have identified four tasks which must be completed by the mother of a premature infant in order to prevent the parenting problems described. The first task, that of *anticipatory grief*, involves a withdrawal from the relationship already established with the child so that she still hopes the baby will survive but simultaneously prepares for his death. Second, she must *face and acknowledge her maternal failure to deliver a normal full-term baby*. The grief and depression are signs that she is struggling with these tasks. These are healthy responses and usually last until the baby's chances for survival seem secure. The remaining tasks need to be performed while baby is recovering. The third task involves *resumption of the previously interrupted process of relating to the baby*. In the case of the premature infant, the mother has not had the same length of time to prepare for the mothering role which is afforded the mother of the full-term infant.

The mother had been preparing herself for a loss, but as the baby begins to improve, she must respond with hope and anticipation of his recovery. There is usually a point at which the mother really believes her baby will survive. This turning point may be related to a change in baby's weight, his feeding pattern or activity, or even a change in the nurse's manner.

In the fourth task, the mother must *understand how this baby differs in relation to special needs and growth patterns*. It is also important that she see these special needs as being temporary and that they will yield in time to more normal patterns.

It is felt that each of these tasks must be accomplished in the order in which they are listed: A successful outcome is considered to be one in which the mother regards the baby as potentially normal, gives him realistic care, and takes pride and satisfaction in that care.[3]

Although these tasks have been specifically identified for the mother of the premature infant, we feel that there is some applicability to both parents and that the situation could relate to any infant in a vulnerable condition. It is the nurse's role to help parents accomplish these tasks.

Often, in the case of the high-risk infant, the mother is discharged from the hospital some time before the baby is ready to go. What is the effect upon siblings when mother returns home without the promised baby? Our response to this question is based largely upon experiences. In those instances in which parents have not been able to cope successfully with the threat to their child's life, their over-attentiveness to this baby may limit the time and energies available for other children. This can then set the stage for jealousy and rivalry. On the other hand, parents who are able to accomplish Kaplan and Mason's four tasks seem to be able to use the time alone with their children to prepare them for baby's homecoming.

REFERENCES

1 Nelson, Waldo E., Victor C. Vaughan, and R. James McKay: *Textbook of Pediatrics*, 9th ed., Saunders, Philadelphia, 1969, p. 360.
2 Fitzpatrick, Elise, Sharon Reeder, and Luigi Mastroianni, Jr.: *Maternity Nursing*, 12th ed., Lippincott, Philadelphia, 1971, p. 416.
3 Kaplan, David M., and Edward A. Mason: "Maternal Reactions to Premature Birth Viewed as an Acute Emotional Disorder," in Howard J. Parad (ed.), *Crisis Intervention: Selected Readings*, Family Service Association of America, New York, 1965, pp. 124–125.

BIBLIOGRAPHY

Babson, S. Gorham, and Ralph C. Benson: *Management of High Risk Pregnancy and Intensive Care of the Neonate*, Mosby, St. Louis, 1971.
Barnett, C. R., Herbert P. Leiderman, Rose Grobstein, and Marshall Klaus: "Neonatal Separation: The Maternal Side of Interactional Deprivation," *Pediatrics*, 45:197, February 1970.
Brann, Alfred W., Jr., and Jose M. Montalvo: Barbiturates and Asphyxia, *Pediatric Clinics of North America*, 17:851, November 1970.
Cohen, Sanford N., and William A. Olson: "Drugs that Depress the Newborn Infant," *Pediatric Clinics of North America*, 17:835, November 1970.
Erikson, Erik H.: *Childhood and Society*, 2d ed., Norton, New York, 1963.
Fitzpatrick, Elise, Sharon Reeder, and Luigi Mastroianni, Jr.: *Maternity Nursing*, 12th ed., Lippincott, Philadelphia, 1971.
Gluck, Louis, et al.: "Perinatal Prediction of Respiratory Distress Syndrome," The American Academy of Pediatrics Society, Inc., 81st Annual Meeting, *Program and Abstracts*, Atlantic City, May 1971, p. 14.
Green, Morris, and Albert J. Solnit: "Reactions to the Threatened Loss of a Child: A Vulnerable Child Syndrome," *Pediatrics*, 34:58, 1964.
Greenbaum, Edward I., et al.: "Rectal Thermometer Induced Pneumoperitoneum in the Newborn," *Pediatrics*, pp. 539–542, October 1969.
Hall, Calvin, and Gardner Lindzey (eds.): *Theories of Personality*, Wiley, New York, 1957.
Hathaway, William: "Coagulation Problems in the Newborn," *Pediatric Clinics of North America*, 17:929, November 1970.
Hill, Reba M., and Murdina Desmond: "Management of the Narcotic Withdrawal Syndrome in the Neonate," *Pediatric Clinics of North America*, 10:67–85, 1963.
Hosack, Alice Marie: "A Comparison of Crises: Mothers' Early Experiences with Normal and Abnormal First Born Infants," unpublished doctoral thesis, Harvard University, 1968.

Kahn, Eric, Lois Neumann, and Gene-Ann Polk: "The Course of the Heroin Withdrawal Syndrome in Newborn Infants Treated with Phenobarbital or Chlorpromazine," *Journal of Pediatrics*, 75:495–500, September 1969.

Kaplan, David M., and Edward A. Mason: "Maternal Reactions to Premature Birth Viewed as an Acute Emotional Disorder," *American Journal of Orthopsychiatry*, 30:118–128, July 1960.

Kitterman, Joseph A., Roderic H. Phibbs, and William H. Tooley: "Catheterization of Umbilical Vessels in Newborn Infants," *Pediatric Clinics of North America*, 17:4, November 1970.

Klaus, Marshall H., and John Kennell: "Mothers Separated from Their Newborn Infants," *Pediatric Clinics of North America*, 17:1015, November 1970.

Kumpe, Mary, and Leonard Kleinman: "Care of the Infant with Respiratory Distress Syndrome," *Nursing Clinics of North America*, 6:25–37, March 1971.

Lindemann, Erich: "Symptomatology and Management of Acute Grief," *American Journal of Psychiatry*, 101:141–148, 1944.

Lubchenco, Lula O.: "Assessment of Gestational Age and Development at Birth," *Pediatric Clinics of North America*, 17:125, February 1970.

Lutz, Linda, and Paul H. Perlstein: "Temperature Control in Newborn Babies," *Nursing Clinics of North America*, 6:15–23, March 1971.

Marlow, Dorothy: *Textbook of Pediatric Nursing*, Saunders, Philadelphia, 1969.

Nelson, Nicholas M.: "On the Etiology of Hyaline Membrane Disease," *Pediatric Clinics of North America*, 17:943, November 1970.

Nelson, Waldo E., Victor C. Vaughan, and R. James McKay: *Textbook of Pediatrics*, 9th ed., Saunders, Philadelphia, 1969.

O'Brien, Richard, and Howard Pearson: "Physiologic Anemia of the Newborn Infant," *Journal of Pediatrics*, 79:132–138, July 1971.

Ortho Diagnostics: *Blood Group Antigens and Antibodies as Applied to Hemolytic Disease of the Newborn*, Ortho Diagnostics, Raritan, N. J., 1968.

Owens, Charlotte: "Parents' Reactions to Defective Babies," in Nancy A. Lytle (ed.): *Maternal Health Nursing*, Brown, Dubuque, Iowa, 1967.

Parad, Howard J. (ed.): *Crisis Intervention: Selected Readings*, Family Service Association of America, New York, 1965.

Perlmutter, J. F.: "Drug Addiction in Pregnant Women," *American Journal of Obstetrics and Gynecology*, 99:569, 1969.

Segal, Sydney: "Oxygen: Too Much, Too Little," *Nursing Clinics of North America*, 6:39–53, March 1971.

Sinclair, John C., John M. Driscoll, Jr., William C. Heird, and Robert W. Winters: "Supportive Management of the Sick Neonate: Parenteral Calories, Water, and Electrolytes," *Pediatric Clinics of North America*, 17:4, November 1970.

Sisson, T. R., et al.: "Retinal Changes Produced by Phototherapy," *Journal of Pediatrics*, 77:221–227, August 1970.

Tahernia, C.: "Cardiac Arrests in Infants and Children," *Pediatric Nursing Currents*, 17:4, July–August 1970.

Wallace, Helen M. (ed.): *Health Services for Mothers and Children*, Saunders, Philadelphia, 1962.

White, Mary, and William J. Keenan: "Recognition and Management of Hypoglycemia in the Newborn Infant," *Nursing Clinics of North America*, 6:1, March 1971.

35 | INTRAUTERINE GROWTH DEVIATIONS

Katharine A. McCarty and Gladys M. Scipien

In a society in which physical and intellectual attainment is an ideal, the birth of a defective infant is a tragic event for the individual, family, and society. A pregnant woman plans for the arrival of her infant both physically and psychologically. Physically she is concerned about the changes within her own body. Her doctor's visits are generally centered around her blood pressure, her weight, her urine, and the fetal heart beat. She may or may not begin to purchase articles for her infant early in pregnancy. Psychologically many changes are also occurring. She is concerned about her changing body image and whether she will regain her normal figure. Will changes need to be made in her family living situation? Will there be alterations in relationships between her and her husband and among the other children?

The fear of having a defective infant is a periodic concern of many pregnant women. She may express her concern and question openly when she states, "My niece is having corrective surgery for a harelip. What are the chances of this happening to my baby?" Or her fears may not be overtly expressed. Frequently clues to her fears are expressed in the form of, "I don't care what I have as long as the baby is healthy and normal." At the time of delivery one of the first questions a mother asks is, "Is my baby normal?"

Regardless of what the doctor or nurse says to her, she will want to examine her infant and see for herself that her infant is normal.

The birth of a defective infant is a crisis for the mother and the family. A crisis manifests itself when the normal course of living is upset. In a state of crisis, the usual patterns of solving problems are not adequate, and nursing intervention can be meaningful. Each mother reacts differently to a defective infant. This reaction may be demonstrated by her refusal to talk about the infant, her silences, her outbursts of tears, or casualness about the infant. Her reaction will be influenced by her own past experiences with her parents and siblings as well as by other significant events in her life.[1]

A nurse's reaction to the birth of a defective infant will *also* be influenced by the degree and extent of the abnormality as well as her own past experiences with her family and community. A nurse, as a person, will often have thoughts and concerns about what kind of a mother she will be and whether she will rear her child differently from her own experiences. Through mass media, nurses are constantly reminded of the rights and place of the physically and mentally handicapped in society.

Predictions of genetic engineering and the ethical questions that arise are subjects of many newspaper and magazine articles. Nurses, too, think about their own reproductive ability and the possibility of bearing a defective infant. Facing the crisis of the birth of a defective infant is upsetting. Negative feelings of disgust and physical withdrawal from the infant are normal reactions. Many questions arise: Did the mother or father do or take something that predetermined the defect? Is an extensive, costly rehabilitation period worthwhile? In the case of some defects, the repulsion of seeing the infant is so overwhelming to the entire personnel involved in the care of the baby that the mother is left isolated from all but minimal care. A cognitive approach to the understanding of intrauterine defects is an essential basis for a nursing care plan. An understanding of the feelings that arise within nurses, the family, and ward personnel is essential before nursing intervention can be considered. Feelings about defective infants are a part of everyone and need to be expressed and discussed. The feelings of the nurse need to be overtly expressed in order for the parents and family to receive the help which they need.

Interdisciplinary Team Approach

An interdisciplinary team approach to the care of the infant and his family is primary. Frequently intensive, supportive medical, and/or surgical care may be needed over a period of years. The availability of nutritional, physical therapy, social, and nursing care services must be provided for the infant and his family in the hospital and the community. Each member of the team can contribute toward total care when there is mutual respect among the team members. The family in its initial shock and grief may reach out to or withdraw from the individual team members. Sensitivity to what is happening to the mother and family is of prime importance in assessing the needs of the family at this time. Individual team members also can derive support from each other in order to help the family.

The Nurse as a Member of the Interdisciplinary Team

The nurse is often in an enviable position in relation to patient care and may be the only member of the team who gives direct nursing care to the infant, his mother, and father. Observation, formulation, implementation, and evaluation of a nursing care plan for the mother and infant are essential. Elements of the nursing care plan for the infant can be demonstrated and discussed with the mother. Initially, the mother will be timid about the care of her infant. Her concerns about the physical appearance and care of her baby may intensify her feelings about producing a defective infant. She will need patience and understanding from the nurse and repeated demonstrations of care. As a team member, the nurse will have knowledge of the condition of the infant and the mother may need help in cognitively grasping what is wrong with her infant. An initial explanation about the infant's condition may not have been heard or understood by the mother and family. Repeated explanations are often necessary. The mother must be allowed the opportunity to express her fears and concerns about the infant. Misinformation can be cleared up and added information can be given. As a helping person, the nurse must be prepared for the negative responses and irrational attitudes of the mother and family. These expressions need to be placed in a rational context by understanding and clarifying the issues.

In times of crisis, people reach out to others for comfort and support. The ways in which mothers reach out at this time may differ from mother to mother. She may, in turn, accept and reject those who are helping her. Understanding what the mother is experiencing at the time will enable the nurse to provide the supportive nursing care needed. As a member of the team, the nurse's caring role will be an essential ingredient in providing humanistic care to the mother, infant, and the family.

INTRAUTERINE GROWTH DEVIATIONS WHICH AFFECT STRUCTURE OR FUNCTION

The birth of a child is never an isolated, solitary event. As the umbilical cord is cut, it is replaced by other ties that bind each infant to his parents, the community, and society. This is particularly true in the case of a child born with a birth defect or anomaly.

There are about 250,000 infants born each year with significant intrauterine growth deviations which affect structure as well as function, and these defects are second only to accidents as a cause of death in childhood. It is a significant public health problem when one considers the rehabilitation, education, and the sequential surgical procedures these infants and children undergo in the process of survival. They spend approximately 6 million days in hospitals each year, at costs exceeding $180,000,000.

Indeed, our society faces a tremendous dilemma. As sophisticated diagnostic tools identify severe defects more readily, surgical interventions improve technically, and antibiotic therapy expands, the survival rate has increased. Although medically or surgically complicated at intervals, now these infants and children can live useful, productive lives. The demands made and the challenges presented to nurses and other members of a health team are overwhelming, but the rewards and satisfactions experienced in working with these children and their parents are most gratifying.

It is important to remember that the prognosis of these infants and children has changed drastically. For verification one need only review the mortality figures of 10 or 15 years ago. A contributing factor in reducing the death rate has been the mobilization of an interdisciplinary team approach. Another issue which has been identified is the interaction of the financial, social, and psychological problems of handicapping. They are no longer ignored or dismissed, for they affect each member of the family in some way. The interdisciplinary team can greatly enhance resolution through realistic guidance, support, and understanding. The nurse who works so closely with these infants and their families is a logical coordinator of team-related activities.

Unfortunately these particular intrauterine growth deviations occur frequently and contribute substantially to infant morbidity and mortality. Prevention, detection, and management appear to be of paramount importance. Better health care, a more effective, coordinated team approach, and more realistic operational long-term planning are imperative in meeting the needs of these children, their parents, and society.

For the purposes of clarity the authors wish to define a congenital anomaly as a defect of body structure or function present at birth and noted upon the routine inspection of an infant in the delivery room or newborn nursery. In utilizing this definition particular abnormalities such as the inborn errors of metabolism, mental retardation, or those anomalies which manifest themselves later in life have been purposefully excluded. However, in view of current practice in newborn nurseries, it is essential that phenylketonuria be discussed.

Birth defects or congenital anomalies may be divided into two categories. A major anomaly is one serious enough to cause death or result in severe handicapping of the infant, and examples are meningomyeloceles or a severe form of cyanotic congenital heart disease such as transposition of the great vessels. On the other hand, a minor anomaly such as a club foot or syndactyly will not prove to be a serious impediment to a normal life or the realization of a full life expectancy.

The Known Causes of Birth Defects

Most human malformations are believed to be due to an interaction of both genetic and environmental influences—a combination of all internal factors present in the fertilized egg, and all external factors which may affect its growth in utero. At the present time 1 percent of the causes of these abnormalities can be attributed to specific teratogenic agents (viruses, irradiation, drugs), while gross chromosomal abnormalities account for 9 percent of the total. This leaves 90 percent that cannot be explained. It is staggering to imagine that a quarter of a million infants are born with anomalies each year and that the cause is known in only 10 percent of the cases.

It is important to remember that developmentally the fetus is most susceptible to teratogenesis at three crucial stages. The first is during oogenesis; the second is during the period of late blastula and early gastrula formation when the initial differentiation of presumptive organ regions is made and the three germ layers (endodermal, mesodermal, and ectodermal) are established. The last critical stage is whenever a major organ or system is being developed.

There is intense intracellular metabolic activity during these phases. Any harmful agents introduced which do not destroy the entire embryo exert some effect upon the anatomic or physiological processes being developed.

VIRAL INFECTIONS

Rubella

The role of viruses as possible teratogenic agents first became evident in 1941 during an epidemic in Australia when Gregg reported large numbers of children born with certain abnormalities to mothers who had had rubella early in their pregnancies. According to the National Foundation, the rubella epidemic which swept across the United States in 1964 caused some 50,000 abnormal pregnancies, resulting in some 20,000 live-born babies with birth defects and about 30,000 fetal deaths.

These pregnant women who had rubella during their first trimester gave birth to infants with congenital heart disease, cataracts, deafness, and developmental brain anomalies as well as mental retardation. With the isolation of the rubella virus from human fetal tissue in 1963, subsequent research has indicated the persistence of the virus in a chronic state in the newborn infant. It has continued to be isolated from urine and conjunctival smears from 18 months to 2 years after an infant's birth. Such information has grave implications for pregnant women with whom these infants may come in contact as well as for pediatric areas and personnel caring for them during hospitalization.

The effect of the rubella virus upon the embryo has been confirmed and conclusively demonstrates its lethal character. Yet to be proven or disproven is the theory proposed by some investigators that infants conceived 1 year or more after their mothers had been infected by rubella were born malformed.[2] Is there a rubella carrier state mothers assume which is hazardous to subsequent pregnancies? Some physicians advise women not to become pregnant until 18 months after exposure.

Cytomegalovirus

Another virus which is associated with chronic infection in man is the cytomegalovirus, which crosses the placental barrier and initiates a chronic infection in the developing fetus. There is no definitive evidence to indicate the period in pregnancy when the embryo is most susceptible.

Cytomegalovirus has been known to cause hydrocephalus, microcephalus, focal cerebral dysfunctions, mental retardation, deafness, and optic atrophy in addition to visceral and skeletal malformation. Very little is known of transmission. Cytomegalic inclusion disease is more common than rubella but is probably not as devastating to the fetus.

Coxsackie Virus

A longitudinal study in Michigan has most recently pointed to the hazards of Coxsackie virus infections during the first trimester of a pregnancy. Mothers who demonstrated Coxsackie virus, Type B in serological studies delivered offspring with various cardiovascular anomalies.[3] At this time it appears that the cardiovascular system is the only one affected.

The rubella virus and cytomegalovirus have been repeatedly documented as influencing forces upon the developing embryo. The results of the Michigan study implicating the Coxsackie virus are being accepted as valid and reliable. Although other viruses such as mumps and influenza have also been linked with deformities, this has not been absolutely proven.

Knowledge regarding malformations due to viral infections is meager. There are many questions still to be answered. Why do certain viruses cross placental barriers to produce these intrauterine growth deviations? How can a virus as innocuous as rubella be responsible for such devastating handicaps? How are they able to produce chronic infections in the presence of antibodies in the fetus and newborn?

CONGENITAL SYPHILIS

Syphilis continues to be a major concern for those interested in and responsible for community health. Congenital syphilis is passed from the pregnant woman to the fetus through the placenta. Transplacental infection by *Treponema pallidum* before the sixteenth week has not been documented; therefore, it is believed that this fetal infection occurs after the midgestational period. Although there is a greater incidence of abortions in infected pregnant women, it is also important to note that these women have eight times the normal number of stillborns.[4] Penicillin is the most frequently used drug for treatment of syphilis. Treatment of the pregnant woman through the second trimester effects the cure of the fetus, and results in the third trimester are almost always excellent. Most states require serologic examinations of all pregnant women. An important step in eradication is to check pregnant women not only in early pregnancy but in the last trimester.

There are two clinical forms of congenital syphilis—early in children under two years, and *late*, beyond the age of two. Early congenital syphilis is often characterized by cutaneous or mucous membrane lesions, often vesicular or bullous, particularly involving the palms of the hands and the soles of the feet. Hepatosplenomegaly, pseudoparalysis or painful limbs, anemia, jaundice, and rhinitis are some of the most common symptoms presented by a newborn with congenital syphilis.

It is apparent that early treatment of the pregnant woman with syphilis can eradicate the problem of congenital syphilis.

DRUGS

In 1961–1962, thousands of German infants were born with gross abnormalities involving all extremities, as extensive as total absence of limbs, complete phocomelia, or any variation thereof. Subsequent investigations revealed that practically all the mothers who delivered these children had taken the sedative Thalidomide during the early part of their pregnancies. In this instance the relationship between the medication and the deformities was conclusive. As a result of this tragedy the United States Food and Drug Administration tightened regulations pertaining to drug approval. The most important lesson learned was that no pregnant woman should take any drugs without the approval of her physician.

There are investigations regarding the use of hallucinogenic substances in pregnancy and the delivery of a deformed infant; however, the published reports are conflicting in the conclusions reached. Zellweger et al. have reported chromatid breaks in peripheral white cells of LSD (lysergic acid diethylamide) users and the delivery of babies with malformed legs.[5] On the other hand, Gardner et al. have collected data which reveal no damage to chromosomes of mothers who admitted using LSD and who also delivered infants with abnormalities.[6] It appears that the collection and careful analysis of data on lysergic acid intake in relation to the condition of the infant at birth are needed before the question of whether LSD has teratogenic properties in man can be answered. At this time, the information, the observations, the data are too scanty to be considered reliable.

Most of the studies related to the use of methamphetamines and the incidence of anomalies have been confined to animal research in which a causal relationship has been demonstrated. One group of investigators revealed a 38 percent frequency of anomalies, including defects of the heart, central nervous system, skeletal system, and face. Nora et al. in 1967 clearly stated there was no causal relationship between maternal dexamphetamine ingestion and congenital heart disease, but in continuing their study at Baylor they have reconsidered their statement and now urge a large-scale investigation of the drug and its effects. They appear to have doubt regarding the nonexistence of a relationship.[7]

It should be obvious that the investigation of teratogenic agents is extraordinarily difficult. An additional explanation for the lack of clear-cut evidence regarding the influence of a drug upon the developing embryo and fetus is that the possible teratogen may also produce an abnormality only in an individual with a hereditary predisposition. Evidence must support a causal relationship between the drug taken in pregnancy and its adverse effect upon the infant delivered.

RADIATION

There is absolutely no doubt that radiation causes somatic damage to the embryo and fetus. There is an extreme susceptibility to the effects of radiation, particularly in the earliest phases of neural development, for this is the period of major organogenesis. The period from 2 to 6 weeks is probably the most damaging, but unfortunately this is also the period during which the pregnancy may be unsuspected. A classic study frequently referred to in the literature found that 11 of 11 fetuses irradiated in the first 2 months of a pregnancy showed extensive damage; 7 of 11 irradiated between 3 and 5 months demonstrated defects, and 3 out of 13 fetuses exposed between the sixth and ninth months were abnormal at delivery. It should be apparent that exposure at later stages of gestation may cause less obvious deviations.

Among the most common kinds of growth deviations noted in infants irradiated in utero include microcephaly, anencephaly, microphthalmia, cataracts, mental retardation, midline defects of the central nervous system such as meningoceles, and other diverse skull malformations.

These grave consequences should be considered when radiation procedures are carried out upon a pregnant woman. For example, radioisotope studies should not be done during the second half of a menstrual cycle because of the possibility of an unsuspected early pregnancy. Husbands may also experience chromosomal damage. If a physician is conscious of severe fetal damage which might have occurred, his patient should be advised. Her right to a therapeutic abortion should be respected.[8]

Environmental irradiation or radiocontamination also contributes to concern regarding the causes of deformities. This is a frustrating area, for there is little human control over atmospheric contamination which occurs after testing nuclear weapons or nuclear accidents. The anomalous effects of environmental radiocontamination have been most dramatically documented since the Nagasaki and Hiroshima nuclear blasts.

Identifiable Intrauterine Growth Deviations Involving the Nervous System

When one considers the various internal and external forces which influence the embryo, in addition to the complexities associated with the differentiation of tissue, it is no wonder that intrauterine growth deviations occur. Midline anomalies of the central nervous system are usually identified as major birth defects. The most commonly seen are spina bifida occulta, meningocele, myelomeningocele (meningomyelocele), and myelocele.

The etiology of these developmental defects is unknown. Since the closure of the neural tube is completed in the embryo by the fourth week of gestation, these midline neurological conditions must occur at that time.

SPINA BIFIDA

Spina bifida occulta results from the incomplete fusion of the spines and laminae which constitute the neural arch of the vertebrae, without an external protrusion of the intraspinal contents. They are most commonly found in the lower segment of the back, although they may occur anywhere along the vertebral column.

A protrusion through the spina bifida which forms a soft, sac-like appearance along the spinal axis is a meningocele which contains cerebrospinal fluid and meninges within the sac. An even more severe defect is a myelomeningocele (meningomyelocele) which is also an external protrusion including fluid and meninges in addition to the spinal cord and/or nerve roots. (See Figure 35-1.)

Meningoceles and myelomeningoceles are covered by a thin, transparent membrane and a thicker, irregular epithelium or normal skin. The neurological manifestations accompanying a meningocele are generally slight, but the symptoms associated with a meningomyelocele vary, depending upon the extent of the defect as well as the site of the mass. Observing an infant with a meningomyelocele a nurse notices the constant dribbling of urine, the absence of sphincter control, and deformities of the feet, indicative of extensive damage.

The location of the deviation determines the extent of neuromuscular involvement, particularly of the lower extremities. There may be paralysis, flaccidity, spasticity, or no involvement whatsoever. Differentiating a meningocele from a meningomyelocele may be dependent upon the nurse's astute observation of symptoms being presented by the newborn. (See Figure 35-2.)

A myelocele, the most severe of defects associated with spina bifida occulta, is a mass of nervous tissue representative of underdeveloped embryonic

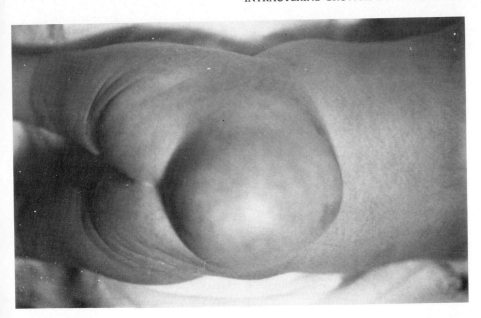

FIGURE 35-1
Sacral meningocele. *(Courtesy of The University of Colorado Medical Center, Denver, Colorado)*

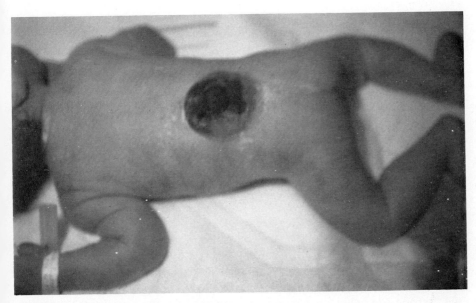

FIGURE 35-2
Lumbar myelomeningocele. *(Courtesy of The University of Colorado Medical Center, Denver, Colorado)*

tissue, which appears as a disorganized, protuberant ulceration along the back. Although it is surgically correctable, it may be incompatible with life.

Nursing Responsibilities

These neurological conditions, if amenable to surgery, are corrected in the early days of life. In the period before correction, the infant must be handled most cautiously. Rupture, infection, irritation or leakage from the sac are all possible, and as such, they are life-threatening to the newborn. Careful handling and avoiding any pressure over the mass as well as positioning become extremely important measures for nursery personnel to perform conscientiously.

Head circumference is taken and recorded daily. The anterior fontanel should be checked frequently for symptoms of increasing tension, indicative of developing hydrocephalus. Neurological evaluation of sphincter control can be realized through observation and by recording the character and number of voidings and stools. These infants' nutritional needs must also be met, but whether the baby may be held for feedings will depend upon the physician's preference and the nurse's confidence in her handling ability.

Skin care is important, too, particularly around the sac and surrounding skin. The specific care associated with the deformity and the use of a dressing or a topical ointment will again depend upon the neurosurgeon's orders.

HYDROCEPHALUS

Another neurological abnormality noted at delivery is hydrocephalus, which is characterized by an abnormal increase in cerebrospinal fluid volume within the intracranial cavity. (See Figure 35-3.) Unless otherwise stipulated, hydrocephalus refers to internal hydrocephalus in which the fluid accumulates under pressure within the ventricles.

There are two differentiations which must be made for the sake of clinical clarity. Noncommunicating, or obstructive, internal hydrocephalus is an obstruction within the ventricles which prevents the fluid from entering the subarachnoid space. Communicating internal hydrocephalus occurs when the obstruction is located in the subarachnoid cisterns at the base of the brain and/or within the subarachnoid space.

The head of an infant with this growth deviation may be normal or just slightly enlarged at birth. The suture lines are wide, and the anterior fontanel, which may be bulging, is also broader and wider than usually felt in the newborn. The bridge of the nose may also be flat and broad in addition to the forehead having a bulging appearance. As the fluid increases there may be a downward displacement of the eyes, which is frequently referred to as the "setting sun" sign. In severe form, the head size increases rapidly, the infant's cry is shrill and high-pitched, and the baby is irritable and restless. In

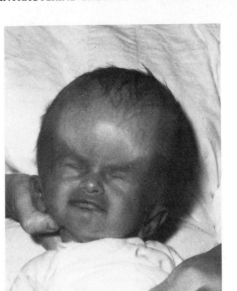

FIGURE 35-3
Hydrocephalus. (*Courtesy of The University of Colorado Medical Center, Denver, Colorado*)

some instances, increase in head circumference can be arrested through a successful ventricular shunt.

Nursing Responsibilities

As in the case of infants with other neurological problems, careful observation is imperative. Head circumference measurements and size and fullness of the anterior fontanel should be recorded, and any changes in behavior should be reported.

An adequate nutritional intake is essential, but when an infant is irritable or vomiting, feedings may become a problem. In such instances techniques should vary and be flexible in meeting the needs of the individual baby. Small, frequent feedings are sometimes much more effective than adhering to rigid nursery routines.

Positioning may be a potential problem, particularly when the head is growing rapidly, and the infant is prone to developing bed sores. Frequent changes, a meticulously dry and clean bassinet, and the use of lamb's wool will deter skin breakdown. It is also important that the infant be turned cautiously, for the increase in head size can place an additional strain on the baby's neck.

All of these infants have very specific needs, and in meeting them nurses occasionally become involved in the management of care. These newborns have very definite emotional needs which are sometimes overlooked, particularly if the defect is large, and the nurse is hesitant in handling the baby. Dexterity comes through experience, and the physical contact the infant may enjoy when being held in one's lap or in being cuddled is so important. Such an endeavor may support and encourage others to do likewise.

Identifiable Intrauterine Growth Deviations Involving the Gastrointestinal System

CLEFT LIP AND PALATE

Cleft lip or a cleft palate is one of the more frequently seen anomalies which involves the upper lip or palate. The fusion of maxillary or premaxillary processes normally occurs between the fifth and the eighth weeks of embryonic development. The palatal processes fuse about 1 month later. Incomplete fusion results in a cleft lip, a cleft palate, or both (Figures 35-4 and 35-5).

The incidence of this impaired fusion is about 1 in 800 births. As with other growth deviations, the specific cause is unknown; however, some studies indicate a strong genetic influence.

A cleft lip (harelip) is seen more frequently in males, varying in severity from a small notch to a total separation extending into the floor of the nose.

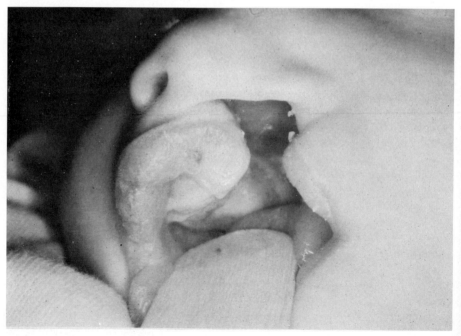

FIGURE 35-4
Unilateral cleft lip and palate.

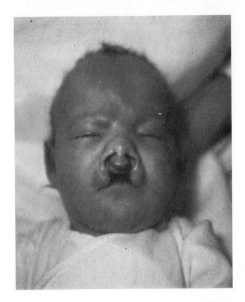

FIGURE 35-5
Bilateral cleft lip and palate. *(Courtesy of
The University of Colorado Medical Cen-
ter, Denver, Colorado)*

Unilateral or bilateral, these clefts usually involve the dental ridges, hence
additional anomalies of deformed, supernumerary, or absent teeth present
themselves later in a child's development.

A cleft palate occurring alone or in association with a cleft lip is seen
more frequently in females. This malformation may involve only the uvula or
may extend into or through the soft and hard palates. When seen with a cleft
lip the defect may involve the midline of the soft palate and extend into the
hard palate, exposing one or both sides of the nasal cavities, depending on
whether it is a unilateral or bilateral cleft palate.

Nursing Responsibilities

The role of the nursery nurse in caring for an infant with these problems is
defined by the plastic surgeon who will be repairing the lip or palate. Maintenance of an adequate nutritional state is the most immediate problem. If
only the lip is involved, surgical repair may be done soon after birth. Should
the anomaly be extensive, however, surgery may be delayed and the lip repaired at 6 to 8 weeks of age, while the palate may not be repaired for 12 to
15 months or longer. The operative schedule depends upon the infant's physical status and the surgeon's preference. (See Figure 35-6.)

An important aspect of newborn care then will be teaching the parents
how to feed their baby. It is best to feed these infants in a sitting position
with any one of the several varieties of nipples or syringes available. These
include a soft, cross-cut rubber nipple, a cleft palate nipple, or a "duck bill"

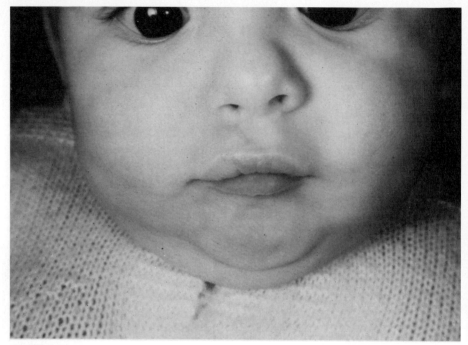

FIGURE 35-6
Successful repair of right unilateral cleft lip.

nipple. Some plastic surgeons prefer to use a rubber-tipped syringe or medicine cup at least until the lip is repaired. Should a syringe or medicine cup be used, it is important to remember to direct the flow of formula toward the side of the mouth, thereby decreasing the possibility of aspiration. Since these babies cannot create suction, they tend to become irritable and frustrated in their attempts to feed. Regardless of the feeding method used, the rate of flow of the formula must be adjusted to each individual baby.

Since these infants characteristically swallow large amounts of air, frequent burping is essential. Rest periods should be provided in order to avoid tiring the infant. When a mother begins to feed her baby, reassurance, patience, and the understanding of nursery personnel are important components of this learning situation. A mother frequently finds herself "all thumbs"—frightened at the prospect of feeding her baby, and yet she must learn, for feeding will be her responsibility at discharge. The initial clumsiness will be overcome once the infant's sucking attempts are coordinated with the formula being given, and the mother will become more comfortable and more confident in her ability to care for the baby. Praise and encouragement from the nurse will help reduce the parents' anxiety.

TRACHEOESOPHAGEAL FISTULA

A problem detected before or at the time an infant is given his first fluids by mouth is a tracheoesophageal fistula, possibly accompanied by an esophageal atresia. In the embryo, by the fourth week the laryngotracheal groove develops into the larynx, trachea, and primordial lung tissue, while the esophagus is elongated as the heart and lungs push the stomach caudally. By the eighth week the esophageal lumen is formed. Various anomalies occur as a result of the failure of these processes to be completed correctly.

The most common form of esophageal atresia and tracheoesophageal fistula seen in about 90 percent of the cases is the upper portion of the esophagus ending in a blind pouch at or just above the bifurcation of the trachea, while the lower portion from the stomach is connected to the trachea by a short, fistular tract.

Tracheoesophageal fistula is sometimes associated with polyhydramnios which alerts personnel to observe these infants more closely.

Nursing Responsibilities

One of the nurse's primary responsibilities in caring for newborn infants is accurate astute observation and being able to differentiate normal from pathological conditions.

Some of the symptoms indicative of a tracheoesophageal fistula which the nurse can observe are excessive mucus or constant drooling from the corner of the mouth. When the infant is fed for the first time, the nurse notes that the first swallow or two is normal, but suddenly the fluid returns through his nose and mouth, the baby is coughing, gagging, cyanotic, and struggling for breath. He may even stop breathing. A second attempt to feed results in the same sequence of events.

Since early diagnosis is imperative and surgical intervention is the only definitive treatment, early nursing assessment of the infant's status is essential. Even though immediate surgery is desirable, complications such as pnuemonia, dehydration, or electrolyte imbalance may delay action until the surgical risk is reduced.

The baby is kept in an upright position to avoid leaking of gastric juices into the trachea and lungs. Gentle suctioning is used to remove mucus from the mouth and esophagus. These infants are usually placed in incubators and receive humidified oxygen. The episodes of respiratory difficulty can be relieved, and the viscosity of the secretions be decreased. Antibiotics and intravenous therapy are initiated in the preoperative period.

The uneventful recovery of these infants depends upon cooperative planning and skill of the health team.

IMPERFORATE ANUS

Abdominal distention or the absence of meconium may be indicative of an obstruction of the intestinal tract. Embryologically the differentiation of tissue and the separation into two closed systems, dorsally the rectum and ventrally the bladder and urethra, occur by the eighth week. Interference with development of the anal-rectal structures gives rise to a variety of anomalies. Although the true incidence of imperforate anus is unknown, it is estimated that about 1 in 1,000 infants needs some major surgical correction. (See Figure 35-7.)

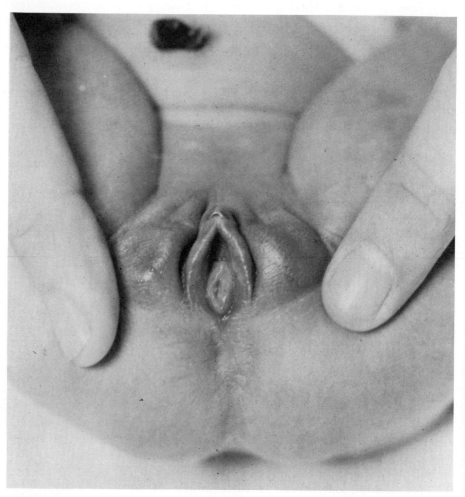

FIGURE 35-7
Imperforate anus.

The diagnosis is made when no anal opening is found, there is no passage of meconium, the nurse cannot insert a small gloved finger into the rectal canal, or she feels the "blind pouch" of the cavity. Later abdominal distention develops. It is not uncommon for a tracheoesophageal fistula to be accompanied by an imperforate anus.

Nursing Responsibilities

The diagnosis can be made by observation, insertion of a thermometer, or by digital examination. Observation of the newborn permits the detection of the anomaly, unless it is the simple type, having a thin membrane covering the anal orifice, which can be diagnosed on delivery.

Occasionally a nurse does not suspect an obstruction for a day or two after delivery. This gross oversight can be prevented through a thorough digital examination at birth. The absence of meconium coupled with some abdominal distention may be the first clues given by the infant to indicate some intestinal obstruction. X rays reveal the extent of the malformation and permit the surgeon to plan the most appropriate intervention.

OMPHALOCELE

Occasionally, on delivery an infant appears to have a protrusion of abdominal contents into the base of the umbilical cord at the point of juncture of the umbilical cord and the abdomen. The herniation, which is usually covered with a thin peritoneum is called an omphalocele, and occurs in 1 out of 6,500 deliveries. (See Figure 35-8.)

The persistence of the embryonic stage of development between the seventh and tenth week of fetal life has resulted in varying amounts of abdominal viscera lying within the umbilical cord. The diagnosis is made at delivery, when it is also observed that the abdominal cavity appears to be proportionately small owing to the arrest in development.

Nursing Responsibilities

Careful handling of the omphalocele is one of nursing's most important functions. For survival it is essential that infection, rupture, or drying of the peritoneal sac does not occur.

These infants are usually repaired soon after delivery. Pediatric surgeons frequently pass a nasogastric tube which is attached to low intermittent suction to prevent abdominal distention. There is usually an order to keep the omphalocele covered with sterile towels or sterile sponges (without cotton fill), keeping either one moist with sterile saline solution until the infant is transferred to the operating room. Monitoring vital signs, keeping the involved area covered and moist, and checking the suction apparatus are important nursing procedures.

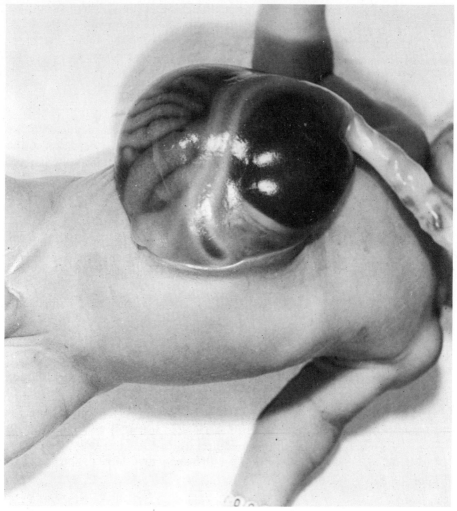

FIGURE 35-8
Omphalocele.

Identifiable Intrauterine Growth Deviations Involving the Genitourinary Tract

Malformations of the genitourinary system are common; however, many of them do not produce any symptoms or disturbances in function during the neonatal period. These are usually demonstrated as the infant grows and develops.

EXSTROPHY OF THE BLADDER

One deviation in intrauterine growth involving the genitourinary tract which is readily identified at birth is exstrophy of the bladder (Figure 35-9). Characterized by an absent anterior wall over the bladder area, there may be a complete or partial exposure of bladder mucosa. The exposed mucosa is bright red, has numerous folds and is most sensitive to touch. In the male, anomalies such as an undescended testes, a short penis, epispadias, and inguinal hernias may also be present. These conditions compound parental concern.

Nursing Responsibilities

The anomaly is obvious at birth. There is urine seepage onto the abdominal wall from the involved structures. Excoriation of the surrounding skin may occur, and there is also the constant odor of urine. Ulceration of the exposed

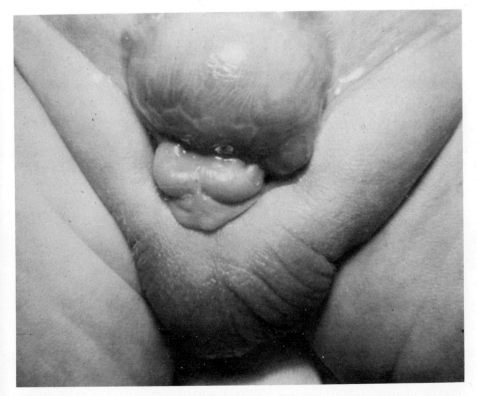

FIGURE 35-9
Exstrophy of the bladder.

bladder mucosa may occur. Good hygiene and good skin care are also necessary to prevent any infections from developing, for such an occurrence may involve the kidneys.

Each infant is different, and depending upon the extent of the deformity as well as the surgical timetable, parents are sometimes taught to care for their infants before the operative procedure is done. Seeing the exstrophy initially, mothers usually become frightened and distressed. Cleansing the skin around the defect may be particularly difficult for them to do. The parents' dexterity in handling the baby as well as their ability to retain their composure whenever viewing the exstrophy comes with experience and time.

For the nurse the emphasis should be on prevention of infections or the formation of ulcerations on the mucosa. This can be accomplished by placing sterile petrolatum gauze dressings over the exposed area. Stool contamination and urine odor retention can be avoided by frequent diaper changes. Diapers should be loosely applied to avoid any pressure over the exposed bladder.

Care given in the nursery and clearly demonstrated to a mother, coupled with a relaxed atmosphere which is conducive to questions, frequently reduces the stress and anxiety experienced by the mother. With the acceptance, encouragement, and understanding of the nurse, a mother begins to feel comfortable in caring for her baby.

HYPOSPADIAS

One of the most common malformations of the male genitourinary system is hypospadias, in which the urethral orifice is ventral and posterior to its normal opening. While the meatus usually occurs near the glans, it may occur anywhere along the shaft of the penis. If the infant should void while he is in the delivery room, the defect could be identified then, otherwise it may go undetected until a voiding is actually observed.

Nursing Responsibilities

The care associated with this intrauterine deviation does not differ from that given to other babies in the nursery. Physical complications may be minimal; however, the social, financial, and psychological implications may be many. The nurse should be prepared to answer parents' questions honestly and realistically so that they can plan for the future welfare of the child.

Identifiable Intrauterine Growth Deviations Involving the Circulatory System

The circulatory system does not escape anomalous formation in utero; however, these defects are not usually noted at birth or in a few days following delivery. Cyanosis may not be manifested until the ductus arteriosus begins to close. Infants at three to six weeks of age may be admitted to pediatric units with rapid respirations, no weight gain, tachycardia, and signs of congestive heart failure.

TRANSPOSITION OF THE GREAT VESSELS

A condition which usually occurs in infants large for gestational age and diagnosed during the first few days of life is transposition of the great vessels. The primary symptom which manifests itself soon after delivery is cyanosis. In transposition of the great vessels the aorta arises from the right ventricle, and the pulmonary arteries from the left ventricle. With the systemic veins returning to the right atrium and the pulmonary veins emptying into the left atrium, two independent circuits are present. This condition is incompatible with life unless the foramen ovale or ductus arteriosus remains open or there is an intraventricular or intraatrial septal defect.

Nursing Responsibilities

Cyanosis may not be present at delivery; therefore, observation of the infant in the nursery is important. The rapid respirations, dyspnea, and cyanosis are the initial symptoms presented. When the infant is fed for the first time the nurse notes that the sucking reflex is poor and that the respirations are rapid and may be in excess of 80 or 100 per minute. The baby's color is dusky and not the pink that is characteristic of newborns. He appears to be so busy breathing, he is unable to eat.

The diagnosis is made early and a septostomy or surgical intervention occurs soon after confirmation. The time spent in the nursery before any procedure is done is most important to that baby's survival. Astute observations are essential, for his condition changes rapidly.

Congestive heart failure may occur, and the nurse should be aware of the manifestations. Poor sucking, rapid respirations, and increasing cyanosis together with sudden weight gain, edema, and retractions and nasal flaring are indicative of the infant's deteriorating condition.

The problem of feeding becomes a major issue for the nurse. The infant tires easily and is utterly exhausted as he attempts to suck. More frequent feedings, a high-calorie formula, and frequent rest periods will permit a more sufficient intake. It will not be unusual for the nurse to take as long as 45 minutes to feed the infant, but it is imperative that she take the time in order to ensure adequate nutrition.

If diuretics are being given, weight should be checked accurately at 8-hour intervals and the urinary output carefully noted, for both will indicate the success of the therapy to the cardiologist. In administering a digitalis preparation in the digitalization process, vital signs should be monitored hourly. These nursing measures are applicable when adjusted and individualized to meet the needs of the infant with other forms of congenital heart disease.

TETRALOGY OF FALLOT

Another cardiac condition which may be present, but which may not necessarily manifest itself in the delivery room or in the newborn nursery, is tetralogy of Fallot. The presence of pulmonary stenosis, a ventricular septal defect, dextroposition of the aorta, and a right ventricular hypertrophy constitute this congenital heart disease.

Hemodynamically, as the right ventricle contracts, resistance at the pulmonary stenosis shunts unoxygenated blood across the ventricular septal defect into the aorta. The persistent arterial unsaturated state results in cyanosis. It is the most common condition accompanied by persistent cyanosis and accounts for three-fourths of the cyanotic congenital heart diseases in children over the age of one year. The nurse should remember, however, that the cyanosis which is characteristic of this disease may not be present at birth, for as long as the ductus arteriosus remains open sufficient blood flows through the lungs to prevent this manifestation.

The great strides made in cardiac surgery, both palliative and total corrective procedures, have resulted in lowering the mortality rate and improving the prognosis.

PULMONARY ATRESIA

In this anomalous condition, cyanosis generally appears soon after birth, and as the heart progressively enlarges, congestive heart failure may occur. The presence of a small right ventricle and tricuspid valve results in blood entering the left atrium via the foramen ovale or an atrial septal defect. Generally the prognosis is poor.

PULMONARY STENOSIS

It is important for the nurse to remember that pulmonary stenosis may exist as a separate entity or with associated defects of the atrial or ventricular septum. In the commonest type of isolated pulmonic stenosis the valve cusps are dome-shaped, with a small central or eccentric opening. The obstruction to the blood flow from the right ventricle to the pulmonary artery results in an increased systolic pressure as well as a hypertrophy of the right ventricle. The symptoms vary according to the degree of stenosis from mild to severe. In the latter, peripheral cyanosis may be present. Prognosis is correlated with the severity of the condition.

The Role of the Nurse in Interhospital Transportation

The special nursing care of a neonate requiring surgery begins when the diagnosis is made and ends when the infant is returned to his parents. Early diagnosis increases the chance for survival, and the nurse's contributions to early detection of an anomaly cannot be underestimated.

Occasionally once the diagnosis is made these infants are transferred to larger, specialized pediatric areas where the surgery may be performed. In these instances, pertinent information should accompany the infant. The nurse who accompanies the baby is expected to share this information with the nursing personnel who will be assuming the responsibility of caring for the baby. Of particular value are the symptoms presented by the baby, the condition at the time of delivery, and the behavior of the baby in the nursery. Fathers who accompany their infants are usually so distraught they cannot be expected to relate information which medical personnel consider essential data.

Should it be impossible for a nurse to accompany the infant, then a detailed, written set of nursery notes sent with the baby will be helpful to the receiving nursing personnel. Still another alternative could be a phone call to the head nurse of the ward to which the child will be admitted. A nursing assessment and evaluation of an infant's condition is gratefully appreciated by those who will be directly involved in caring for the baby. It makes them aware of the infant's status before his arrival and permits the assembly of all necessary equipment essential to his care.

Frequently overlooked in the hurried arrangements for transfer is the operative permit, and the result is that surgery is sometimes delayed until legal permission is obtained. This is true when the father does not accompany the baby. Arrangements for telegram consents or other legal forms acceptable to the receiving hospital will facilitate the interhospital transfer.

Under ideal conditions a nurse accompanying the infant should find a vehicle properly equipped for such transportation. Oxygen and suction should be available and ready for use. The infant should be kept warm, properly positioned, and appropriate measures are taken to maintain fluid balance. His birth, the tests essential for diagnosis, and now his transferral to another hospital are all extremely traumatizing and contribute to his deteriorating physical status. We should never forget what this tiny individual is experiencing in his quest for survival.

Identifiable Intrauterine Growth Deviations Involving the Musculoskeletal System

There are two anomalies of the musculoskeletal system which are commonly seen in the newborn nursery, and they are easily diagnosed. In both instances early recognition and treatment is essential for successful correction.

The longer a condition goes unidentified, the more severe the deformity becomes, the more difficult the repair, and the less favorable the prognosis.

CONGENITAL DISLOCATION OF THE HIP

In the newborn, congenital dislocation of the hip usually exists as a potential dislocation rather than an actual dislocation. The hip joint which develops from mesoderm emerges at about the seventh embryonic week, but at birth the fetal, cartilaginous state persists. The delay in ossification seems to be due to insufficient pressure of the femoral head into the acetabulum during fetal life, thereby delaying ossification of the ball-and-socket joint.

It is found in females six times more frequently than in males, and unilateral dislocations are about twice as common as bilateral dislocations.

On examination of the infant there is an asymmetry of the gluteal and inguinal folds on the affected side. They appear to be higher than the folds on the unaffected side. A shortening of the involved leg is also evident. When the baby moves both legs the observant nurse notes there is less motion in the affected leg because of a limitation of abduction of the affected hip.

CONGENITAL CLUB FOOT

About 95 percent of the infants born with a club foot are of the *equinovarus* type. The entire foot is inverted, the heel is drawn up, and the forefoot is abducted. There is a deep transverse crease that is also seen on the sole of the foot. If the baby were able to walk, he would be walking on his ankle rather than the sole of his foot.

Occurring in 1 in 800 births, it is found twice as frequently in males as in females. This deformity of the foot is identified at birth; however, it must be differentiated from a positional deformity of the foot which can be attributed to an infant's position in utero.

Nursing Responsibilities

A nurse is in a unique position to detect these particular problems in the nursery. As the newborn is cared for the nurse can note the height of the gluteal and inguinal folds, and can also contribute the information necessary to distinguish a positional deformity from a club foot. The parents will need information regarding the anomaly, but the nurse's emphasis should be upon the need for long-term follow-up. Of course, their questions should be answered honestly and in terms readily understandable.

Identifiable Metabolic and Chromosomal Deviations in the Newborn

PHENYLKETONURIA

The disease known as phenylketonuria (PKU) is an inborn error of metabolism which, without treatment, results in mental retardation. Phenylalanine is an essential amino acid present in all protein foods. The primary biochemical defect in PKU is the absence of the liver enzyme phenylalanine hydroxylase which transforms phenylalanine to tyrosine, permitting further metabolism. In a child with PKU, the excessive phenylalanine is unable to be converted to tyrosine, and it builds up in the tissues, including the brain, and spills into the urine as phenylpyruvic acid, phenylacetic acid, orthohydroxyphenylacetic acid, and the excessive phenylalanine.

If this metabolic disorder is present, as a newborn takes in food there should be an accumulation of phenylalanine. A simple blood test which involves a heel puncture permits an early diagnosis. There are also some health care facilities which utilize urine analyses for the detection. Regardless of the method, testing is usually done about the third day, and it is mandatory in most states. This is the example of an instance in which mental retardation can be prevented by preventing phenylalanine intake from infancy. Substitute diets should be implemented immediately after confirmation so that the brain will be permitted to develop normally.

Nursing Responsibilities

The nurse's prime responsibility is to see that the appropriate blood or urine test is done before the baby is discharged from the nursery. Different hospitals have different procedures for collecting the appropriate sample. It is important that the test be done before the infant is discharged from the nursery, and that the infant has had 120 ml. of formula, 20 calories per 30 ml. prior to the blood work. Since this metabolic error is easily detected, it seems imperative that nursery nurses assume the responsibility of verifying the fact that appropriate tests have been done. Dietary management and the prevention of mental retardation can occur only through early detection.

Intrauterine Growth Deviations Affecting Birth Weight

The developing fetus is part of a delicately balanced biological unit which also includes the mother's environment, the mother, and the placenta. Any external and internal factors which affect any component of this integral unit are reflected in the neonate at delivery. Unfortunately, only a few of these adverse conditions are understood and can be associated with growth deviations in utero. These infants, whether small or large for their gestational age, account for the morbidity and mortality of the so-called high-risk infants.

INFANTS SMALL FOR GESTATIONAL AGE

About one-third of all newborns weighing less than 2,500 Gm are considered small for their gestational age and therefore represent another type of intrauterine growth deviation.[9] These are the infants identified in the literature as small for date, demonstrating fetal malnutrition, fetal undergrowth, or intrauterine growth retardation. Some authors term these infants dysmature in an effort to unify the various terms. Although the terminology may be confusing, it is important to remember that most of these infants weigh less than 2,500 Gm, or 5½ pounds. They have failed to achieve expected size for the duration of their gestational period, which may be 38 weeks or longer. The small-for-date infant differs greatly from the premature, who has developed normally but has failed to remain in utero long enough to achieve full-term size.

On visual examination these babies are long and thin, with dry skin and diminished skin turgor. They are much more active and alert than their premature counterparts. They have creases on their soles, and their hair is coarse, straight, and silky compared to the fine, fuzzy hair found in premature infants. The ear cartilage is also very well developed, with sharp ridges, and these small-for-date infants also have firm skull bones. When palpating the area around the anterior fontanel, it is hard and thick right up to the edge of the fontanel, not at all like the soft, cartilaginous feeling of a premature's skull bones. Lanugo is not found in infants demonstrating growth retardation.

Causes of Poor Fetal Growth

The weight of an infant at birth in relation to his gestational age portrays, to some extent, his intrauterine environment and the effects of maternal influences. Factors which affect growth may originate in the fetus, the mother, the placenta, or the mother's environment.

Congenital anomalies, such as congenital heart disease; chromosomal aberrations, such as Down's syndrome; and teratogenic, genetic, and metabolic diseases are frequently associated with reduced growth potentials. A causal relationship has been established between rubella and cytomegalovirus and small-for-date infants.

The pregnant woman's nutritional status has a primary influence upon the developing embryo, although it probably has little effect prior to the third trimester when requirements are relatively low. The most vulnerable women entering pregnancy are adolescents with poor eating habits. Such habits contribute substantially to the increase in severe preeclampsia as well as the increased incidence of small-for-gestational-age infants.[10]

It is important to remember that the fetus receives adequate nutrients from maternal sources during gestation, enabling him to build up stores of glycogen and fat late in pregnancy which will tide him over the period from birth to when he begins to feed. Should these stores be inadequate, an infant's glucose level falls as his available energy sources are mobilized, and hypoglycemia may occur.

Maternal infections which involve the fetus can occur through the placenta (transplacentally) or via the amniotic fluid. The former relates to the presence of the offending organism in the mother's bloodstream, while the latter refers to an ascending type of infection. Bacteria and fungi commonly infect the fetus via the amniotic cavity; viruses, protozoa, and spirochetes usually infect the fetus transplacentally.

Women with hypertensive cardiovascular and/or renal disease also may deliver infants who are small for their gestational age. Pregnant women at either end of the age spectrum tend to deliver smaller babies, as do women who have children at intervals of less than 2 years. Likewise, women who give birth at intervals of 6 years or more tend to deliver infants demonstrating fetal malnutrition.

In utero single infants and twins develop at the same rate until 29 to 32 weeks of gestation when the growth rate of twins slows down.[11] When fetal malnutrition occurs in a twin pregnancy, it usually does so in only one fetus. Such twin sets are of markedly different weights.

A third factor which affects growth is the placenta. Site of the implantation and its development, composition, and metabolism play an important role in fetal development. Some etiologic placental causes which interfere with the main nutritional supply line of the fetus include (1) limitation of uterine blood flow, (2) reduced maternal concentration of essential nutrients, (3) reduced effective area for placental exchange, and (4) impaired diffusion or active transport across placental membrane. All contribute to fetal malnutrition.[12]

There are some placental lesions which are potentially harmful to the developing fetus and result in small-for-date babies. The most common include an abnormal insertion of the cord, an abnormal placental outline, insufficient vascular patterns, and multiple infarctions. However, the ability to identify these causes of impaired placental transfer is most difficult—until the baby is born.

The pregnant woman's environment also exerts its influence upon the developing fetus. Women in low socioeconomic circumstances with little education and little or no antepartal care tend to deliver malnourished infants. Women who smoke as well as women who live at high elevation also tend to deliver infants with growth retardation.

Nursing Responsibilities

An initial nursing problem identified at birth is the limited ability of these infants to conserve heat. They are of small size and have a scanty amount of subcutaneous fat. However, they have a large surface area compared to their weight, they are wet, and the cool air-conditioned surroundings result in heat loss by evaporation, convection, and radiation. These environmental stresses can lead to a slower recovery from birth and an exhaustion of fat and glycogen stores, and increase the risk of hypoglycemia. All efforts must be taken to prevent heat loss.

The nurse should observe these infants carefully, particularly if feedings are not started early or tolerated well. Although active, vigorous babies free of tremors may develop hypoglycemia, generally these infants are jittery, listless, depressed, and occasionally they may have apneic episodes. A knowledge of the consequences of hypoglycemia, the degree of cerebral impairment, and its contribution to infant mortality and morbidity emphasizes the need for close nursing observation.

If the fetal malnutrition has been of long duration, heart failure may present itself after delivery. It is also important to note the number of voidings per day, for there may also be renal failure. Sometimes pediatricians order weights to be done on each nursing shift. It is essential to remember that the general condition of a small-for-gestational age infant is such that physical deterioration has long preceded birth, there are many systems involved, and careful examination is imperative.

Since these infants are usually difficult to feed, they are frequently on 3-hour feeding routines. It is interesting to note that there is an immediate weight gain which characteristically differentiates the malnourished infant from his premature counterpart. It suggests rehydration of a dehydrated state rather than actual tissue growth.

Sometimes these infants are placed on high-calorie formulas. Occasionally, diarrhea may develop because the ability of the intestinal tract to absorb is quite limited during the early days of life.

The nurse has a significant role in preventing complications. Protecting the infant from an initial, devastating heat loss, noting tremors, ensuring an adequate oral intake, and observing any changes in his behavior assist the small-for-gestational age infant in adjusting more satisfactorily to his new environment.

INFANTS LARGE FOR GESTATIONAL AGE

Infants delivered of diabetic mothers tend to be large for gestational age, and demonstrate still another growth deviation—the large-for-date baby. Fetal hyperinsulinism in response to maternal hyperglycemia is postulated as the cause of the large size of these infants. However, it does not explain the large size of babies delivered to prediabetic women. Longitudinal studies have indicated that women who delivered infants weighing 10 pounds or more developed diabetes later in life, and therefore the diabetic and prediabetic states pose a hazard to the developing fetus. Maternal corticotropin has also been suggested as contributing to the largeness and cushingoid features of these infants.

These babies frequently weigh more than 10 pounds, have round "cherub's" cheeks, and are large, plump, puffy looking with buried eyes, short necks, and red skin. Their overweight appearance is deceiving, for the maturity of these babies does not correspond to their actual weight, but to a lower weight.[12]

Mortality rates are quite high, as is the incidence of intrauterine death after 36 weeks. Some studies have indicated that the incidence of congenital anomalies is two to four times the expected rate. Anomalies of the lumbosacral region, such as meningomyelocele, occur most frequently. Interestingly enough, despite their large size, these infants seem to have an increased vulnerability to disease.

In the nursery these babies are restless, jittery, twitching, tremorous, hyperexcitable, and may have some cyanotic episodes. Hypoglycemia, hypocalcemia, respiratory distress, and hyperbilirubinemia are common. The increased perinatal mortality may be secondary to maternal ketosis, hydramnios, preeclampsia, and vascular degeneration, which are more common in the diabetic than the nondiabetic.

Nursing Responsibilities

Sometimes the babies of diabetic mothers are admitted directly to special care nurseries because of the high incidence of respiratory distress syndrome in these infants. In addition to the usual newborn appraisal, the nurse may assist the pediatrician in aspirating gastric contents, a procedure routinely performed on these infants.

Vital signs are monitored at least every hour, and strict attention is given to the physical status of the infant. Tremors, hyperirritability, cyanosis, and restlessness are detected and reported immediately.

Feedings of glucose and water are started 2 to 3 hours after delivery. If seizure activity is noted, intravenous glucose may be started after blood sugar levels are drawn. In these instances intravenous therapy may continue until the baby is taking fluids well by mouth.

These infants are a challenge to the nurse working in a nursery, for the baby's physical status may change rapidly; the happiness enjoyed by a diabetic mother, however, in taking her infant home is the result of the nurses' conscientious efforts.

SUMMARY AND CONCLUSIONS

The authors have presented content relevant to deviations in intrauterine growth. Material presented covered anomalies in structure and function as well as birth weight. The particular deviations presented are those commonly seen in the neonatal period. This is *not* to say that anomalies do not present themselves later on in life. It is imperative that nurses be cognizant of this fact.

Advancements in technology, diagnostic procedures, and the field of genetics have necessitated an exploration of the role of the nurse in antenatal genetics. In view of the legal, moral, and ethical implications of current research, nursing must become conscientiously and actively involved in these considerations.

There has been emphasis on the utilization of an interdisciplinary team method. The advantages of such an approach cannot be underestimated. If the infant is to survive, to grow and develop, and to be accepted as a productive member of society, then he and his family must be provided with the skills, knowledge, and understandings of every discipline striving together to achieve individualized humanistic care.

REFERENCES

1 Solnik, Albert J., and Mary H. Stark: "Mourning and the Birth of a Defective Child," *Psychoanalytic Study of the Child*, 16:525, 1961.

2 Plotkin, S. A., and W. J. Mellman: "Rubella in the Distant Past as a Possible Cause of Congenital Malformations," *American Journal of Obstetrics and Gynecology*, 108(3):387, Oct. 1, 1971.

3 Brown, Gordon: "Maternal Virus Infections and Congenital Anomalies," *Archives of Environmental Health*, 21(3):362–365, September 1970.

4 Caldwell, Joseph G.: "Congenital Syphilis: A Nonvenereal Disease," *American Journal of Nursing*, 79(9):1768, September 1971.

5 Zellweger, Hans, et al.: "Is Lysergic Acid Diethylamide (L.S.D.) a Teratogen?" *Lancet*, 7525:1066, November 18, 1967.

6 Gardner, L. I., Salma Regina Assemany, and Richard L. Nev: "Deformities in a Child Whose Mother Took L.S.D.," *Lancet*, 7659:1290, June 13, 1970.

7 Nora, James T., et al.: "Dexamphetamine: A Possible Trigger in Cardiovascular Malformations," *Lancet*, 7659:1290, June 13, 1970.

8 Chase, H. Peter, et al.: "Intrauterine Undernutrition and Brain Development," *Pediatrics*, 47(3):491, March 1971.

9 Hunscher, Helen A., and Winslow T. Tompkins: "Influence of Maternal Nutrition on the Immediate and Long-term Outcome of Pregnancy," *Clinical Obstetrics and Gynecology*, 13(1):138, March 1970.

10 Cassady, George: "Body Composition in Intrauterine Growth Retardation," *Pediatric Clinics of North America*, 17(1):79, February 1970.

11 Page, Ernest W.: "Pathogenesis and Prophylaxis of Low Birth Weights," *Clinical Obstetrics and Gynecology*, 13(1):82, March 1970.

12 Pederson, Jorgen: *The Pregnant Diabetic and Her Newborn*, Scandinavian University Books, Munksgaard, Copenhagen, Denmark, 1967, p. 61.

BIBLIOGRAPHY

Abramson, Harold: *Symposium on the Functional Physiopathology of the Fetus and Neonate*, Mosby, St. Louis, 1971.

Adamson, Karlis: *Diagnosis and Treatment of Fetal Disorders*, Springer-Verlag, New York, 1968.

Apgar, Virginia, and Gabriel Stickle: "Birth Defects—Their Significance as a Public Health Problem," *Journal of the American Medical Association*, 204(5):371–374, April 29, 1968.

————: "Assessment of Gestational Age and Development at Birth," *Pediatric Clinics of North America*, 17(1):125–130, February 1970.

Austin, R. Lee: "Congenital Malformations," *Postgraduate Medicine*, 46(5):193–195, November 1969.

Bernfeld, Merton R.: "Progress in Birth Defects Research," *California Medicine*, 112(2):26–42.

Cooke, Cynthia W., et al.: "Fetal and Maternal Outcome in Asymptomatic Bacilluria of Pregnancy," *Obstetrics and Gynecology*, 36(6):840–844, December 1970.

Cooper, George, Jr., and Byron, Cooper: "Radiation Hazards to Fetus and Mother," *Clinical Obstetrics and Gynecology*, 9(1):11–21, March 1966.

Davies, Pamela A.: "Bacterial Infection in the Fetus and Newborn," *Archives of Diseases in Childhood*, 46(245):1–27, February 1971.

Drillien, C. M.: "The Small for Date Infant; Etiology and Prognosis," *Pediatric Clinics of North America*, 17(1):9–24, February 1970.

Elizan, Teresita, and Okingele Fabije: "Congenital and Neonatal Anomalies Linked with Viral Infections in Experimental Animals," *American Journal of Obstetrics and Gynecology*, 106(1):147–165, January 1, 1970.

Ferreira, Antonio J.: *Prenatal Environment*, Charles C Thomas, Springfield, Ill., 1969.

Fishbein, Morris: *Birth Defects*, Lippincott, Philadelphia, 1963.

Franciosi, Ralph A.: "Fetal Infection via Amniotic Fluid," *Rocky Mountain Medical Journal*, 67(10):32–34, October 1970.

Fuchs, Fritz, and Lars L. Cedarquist: "Recent Advances in Antenatal Diagnosis by Amniotic Fluid Analysis," *Clinical Obstetrics and Gynecology*, 13(1):178–201, March 1970.

Greene, John W., Jr., and John L. Dukring: "Diabetes and Pregnancy," *Journal of Tennessee Medical Association*, 64(2):113–118, February 1971.

Hecht, Frederick, and Everett W. Lovrien: "Genetic Diagnosis in the Newborn," *Pediatric Clinics of North America*, 17(4):1039–1053, November 1970.

Hendricks, Charles H., and William Brenner: "Toxemia of Pregnancy: Relationships between Fetal Weight, Fetal Survival, and the Maternal State,"

American Journal of Obstetrics and Gynecology, 109(2):225–233, January 15, 1971.

Hughes, Walter T.: "Infection and Intrauterine Growth Retardation," *Pediatric Clinics of North America,* 17(1):119–124, February 1970.

Important Facts about the Diagnosis of Birth Defects in Early Pregnancy, The Genetics Unit, The Walter E. Fernald State School, Waltham, Mass.

Kasirsky, Gilbert, and Martin F. Tansy: "Teratogenic Effects of Methamphetamine in Mice and Rats," *Teratology,* 4(2):131–134, May 1971.

Klein, Jerome, and S. Michael Marcy: "Infection in the Newborn," *Clinical Obstetrics and Gynecology,* 13(2):321–347, June 1970.

Lenz, W.: "How Can the Teratogenic Action of a Factor Be Established in Man?" *Southern Medical Journal,* 64:41–47, February 1971.

———: "Malformations Caused by Drugs in Pregnancy," *American Journal of Diseases of Children,* 112(2):99–106, August 1966.

Lubchenko, Lula, and Harry Bard: "Incidence of Hypoglycemia in Newborn Infants Classified by Birth Weight and Gestational Age," *Pediatrics,* 47(5):831–838, May 1971.

Lugo, G., and George Cassady: "Intrauterine Growth Retardation," *American Journal of Obstetrics and Gynecology,* 109(4):615–622, February 15, 1971.

MacVicar, John: "Chorioamnionitis," *Clinical Obstetrics and Gynecology,* 13(2):272–290, June 1970.

Milunsky, Aubrey, et al.: "Prenatal Genetic Diagnosis, Part I," *New England Journal of Medicine,* 283(25):1370–1381, December 17, 1970.

———: "Prenatal Genetic Diagnosis, Part II," *New England Journal of Medicine,* 283(26):1441–1446, December 24, 1970.

———: "Prenatal Genetic Diagnosis, Part III," *New England Journal of Medicine,* 283(27):1498–1503, December 31, 1970.

Navarrette, V. N., et al.: "Subsequent Diabetes in Mothers Delivered of a Malformed Child," *Lancet,* 2(7681):993–994, 1970.

Nelson, Waldo E., Victor C. Vaughan, III, and R. James McKay: *Textbook of Pediatrics,* 9th ed., Saunders, Philadelphia, 1969.

North, A. Frederick: "Small for Date Neonates," *Pediatrics,* 38(6):1013–1018, December 1966.

O'Brien, John S., et al.: "Tay-Sachs Disease: Prenatal Diagnosis," *Science,* 172(3978):61–64, April 2, 1971.

Parad, Howard J. (ed.): *Crisis Intervention: Selected Readings,* Family Service Association of America, New York, 1970.

Patrick, Marguerite J.: "Influence of Maternal Renal Infection on the Fetus and Infant," *Archives of Diseases of Childhood,* 42(222):208–213, April 1967.

Pederson, Jorgen: *The Pregnant Diabetic and Her Newborn,* Scandinavian University Books, Munksgaard, Copenhagen, Denmark, 1967.

Rubin, Alan (ed.): *Handbook of Congenital Malformations*, Saunders, Philadelphia, 1967.

Rubin, Reva: "Cognitive Style in Pregnancy," *American Journal of Nursing*, 70(3), 1970.

Richards, J. D.: "Congenital Malformations and Environmental Influences in Pregnancy," *British Journal of Preventative and Social Medicine*, 23(4):218–225, November 1969.

Schneck, L., et al.: "Prenatal Diagnosis of Tay-Sachs Disease," *Lancet*, (7647):582–584, March 21, 1970.

Sever, John L.: "Viral Infections and Malformations," *Federation Proceedings*, 30(1):114–117, January–February 1971.

Shanklin, D. R.: "Influence of Placental Lesions on the Newborn Infant," *Pediatric Clinics of North America*, 17(1):25–42, February 1970.

Siegel, Morris, Harold T. Fuerst, and Vincent F. Guinee: "Rubella Epidemicity and Embryopathy," *American Journal of Diseases of Children*, 121(6): 469–473, June 1971.

Sternberg, Joseph: "Irradiation and Radiocontamination during Pregnancy," *American Journal of Obstetrics and Gynecology*, 108(3):490–511, October 1, 1970.

Terris, Milton, and Edwin Gold: "An Epidemiological Study of Prematurity," *American Journal of Obstetrics and Gynecology*, 103(3):358–379, February 1, 1969.

Toledo, T. M., et al.: "Fetal Effects during Cyclophosphomide and Irradiation Therapy," *Annals of Internal Medicine*, 74(1):87–91, January 1971.

Tompkins, Winslow T.: "National Effects to Reduce Perinatal Mortality and Morbidity," *Clinical Obstetrics and Gynecology*, 13(1):44–56, March 1970.

Usher, Robert H.: "Clinical and Therapeutic Aspects of Fetal Malnutrition," *Pediatric Clinics of North America*, 17(1):169–183, February 1970.

Von Schilling, Karin C.: "The Birth of a Defective Child," *Nursing Forum*, 7:424–439, April 1968.

Wallace, Helen: "Factors Associated with Perinatal Mortality and Morbidity," *Clinical Obstetrics and Gynecology*, 13(1):13–43, March 1970.

Yamazaki, James N.: "A Review of the Literature on the Radiation Dosage Required to Cause Manifest Central Nervous System Disturbances from in Utero and Postnatal Exposure," *Pediatrics*, 37(5):877–897, May 1966.

Yeung, C. Y.: "Hypoglycemia in Neonate Sepsis," *Journal of Pediatrics*, 77(5):812–817, November 1970.

GLOSSARY

abortion. Termination of pregnancy prior to viability of the fetus, i.e., less than 20 to 24 weeks' gestational age.

abortorium. An institution in which only abortions are performed.

acrocyanosis. Cyanosis of fingertips and other extremities.

anaerobic catabolism. The breakdown, in the absence of free oxygen, of organized substances into simpler compounds with the resultant release of energy.

anoxia. Absence or deficiency of oxygen, as reduction of oxygen in body tissues below physiologic levels.

autosomes. The chromosomes in the body other than the sex (X and Y) chromosomes.

azoospermic. A condition in which sperm is absent in the semen.

bicornuate uterus. A double uterus.

bilirubin. The orange- or yellow-colored pigment in bile produced by the breakdown of hemoglobin and excreted by the liver cells.

caput succedaneum. Swelling produced on the presenting part of the fetal head during labor.

cephalhematoma. A localized effusion of blood beneath the periosteum of the skull of a newborn infant caused by disruption of the vessels during birth.

choanal atresia. Congenital obstruction of the posterior nares.

chromosome. The microscopic, rod-shaped bodies (46 in man) which develop from cell nucleus material and contain the genes.

colostrum. The "first milk" secreted from the lactiferous glands.

consanguinity. Blood relationship to another person.

deoxyribonucleic acid. A complex protein which is the carrier of genetic information and consists of adenine and guanine, which are purines, and two pyrimadines, thymine and cystosine.

desquamation. Shedding of cells from the skin or mucous membrane.

dilatation of cervix. The enlargement of the external os from an orifice a few millimeters in size to an opening large enough to allow the passage of the infant. A cervical opening approximately 10 cm (4 inches) in diameter is usually considered complete dilatation.

ductus arteriosus. A communicating channel between the aorta and the pulmonary artery of the fetus.

ductus venosus. A fetal blood vessel that connects the umbilical vein and the inferior vena cava.

dyspareunia. Painful sexual intercourse experienced by females.

ecchymosis. Skin discoloration resulting from extravasation of blood into the skin or mucous membrane.

eclampsia. Acute toxemia of pregnancy characterized by convulsions and coma occurring during pregnancy, labor, or the puerperium.

effacement. A thinning and shortening of the cervix which occurs during late pregnancy and/or labor.

effurage. A stroke used in massage.

epicanthus. A fold of skin extending from the root of the nose to the median end of the eyebrow and covering the inner canthus and caruncle. It is a characteristic of the Mongolian race and may occur as a congenital anomaly in Caucasians.

Epstein's pearls. Small, white epithelial cysts along both sides of the median raphe of the hard palate. Commonly found in newborn infants.

erythema toxicum neonatorum. An urticarial condition affecting newborns in the first few days of life. The lesions consist of dead white papules grainy to the touch, with or without surrounding areas of redness.

erythroblastosis fetalis. A blood dyscrasia of the newborn characterized by agglutination and hemolysis of erythrocytes; usually caused by incompatibility between the infant's blood and the mother's.

esophageal atresia. A condition in which the esophagus ends in a blind pouch or narrows into a thin cord; usually occurs between the upper and mid third of the esophagus.

facies. The expression or appearance of the face; certain congenital syndromes present with a specific facial appearance.

fontanel. An unossified space or "soft spot" lying between the cranial bones of the skull of a fetus.

foramen ovale. The septal opening in the fetal heart that provides a communication between the atria.

gene. A factor responsible for the transmission of hereditary characteristics to offspring.

generative. Capable of reproducing.

genotype. The hereditary combination of genes which makes up a person.

gestation period. The number of completed weeks of pregnancy calculated from the first day of the last menstrual period.

gravida. The number of times a woman has been pregnant.

hemoconcentration. An increase in the number of red blood cells resulting from a decrease in the volume of plasma.

hirsutism. The excessive growth of hair, or growth of hair in unusual areas of the body.

homeothermic. Referring to an animal which maintains its internal temperature at a specified level regardless of its environmental temperature.

hydatidiform mole. Cystic proliferation of chorionic villi resembling a cluster of grapes.

hydrocephalus. An excess of cerebrospinal fluid within the ventricular system.

hydrocephalus, communicating. Cerebral fluid that circulates into the lumbar thecal space.

hydrocephalus, noncirculating. Ventricular fluid that does not empty into the lumbar thecal space.

hyperbilirubinemia. An excessive amount of unconjugated bilirubin in the blood.

hyperemesis gravidarum. Excessive vomiting during pregnancy.

hypersonia. Excessive need for sleep.

hypofibrinogenemia. A deficiency of fibrinogen in the blood.

hypospadias. A condition in which the urethral orifice is at some point between the scrotal raphe and the base of the glans penis.

hypoxia. A broad term meaning diminished availability of oxygen to the body tissues.

idiopathic respiratory distress syndrome (hyaline membrane disease). A severe respiratory condition found almost exclusively in preterm infants.

inborn error of metabolism. A hereditary disease caused by a deficiency of a specific enzyme.

jaundice. A condition characterized by a yellow color of the skin, the whites of the eyes, the mucous membranes, and body fluids that is due to deposition of bile pigment resulting from excess bilirubin in the blood.

kernicterus. A clinical syndrome in newborn infants manifested by pathological changes in the central nervous system resulting from deposition of unconjugated bilirubin in certain nuclei of the brain.

lanugo. Fine, downy hair growing over the body of the fetus.

large-for-gestational-age. An infant above the 90th percentile.

lochia. The vaginal discharge during the puerperium, consisting of blood, mucus, and tissue.

lochia alba. The thin, colorless discharge which follows lochia serosa on about the 10th postpartum day and may last from the end of the third to the sixth postpartum week.

lochia rubra. The color description of the red, sanguinous vaginal flow which follows delivery and which lasts two to four days postpartum.

lochia serosa. The serous, pinkish-brown watery discharge which follows lochia rubra and lasts until about the 10th postpartum day.

lysozyme. An enzyme with antiseptic qualities which destroys foreign protein.

meconium. Dark green mucus material in the intestine of the full-term fetus. It constitutes the first stools passed by the newborn infant.

meiosis. The process by which germ cells divide.

milia. Distended sebaceous glands which produce tiny pinpoint papules on the skin of newborn infants. Commonly found over the bridge of the nose, chin, and cheeks.

mitochondrion. A filamentous or granular component (organelle) of cytoplasm, the principle site of oxidative reaction by which the energy in foodstuff is made available for endergonic processes in the cell.

mitosis. The process of somatic cell division by which multicellular organisms multiply.

Mongolian spots. Benign bluish pigmentation over the lower back, buttocks, or occasionally over the extensor surfaces. May be present at birth, particularly in dark-skinned races.

mucus-trap suction apparatus. A type of suction apparatus used in aspirating the nasopharynx and trachea of a newborn infant. It consists of catheter with a mucus trap which prevents mucus from the baby from being drawn into the operator's mouth.

neonatal period. From birth to 28 days.

nursing process. Perceiving, assessing, planning, implementing, and evaluating.

nystagmus. Involuntary rhythmic oscillation of the eyeball—horizontal, vertical, or rotary.

omphalocele. A defect resulting from failure of closure of the abdominal wall or muscles whereby abdominal visera is covered by a thin membrane only.

ophthalmia neonatorum purulent. Infection of the eye of the newborn, usually caused by gonococcus.

parity. The number of viable infants live or dead that a woman has delivered.

perinatalogist. A physician with expertise in fetal and neonatal care.

phenotype. The physical appearance of a person.

phenylketonuria. A congenital disease caused by a defect in the metabolism of the amino acid phenylalanine. The condition is hereditary and results from lack of an enzyme, phenylalanine hydroxylase, necessary for the conversion of the amino acid phenylalanine into tyrosine.

phototherapy. The therapeutic measure used in the treatment of hyperbilirubinemia.

placenta. A disclike vascular structure in the impregnated uterus which nourishes and removes waste products from the fetus.

placenta abruptio. A premature separation of a normally implanted placenta.

placenta dysfunction. A placenta that is failing to meet fetal requirements.

placenta marginal. A condition that exists when the placental edges are not firmly attached to the wall of the uterus.

placenta previa. A placenta which is implanted in the lower uterine segment so that it partially covers the internal os of the cervix.

plethora. A condition marked by vascular turgescence, excess of blood, and fullness of pulse.

premature infant. A liveborn infant of less than 38 weeks' gestation.

pseudocyesis. False pregnancy.

psychological miscarriage. Lack of love for the infant.

resuscitation. Restoration of life or consciousness of one apparently dead or whose respiration has ceased.

retrolental fibroplasia. A condition resulting from high oxygen tension in the arterial blood which may cause retinal vasospasm leading to ischemic injury to the retina.

scaphoid abdomen. An abdomen with a hollowed interior wall.

shirodkar. Operative procedure for correcting an incompetent cervix.

skin turgor. Normal fullness of the tissue.

small-for-gestational-age. An infant who falls below the 10th percentile.

spermatogenesis. The process by which mature spermatozoa are formed and during which the diploid chromosome number is reduced to the haploid.

spina bifida occulta. A congenital defect of the walls of the spinal canal caused by the lack of union between the laminae of the vertebrae.

stillborn. Born without life.

striae gravidarum. Reddish streaks on the abdomen, thighs, and breasts during pregnancy from overstretching; the streaks turn silvertone in time.

surfactant. A substance formed in the lungs that helps to keep the small air sacs extended by virtue of its ability to reduce the surface tension.

telangiectasis. The presence of small, red focal lesions, usually in the skin or mucous membrane, caused by dilation of capillaries, arterioles, or venules.

teratogenic agent. Virus, irradiation, or drugs, the exposure to which can damage the fetus in a pregnant woman.

term infant. A liveborn infant of between 38 and 42 weeks' completed gestation.

tetralogy of Fallot. A common cardiac malformation consisting of pulmonary stenosis, ventricular septal defect, dextroposed aorta, and hypertrophy of the right ventricle.

thermogenesis. The production of heat, especially in the body.

thrombocytopenic purpura. A hematological disorder in the newborn in which the bleeding time is prolonged, platelets are greatly decreased, and there is cell fragility.

thromboembolus. A blood clot in a vein.

thrombophlebitis. Inflammation of a vein developing before the formation of a thrombus.

thrush. Infection of the oral membrane by a fungus, usually *Candida albicans*. It is characterized by white patches on a red, moist, inflamed surface and may occur anywhere in the mouth.

torticollis. Wryneck; stiff neck caused by spasmodic contraction of neck muscles drawing the head to one side with the chin pointing to the other side. Congenital or acquired.

toxemia. Disorders occurring during pregnancy or early puerperium which are characterized by one or all of the following: hypertension, edema, albuminuria, and, in severe cases, convulsions and coma.

tracheoesophageal fistula. A congenital anomaly in which there is an abnormal tubelike passage between the trachea and the esophagus.

vernix caseosa. A cheeselike substance which covers the skin of the fetus.

APPENDIX

STANDARDS OF MATERNAL AND CHILD HEALTH NURSING PRACTICE[*]

INTRODUCTION

Nursing practice is a direct service, goal directed and adaptable to the needs of the individual, family, and community during health and illness. Professional practitioners of nursing bear primary responsibility and accountability for the nursing care clients/patients receive. The purpose of standards of nursing practice is to fulfill the profession's obligation to provide and improve this practice.

The standards focus on practice. They provide a means for determining the quality of nursing which a client/patient receives regardless of whether such services are provided solely by a professional nurse or by a professional nurse and nonprofessional assistants.

The standards are stated according to a systematic approach to nursing practice: assessment of the client's/patient's status, planning nursing actions, implementation of the plan, and evaluation. These specific divisions are not intended to imply that practice consists of a series of discrete steps, taken in strict sequence, beginning with assessment and ending with evaluation. The processes described are used concurrently and recurrently. Assessment, for

* Reprinted with permission of the American Nurses' Association.

example, frequently continues during implementation; similarly evaluation dictates reassessment and replanning.

These standards for nursing practice apply to nursing practice in any setting. Nursing practice in all settings must possess the characteristics identified by these standards if patients are to receive high-quality nursing care. Each standard is followed by a rationale and examples of assessment factors. Assessment factors are to be used in determining achievement of the standard.

Implementation of the standards will be facilitated by use of the standards as a basis for evaluating nursing practice by:

(a) the individual nurse (self-evaluation)
(b) nurses (peer view)
(c) nurses with superior clinical expertise
(d) nurse administrators

In addition to evaluation of nursing practice by nurses, nurses will solicit and be responsive to an evaluation by:

(a) interdisciplinary colleagues
(b) clients/patients
(c) official and voluntary accrediting agencies
(d) community representatives

DEFINITION

Maternal and child nursing practice is a direct service to individuals, their families, and the community during childbearing and childrearing phases of the life cycle. It is a dynamic process involving specific activities which are goal directed and adapted to the needs of individuals and families during health and illness. The primary responsibility and accountability for nursing care clients/patients receive is that of the maternal child nurse. It is given independently and in collaboration with nursing colleagues and/or with members of other health disciplines.

PHILOSOPHY

Maternal and child nursing practice is based on nursing knowledge, principles, and concepts drawn from the biological, physical, and social sciences and from the humanities. These principles and concepts are selected and synthesized into the theoretical basis for maternal and child nursing practice. Regardless of the setting in which nursing is practiced (hospital, home, school, community, etc.), basic concepts and principles are used to describe, explain, and predict human development and behavior potential. A thorough understanding of the interrelatedness of the cultural, psychosocial, spiritual and physiological influence on the individual and the family is essential to effective practice.

Maternal and child nursing practice includes independent, dependent and interdependent functions. Independent functions are those activities performed by the nurse which are not prescribed nor subject to the control of nonnurse personnel. Dependent functions are those delegated by another member of the health team. Interdependent functions are derived from collaboration with members of the interdisciplinary team.

The health plan for care and cure evolves from the assessment and evaluation made by each member of the health team. Responsibility for the development of total health services for the entire community is shared with all health-related disciplines. Such comprehensive care should be geared to economic efficiency and intelligent use of personnel.

SKILLS

The skills needed in maternal and child nursing practice are multiple: intellectual communication, observation, and manual (technical). Intellectual skills are essential in making judgments, assessing success and failure, developing new concepts, developing goals and plans for the future, seeking new knowledge, and scientifically investigating clinical problems. Communication skills are important in interviewing, teaching, guidance, and counseling. They are also necessary for effective collaboration with health team members and with the family. Observational skills are important to the assessment and evaluation of the health status. Manual skills are an essential part of the total nursing process and must be used in conjunction with other skills. All of these skills are essential to planning, implementing, and evaluating nursing care during the preconceptual, conceptual, childbearing, childrearing, and childhood phases of the life cycle.

The way in which the nurse utilizes knowledge and skills is contingent upon her awareness and understanding of self as a therapeutic agent, as well as upon her ability to weld these knowledges and skills into effective practice.

A systematic approach to assessment, interpretation, planning, implementation, evaluation, and reassessment of care is inherent in this process.

Effective practice is planned and evaluated independently and in collaboration with nurse colleagues, others on the interdisciplinary health team and with representatives of the community.

PREMISES

Maternal and child nursing practice is based on the following premises:
1 Survival and the level of health of a society is inextricably bound to maternal and child health.
2 Maternal and child nursing practice respects the human dignity and rights of individuals.
3 Maternal and child nursing practice is family-centered.

4 Maternal and child nursing practice focuses on the childbearing/ childrearing phases of the life cycle which include the development of sexuality, family planning, interconceptual care, and child health from conception through adolescence.

5 Maternal and child nursing makes a significant difference to society in achieving its health goals.

6 Man is a total human being: his psychosocial and biophysical self are interrelated.

7 Human behavior shapes and is shaped by environmental forces and as such sets into motion a multitude of reciprocal responses.

8 Through his own process of self-regulation the human being attempts to maintain equilibrium amidst constant change.

9 All behavior has meaning and is influenced by past experiences, the individual(s) perception of those experiences, and forces impinging upon the present.

10 Growth and development is ordered and evolves in sequential stages.

11 Substantive knowledge of the principles of human growth and development, including normative data, is essential to effective maternal and child nursing practice.

12 Periods of developmental and traumatic crises during the life cycle pose internal and external stresses and may have a positive or negative effect.

13 Maternal and child nursing provides for continuity of care and is not bound by artificial barriers and exclusive categories which tend to restrict and delimit practice.

14 *All* people have a right to receive the benefit of the delivery of optimal health services.

GOALS

Maternal and child nursing practice is aimed at:

1 Promoting and maintaining optimal health of each individual and the family unit

2 Improving and/or supporting family solidarity

3 Early identification and treatment of vulnerable families

4 Preventing environmental conditions which block attainment of optimal health

5 Prevention and early detection of deviations from health

6 Reducing stresses which interfere with optimal functioning

7 Assisting the family to understand and/or cope with the developmental and traumatic situations which occur during childbearing and childrearing

8 Facilitating survival, recovery, and growth when the individual is ill or needs health care

9 Reducing reproductive wastage occurring at any point on the continuum

10 Continuously improving the quality of care in maternal and child nursing

11 Reducing inequalities in the delivery of health care services

REASONS FOR STANDARDS

Standards prepared for the profession exceed the minimum requirements for licensure.

1 To assist the profession in evaluating the quality of practice in any setting

2 To serve as a tool for self-evaluation

3 To provide a common base for practitioners to coordinate and unify their efforts in the improvement of practice

4 To provide a common base for practitioners and others concerned to coordinate their efforts in the improvement of health care

5 To identify the elements of independent, dependent, and interdependent functions of practice

6 To provide one of the bases for planning and evaluating educational programs preparing practitioners

7 To help employers understand what to expect of the practitioner

8 To inform society of our concern for the improvement of practice

9 To assist the public in understanding what to expect from practice

10 To provide one measure by which eligibility for certification of individual practitioners can be determined by the Division on Maternal and Child Health Nursing Practice

11 To encourage a philosophy of comprehensive rather than compartmentalized maternal and child care

12 To develop a measure by which the achievement of maternal and child nursing goals can be evaluated

STANDARDS OF MATERNAL AND CHILD HEALTH NURSING PRACTICE

I Maternal and child nursing practice is characterized by the continual questioning of the assumptions upon which practice is based, retaining those which are valid and searching for and using new knowledge.

II Maternal and child nursing practice is based upon knowledge of the biophysical and psychosocial development of individuals from conception through the childrearing phase of development and upon knowledge of the basic needs for optimum development.

III The collection of data about the health status of the client/patient is systematic and continuous; the data are accessible, communicated, and recorded.

IV Nursing diagnoses are derived from data about the health status of the client/patient.

V Maternal and child nursing practice recognizes deviations from expected patterns of physiologic activity and anatomic and psychosocial development.

VI The plan of nursing care includes goals derived from the nursing diagnoses.

VII The plan of nursing care includes priorities and the prescribed nursing approaches or measures to achieve the goals.

VIII Nursing actions provide for client/patient participation in health promotion, maintenance, and restoration.

IX Maternal and child nursing practice provides for the use and coordination of all services that assist individuals to prepare for responsible sexual roles.

X Nursing actions assist the client/patient to maximize his health capabilities.

XI The client's/patient's progress or lack of progress toward goal achievement is determined by the patient/client and the nurse.

XII The client's/patient's progress or lack of progress toward goal achievement directs reassessment, reordering of priorities, new goal setting and revision of the plan of nursing care.

XIII Maternal and child nursing practice evidences active participation with others in evaluating the availability, accessibility, and acceptability of services for parents and children and cooperating and/or taking leadership in extending and developing needed services in the community.

STANDARD I

Maternal and child nursing practice is characterized by the continual questioning of the assumptions upon which practice is based, retaining those which are valid and searching for and using new knowledge.

Rationale: Since knowledge is not static, all assumptions are subject to change. Assumptions are derived from knowledge or findings of research which are subject to additional testing and revision. They are carefully selected and tested and reflect utilization of present and new knowledge. Effective utilization of these knowledges stimulates more astute observations and provides new insights into the effects of nursing upon the individual and family. To question assumptions implies that nursing practice is not based on stereotyped or ritualistic procedures or methods of intervention; rather practice exemplifies an objective, systematic, and logical investigation of a phenomenon or problem.

Assessment factors:
Therefore in
practice, the MCN:

1 Critically examines and questions accepted modes of practice rather than relying on ritualistic or routinized modes of practice

2 Utilizes current and new knowledge in identifying and questioning the validity of the assumptions which form the bases of nursing practice

3 Continuously expands and improves nursing practice by utilizing theories and research findings in search for alternative solutions

4 Actively shares new knowledge and approaches with colleagues and others in the community

STANDARD II

Maternal and child nursing practice is based upon knowledge of the biophysical and psychosocial development of individuals from conception through the childrearing phase of development and upon knowledge of the basic needs for optimum development.

Rationale:

A knowledge and understanding of the principles and normal ranges in human growth, development, and behavior are essential to MCN practice. Concomitant with this knowledge is the recognition and consideration of the psychosocial, environmental, nutritional, spiritual, and cognitive factors that enhance or deter the biophysical and psychological maturation of the individual and his family.

Assessment factors:
Therefore in
practice, the MCN:

1 Observes, assesses, and describes the developmental level and/or needs of the individual within the family before performing any actions

2 Involves the individual and family in the assessment and planning of care

3 Works with individuals and groups utilizing knowledge of the psychosocial, environmental, nutritional, spiritual, and cognitive factors inherent in the family or group environment.

STANDARD III

The collection of data about the health status of the client/patient is systematic and continuous; the data are accessible, communicated, and recorded.

Rationale: Comprehensive care requires complete and ongoing collection of data about client/patient to determine the nursing care needs and other health care needs of the client/patient; all health status data about the client/patient must be available for all members of the health care team.

Assessment factors:

1 Health status data includes:
   (a) growth and development
   (b) biophysical status
   (c) emotional status
   (d) cultural, religious, socioeconomic background
   (e) performance of activities of daily living
   (f) patterns of coping
   (g) interaction patterns
   (h) clients/patients perception and satisfaction with his health status
   (i) client/patient health goals
   (j) environment (physical, social, emotional, ecological)
   (k) available and accessible human and material resources

2 Data are collected from:
   (a) client/patient, family, significant others
   (b) health care personnel
   (c) individuals within the immediate environment and/or the community

3 Data are obtained by:
   (a) interview
   (b) examination
   (c) observation
   (d) reading records, reports, etc.

4 Format for the collection of data:
   (a) provides for a systematic collection of data
   (b) facilitates the completeness of data collection

5 Continuous collection of data is evident by:
   (a) frequent updating
   (b) recording of changes in health status

6 The data are:
   (a) accessible on the client/patient records

(b) retrievable
(c) confidential

STANDARD IV

Nursing diagnoses are derived from data about the health status of the client/patient.

Rationale: The health status of the client/patient is the basis for determining the nursing care needs. The data are analyzed and compared to norms.

Assessment factors:
1 The client's/patient's health status is compared to the norm to determine if there is a deviation, the degree and direction of deviation.
2 The client's/patient's capabilities and limitations are identified.
3 The nursing diagnoses are related to and comparable with the totality of the client's/patient's health care.

STANDARD V

Maternal and child nursing practice recognizes deviations from expected patterns of physiologic activity and anatomic and psychosocial development.

Rationale: Early detection of deviations and therapeutic intervention are essential to the prevention of illness, to facilitating growth and developmental potential, and to the promotion of optimal health for the individual and the family.
Early detection requires that minute deviations be recognized, often before the individual or his family is aware that such deviations exist. The nurse has a unique opportunity to observe and assess the patient and his family, particularly in the community setting.

Assessment factors:
Therefore in
practice, the MCN:
1 Demonstrates a thorough understanding of the range of normal body structure and function by detecting signs and symptoms which are not within normal limits
2 Identifies the variety of coping mechanisms which may serve an adaptive function or represent maladaptive patterns of response

3 Searches for improved means of detecting impairment of physical and emotional function

4 Searches for improved means of detecting physical, psychological, or environmental situations which may lead to impaired functioning

5 Instructs the individual and family in recognizing and understanding deviations

STANDARD VI

The plan of nursing care includes goals derived from the nursing diagnoses.

Rationale: The determination of the desired results from nursing actions is an essential part of planning care.

Assessment factors:
1 Goals are mutually set with the client/patient and significant others:
   (*a*) They are congruent with other planned therapies.
   (*b*) They are stated in realistic and measurable terms.
   (*c*) They are assigned a time schedule for achievement.
2 Goals are established to maximize functional capabilities and are congruent with:
   (*a*) growth and development
   (*b*) biophysical status
   (*c*) behavioral patterns
   (*d*) human and material resources

STANDARD VII

The plan of nursing care includes priorities and the prescribed nursing approaches or measures to achieve the goals.

Rationale: Nursing actions are planned to promote, maintain, and restore the client's/patient's well-being.

Assessment factors:
1 Physical measures are planned to manage (prevent or control) specific client/patient problems and clearly relate to the nursing diagnosis and goals of care, e.g., ADL, use of self-help devices, etc.
2 Psychosocial measures are specific to the client's/patient's nursing care needs and to the nursing care goals, e.g., techniques to control aggression.
3 Teaching-learning principles are incorporated into the plan of care and objectives for learning stated in

behavioral terms, e.g., specification of content for learner's level, reinforcement, readiness, etc.

4 Approaches are planned to provide for a therapeutic environment:

(a) physical environmental factors, e.g., control of noise, control of temperature, etc.

(b) psychosocial measures are used to structure the environment for therapeutic ends, e.g., paternal participation in all phases of the maternity experience.

(c) group behaviors are used to structure interaction and influence the therapeutic environment, e.g., conformity, territorial rights, locomotion, etc.

5 Approaches are specified for orientation of client/patient to:

(a) new roles and relationships

(b) relevant health (human and material) resources

(c) modifications in plan of nursing care

(d) relationship of modifications in nursing care plan to the total care plan

6 The plan includes the utilization of available and appropriate resources:

(a) human resources—other health professionals

(b) material resources

(c) community

7 The plan is an ordered sequence of proposed nursing actions.

8 Nursing approaches are planned on the basis of current knowledge.

STANDARD VIII

Nursing actions provide for client/patient participation in health promotion maintenance and restoration.

Rationale: The client/patient and family is provided the opportunity to participate in the nursing care. Such provision is made based upon theoretical and experiential evidence that participation of client/patient and family may foster growth.

Assessment factors: 1 The client/patient and family are kept informed about:

(a) current health status

(b) changes in health status

      (c) the total health care plan
      (d) the nursing care plan
      (e) roles of health care personnel
      (f) health care resources

2 The client/patient and family is provided with the information needed to make decisions and choices about:
      (a) promoting, maintaining, and restoring health
      (b) seeking appropriate health care personnel
      (c) maintaining and using health care resources

STANDARD IX

Maternal and child nursing practice provides for the use and coordination of all services that assist individuals to prepare for responsible sexual roles.

Rationale:

People are prepared for sexual roles through a process of socialization that takes place from birth to adulthood. This process of socialization, to a large extent, is carried out within the family structure. Social control over child care increases in importance as humans become increasingly dependent on the culture rather than upon the family unit. The culture of any society is maintained by the transmission of its specific values, attitudes, and behaviors from generation to generation. Attitudes and values concerning male and female roles develop as part of the socialization process. Attitudes toward self, the opposite sex, and toward parents will influence the roles each individual assumes in adulthood and the responsibilities accepted.

Assessment factors:
Therefore in
practice, the MCN:

1 Utilizes resources available in the social and behavioral sciences to help her understand the attitudes and values of individuals and families with whom she is working

2 Utilizes opportunities available to her to promote those attitudes and values conducive to emotional and physical health and family solidarity, without imposing her own value system

3 Encourages society to provide the resources needed to help people prepare for responsible sexual roles

4 Interprets to other health personnel the needs of individuals and families as she sees them and attempts

to understand the needs as seen by other health personnel

5 Works with other health personnel to develop services which promote optimal health and family solidarity

STANDARD X

Nursing actions assist the client/patient to maximize his health capabilities.

Rationale: Nursing actions are designed to promote, maintain, and restore health. A knowledge and understanding of the principles and normal ranges in human growth, development, and behavior are essential to MCN practice.

Assessment factors: 1 Nursing actions:
    (*a*) are consistent with the plan of care
    (*b*) are based on scientific principles
    (*c*) are individualized to the specific situation
    (*d*) are used to provide a safe and therapeutic environment
    (*e*) employ teaching-learning opportunities for client/patient
    (*f*) include utilization of appropriate resources
2 Nursing actions are directed to the physical, psychological, and social behavior associated with:
    (*a*) ingestion of food, fluid, and nutrients
    (*b*) elimination of body wastes
    (*c*) locomotion, exercise
    (*d*) temperature and other regulatory mechanisms
    (*e*) relating with others
    (*f*) self fulfillment

STANDARD XI

The client's/patient's progress or lack of progress toward goal achievement is determined by the patient/client and the nurse.

Rationale: The quality of nursing care depends upon comprehensive and intelligent determination of the impact of nursing upon the health status of the client. The client is an essential part of this determination.

Assessment factors: 1 Current data about the client are used to measure his progress toward goal achievement.

2 Nursing actions are analyzed for their effectiveness in goal achievement of the client.

3 The client/patient evaluates nursing actions and goal achievement.

4 Provision is made for nursing follow-up of particular patients to determine the long term effects of nursing care.

STANDARD XII

The client's/patient's progress or lack of progress toward goal achievement directs reassessment, reordering of priorities, new goal setting, and revision of the plan of nursing care.

Rationale: The nursing process remains the same but the input of new information may dictate new or revised approaches.

Assessment factors: 1 Reassessment is directed by goal achievement or lack of goal achievement.

2 New priorities and goals are determined and additional nursing approaches are prescribed appropriately.

3 New nursing actions are accurately and appropriately initiated.

STANDARD XIII

Maternal and child nursing practice evidences active participation with others in evaluating the availability, accessibility, and acceptability of services for parents and children and cooperating and/or taking leadership in extending and developing needed services in the community.

Rationale: Knowledge of services presently offered to parents and children is the first step in determining the effectiveness of health care to all in the community. When it is recognized that needed services are not available, accessible or acceptable, the nurse takes leadership in working with consumers, other health disciplines, the community, and governmental agencies in extending and/or developing these services. Services must be continually evaluated, expanded, and changed if they are to improve the health and well-being of all parents and children within our society.

Assessment factors:
Therefore in
practice, the MCN:

1 Applies and shares the cultural and socioeconomic concepts which help her understand the differences in the unique needs of individuals and families
2 Recognizes the need for available health services for all parents and children in the community
3 Utilizes the services and resources presently available
4 Works with consumers, nurse colleagues, other health disciplines, the community and governmental agencies in evaluating the availability, accessibility and acceptability of services to all parents and children in the community
5 Participates actively with significant others in initiating changes in the delivery of health services and/or developing new services to enable each individual in the family to function at his optimum capacity and to enhance family unity

INDEX

Page references in **boldface** indicate tables or figures.